The Hospital for Sick Children Handbook of Pediatrics

Eleventh Edition

Expert | CONSULT

Online + Print

Online access activation instructions

This Expert Consult title comes with access to the complete contents online. **Activate your access today** by following these simple instructions:

1. Gently scratch off the surface of the sticker below, using the edge of a coin, to reveal your **activation code**.

2. Visit **www.expertconsultbook.com** and click on the **"Register"** button.

3. **Enter your activation code** along with the other information requested... and begin enjoying your access.

It's that easy! For technical assistance, email **online.help@elsevier.com** or call **800-401-9962** (inside the US) or **+1-314-995-3200** (outside the US).

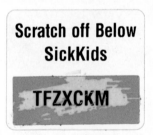

**Scratch off Below
SickKids**

TFZXCKM

SAUNDERS
ELSEVIER

**Copyright © 2009 Elsevier Canada, a division
of Reed Elsevier Canada, Ltd.**

Library and Archives Canada Cataloguing in Publication

The Hospital for Sick Children handbook of pediatrics/editors, Anne I. Dipchand ... [et al.]. — 11th ed.

Includes index.
Previous edition published under title The HSC handbook of pediatrics.
ISBN 978-1-897422-04-5

1. Pediatrics—Handbooks, manuals, etc. I. Dipchand, Anne I
II. Hospital for Sick Children   III. Title: Handbook of pediatrics.

RJ48.H78 2009   618.92   C2008-904048-1

Vice President, Publishing: Ann Millar
Managing Developmental Editor: Martina van de Velde
Developmental Editor: Sondra Greenfield
Managing Production Editor: Rohini Herbert
Copy Editor: Susan Anglin
Cover Design: Monica Kompter/Louis Forgione
Interior Design: Monica Kompter
Typesetting and Assembly: Jansom
Printing and Binding: Transcontinental

Elsevier Canada
905 King Street West, 4th Floor
Toronto, ON, Canada M6K 3G9
Phone: 1-866-896-3331
Fax: 1-866-359-9534

Printed in Canada

2 3 4 5   13 12 11 10 09

The Hospital for Sick Children Handbook of Pediatrics

Eleventh Edition

EDITORS

Anne I. Dipchand, MD, FRCPC
Head, Heart Transplant Program
and Staff Cardiologist, Labatt
Family Heart Centre
Associate Director, SickKids
Transplant Centre
Department of Pediatrics, The
Hospital for Sick Children
Associate Professor, Faculty
of Medicine, University of
Toronto

Jeremy N. Friedman, MB, ChB, FRCPC, FAAP
Head, Division of Pediatric
Medicine
Department of Pediatrics,
The Hospital for Sick Children
Associate Professor, Faculty
of Medicine, University of
Toronto

Zia Bismilla, MEd, MD, FRCPC
Pediatric Medicine Fellow
Department of Pediatrics,
The Hospital for Sick Children

Sumit Gupta, MD
Resident
Department of Pediatrics,
The Hospital for Sick Children

Catherine Lam, MD
Hematology/Oncology Fellow
Department of Pediatrics,
The Hospital for Sick Children

SickKids

SAUNDERS
ELSEVIER

Notice

This book is a general guide only and should never be a substitute for the skill, knowledge, and experience of a qualified medical professional dealing with the facts, circumstances, and symptoms of a particular case. Neither the Publisher nor the Authors assume any responsibility for any loss or injury and/or damage to persons or property arising out of or related to any use of the material contained in this book. It is the responsibility of the treating practitioner, relying on independent expertise and knowledge of the patient, to determine the best treatment and method of application for the patient.

– The Hospital for Sick Children

Knowledge and best practice in this field are constantly changing. As new research and experience broaden our knowledge, changes in practice, treatment, and drug therapy may become necessary or appropriate. Readers are advised to check the most current information provided (i) on procedures featured or (ii) by the manufacturer of each product to be administered, to verify the recommended dose or formula, the method and duration of administration, and contraindications. It is the responsibility of the practitioners, relying on their own experience and knowledge of the patients, to make diagnoses, to determine dosages and the best treatment for each individual patient, and to take all appropriate safety precautions. To the fullest possible extent of the law, neither the Publisher nor the Editors assume any liability for any injury and/or damage to persons or property arising out of or related to any use of the material contained in this book.

– The Publisher

Dedication

To...
Lauren, Rachel, and Emma for sharing their "mommy time" so that this book could become a reality, and to Jake for his unconditional love and support. **AID**

To...
all the children and families that I have had the privilege of looking after and from whom I have learned so much, and to Shelley, Sam, and Danielle. **JNF**

To...
my family and to Karanpal Samra and his family. **ZB**

To...
the Anglins, who first started me down the road to pediatrics; to my family, who got me to the point where I could make that choice; and to the friends who have kept me sane since. **SG**

To...
my loving parents, my brother Cedric, and my sister Chris. **CL**

Contents

Foreword to the 11th Edition

For more than 50 years now, *The Hospital for Sick Children Handbook of Pediatrics* has been a mainstay quick-reference text for Canadian, American, and international medical students, residents, and fellows, as well as other health care professionals involved in the day-to-day care of neonates, infants, children, and youth. In the past, the handbook could be seen bulging out of the pockets of white coats all over The Hospital for Sick Children (SickKids) as well as other hospitals. In more recent times, as the white coat is being steadily phased out, the handbook is now seen attached to clipboards, kept in diagnostic bags, and even chained to desktops on wards and outpatient units.

The major purpose of *The Hospital for Sick Children Handbook of Pediatrics,* 11th edition, is to provide "frontline" pediatric health care providers with the essential, up-to-date information required to meet the needs of the individual child and family in their care: assistance in making the diagnosis, ordering the appropriate tests, and developing the appropriate management strategy for both acute and chronic disorders of childhood. The development of the handbook was the result of the close collaboration between the residents or fellows and the staff pediatricians or pediatric subspecialists in SickKids who wrote the various chapters. The 11th edition has a state-of-the-art approach to pediatrics based on the knowledge and experience of pediatricians from one of the largest and best-known freestanding children's hospitals in the world (*www.sickkids.ca*).

Each year, SickKids cares for over 50,000 children and youth in its Emergency Department; more that 13,000 admissions are made to the in-patient services; and over 175,000 make ambulatory care visits. These children present with a wide range of childhood disorders—from the common to the exceedingly rare, and from the simple to the inordinately complex.

The 11th edition of *The Hospital for Sick Children Handbook of Pediatrics* is the direct result of the dedication, skills, and leadership of its five Chief Editors—two of them faculty members and three trainees. Our enormous thanks are extended to them for producing such an outstanding edition, as well as to all of their section authors, both faculty and trainees. Soon work will begin on the 12th edition!

Denis Daneman MB, BCh, FRCPC
Chair, Department of Pediatrics – University of Toronto
Pediatrician-in-Chief, The Hospital for Sick Children
RS McLaughlin Foundation Chair in Pediatrics
at The Hospital for Sick Children

Preface

Welcome to the new and improved 11th edition of the *The Hospital for Sick Children Handbook of Pediatrics*! The Hospital for Sick Children in Toronto, Canada, affectionately known as "SickKids," was established in 1875 and has become one of the top pediatric academic health science centers in the world, with an international reputation for excellence in health care, research, and education. The first 10 editions of the *Handbook* have set a high standard, which we hope that we have not only continued but also built upon to produce this 11th edition.

We know that the reader needs succinct, easily accessible, and evidence-based answers to the problems we all see regularly in pediatrics. Our goal in this edition of the *Handbook* is to provide practical, algorithmic, and system-based approaches to a wide range of pediatric diagnoses and scenarios. Every chapter has been extensively revised to reflect up-to-date diagnostic and therapeutic approaches to pediatric clinical problems, using evidence-based guidelines wherever possible. A wide range of topics spanning primary to quaternary care pediatric medicine have been included, making this handbook an important reference for medical students and residents, practicing pediatricians, family doctors, emergency department physicians, nurses, and other interdisciplinary practitioners providing care to children.

We have reorganized and revised all urgent and emergent clinical scenarios, creating a *new* section on Acute Care covering key pediatric emergencies (e.g., anaphylaxis, status epilepticus, and status asthmaticus) and relocating this important section to the front of the *Handbook* for easy reference. Updated comprehensive chapters include *Resuscitation, Emergency Medicine, Pain and Sedation, Poisonings and Toxicology, Anesthesia,* and *Procedures.* We have also made readily accessible the key information for urgent situations, including all new Pediatric Advanced Life Support (PALS) algorithms, as well as new topics like substance abuse, psychiatric emergencies, and the acute presentation of eating disorders. Common resuscitation drugs and useful calculations have been incorporated inside the front and back covers for rapid access.

In this edition of the *Handbook*, you will find several *new* chapters: *Diagnostic Imaging and Interventional Radiology*, with practical approaches to ordering and interpreting imaging in key scenarios; *Immunoprophylaxis*, with comprehensive information on vaccinations and chemoprophylaxis; and *Child Maltreatment*, with vital points for the recognition and management of these difficult situations. Throughout the *Handbook* we have added all important *normal* reference values, including heart rate, respiratory rate, blood pressure, ECG parameters, and body mass index, for the spectrum of ages and sizes making up the pediatric patient population.

Extensively revised chapters include *Cardiology*, with a more problem-oriented approach to common presenting complaints such as tachycardia and cyanosis; *Fluids and Electrolytes*, with user-friendly guidelines for maintenance fluid requirements and electrolyte disturbances; *Genetics*, with new diagnostic algorithms for common presenting problems (e.g., cleft lip and palate, microcephaly, and ear anomalies); *Growth and Nutrition*, including normal dietary intake and a guide to total parenteral nutrition; *Hematology*, with expanded sections on thrombosis, bleeding disorders, and transfusion medicine; *Neurology and Neurosurgery*, including a succinct guide to the pediatric neurologic examination; and *Transplantation*, with easy-to-refer-to tables for early recognition and management of post-transplant complications.

Included in the *Handbook* are multiple new algorithms for bedside diagnosis (e.g., thrombocytopenia, limping, and metabolic acidosis) and management of various urgent scenarios (e.g., increased intracranial pressure, febrile neutropenia, and head injury). Figures have been added to highlight both pathology (e.g., cardiomegaly, mediastinal masses, hypospadias) and normal landmarks (e.g., for tympanic membranes and chest X-rays). Multiple new tables, designed for ease of information retrieval, either outline practical diagnostic approaches (e.g., syncope, oncologic presentations, and immunodeficiencies) or contain easy side-by-side comparisons of differential diagnoses (e.g., common ocular complaints and congenital infections).

The comprehensive sections on *The Hospital for Sick Children Formulary and Laboratory Reference Values* have been thoroughly updated to reflect changing knowledge and clinical practice. We have included key Web sites so that the most up-to-date diagnostic methodology and interpretation of results can be readily accessed by the user (e.g., serologic testing). Along with the Useful Web Sites section, we have also included an expanded Further Readings section at the end of each chapter.

We trust that the 11th edition of the *The Hospital for Sick Children Handbook of Pediatrics* will be an essential resource for many health care practitioners for years to come.

Anne I. Dipchand
Jeremy N. Friedman
Zia Bismilla
Sumit Gupta
Catherine Lam

Acknowledgements

So many people have helped make the 11th edition of *The Hospital for Sick Children Handbook of Pediatrics* a reality. In particular, we would like to acknowledge Drs. Susan Tallett and Adelle Atkinson, the previous and present Directors of Postgraduate Medicine at The Hospital for Sick Children for the facilitation of the process, wise insight, and support; Susana Andres and Heidi Falkh, from the The Hospital for Sick Children Corporate Development office, for their ongoing help with the contracts and ensuring smooth communication with the publishers; and Diva Mendes and Tracey Clatworthy for their invaluable administrative support. Many thanks go to Ann Millar, Vice President, Publishing, Elsevier Canada, for assistance with getting the whole process of a new edition started. Special thanks go to our editors at different stages, Martina van de Velde, Sondra Greenfield, and Rohini Herbert, for being a tremendous source of advice and support throughout the production process. Finally, we would like to thank all of the chapter authors—both trainees and staff—for their dedication and hard work culminating in the 11th edition of the *The Hospital for Sick Children Handbook of Pediatrics*.

Anne I. Dipchand
Jeremy N. Friedman
Zia Bismilla
Sumit Gupta
Catherine Lam

Resident Authors

Fatma Al-Jasmi, MBBS, FRCPC
Fellow
Clinical and Metabolic Genetics
Chapter 25: Metabolic Disease

Dalia Alabdulrazzaq, MD, BMBCh
Resident
Pediatric Medicine
Chapter 21: Gynecology

Fatoumah M.Y.M. Alabdulrazzaq,
BMedSc, BMBCh
Resident
Pediatric Medicine
Section III: Laboratory Reference Values

Daniela S. Ardelean, MD
Fellow
Rheumatology
Chapter 19: Genetics

Sowmya Balasubramanian, MD, MSc
Resident
Pediatric Medicine
Chapter 3: Emergency Medicine

Ereny Bassilious, BSc.PT, MD
Resident
Pediatric Medicine
Chapter 11: Dentistry

Michelle Batthish, BSc(Hon),
MSc, MD
Resident
Pediatric Medicine
Chapter 35: Rheumatology

Glenda N. Bendiak, BSc(Hon), MD
Resident
Pediatric Medicine
Chapter 18: General Surgery

Elizabeth Berger, BA, MD
Fellow
Nephrology
Chapter 27: Nephrology

Teresa D. Berger, HBSc, DDS
Resident
Dentistry
Chapter 11: Dentistry

Nirit Bernhard, MSc, MD, FRCPC
Associate Staff Physician/Chief
Resident
Pediatric Medicine
Chapter 1: Resuscitation

Vicky R. Breakey, BSc, MD, FRCPC
Fellow
Hematology/Oncology
Chapter 22: Hematology

Michelle Bridge, BSc, MD
Resident
Pediatric Medicine
Chapter 24: Infectious Diseases

Fabio Ferri-de-Barros, MD, FSBOT
Fellow
Orthopedic Surgery
Chapter 31: Orthopedics

Sloane J. Freeman, MSc, MD
Resident
Pediatric Medicine
Chapter 24: Infectious Diseases

Sharan Goobie, MSc, MD
Resident
Clinical and Metabolic Genetics
Chapter 19: Genetics

Joelene F. Huber, MD, MSc(A),
SLP(c), PhD
Resident
Pediatric Medicine
Chapter 13: Development

Clare Hutchinson, MDCM
Fellow
Rheumatology
Chapter 6: Procedures

Marissa O. Joseph, MD
Resident
Dermatology
Chapter 12: Dermatology

Alisha Kassam, BEng, MD
Resident
Pediatric Medicine
Chapter 22: Hematology

Vy Hong-Diep Kim, HBSc, MD
Resident
Immunology and Allergy
Chapter 8: Allergy and Immunology

Radha P. Kohly, MD, PhD
Resident
Ophthalmology
Chapter 30: Ophthalmology

Ganesh Krishnamurthy, MD
Fellow
Interventional Radiology
Chapter 14: Diagnostic Imaging and
    Interventional Radiology

Mathieu Lemaire, MSc, MDCM
Resident
Nephrology
Chapter 16: Fluids, Electrolytes, and Acid–Base

Nadia Luca, HBSc, MD
Resident
Pediatric Medicine
Chapter 4: Poisonings and Toxicology

Melanie M. Makhija, BSc, MD,
    MSc Epi
Resident
Pediatric Medicine
Chapter 23: Immunoprophylaxis

Arif Manji, MD, B Arts Sc
Resident
Pediatric Medicine
Chapter 14: Diagnostic Imaging and
    Interventional Radiology

Caroline McLaughlin, MSc, MD
Resident
Pediatric Medicine
Chapter 15: Endocrinology

Shruti Mehrotra, HBSc, MD
Resident
Pediatric Medicine
Chapter 28: Neurology and Neurosurgery

Briseida Mema, MD
Resident
Pediatric Medicine
Chapter 37: Urology

Sharon Naymark, MD, FRCPC
Associate Staff Physician/Chief
    Resident
Pediatric Medicine
Chapter 10: Child Maltreatment

Melissa J. Parker, MD, MSc, FRCPC,
    FAAP
Fellow
Emergency and Critical Care Medicine
Chapter 3: Emergency Medicine

Seetha Radhakrishnan, MDCM
Fellow
Nephrology
Chapter 16: Fluids, Electrolytes, and
    Acid–Base

Tania Samanta, BSc(Hon), MD
Resident
Respiratory Medicine
Chapter 34: Respirology

Gagan Saund, BSc, MD
Resident
Pediatric Medicine
Chapter 26: Neonatology

Deena Savlov, BSc, MD
Resident
Pediatric Medicine
Chapter 20: Growth and Nutrition

Rayzel M. Shulman, BSc, MD
Fellow
Endocrinology
Chapter 15: Endocrinology

Ewurabena A. Simpson, BSc(Hons),
    MDCM
Resident
Pediatric Medicine
Chapter 17: Gastroenterology and
    Hepatology

Ksenia Slywynska, BASc, MD
Resident
Pediatric Medicine
Chapter 33: Plastic Surgery

Gordon S. Soon, BSc, MD
Resident
Pediatric Medicine
Chapter 32: Otolaryngology

Joanna Swinburne, MD, BSc
Resident
Respiratory Medicine
Chapter 34: Respirology

Lindsay Teskey, MD, FRCPC
Fellow
Nephrology
Chapter 36: Transplantation

Mark O. Tessaro, MDCM, BSc
Resident
Pediatric Medicine
Chapter 5: Pain and Sedation

Nisha Thampi, BASc, MD
Resident
Pediatric Medicine
Chapter 22: Hematology

Alène A. Toulany, BSc(Hons), MD
Resident
Pediatric Medicine
Chapter 20: Growth and Nutrition

Tony H. Truong, MD, FRCPC
Fellow
Hematology/Oncology
Chapter 29: Oncology

Ellie Vyver, MD, FRCPC
Fellow
Adolescent Medicine
Chapter 7: Adolescent Medicine

Catharine M. Walsh, MD, FRCPC
Fellow
Gastroenterology, Hepatology and
    Nutrition
Chapter 17: Gastroenterology and
    Hepatology

Andrea Wan, BSc, MD
Resident
Pediatric Medicine
Chapter 9: Cardiology

Kevin Weingarten, MD
Resident
Pediatric Medicine
Chapter 29: Oncology

Constance Williams, MD, FRCPC
Fellow
Neonatology
Chapter 26: Neonatology

Derek Wong, FRCPC, FAAP, MD
Fellow
Cardiology
Chapter 9: Cardiology

Gail K. Wong, MBBS, BSc(Med),
    FANZCA
Associate Staff
Anesthesia
Chapter 2: Anesthesia

Staff Authors

Oussama Abla, MD
Staff Physician
Hematology/Oncology
Chapter 29: Oncology

Khosrow Adeli, PhD, FCACB, DABCC
Head, Clinical Biochemistry Division
Pediatric Laboratory Medicine
Section III: Laboratory Reference Values

Lisa M. Allen, MD, FRCSC
Staff Surgeon; Head, Department of
    Pediatric and Adolescent
    Gynecology
Pediatric and Adolescent Gynecology
Chapter 21: Gynecology

Adelle R. Atkinson, MD, FRCPC
Staff Physician; Immunology and
    Allergy
Director of Postgraduate Medical
    Education Pediatrics
Chapter 8: Allergy and Immunology

Georges Azzie, MD, FRCSC
Staff Surgeon
General Surgery
Chapter 18: General Surgery

Darius J. Bagli, MDCM, FRCSC,
    FAAP, FACS
Staff Surgeon
Urology
Chapter 37: Urology

Ross Barlow, MD, FRCPC
Staff Physician
Anesthesia
Chapter 2: Anesthesia

Stacey Bernstein, MD, FRCPC
Staff Physician; Director of
    Undergraduate Medical Education
Pediatric Medicine
Chapter 20: Growth and Nutrition

Ari Bitnun, MD, MSc, FRCPC
Staff Physician
Infectious Diseases
Chapter 24: Infectious Diseases

Paolo Campisi, MSc, MD, FRCSC,
    FAAP
Staff Surgeon
Otolaryngology
Chapter 32: Otolaryngology

Bairbre Connolly, MB, DCH, FRCSI,
    MCh, FFRRCSI, FRCPC
Staff Physician
Diagnostic Imaging and Interventional
    Radiology
Chapter 14: Diagnostic Imaging and
    Interventional Radiology

Emma Cory, MD, FRCPC
Associate Staff Physician
Pediatric Medicine
Chapter 10: Child Maltreatment

Christopher R. Forrest, MD, MSc,
    FRCSC, FACS
Staff Surgeon; Medical Director,
    Craniofacial Program; Head,
    Plastic Surgery
Plastic Surgery
Chapter 33: Plastic Surgery

Fraser Golding, MD, FRCPC
Staff Physician
Cardiology
Chapter 9: Cardiology

Hartmut Grasemann, MD, PhD
Staff Physician
Respiratory Medicine
Chapter 34: Respirology

Andrew W. Howard, MD, MSc, FRCSC
Staff Surgeon
Orthopedic Surgery
Chapter 31: Orthopedics

Elizabeth A. Jimenez, BSc, MD, FRCPC
Staff Physician
Developmental Pediatrics
Chapter 13: Development

Miriam Kaufman, BSN, MD, FRCPC
Staff Physician
Adolescent Medicine
Chapter 7: Adolescent Medicine

Melanie-Ann Kirby, MBBS, FRCPC
Staff Physician
Hematology/Oncology
Chapter 22: Hematology

Amina Lalani, MD, FRCPC, FAAP
(PEM)
Staff Physician
Emergency Medicine
Chapter 3: Emergency Medicine

Valerie Langlois, MD, FRCPC
Staff Physician
Nephrology
Chapter 27: Nephrology

Elaine Lau, BScPhm, PharmD, MSc,
RPh
Coordinator, Drug Information Service
Pharmacy
Section IV: Pediatric Drug Dosing Guidelines

Wendy Lau, MBBS, FRCPC
Director, Transfusion Medicine
Pediatric Laboratory Medicine
Section III: Laboratory Reference Values

Christoph Licht, MD, FASN
Staff Physician
Nephrology
Chapter 16: Fluids, Electrolytes,
and Acid–Base

Bruce A. Macpherson, MD, FRCPC
Staff Physician
Anesthesia
Chapter 1: Resuscitation

Shonna L. Masse, HBSc, DDS, MS,
FRCDC
Staff Pediatric Dentist
Dentistry
Chapter 11: Dentistry

Roberto Mendoza-Londono, MD,
MSc, FACMG, FCCMG
Staff Physician
Clinical and Metabolic Genetics
Chapter 19: Genetics

Aideen Moore, MB, BCh, BAO, MD,
MRCPI, MHSc, FRCPC
Staff Physician
Neonatology
Chapter 26: Neonatology

Basem Naser, MBBS, FRCPC
Staff Physician; Director, Acute Pain
Service
Anesthesia
Chapter 5: Pain and Sedation

Vicky Lee Ng, MD, FRCPC
Staff Physician
Gastroenterology, Hepatology and
Nutrition
Chapter 36: Transplantation

Kusiel Perlman, BSc(Med), MD, FRCPC
Staff Physician
Endocrinology
Chapter 15: Endocrinology

Jonathan Pirie, MD, MEd, FRCPC,
FAAP(PEM)
Staff Physician
Emergency Medicine
Chapter 6: Procedures

Elena Pope, MSc, FRCPC
Staff Physician; Head, Dermatology
Pediatric Medicine
Chapter 12: Dermatology

Julian A.J. Raiman, MBBS, MSc,
MRCP(Lond)
Staff Physician
Clinical and Metabolic Genetics
Chapter 25: Metabolic Disease

Teesta Soman, FAAP, DABPN, MBA
Staff Physician
Neurology
Chapter 28: Neurology and Neurosurgery

Nasrin Najm Tehrani, MBBCh, MSc,
FRCS Ed(Ophth)
Staff Physician
Ophthalmology
Chapter 30: Ophthalmology

Margaret Thompson, MD, FRCPC,
FACMT
Medical Director, Ontario Poison
Centre
Chapter 4: Poisonings and Toxicology

Dat J. Tran, MD, MS, FAAP, FRCPC
Staff Physician
Infectious Diseases
Chapter 23: Immunoprophylaxis

Shirley M.L. Tse, MD, FRCPC
Staff Physician
Rheumatology
Chapter 35: Rheumatology

Mary Zachos, MD, FRCPC
Staff Physician
Gastroenterology, Hepatology and
Nutrition
Chapter 17: Gastroenterology and
Hepatology

Chapter Authors

Section I:
ACUTE CARE PEDIATRICS

Chapter 1: Resuscitation

Nirit Bernhard, MSc, MD, FRCPC
Associate Staff Physician/Chief
    Resident
Pediatric Medicine

Bruce A. Macpherson, MD, FRCPC
Staff Physician
Anesthesia

Chapter 2: Anesthesia

Gail K. Wong, MBBS, BSc(Med),
    FANZCA
Associate Staff Physician
Anesthesia

Ross Barlow, MD, FRCPC
Staff Physician
Anesthesia

Chapter 3: Emergency Medicine

Sowmya Balasubramanian, MD,
    MSc
Resident
Pediatric Medicine

Melissa J. Parker, MD, MSc, FRCPC
Fellow
Emergency and Critical Care Medicine

Amina Lalani, MD, FRCPC,
    FAAP(PEM)
Staff Physician
Emergency Medicine

Chapter 4: Poisonings and Toxicology

Nadia Luca, HBSc, MD
Resident
Pediatric Medicine

Margaret Thompson, MD, FRCPC,
    FACMT
Medical Director
Ontario Poison Centre

Chapter 5: Pain and Sedation

Mark O. Tessaro, MDCM, BSc
Resident
Pediatric Medicine

Basem Naser, MBBS, FRCPC
Staff Physician; Director, Acute Pain
    Service
Anesthesia

Chapter 6: Procedures

Clare Hutchinson, MDCM
Fellow
Rheumatology

Jonathan Pirie, MD, MEd, FRCPC,
    FAAP(PEM)
Staff Physician
Emergency Medicine

Section II:
SUBSPECIALTY
PEDIATRICS

Chapter 7: Adolescent Medicine

Ellie Vyver, MD, FRCPC
Fellow
Adolescent Medicine

Miriam Kaufman, BSN, MD, FRCPC
Staff Physician
Adolescent Medicine

Chapter 8: Allergy and Immunology

Vy Hong-Diep Kim, HBSc, MD
Resident
Immunology and Allergy

Adelle R. Atkinson, MD, FRCPC
Staff Physician, Immunology and
    Allergy
Director of Postgraduate Medical
    Education, Pediatrics

Chapter 9: Cardiology

Andrea Wan, BSc, MD
Resident
Pediatric Medicine

Derek Wong, FRCPC, FAAP, MD
Fellow
Cardiology

Fraser Golding, MD, FRCPC
Staff Physician
Cardiology

Chapter 10: Child Maltreatment

Sharon Naymark, MD, FRCPC
Associate Staff Physician/Chief
Resident
Pediatric Medicine

Emma Cory, MD, FRCPC
Associate Staff Physician
Pediatric Medicine

Chapter 11: Dentistry

Ereny Bassilious, BSc.PT, MD
Resident
Pediatric Medicine

Teresa D. Berger, HBSc, DDS
Dental Resident
Dentistry

Shonna L. Masse, HBSc, DDS, MS,
FRCDC
Staff Pediatric Dentist
Dentistry

Chapter 12: Dermatology

Marissa O. Joseph, MD
Resident
Dermatology

Elena Pope, MSc, FRCPC
Staff Physician; Head, Dermatology
Pediatric Medicine

Chapter 13: Development

Joelene F. Huber, MD, MSc(A),
SLP(c), PhD
Resident
Pediatric Medicine

Elizabeth A. Jimenez, BSc, MD,
FRCPC
Staff Physician
Developmentlal Pediatrics

Chapter 14: Diagnostic Imaging and Interventional Radiology

Arif Manji, MD, B Arts Sc
Resident
Pediatric Medicine

Ganesh Krishnamurthy, MD
Interventional Fellow
Diagnostic Imaging and Interventional
Radiology

Bairbre Connolly, MB, DCH, FRCSI,
MCh, FFRRCSI, FRCPC
Staff Physician
Diagnostic Imaging and Interventional
Radiology

Chapter 15: Endocrinology

Caroline McLaughlin, MSc, MD
Resident
Pediatric Medicine

Rayzel M. Shulman, BSc, MD
Fellow
Endocrinology

Kusiel Perlman, BSc(Med), MD,
FRCPC
Staff Physician
Endocrinology

Chapter 16: Fluids, Electrolytes, and Acid–Base

Mathieu Lemaire, MSc, MDCM
Resident
Nephrology

Seetha Radhakrishnan, MDCM
Fellow
Nephrology

Christoph Licht, MD, FASN
Staff Physician
Nephrology

Chapter 17: Gastroenterology and Hepatology

Catharine M. Walsh, MD, FRCPC
Fellow
Gastroenterology, Hepatology
and Nutrition

Ewurabena A. Simpson, BSc(Hons),
MDCM
Resident
Pediatric Medicine

Mary Zachos, MD, FRCPC
Staff Physician
Gastroenterology, Hepatology and
    Nutrition

Chapter 18: General Surgery

Glenda N. Bendiak, BSc(Hon), MD
Resident
Pediatric Medicine

Georges Azzie, MD, FRCSC
Staff Surgeon
General Surgery

Chapter 19: Genetics

Daniela S. Ardelean, MD
Fellow
Rheumatology

Sharan Goobie, MSc, MD
Resident
Clinical and Metabolic Genetics

Roberto Mendoza-Londono, MD,
    MSc, FACMG, FCCMG
Staff Physician
Clinical and Metabolic Genetics

Chapter 20: Growth and Nutrition

Deena Savlov, BSc, MD
Resident
Pediatric Medicine

Alène A. Toulany, BSc(Hons), MD
Resident
Pediatric Medicine

Stacey Bernstein, MD, FRCPC
Staff Physician; Pediatric Medicine
Director of Undergraduate Medical
    Education

Chapter 21: Gynecology

Dalia Alabdulrazzaq, MD, BMBCh
Resident
Pediatric Medicine

Lisa M. Allen, MD, FRCSC
Staff Surgeon; Head, Department
    of Pediatric and Adolescent
    Gynecology
Pediatric and Adolescent Gynecology

Chapter 22: Hematology

Vicky R. Breakey, BSc, MD, FRCPC
Fellow
Hematology/Oncology

Alisha Kassam, BEng, MD
Resident
Pediatric Medicine

Nisha Thampi, BASc, MD
Resident
Pediatric Medicine

Melanie-Ann Kirby, MBBS, FRCPC
Staff Physician
Hematology/Oncology

Chapter 23: Immunoprophylaxis

Melanie M. Makhija, BSc, MD, MSc Epi
Resident
Pediatric Medicine

Dat J. Tran, MD, MS, FAAP, FRCPC
Staff Physician
Infectious Diseases

Chapter 24: Infectious Diseases

Michelle Bridge, BSc, MD
Resident
Pediatric Medicine

Sloane J. Freeman, MSc, MD
Resident
Pediatric Medicine

Ari Bitnun, MD, MSc, FRCPC
Staff Physician
Infectious Diseases

Chapter 25: Metabolic Disease

Fatma Al-Jasmi, MBBS, FRCPC
Fellow
Clinical and Metabolic Genetics

Julian A.J. Raiman, MBBS, MSc,
    MRCP(Lond)
Staff Physician
Clinical and Metabolic Genetics

Chapter 26: Neonatology

Gagan Saund, BSc, MD
Resident
Pediatric Medicine

Constance Williams, MD, FRCPC
Fellow
Neonatology

Aideen Moore, MB, BCh, BAO, MD,
    MRCPI, MHSc, FRCPC
Staff Physician
Neonatology

Chapter 27: Nephrology

Elizabeth Berger, BA, MD
Fellow
Nephrology

Valerie Langlois, MD, FRCPC
Staff Physician
Nephrology

Chapter 28: Neurology and Neurosurgery

Shruti Mehrotra, HBSc, MD
Resident
Pediatric Medicine

Teesta Soman, FAAP, DABPN, MBA
Staff Physician
Neurology

Chapter 29: Oncology

Tony H. Truong, MD, FRCPC
Fellow
Hematology/Oncology

Kevin Weingarten, MD
Resident
Pediatric Medicine

Oussama Abla, MD
Staff Physician
Hematology/Oncology

Chapter 30: Ophthalmology

Radha P. Kohly, MD, PhD
Resident
Ophthalmology

Nasrin Najm Tehrani, MBBCh, MSc, FRCS Ed(Ophth)
Staff Physician
Ophthalmology

Chapter 31: Orthopedics

Fabio Ferri-de-Barros, MD, FSBOT
Fellow
Orthopedic Surgery

Andrew W. Howard, MD, MSc, FRCSC
Staff Surgeon
Orthopedic Surgery

Chapter 32: Otolaryngology

Gordon S. Soon, BSc, MD
Resident
Pediatric Medicine

Paolo Campisi, MSc, MD, FRCSC, FAAP
Staff Surgeon
Otolaryngology

Chapter 33: Plastic Surgery

Ksenia Slywynska, BASc, MD
Resident
Pediatric Medicine

Christopher R. Forrest, MD, MSc, FRCSC, FACS
Staff Surgeon; Medical Director, Craniofacial Program; Head, Plastic Surgery
Plastic Surgery

Chapter 34: Respirology

Tania Samanta, BSc(Hon), MD
Resident
Respiratory Medicine

Joanna Swinburne, MD, BSc
Resident
Respiratory Medicine

Hartmut Grasemann, MD, PhD
Staff Physician
Respiratory Medicine

Chapter 35: Rheumatology

Michelle Batthish, BSc(Hon), MSc, MD
Resident
Pediatric Medicine

Shirley M.L. Tse, MD, FRCPC
Staff Physician
Rheumatology

Chapter 36: Transplantation

Lindsay Teskey, MD, FRCPC
Fellow
Nephrology

Vicky Lee Ng, MD, FRCPC
Staff Physician
Gastroenterology, Hepatology and Nutrition

Chapter 37: Urology

Briseida Mema, MD
Resident
Pediatric Medicine

Darius J. Bagli, MDCM, FRCSC, FAAP, FACS
Staff Surgeon
Urology

Section III:
LABORATORY REFERENCE VALUES

Fatoumah M. Y. M. Alabdulrazzaq, BMedSc, BMBCh
Resident
Pediatric Medicine

Khosrow Adeli, PhD, FCACB, DABCC
Head, Clinical Biochemistry Division
Pediatric Laboratory Medicine

Wendy Lau, MBBS, FRCPC
Director, Transfusion Medicine
Pediatric Laboratory Medicine

Section IV:
PEDIATRIC DRUG DOSING GUIDELINES

Elaine Lau, BScPhm, PharmD, MSc, RPh
Coordinator, Drug Information Service
Pharmacy

Chapter 1 Resuscitation

Nirit Bernhard

Bruce A. Macpherson

Chapter 1   Resuscitation

COMMON ABBREVIATIONS

ABC	airway, breathing, circulation
ABG	arterial blood gas
BVM	bag valve mask
CPAP	continuous positive airway pressure
ETT	endotracheal tube
IO	intraosseous
LMA	laryngeal mask airway
PALS	Pediatric Advanced Life Support
PEA	pulseless electrical activity
PICU	pediatric intensive care unit

RESUSCITATION DRUGS IN INFANTS AND CHILDREN

- See table inside front cover, Resuscitation Drugs in Infants and Older Children—Intermittent Doses
- See Table 1.1 for continuous infusions
- See inside back cover for infusion calculations and common resuscitation IV infusions

Table 1.1	Resuscitation Drugs in Infants and Older Children—Infusions	
Supplied	**Dose**	**Comments**
Alprostadil (prostaglandin E_1) Injection: 500 mcg/mL	0.01–0.1 mcg/kg/min IV as a continuous infusion	250 mcg in 80 mL D5W at 1 mL/kg/h = 0.05 mg/kg/min 500 mcg in 80 mL D5W at 1 mL/kg/h = 0.1 mcg/kg/min Caution: may cause apnea
Amiodarone Injection: 150 mg/3 mL ampule 50 mg/mL	5–15 mcg/kg/min IV as a continuous infusion	Use non-PVC tubing 15 × weight (kg) = dose (mg) added to 50 mL D5W An infusion of 1 mL/h = 5 mcg/kg/min CVL administration preferred; watch site with peripheral line administration
Dopamine* Injection: 800 mcg/mL (200 mg/250 mL) OR 3200 mcg/mL (800 mg/250 mL)	5–20 mcg/kg/min IV/IO as a continuous infusion	15 × weight (kg) = dose (mg) added to 50 mL crystalloid to make 1 mL/h = 5 mcg/kg/min

(continued)

Table 1.1 — Resuscitation Drugs in Infants and Older Children—Infusions (continued)

Supplied	Dose	Comments
Epinephrine Injection: 1:1000 1 mg/mL ampule, 30 mg/30 mL vial 1 mg/mL	0.1–1 mcg/kg/min IV/IO as a continuous infusion	0.3 × weight (kg) = dose in mg added to 50 mL crystalloid to make 1 mL/h = 0.1 mcg/kg/min
Insulin (regular) Injection: 100 units/mL	DKA : 0.1 units/kg/h Hyperkalemia: 1 unit per 5 g of IV dextrose	Dilute 25 units in 250 mL of 0.9% NaCl to make 1 mL/kg/h = 0.1 units/kg/h Use 5 units insulin in 50 mL of D50W at a dose of 1 mL/kg (give as a bolus)
Isoproterenol Injection: 1 mg/5 mL 0.2 mg/mL	0.025–0.1 mcg/kg/min IV as a continuous infusion Titrate to heart rate	0.15 × weight (kg) = dose in mg added to 50 mL crystalloid to make 1 mL/h = 0.05 mcg/kg/min
Labetalol Injection: 100 mg/20 mL 5 mg/mL	1–3 mg/kg/h	50 × weight (kg) = dose in mg added to 50 mL crystalloid to make 1mL/h = 1 mg/kg/h Maximum concentration: 250 mg/50 mL undiluted solution
Lidocaine 2% Injection: 100 mg/5 mL syringe, 100 mg/5 mL vial; 20 mg/mL	20–50 mcg/kg/min IV as a continuous infusion	60 × weight (kg) = dose in mg added to 50 mL crystalloid to make 1 mL/h = 20 mcg/kg/min
Procainamide Injection: 1 g/10 mL 100 mg/mL	20–80 mcg/kg/min IV as a continuous infusion Maximum 20 mg/min IV infusion up to total maximum dose 17 mg/kg	60 × weight (kg) = dose in mg added to 50 mL crystalloid to make 1 mL/h = 20 mcg/kg/min

IV, intravenous; *IO*, intraosseous; *CVL*, central venous line; *DKA*, diabetic ketoacidosis.
*Dobutamine is same dose and administration.
© The Hospital for Sick Children. Adapted from Griffiths K, ed. *The Hospital for Sick Children Drug Formulary, 2006–2007*, 25th ed. Toronto, Ontario: The Hospital for Sick Children.

PEDIATRIC VITAL SIGNS

- See inside back cover for normal vital signs
- See Table 1.2 for abnormal vital sign parameters

Table 1.2	Abnormal Vital Signs in Children—Age-Specific Parameters		
Age	Heart Rate (beats/min)	Respiratory Rate (breaths/min)	Systolic Blood Pressure* (mmHg)
Newborn-3 mo	<80 or >200	<30 or >60	<60
3-12 mo	<80 or >180	<24 or >50	<65
1-10 yr	<60 or >150	<22 or >40	<70 + (2 × age [yr])
>10 yr	<60 or >120	<12 or >30	<90

*Systolic BP is 5th percentile for age.
Adapted from *Pediatric Advanced Life Support Pocket Reference Card.* American Heart Association; 2006.

INFANT AND CHILD CARDIOPULMONARY RESUSCITATION

AIRWAY

- See Figure 1.1 for an approach to airway management
- See Table 1.3 for intubation equipment sizing
- See Table 1.4 for drugs used for intubation
- See Boxes 1.1, 1.2, and 1.3

Figure 1.1 Airway

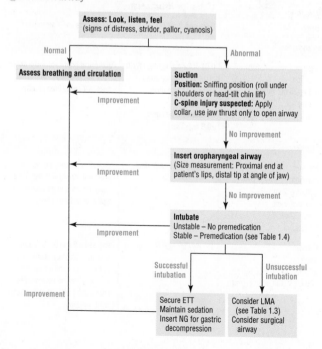

Table 1.3 — Intubation Equipment Sizing by Age and Weight

Age	Avg Wt (kg)	ETT (mm)	Blade	LMA	Suction (F)
Birth	3.5	2.5-3.5	0 straight	1-1.5	6-8
6 mo	7.5	3.5	1 straight	1.5-2	8
1 yr	10	4.0	1 straight	1.5-2	8
2 yr	12	4.5	2 straight	2	8
3 yr	14	4.5-5	2 straight	2	8-10
4 yr	16	5.0	2 straight	2	10
6 yr	20	5.5	2 or 3 curved	2-2.5	10
8 yr	24	6.0 C	3 curved	2.5	12
9-12 yr	27-40	6.0 C	3 curved	3-4	12

C, cuffed endotracheal tube.
Adapted from Shann A. *Drug Doses*, 13th ed. Melbourne, Australia: Collective Pty Ltd; 2005.

Table 1.4 — Drugs* Used for Intubation

Drug	Dose and Route	Side Effects and Comments
Preinduction		
Atropine Premedication Injection: 0.5 mg/5 mL syringe 0.1 mg/mL	0.01-0.02 mg/kg/dose IV/IO (0.1-0.2 mL/kg/dose) Minimum single dose: 0.1 mg (1 mL) Maximum single dose: 0.3 mg (3 mL)	Paradoxical bradycardia with dose <0.1 mg, pupillary dilation (but does NOT cause fixed pupils)
Induction		
Fentanyl Injection: 100 mcg/2 mL 250 mcg/5 mL 1 mg/20 mL 50 mcg/mL	2-4 mcg/kg/dose IV slowly	Respiratory depression, hypotension, chest wall rigidity with high-dose rapid infusions, in addition to typical opioid side effects
Ketamine Injection: 200 mg/20 mL = 10 mg/mL 500 mg/10 mL = 50 mg/mL	1-2 mg/kg/dose IV	Increased ICP and BP, increased secretions and laryngospasm, hallucinations and emergence reactions (can be decreased by concomitant use with midazolam) Useful in asthma

(continued)

Table 1.4   Drugs* Used for Intubation (continued)

Drug	Dose and Route	Side Effects and Comments
Lidocaine 2% Injection: 100 mg/5 mL syringe/vial 20 mg/mL	1–2 mg/kg/dose IV (0.05–0.1 mL/kg/dose)	Myocardial and CNS depression with high doses and possible seizures with repeated doses Useful with raised ICP
Midazolam Injection: 5 mg/mL, 50 mg/10 mL 5 mg/mL	0.05–0.2 mg/kg/dose over 3–5 min IV	Respiratory depression, hypotension, especially when combined with narcotic Not an analgesic agent
Propofol Injection: 200 mg/20 mL 10 mg/mL	2–5 mg/kg/dose IV	Respiratory depression and hypotension, especially with underlying hypovolemia
Thiopental Injection: 1g/vial Reconstitute with 40 mL sterile water for injection = 25 mg/mL	2–4 mg/kg/dose IV	Hypotension, decreases ICP, negative inotropic effects and potentiates respiratory depression of narcotics and benzodiazepines Not an analgesic agent
Muscle Relaxants		
Rocuronium Injection: 50 mg/5 mL 10 mg/mL	0.6–1.2 mg/kg/dose IV/IO	Neuromuscular blocking agent Minimal cardiovascular side effects with rapid onset of action; duration of action 30–60 min
Succinylcholine Injection: 200 mg/10 mL 20 mg/mL	1–2 mg/kg/dose IV Give single dose and avoid repeated dosing	Neuromuscular blocking agent Contraindicated in myopathies, raised intraocular pressure, hyperkalemia, renal failure Can cause muscle fasciculations and hyperkalemia

*These agents are to be used by medically trained individuals skilled in advanced airway management.
© The Hospital for Sick Children. Adapted from Griffiths K, ed. *The Hospital for Sick Children Drug Formulary, 2006–2007*, 25th ed. Toronto, Ontario: Hospital for Sick Children.

Box 1.1   Estimation Guidelines for Children Aged 1–10 Years

Weight:	$(2 \times [age]) + 8$
ETT size:	Uncuffed ETT: age/4 + 4
	Cuffed ETT: age/3 + 4
ETT depth (cm):	Measured at mouth: $3 \times$ ETT size

Length-based resuscitation tapes such as the Broselow tape are available for children up to approximately 35 kg and should be used when available.

From American Heart Association. 2005 American Heart Association Guidelines for Cardiopulmonary Resuscitation and Emergency Cardiovascular Care: Pediatric Advanced Life Support. *Circulation.* 2005;112(suppl 1, pt 12):IV–169.

Box 1.2 Verification of ETT Placement

- Direct laryngoscopy (gold standard)
- Equal chest movement/breath sounds bilaterally
- Pulse oximetry
- End-tidal CO_2 monitor
- CXR

Box 1.3 Causes of Deterioration in an Intubated Patient (DOPE)

- **D**isplacement of ETT
- **O**bstruction of ETT
- **P**neumothorax
- **E**quipment failure

From American Heart Association. 2005 American Heart Association Guidelines for Cardiopulmonary Resuscitation and Emergency Cardiovascular Care: Pediatric Advanced Life Support. *Circulation*. 2005;112(suppl 1, pt 12):IV–169.

BREATHING

- See Figure 1.2

Figure 1.2 Breathing

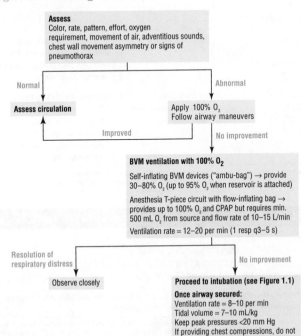

Assess
Color, rate, pattern, effort, oxygen requirement, movement of air, adventitious sounds, chest wall movement asymmetry or signs of pneumothorax

Normal → **Assess circulation**

Abnormal → Apply 100% O_2
Follow airway maneuvers

Improved

No improvement

BVM ventilation with 100% O_2

Self-inflating BVM devices ("ambu-bag") → provide 30–80% O_2 (up to 95% O_2 when reservoir is attached)

Anesthesia T-piece circuit with flow-inflating bag → provides up to 100% O_2 and CPAP but requires min. 500 mL O_2 from source and flow rate of 10–15 L/min

Ventilation rate = 12–20 per min (1 resp q3–5 s)

Resolution of respiratory distress → Observe closely

No improvement →

Proceed to intubation (see Figure 1.1)
Once airway secured:
Ventilation rate = 8–10 per min
Tidal volume = 7–10 mL/kg
Keep peak pressures <20 mm Hg
If providing chest compressions, do not pause compressions during ventilation

CIRCULATION

- See Figure 1.3

Figure 1.3 Circulation

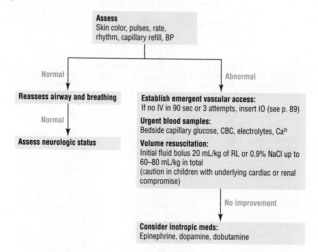

PEDIATRIC ADVANCED LIFE SUPPORT ALGORITHMS

TACHYCARDIA

- See Figure 1.4

BRADYCARDIA

- See Figure 1.5

PULSELESS ARREST (PEA)

- See Figure 1.6
- Indications for chest compressions: HR <60 beats/min and evidence of poor systemic circulation, OR no palpable femoral or brachial pulse; goal is to "push hard and push fast"
- Cardiac compression to ventilation ratios: 15:2 for two rescuers, 30:2 for single rescuer. Goal is 100 compressions/min with full recoil after each compression and minimal interruptions
- Landmarking and chest compression technique: two finger spaces above xyphoid or at nipple line and depress ⅓ to ½ AP chest wall diameter
- Place firm surface (backboard) under patient, extending from shoulders to waist

Figure 1.4 Tachycardia

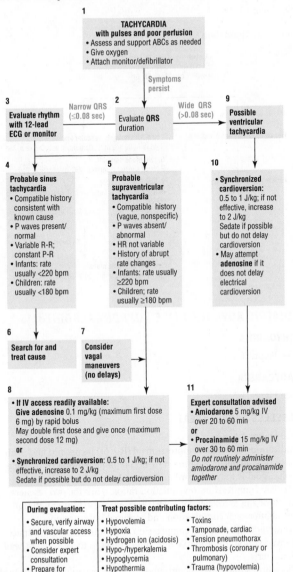

1

**TACHYCARDIA
with pulses and poor perfusion**
- Assess and support ABCs as needed
- Give oxygen
- Attach monitor/defibrillator

Symptoms persist

2

Evaluate **QRS** duration

Narrow QRS (≤0.08 sec)

3

Evaluate rhythm with 12-lead ECG or monitor

Wide QRS (>0.08 sec)

9

Possible ventricular tachycardia

4

Probable sinus tachycardia
- Compatible history consistent with known cause
- P waves present/normal
- Variable R-R; constant P-R
- Infants: rate usually <220 bpm
- Children: rate usually <180 bpm

5

Probable supraventricular tachycardia
- Compatible history (vague, nonspecific)
- P waves absent/abnormal
- HR not variable
- History of abrupt rate changes
- Infants: rate usually ≥220 bpm
- Children; rate usually ≥180 bpm

10

- **Synchronized cardioversion:** 0.5 to 1 J/kg; if not effective, increase to 2 J/kg Sedate if possible but do not delay cardioversion
- May attempt **adenosine** if it does not delay electrical cardioversion

6

Search for and treat cause

7

Consider vagal maneuvers (no delays)

8

- If IV access readily available:
Give adenosine 0.1 mg/kg (maximum first dose 6 mg) by rapid bolus
May double first dose and give once (maximum second dose 12 mg)
or
- **Synchronized cardioversion:** 0.5 to 1 J/kg; if not effective, increase to 2 J/kg
Sedate if possible but do not delay cardioversion

11

Expert consultation advised
- **Amiodarone** 5 mg/kg IV over 20 to 60 min
or
- **Procainamide** 15 mg/kg IV over 30 to 60 min
Do not routinely administer amiodarone and procainamide together

During evaluation:	Treat possible contributing factors:	
• Secure, verify airway and vascular access when possible • Consider expert consultation • Prepare for cardioversion	• Hypovolemia • Hypoxia • Hydrogen ion (acidosis) • Hypo-/hyperkalemia • Hypoglycemia • Hypothermia	• Toxins • Tamponade, cardiac • Tension pneumothorax • Thrombosis (coronary or pulmonary) • Trauma (hypovolemia)

Figure 1.5 **Bradycardia**

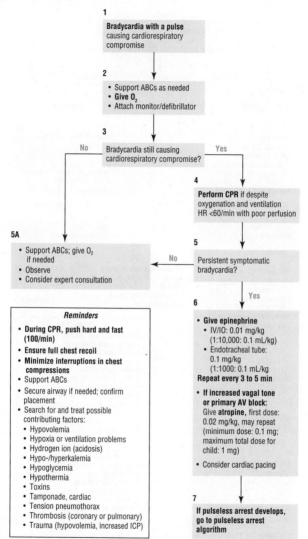

1

Bradycardia with a pulse
causing cardiorespiratory
compromise

2

• Support ABCs as needed
• **Give O₂**
• Attach monitor/defibrillator

3

No   Bradycardia still causing   Yes
cardiorespiratory compromise?

4

Perform CPR if despite
oxygenation and ventilation
HR <60/min with poor perfusion

5A

• Support ABCs; give O₂
 if needed
• Observe
• Consider expert consultation

5

No   Persistent symptomatic
bradycardia?

Yes

6

• **Give epinephrine**
 • IV/IO: 0.01 mg/kg
  (1:10,000: 0.1 mL/kg)
 • Endotracheal tube:
  0.1 mg/kg
  (1:1000: 0.1 mL/kg)
 Repeat every 3 to 5 min

• **If increased vagal tone
 or primary AV block:**
 Give **atropine**, first dose:
 0.02 mg/kg, may repeat
 (minimum dose: 0.1 mg;
 maximum total dose for
 child: 1 mg)

• Consider cardiac pacing

7

**If pulseless arrest develops,
go to pulseless arrest
algorithm**

Reminders

• **During CPR, push hard and fast
 (100/min)**
• **Ensure full chest recoil**
• **Minimize interruptions in chest
 compressions**
• Support ABCs
• Secure airway if needed; confirm
 placement
• Search for and treat possible
 contributing factors:
 • Hypovolemia
 • Hypoxia or ventilation problems
 • Hydrogen ion (acidosis)
 • Hypo-/hyperkalemia
 • Hypoglycemia
 • Hypothermia
 • Toxins
 • Tamponade, cardiac
 • Tension pneumothorax
 • Thrombosis (coronary or pulmonary)
 • Trauma (hypovolemia, increased ICP)

Figure 1.6 Pulseless Arrest

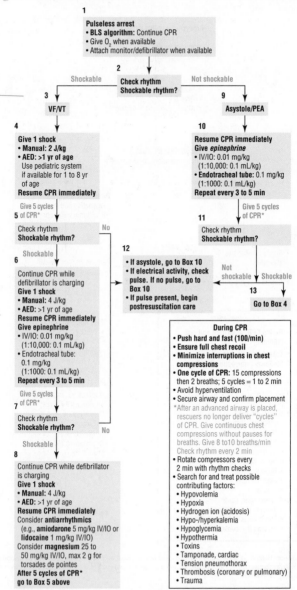

1
Pulseless arrest
- **BLS algorithm:** Continue CPR
- Give O_2 when available
- Attach monitor/defibrillator when available

2
Shockable ← **Check rhythm**
Shockable rhythm? → Not shockable

3
VF/VT

9
Asystole/PEA

4
Give 1 shock
- **Manual:** 2 J/kg
- **AED:** >1 yr of age
  Use pediatric system
  if available for 1 to 8 yr
  of age
Resume CPR immediately

Give 5 cycles
5 of CPR*

10
Resume CPR immediately
Give *epinephrine*
- **IV/IO:** 0.01 mg/kg
  (1:10,000: 0.1 mL/kg)
- **Endotracheal tube:** 0.1 mg/kg
  (1:1000: 0.1 mL/kg)
Repeat every 3 to 5 min

Give 5 cycles
of CPR*

5
Check rhythm
Shockable rhythm? — No

6
Shockable
Continue CPR while
defibrillator is charging
Give 1 shock
- **Manual:** 4 J/kg
- **AED:** >1 yr of age
Resume CPR immediately
Give epinephrine
- **IV/IO:** 0.01 mg/kg
  (1:10,000: 0.1 mL/kg)
- **Endotracheal tube:**
  0.1 mg/kg
  (1:1000: 0.1 mL/kg)
Repeat every 3 to 5 min

Give 5 cycles
7 of CPR*

11
Check rhythm
Shockable rhythm?

12
- If asystole, go to Box 10
- If electrical activity, check
  pulse. If no pulse, go to
  Box 10
- If pulse present, begin
  postresuscitation care

Not shockable ← | → Shockable

13
Go to Box 4

7
Check rhythm
Shockable rhythm? — No

8
Shockable
Continue CPR while defibrillator
is charging
Give 1 shock
- **Manual:** 4 J/kg
- **AED:** >1 yr of age
Resume CPR immediately
Consider antiarrhythmics
(e.g., **amiodarone** 5 mg/kg IV/IO or
lidocaine 1 mg/kg IV/IO)
Consider **magnesium** 25 to
50 mg/kg IV/IO, max 2 g for
torsades de pointes
After 5 cycles of CPR*
go to Box 5 above

During CPR
- **Push hard and fast (100/min)**
- **Ensure full chest recoil**
- **Minimize interruptions in chest
  compressions**
- **One cycle of CPR:** 15 compressions
  then 2 breaths; 5 cycles = 1 to 2 min
- Avoid hyperventilation
- Secure airway and confirm placement
- *After an advanced airway is placed,
  rescuers no longer deliver "cycles"
  of CPR. Give continuous chest
  compressions without pauses for
  breaths. Give 8 to 10 breaths/min
  Check rhythm every 2 min
- Rotate compressors every
  2 min with rhythm checks
- Search for and treat possible
  contributing factors:
  - Hypovolemia
  - Hypoxia
  - Hydrogen ion (acidosis)
  - Hypo-/hyperkalemia
  - Hypoglycemia
  - Hypothermia
  - Toxins
  - Tamponade, cardiac
  - Tension pneumothorax
  - Thrombosis (coronary or pulmonary)
  - Trauma

From American Heart Association. 2005 American Heart Association Guidelines for Cardiopulmonary Resuscitation
and Emergency Cardiovascular Care: Pediatric Advanced Life Support. *Circulation.* 2005;112(suppl 1, pt 12):IV–173.
Reprinted with permission.

Resuscitation

1

FOLLOW-UP AND CONTINUING SUPPORT

- Goals of postresuscitation stabilization: preserve brain function, prevent secondary hypoxic organ injury, facilitate transfer if necessary
- Constant cardiorespiratory monitoring essential; ABG 10–15 min after initially establishing ventilator settings, correlate with exhaled CO_2 monitors
- Treat pain with analgesia (opiates [e.g., fentanyl]) and keep child sedated (benzodiazepines [e.g., midazolam]); consider neuromuscular blockade (e.g., pancuronium) in addition to benzodiazepines if patient is very agitated
- Constantly re-evaluate circulatory status and provide volume resuscitation and inotropic support as needed
- Prevent secondary neuronal injury by maintaining good ventilation, good perfusion, and normal or lower-than-normal body temperatures
- Postresuscitation care ideally occurs in a pediatric intensive care facility; contact one as early as possible
- Coordinate transport to a tertiary care facility with appropriate personnel and equipment
- Family presence during resuscitation is important: strong parental preference to be present
- Deciding to terminate resuscitative efforts is complex: no reliable predictors; therefore, no definitive criteria for when to cease resuscitation

FURTHER READING

American Heart Association. 2005 American Heart Association Guidelines for Cardiopulmonary Resuscitation and Emergency Cardiovascular Care: Pediatric Advanced Life Support. *Circulation*. 2005;112(suppl 1, pt 12):IV-167–IV-187.

Guidelines for the transfer of critically ill patients. Guidelines Committee of the American College of Critical Care Medicine; Society of Critical Care Medicine and American Association of Critical-Care Nurses Transfer Guidelines Task Force. *Crit Care Med*. 1993;21:931–937.

Lalani A, Schneeweiss S, eds. *The Hospital for Sick Children Handbook of Pediatric Emergency Medicine*. Sudbury, Mass: Jones & Bartlett Publishers; 2008.

Young KD, Seidel JS. Pediatric cardiopulmonary resuscitation: a collective review. *Ann Emerg Med*. 1999;33:195–205.

Resuscitation

1

Chapter 2 Anesthesia

Gail K. Wong
Ross Barlow

Chapter 2   Anesthesia

COMMON ABBREVIATIONS

ETT   endotracheal tube
LMA   laryngeal mask airway
MAC   minimum alveolar concentration

AIRWAY ANATOMY

CLINICAL IMPLICATIONS OF PEDIATRIC AIRWAY ANATOMY

- See Table 2.1

Table 2.1	Complicating Anatomic Features in the Pediatric Airway
Anatomic Feature	**Clinical Implications**
Narrow nasal passages	· Nasal obstruction (secretions/edema/choanal atresia) may compromise airway · Neonates are obligate nose breathers
Occipital prominence	· Head flexes forward when lying supine, potentially obstructing airway · Slight extension (e.g., with shoulder roll) may improve airway
Large tongue (relative to oropharynx)	· Increased risk of airway obstruction · Difficult mask ventilation/intubation
High anterior glottis	· At level of C4 instead of C5 · Difficult laryngoscopy · "Sniffing" position more helpful in older children
Long, angulated epiglottis	· Difficult laryngoscopy · Consider straight blade; tip used to elevate epiglottis
Airway narrow at cricoid cartilage (vs. vocal cords)	· ETT may be too large distally (past vocal cords), increasing risk of subglottic stenosis with prolonged intubation · Uncuffed tubes with small leak preferred if <8 yr
Short trachea	· 4-5 cm long in neonate · Increased risk of endobronchial intubation

AIRWAY ASSESSMENT

PREDICTORS OF THE DIFFICULT AIRWAY

- Known history of difficult ventilation or intubation
- Present or impending upper airway obstruction (e.g., epiglottitis, airway burns/trauma/tumor/abscess, angioedema)

15

Anatomic Features

- Macroglossia (e.g., Down syndrome, Beckwith-Wiedemann)
- Retrognathia or micrognathia (e.g., Pierre Robin, Crouzon, Apert)
- Craniofacial dysostosis (e.g., Goldenhar, Treacher Collins, Pfeiffer)
- Limited mouth opening, poor TMJ function (e.g., rheumatoid arthritis)
- Limited cervical spine mobility (e.g., Klippel-Feil, mucopolysaccharidoses)
- Protruding upper incisors

Mallampati Classification

- See Figure 2.1
- May be useful in children >9 yr; not helpful in small children
- Grades I and II may predict a relatively easy intubation; grades III and IV may predict a difficult or impossible intubation

Figure 2.1 **Mallampati Classification**

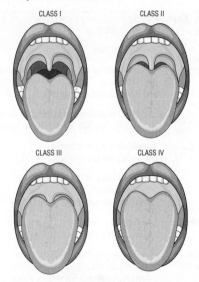

Classification of the pharyngeal view when performing the Mallampati test. The patient must fully extend the tongue during maximal mouth opening. Class I: pharyngeal pillars, soft palate, uvula visible. Class II: only soft palate, uvula visible. Class III: only soft palate visible. Class IV: soft palate not visible.
From Aitkenhead AR, Smith G, Rowbotham DJ. *Textbook of Anaesthesia.* 5th ed. London, England.: Churchill Livingstone/Elsevier; 2006.

AIRWAY MANAGEMENT

MASK VENTILATION

Indication

- Absent or ineffective spontaneous ventilation resulting in hypoxia or hypercarbia

Airway Maneuvers and Devices

- Aim: to improve airway patency in the presence of obstructed/ partially obstructed airway
- Maneuvers: head tilt, chin lift, jaw thrust
- Devices:
  1. Oropharyngeal airway (e.g., Guedel airway)
  2. Nasopharyngeal airway (e.g., nasal trumpet): useful if unable to open mouth because of trismus; better tolerated in a semi-conscious patient; beware of epistaxis
  3. LMA: should only be used by trained personnel; not a secure airway but can provide effective airway if mask ventilation is difficult

INTUBATION

Indications

- Protect airway from aspiration of gastric contents
- Provide adequate ventilation in patients with decreased level of consciousness, loss of airway patency, poor respiratory effort
- Enable suctioning of trachea and larger bronchi

Equipment

- See Table 1.3, p. 6

Endotracheal Tube (ETT)

- General guidelines:
  Sizing (internal diameter in mm) for 1–10 yr: Age/4 + 4
  Depth (>2 yr): length (cm) at lip = Age/2 + 12 or 3 × size of ETT
  length (cm) at nose = Age/2 + 15
  Suction catheter: 2 × ETT size = suction catheter size in French

Laryngoscope Blades
- See Figure 2.2

AIDS TO INTUBATION

- Head and neck in the "sniffing position": atlantoaxial extension, lower cervical flexion
- See Figures 2.3 and 2.4
- Suction equipment to remove airway secretions/blood
- External laryngeal manipulation with "BURP" maneuver: **B**ackward, **U**pward, **R**ightward **P**ressure on the thyroid cartilage
- Bougie or ETT introducer or stylet

POSTINTUBATION

Tube Check

To confirm endotracheal placement and position:
- Look for condensation in ETT and chest movement
- Listen for bilateral breath sounds; listen over stomach for gastric inflation if ETT is esophageal
- Confirm presence of CO_2 via capnography or chemical CO_2 detectors

Figure 2.2 Laryngoscopy With Curved and Straight Blades

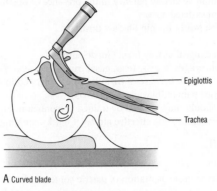

A Curved blade

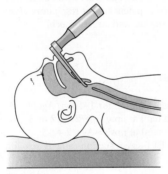

B Straight blade

Use of the laryngoscope. A, Curved blades (older children): tip placed in vallecula (between base of tongue and epiglottis). B, Straight blades: tip advanced beneath epiglottis to lift it off posterior pharyngeal wall.
From Aitkenhead AR, Smith G, Rowbotham DJ. *Textbook of Anaesthesia*. 5th ed. London, England: Churchill Livingstone/Elsevier; 2006.

Ventilation

- Intermittent positive pressure ventilation by hand or with ventilator
- Tidal volumes: 7–10 mL/kg
- Peak pressures: Keep <25 cm H_2O

Conventional Ventilator Respiratory Rates

- Neonate: 30–40 breaths/min
- 6 mon: 20–30 breaths/min
- 1–5 yr: 15–25 breaths/min
- >5 yr: 12–15 breaths/min

Figure 2.3 Cormack and Lehane Grades of Difficulty of Endotracheal Intubation Based on Best View at Laryngoscopy

GRADE I GRADE II GRADE III GRADE IV

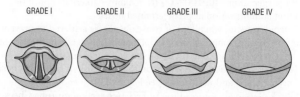

Grading of the laryngoscopic view. Grade I: vocal cords visible. Grade II: arytenoid cartilages and posterior part of vocal cords visible. Grade III: epiglottis visible. Grade IV: epiglottis not visible. Note: The pharyngeal view is a clinical guide to the likely laryngoscopic view.
From Aitkenhead AR, Smith G, Rowbotham DJ. *Textbook of Anaesthesia*. 5th ed. London, England: Churchill Livingstone/Elsevier; 2006.

Figure 2.4 Sniffing Position: Exposure of the Glottic Opening by Closer Alignment of Oral and Laryngeal Axes

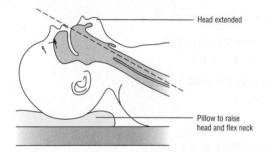

Head extended

Pillow to raise head and flex neck

Head position for laryngoscopy.
From Aitkenhead AR, Smith G, Rowbotham DJ. *Textbook of Anaesthesia*. 5th ed. London, England: Churchill Livingstone/Elsevier; 2006.

Anesthesia

2

RAPID SEQUENCE INDUCTION

INDICATION

- Rapid securing of the airway with minimal risk of aspiration, usually in context of an unfasted patient (e.g., acute abdomen, trauma, cardiorespiratory arrest)

TECHNIQUE

- Preparation of drugs (induction agent and muscle relaxant, usually succinylcholine) and equipment (suction, laryngoscope and blade, various ETT sizes, introducer/stylet)

- Apply appropriate monitoring (ECG, pulse oximetry, BP cuff, capnography or CO_2 detector)
- Preoxygenation with 100% O_2 (to maximize tolerable apnea time)
- Drug administration at predetermined doses
- Cricoid pressure when loss of consciousness is achieved to prevent aspiration by compression of esophagus with the cricoid ring (Sellick maneuver—efficacy controversial, but still widely practiced)
- No mask ventilation after induction to reduce risk of gastric distension
- Laryngoscopy and intubation (see Figure 2.2)
- Check placement and position of ETT (see section on Tube Check and Box 1.2, p. 8)
- Secure ETT at a corner of the mouth with strong adhesive tape; cut long slit into tape ("trouser legs"); stick intact end to one side of mouth; encircle slits around the tube and onto the skin above and below the lips
- Ventilate (see section on Conventional Ventilator Respiratory Rates, p. 18)

DRUGS IN ANESTHESIA

INTUBATION MEDICATIONS
- See Table 1.4, p. 7

INHALATION ANESTHETIC AGENTS
- See Table 2.2

FASTING GUIDELINES FOR ELECTIVE OR SEMIURGENT SURGERY

- See Table 2.3
- Depending on urgency of surgery, fasting guidelines may need to be ignored

MALIGNANT HYPERTHERMIA

- Potentially fatal autosomal dominant inherited disorder of skeletal muscle
- Hypermetabolic state secondary to loss of calcium homeostasis

TRIGGERS
- Volatile anesthetic agents (halothane, isoflurane, sevoflurane, desflurane)
- Succinylcholine

Table 2.2 Inhalational Anesthetic Agents

Drug	MAC*	Comments
Halothane	Neonate 0.9 Infant 1.2 Child 0.9 Adult 0.8	· Slow onset/offset; older agent; not irritating to airway · Used for inhalational induction · May cause bradycardia, myocardial depression, arrhythmias (especially with exogenous catecholamines [e.g., injected epinephrine]) · Halothane hepatitis rarer in children than in adults
Isoflurane	Neonate 1.6 Infant 1.8 Child 1.6 Adult 1.2	· Moderately fast onset/offset; irritating to airway in conscious or semiconscious patient; may precipitate coughing, laryngospasm, breath holding · May cause hypotension, hypoventilation
Sevoflurane	Neonate 3.2 Infant 3.2 Child 2.5 Adult 1.8	· Fast onset/offset; not irritating to airway · Commonly used for inhalational induction · May cause hypotension, hypoventilation · Associated with increased emergence delirium
Desflurane	Neonate 9.1 Infant 9.4 Child 8.5 Adult 6.6	· Fast onset/offset; significantly irritating to airway in conscious or semiconscious patient · Not suited for inhalational inductions · May cause hypotension, hypoventilation · Associated with increased emergence delirium
Nitrous oxide	Neonate N/A Infant N/A Child N/A Adult 104	· Fast onset/offset · Used for brief sedation, as adjunct to inhalational induction, and supplement to maintenance of anesthesia · Can cause expansion of closed gas spaces (e.g., inner ear, bowel, pneumothorax); inactivates vitamin B_{12} and impairs B_{12}-dependent enzyme systems (may cause megaloblastic anemia, agranulocytosis, neuropathy); increases ICP · Associated with postoperative nausea and vomiting

*MAC is the percent of an inhalational anesthetic that will cause immobility in response to a surgical stimulus in 50% of subjects. MAC requirements tend to be greatest in infants, followed by older children, then neonates and adults.

Table 2.3 Recommended Fasting Times Before Elective or Semiurgent Surgery

Food/Fluid Type	Recommended Fasting Time
Clear fluids (residue free [e.g., water, clear apple juice])	2 h
Breast milk	4 h
Formula or cow's milk	6 h
Solids	8 h

Anesthesia

2

CLINICAL MANIFESTATIONS

- Early (nonspecific): hypercarbia, tachycardia, tachypnea, muscle rigidity
- Late: skin flushing, cyanosis, hyperthermia, mixed respiratory and metabolic acidosis, arrhythmias, hyperkalemia, raised CK, myoglobinuria
- Complications: acute renal failure, disseminated intravascular coagulation, acute lung injury, cerebral edema, seizures

TREATMENT

- Cease administration of trigger drug
- 100% O_2
- Dantrolene 2.5 mg/kg rapidly IV, given repeatedly until clinical improvement (decreasing temperature, heart rate, muscle rigidity) or up to cumulative dose of 10 mg/kg (though more may be needed under advisement of an experienced practitioner)
- Active cooling (ice bags, cold water lavage, cold IV 0.9% NaCl)
- Correct fluid and electrolyte disturbance; treat acidosis, arrhythmias, rhabdomyolysis, and coagulopathy, as required
- Close monitoring (intensive care unit), support ventilation

FURTHER READING

Bissonnette B, Dalens B. *Pediatric Anesthesia: Principles and Practice*. New York, NY: McGraw-Hill; 2000.

Steward D, Lerman J. *Manual of Pediatric Anesthesia*. London, England: Churchill Livingstone; 2001.

Barash P, Cullen B, Stoelting R. *Clinical Anesthesia*. 5th ed. Philadelphia, Pa: Lippincott-Raven; 2005.

Allman K, Wilson I. *Oxford Handbook of Anaesthesia*. 2nd ed. Oxford University Press; 2006.

USEFUL WEB SITES

Malignant Hyperthermia Association of the United States. Available at: http://www.mhaus.org.

Chapter 3 Emergency Medicine

Sowmya Balasubramanian
Melissa J. Parker
Amina Lalani

COMMON ABBREVIATIONS

ABCs	airway, breathing, and circulation
ABG	arterial blood gas
ACE	angiotensin-converting enzyme
CBC	complete blood cell count
CPP	cerebral perfusion pressure
ECMO	extracorporeal membrane oxygenation
ETT	endotracheal tube
GCS	Glasgow Coma Scale
HIV	human immunodeficiency virus
ICP	intracranial pressure
INR	international normalized ratio
LFTs	liver function tests
LOC	level of consciousness
MAP	mean arterial pressure
NSAIDs	nonsteroidal anti-inflammatory drugs
PPV	positive pressure ventilation
PTT	partial thromboplastin time
RR	respiratory rate
SBP	systolic blood pressure
SLE	systemic lupus erythematosus
T_4	thyroxine
TSH	thyroid-stimulating hormone

ANAPHYLAXIS

DEFINITION

- Immediate hypersensitivity reaction that can lead to life-threatening cardiorespiratory decompensation
- Due to IgE-mediated release of vasoactive amines from inflammatory cells upon re-exposure to an antigen
- Involvement of ≥ 2 organ systems

DESCRIPTION

- Reactions usually uniphasic; onset of symptoms typically within 30 min of antigen exposure, can be up to 2 h (especially for ingested antigen)
- Biphasic reactions in 15–30%; initial symptoms resolve but recur in 4–24 h
- Symptoms may persist for weeks, despite treatment in protracted reactions

- Non–IgE-mediated anaphylactoid reactions: indistinguishable from anaphylaxis; caused by direct activation of mast cells (e.g., contrast material), changes in arachidonic acid metabolism (e.g., aspirin), cytotoxic reactions (e.g., transfusions), and complement activation by immune protein complexes

ETIOLOGY

- Most common cause: food ingestion (e.g., peanuts, shellfish)
- Other causes:
  - Insect venom: Hymenoptera (e.g., hornet, wasp, honeybee, fire ant)
  - Medications (e.g., antibiotics, aspirin, NSAIDs, insulin)
  - Vaccines, latex, exercise, immunotherapy, idiopathic

CLINICAL MANIFESTATIONS

- Airway: stridor, oropharyngeal and/or laryngeal edema, voice change/hoarseness
- Breathing: wheezing, coughing, ↑RR, chest tightness, shortness of breath, dyspnea
- Circulation: tachycardia, hypotension, arrhythmias
- Dermatologic: flushing, erythema, pruritus, urticaria, angioedema
- Gastrointestinal: nausea, vomiting, abdominal cramps, diarrhea
- Other: anxiety, weakness, feeling of impending doom, dizziness, headache, conjunctival injection, lacrimation, mouth burning

DIFFERENTIAL DIAGNOSES

- Acute asthma exacerbation
- Vasovagal reactions (usually manifest with bradycardia; cool and clammy extremities)
- Flushing syndromes (e.g., alcohol ingestion, sulfonylureas, pheochromocytoma)
- Panic attacks
- Systemic mastocytosis, urticaria pigmentosa, hereditary angioedema

MANAGEMENT

- Maintain ABCs (see pp. 5, 8, and 9)
- Treat at first suspicion of anaphylaxis: 1:1000 epinephrine 0.01 mg/kg (0.01 mL/kg) IM in the upper limb; do not wait for evolution of symptoms and signs
- Discontinue any IV medications or blood products
- Administer O_2; obtain IV access
- If hemodynamic involvement, give 0.9% NaCl (20 mL/kg) IV bolus, repeat as needed
- Treat bronchospasm with bronchodilators
- Give IV steroids (Table 3.1) and diphenhydramine; consider IV histamine (H)$_2$ blocker (e.g., ranitidine)

- Observe for recurrence of symptoms over 4–6 h
- Discharge with EpiPen prescription, EpiPen teaching, Medic Alert bracelet application, and follow-up with an allergist
- EpiPen Junior (0.15 mg) for children <15 kg; EpiPen (0.3 mg) for children >15 kg

Table 3.1	Pharmacologic Management of Anaphylaxis	
Medications	**Dose**	**Comments**
Epinephrine	0.01 mg/kg (0.01 mL/kg of 1:1000), SC/IM; min 0.1 mL/dose; max 0.5 mL/dose	May repeat every 5 min
Diphenhydramine	1–2 mg/kg IV (max 50 mg/dose)	H_1 receptor antagonist
Ranitidine	2–6 mg/kg/d IV ÷ q6–12h	H_2 receptor antagonist
Hydrocortisone	5–10 mg/kg IV q4–6h	Helps prevent late phase of allergic response

HYPOTHERMIA

DEFINITION

- Core temperature <35°C
- Cannot pronounce death in hypothermic patients with absent vital signs until rewarmed to >32°C with no response to resuscitation; important to consider clinical context when making a decision about *initiating* resuscitation efforts (e.g., time without breathing and circulation, signs of lividity, etc.)
- Predisposing factors: endocrine or metabolic abnormalities (e.g., hypoglycemia), infection, alcohol or drug ingestion, intracranial pathology (e.g., trauma), near drowning
- See Table 3.2

INVESTIGATIONS

- CBC, electrolytes, urea, creatinine, glucose (especially in neonates); LFTs; amylase and ABG; drug screen, coagulation screen, thyroid function tests, CXR, ECG

MANAGEMENT

- Maintain ABCs; arrhythmias may be resistant to cardioversion until patient is rewarmed
- Fluid resuscitation with warmed (43°C/109°F) IV fluids (patients are volume depleted)
- Monitor core temperature, BP, ECG, urine output, temperature of inspired gases

Table 3.2	Clinical Manifestations of Hypothermia
Cardiac	Initial: ↑BP and HR Prolonged cooling: ↓HR; complete vasomotor paralysis at 30°C ECG: prolongation of all phases of cardiac cycle, J wave at 32–33°C; sinus bradycardia/atrial fibrillation at 30°C, ventricular fibrillation at 26–28°C
Respiratory	Initial hyperventilation, then normoventilation from 33–35°C Hypoventilation or apnea (especially in premature neonates) at lower temperatures
Neurologic	Slurred speech, mild incoordination at 32–35°C Progressive ↓LOC Coma occurs at 28–30°C Fixed dilated pupils at <25°C
Muscular	Early shivering and thermogenesis, then loss of ability to shiver and progressive rigidity at 28–32°C
Renal	"Cold diuresis," acute tubular necrosis, hypokalemia/hyperkalemia
Metabolic	Lactic acidosis

Emergency Medicine

Rewarming

- Mild hypothermia (33–35°C): passive external rewarming (remove from exposure, remove wet clothing, cover with warm blankets)
- Moderate hypothermia (30–33°C):
  - Active external rewarming: heated water mattress, immersion in warm (37–40°C) water if practical; careful use of radiant heater (avoid burning)
  - Active core rewarming: warm humidified O_2 (40–45°C by mask; 40°C if intubated) and warm IV fluids (0.9% NaCl at 43°C/109°F)
- Severe hypothermia:
  - Additional core rewarming (warm gastric lavage or colonic irrigation with warm 0.9% NaCl), bladder irrigation with warm 0.9% NaCl, peritoneal lavage with warm 0.9% NaCl; can consider use of cardiopulmonary bypass or ECMO (special circumstances)

FROSTBITE

CLINICAL MANIFESTATIONS

- May accompany hypothermia or occur independently
- Usually restricted to head and extremities; frozen part is white and firm

MANAGEMENT

- After core temperature normalized, rapidly rewarm extremity with moist gauze or cloths soaked in water at 37.8–40°C
- Nonviable tissue must be clearly demarcated before considering excision
- Refer to plastic surgeon if extensive area of involvement

3

DEFINITION

- ↑ Body temperature; spectrum ranges from mild heat edema to potentially fatal heat stroke

ETIOLOGY

- Predisposing factors: fever, young age, infection, dehydration, excess clothing, lack of acclimatization, exercise, excess sweating, cystic fibrosis, Riley-Day syndrome (familial dysautonomia), skin abnormalities
- Thyroid storm, malignant hyperthermia, neuroleptic malignant syndrome
- See Table 3.3

COMPLICATIONS

- Seizures: treat with benzodiazepines (see p. 39)
- Hypotension: treat with volume ± inotropes
- Myoglobinuria: treat by alkalinization of urine (see p. 58) and hyperhydration (1.5 × maintenance fluids)
- Renal failure
- Arrhythmias (e.g., ventricular tachycardia, ventricular fibrillation: usually reversed with cooling)

ACUTE HYPERTENSION

DEFINITION

- See Table 27.5 for age- and sex-appropriate normal BP values

ETIOLOGY

- Medication/ingestion, cardiovascular, renovascular, renal parenchymal, endocrine, CNS

INITIAL ASSESSMENT

History

- Symptoms of visual, cerebral, cardiac, and/or renal dysfunction
- Prior history of ↑BP and/or antihypertensive use, renal disease, head injury
- Drug ingestion (e.g., cocaine)

Physical Examination

- Airway: airway patency, stability
- Breathing: RR, effort
- Circulation: BP × 3 with appropriate-sized cuff, four-limb BP, HR, perfusion; assess for congestive heart failure
- GCS, neurologic examination, fundoscopic examination
- Hydration status, edema (peripheral and pulmonary)
- Bruits, abdominal masses

3

Table 3.3	Clinical Spectrum of Hyperthermia and Management Guidelines	
Type	**Clinical Manifestation**	**Treatment**
Heat edema	Minor edema of hands and feet in first few days of exposure to hot environment	Cooler environment
Heat cramps	Muscle cramps after exertion; usually due to replacing fluid losses with hypotonic fluids, resulting in salt depletion	Cooler environment, rest, oral electrolyte solution or IV fluids, salt replacement
Heat syncope	Syncopal episode in unacclimatized patient in early stages of exposure to hot environment	Cooler environment, Trendelenburg position, oral electrolyte solution or IV fluids
Heat exhaustion	Temperature >39°C; water depletion with lethargy, thirst, headache, vomiting, ↑HR, ↑Na$^+$, ↑ urine specific gravity Salt depletion may predominate with similar features, as well as weakness, fatigue, muscle cramps, ↓Na$^+$, ↑ urinary Na$^+$ Neurologic status remains intact	Cooler environment, monitor vital signs, IV rehydration (bolus, then estimate deficit and ongoing losses); do not correct ↓/↑Na$^+$ too rapidly (see p. 289) *Investigations:* CBC, electrolytes, urea, creatinine, urinalysis Observe in hospital until temperature normalizes If in doubt, treat as heat stroke
Heat stroke	Life-threatening emergency; rectal temperature >41°C; neurologic dysfunction (due to cerebral edema): confusion, delirium, seizures, coma; vomiting/diarrhea; hot skin (sweating may stop); ↑HR, ↑RR, ↓BP; circulatory collapse; risk of rhabdomyolysis, acute tubular necrosis, DIC, hepatocellular degeneration; normal or ↑Na$^+$ levels, ↑CPK, Ca^{2+}	Maintain ABCs Active cooling (aim for 39°C): remove clothing; air-conditioned room; spray water over body surface; ice packs to head, groin, axilla; consider immersion in ice bath (difficult with unstable patient) IV fluid replacement with crystalloid to maintain perfusion and urine output (place Foley catheter, consider central venous line placement) *Investigations:* CBC, ABG, electrolytes, urea, creatinine, glucose, Ca^{2+}, LFTs, coagulation studies, CPK, blood culture (if sepsis suspected), urinalysis

Note: For malignant hyperthermia, treat with dantrolene (2.5–10 mg/kg/dose) and supportive measures in ICU setting (see p. 20).

CLINICAL MANIFESTATIONS

- ↑BP, ± ↑HR, ± ↑RR
- Headache, visual complaints, hypertensive retinopathy
- Left ventricular hypertrophy, congestive heart failure
- Seizures, encephalopathy, hemiplegia, facial palsy, cranial bruits

INVESTIGATIONS

- Measurement of ABG, electrolytes, glucose, urea, creatinine; CBC, blood film
- Urinalysis, toxicology screen, if indicated
- ECG, CXR
- Consider levels of plasma renin (before initiating therapy), urinary catecholamines, TSH, T_4

MANAGEMENT

- Maintain ABCs
- Exclude ↑BP due to ↑ICP (clinical history and examination)
- Initial reduction in BP to stabilize symptomatic patient (e.g., seizures), followed by gradual decrease (decrease BP by ⅓ over first 6 h, then slowly decrease over 3–4 d)
- Careful BP management if elevated in response to ↑ICP (need ↑MAP to sustain CPP; do not drop BP too quickly)

Medications

- See Table 3.4 for pharmacologic management of acute hypertension

Table 3.4	Pharmacologic Management of Acute Hypertension	
Medications	**Doses**	**Comments**
Continuous Infusion in Hypertensive Emergencies		
Labetalol	1 mg/kg/h IV Dose limit: 3 mg/kg/h	Contraindicated in asthma *Adverse effects* Nausea/vomiting, dizziness, scalp tingling, heart block, burning throat sensation, liver toxicity
Nitroprusside	0.5–10 mcg/kg/min IV Dose limit: 2.5 mg/kg/d (cumulative dose)	Avoid if ↑ICP or renal failure; medication is photosensitive *Adverse effects* Nausea/vomiting, diaphoresis, muscle twitching
Intermittent Dosing in Acute Hypertension		
Nifedipine	Initial dose: 0.5 mg/kg/d PO ÷ q8h; (min 1.25 mg/dose) prn dose: 0.125–0.25 mg/kg/dose PO q4h	Give with food or milk Do not use in neonates
Hydralazine	Initial dose: 0.15–0.8 mg/kg/dose IV q4-6h Dose limit: 20 mg/dose IV	Adjustment in renal impairment; associated with drug-induced lupus

Monitoring

- Response to vasoactive antihypertensives best monitored with arterial line in the acute care setting
- Where arterial line is not available, adjust rate of infusion after a minimum of two consecutive BP readings and use such agents with caution
- Monitor BP q5–10min while running infusion
- If BP falls below specified goal, stop infusion and consider 10 mL/kg 0.9NaCl bolus until BP recovers; restart infusion at slightly lower rate

SHOCK

DEFINITION

- Impaired delivery of O_2 and nutrients to tissues at a cellular level
  - Compensated: endogenous compensatory mechanisms allow for adequate delivery of O_2 and nutrients
  - Decompensated: O_2 and nutrient requirements not met by endogenous compensatory mechanisms
- Early recognition is critical; rapid intervention may prevent progression to irreversible shock and/or cardiopulmonary arrest

CLINICAL MANIFESTATIONS

- See Chapter 16 for assessment of fluid status
- Classic symptoms, signs often absent early because of compensatory mechanisms
- Early symptoms: poor feeding, lethargy/irritability, fever, ↓ urine output
- Early signs: ↑HR and/or ↑RR, normal SBP, narrowed or widened pulse pressure, mottling, cool or warm extremities, delayed or flash capillary refill time
- Early laboratory signs: metabolic or mixed acidemia with ↑ lactate level, hyperglycemia, or hypoglycemia, leukocytosis or leukopenia
- Type-specific clinical features (Table 3.5)
- Hypotension: SBP <5th percentile for age or documented decrease of 30% from preshock state
  - 5th percentile SBP: <80 mmHg systolic 6 wk–6 yr; (70 mmHg) + $(2 \times age)$ after 6 yr
  - 50th percentile SBP: (80 mmHg) + $(2 \times age)$
- ↑HR
- Altered peripheral perfusion: weak peripheral pulses, cool extremities, mottled skin, ↑ capillary refill time (cold shock) OR bounding pulses, warm extremities, flash capillary refill (warm shock)
- Renal: ↓ urine output (<1 mL/kg/h)
- CNS: altered mental state (lethargy, confusion, combativeness, coma)

Table 3.5	General Classification of Shock		
Type	Primary Circulatory Derangement	Common Causes	Specific Clinical Features
Hypovolemic	↓ Intravascular volume	Hemorrhage, trauma, fluid loss, gastroenteritis	↑HR ↓BP
Distributive	Vasodilation → venous pooling → ↓ preload Maldistribution of regional blood flow	Sepsis, anaphylaxis, CNS or spinal injury, drug intoxication	Septic shock: hyperdynamic "warm" phase (widened pulse pressure) Neurogenic shock: ↓BP without ↑HR or ↓ peripheral perfusion
Cardiogenic	↓ Myocardial contractility	Cardiomyopathy, heart surgery, congenital heart disease, arrhythmias, hypoxia, ischemia, myocarditis, pericarditis	Gallop rhythm with hepatomegaly, cardiomegaly, or dilated neck veins
Obstructive	Mechanical obstruction to ventricular inflow or outflow	Cardiac tamponade, tension pneumothorax, coarctation	↑HR, ↓BP, decreased pulse pressure, distended neck veins; muffled heart sounds in pericardial effusion; tracheal deviation and narrow pulse pressure in tension pmeumothorax
Dissociative	O_2 not released from hemoglobin	Carbon monoxide poisoning, methemoglobinemia	

Adapted from Witte MK, Hill JH, Blumer JL. Shock in the pediatric patient. In: Barness, Bongiovanni, Morrow, Oski, Rudolph, eds. *Advances in Pediatrics*. Vol 34. St. Louis, Mo: Year Book Medical Publishers; 1987:139–174.

INVESTIGATIONS

- CBC; coagulation screen; ABG; electrolytes, glucose, urea, creatinine, Ca^{2+}, lactate; LFTs
- Blood culture, cross-match, sepsis workup (if appropriate)
- CXR

MANAGEMENT

- See Figure 3.1

Monitoring

Noninvasive
- Vital signs every 5–15 min initially, including BP
- Cardiorespiratory monitoring, pulse oximetry
- Bladder catheterization for urine output
- ABG if oximetry is not available

Figure 3.1 Approach to Pediatric Shock

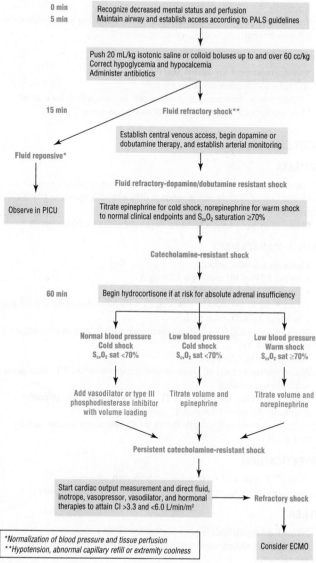

0 min
5 min
Recognize decreased mental status and perfusion
Maintain airway and establish access according to PALS guidelines

Push 20 mL/kg isotonic saline or colloid boluses up to and over 60 cc/kg
Correct hypoglycemia and hypocalcemia
Administer antibiotics

15 min

Fluid refractory shock**

Establish central venous access, begin dopamine or dobutamine therapy, and establish arterial monitoring

Fluid reponsive*

Observe in PICU

Fluid refractory-dopamine/dobutamine resistant shock

Titrate epinephrine for cold shock, norepinephrine for warm shock to normal clinical endpoints and $S_{cv}O_2$ saturation ≥70%

Catecholamine-resistant shock

60 min

Begin hydrocortisone if at risk for absolute adrenal insufficiency

| Normal blood pressure Cold shock $S_{cv}O_2$ sat <70% | Low blood pressure Cold shock $S_{cv}O_2$ sat <70% | Low blood pressure Warm shock $S_{cv}O_2$ sat ≥70% |

Add vasodilator or type III phosphodiesterase inhibitor with volume loading

Titrate volume and epinephrine

Titrate volume and norepinephrine

Persistent catecholamine-resistant shock

Start cardiac output measurement and direct fluid, inotrope, vasopressor, vasodilator, and hormonal therapies to attain CI >3.3 and <6.0 L/min/m² → **Refractory shock**

Consider ECMO

*Normalization of blood pressure and tissue perfusion
**Hypotension, abnormal capillary refill or extremity coolness*

Dellinger RP, Levy MM, Carlet JM, et al. Surviving Sepsis Campaign: International guidelines for management of severe sepsis and septic shock: 2008. *Intensive Care Med*, 2008; 34(1):17–60 (p. 42, Fig. 1). © Society of Critical Care Medicine, 2007. With kind permission of Springer Science + Business Media.

Emergency Medicine

3

- Central venous line (see p. 91) for central venous pressure and blood sampling
- Arterial line (see p. 95) for repeated blood sampling and continuous BP monitoring

Further Management
- Specific treatment for underlying illness
- NG tube to decompress stomach
- Diuretics (e.g., furosemide), if necessary, to promote urine output
- Monitor for multiorgan failure and secondary complications

ACUTE STROKE

CRITERIA
- Focal neurologic deficit: unilateral weakness or sensory change, vision loss or double vision, speech difficulty, dizziness, or trouble walking
- Onset of symptoms <5 h; worsening problem or sudden onset

INITIAL MANAGEMENT
- Maintain normotension:
  - Target SBP of 80 mmHg + (2 × age)
  - Treat ↓BP with 0.9NaCl ± vasopressors
  - Treat ↑BP (>90 mmHg + [3 × age]) with labetalol or ACE inhibitor to lower by 25% over 24 h
- Normovolemia: 0.9NaCl at maintenance with bolus, as needed; keep head of bed flat
- Normalize O_2, CO_2, pH
- Normothermia: treat all patients with temperature >37°C with acetaminophen ± cooling
- Normoglycemia: no glucose in IV unless hypoglycemic, consider insulin if glucose >10 mmol/L, keep NPO
- Seizure control: antiepileptic drugs if any suspected seizure activity (see p. 39)

INVESTIGATIONS
- INR, PTT, type and screen, CBC, fibrinogen, glucose
- Imaging: MRI, CT scan/CT angiogram (if MRI unavailable)

OTHER
- Neurology consultation
- Discuss indications/contraindications for thrombolytics at tertiary care center

DEFINITION

- Altered LOC: decreased awareness of self and environment
- Coma: state of deep unresponsiveness
- Useful mnemonics to remember the important causes in children are TIPS and AEIOU (Table 3.6)

Table 3.6	Causes of Coma: TIPS and AEIOU
TIPS	**AEIOU**
Trauma	**A**lcohol abuse
Insulin/hypoglycemia	**E**lectrolyte abnormalities
Intussusception	**E**ncephalopathy
Inborn errors of metabolism	**E**ndocrinopathy
Psychiatric	**I**nfection
Seizures	**O**verdose/ingestion
Stroke	**U**remia
Shock	
Shunt malfunction	

Emergency Medicine

3

MANAGEMENT

Primary Survey

- Maintain ABCs with cervical spine (C-spine) precautions; intubate if no gag or cough reflex or low GCS (usually <8)
- Modified GCS (Table 3.7)
- Measure temperature
- Check for obvious evidence of trauma
- Hypoglycemia: give glucose 0.5 g/kg (5 mL/kg of D10W IV) empirically or if glucose low on Glucometer
- Check pupils; give naloxone 0.1 mg/kg IV/ETT empirically if small or pinpoint

Secondary Survey

- History: known underlying illness, acute fever, trauma, ingestion
- General and neurologic examination (Tables 3.8 and 3.9)
- Motor responses (focal signs), oculomotor movements, fundi (retinal hemorrhages), fontanelle, nuchal rigidity, bruits
- Breathing pattern abnormalities
- Look for evidence of infection, intoxication, metabolic disease, trauma

Table 3.7 — Modified Glasgow Coma Scale

Area Assessed	Infants	Children	Score*
Eye opening	Open spontaneously	Open spontaneously	4
	Open in response to verbal stimuli	Open in response to verbal stimuli	3
	Open in response to pain only	Open in response to pain only	2
	No response	No response	1
Verbal response	Coos and babbles	Oriented, appropriate	5
	Irritable cries	Confused	4
	Cries in response to pain	Inappropriate words	3
	Moans in response to pain	Incomprehensible words or nonspecific sounds	2
	No response	No response	1
Motor response	Moves spontaneously and purposefully	Obeys commands	6
	Withdraws to touch	Localizes painful stimulus	5
	Withdraws in response to pain	Withdraws in response to pain	4
	Responds to pain with decorticate posturing (abnormal flexion)	Responds to pain with decorticate posturing (abnormal flexion)	3
	Responds to pain with decerebrate posturing (abnormal extension)	Responds to pain with decerebrate posturing (abnormal extension)	2
	No response	No response	1

Adapted from Davis RJ et al. Head and spinal cord injury. In: Rogers MC, ed. *Textbook of Pediatric Intensive Care*. Baltimore, Md: Williams & Wilkins; 1987; from James H, Anas N, Perkin RM. *Brain Insults in Infants and Children*. New York, NY: Grune & Stratton; 1985; and from Morray JP et al. Coma scale for use in brain-injured children. *Crit Care Med*. 1984;12:1018.

Table 3.8 — Distinguishing Diffuse Versus Focal Causes of Coma

	Diffuse	Focal
History	Previous illness	± Previous illness
Consciousness	Gradual ↓	Rapid ↓
General physical examination	Abnormal breathing, odor, skin color	Evidence of trauma
Progression	Affects different levels simultaneously	Rostral → caudal changes
Breathing	↑RR, then ↓RR	Irregular
Pupils	Small, equal, and reactive	Unequal and/or unreactive
Focal signs	Less common	Common
Motor	Myoclonic jerks Multifocal seizures Symmetrically decorticate or decerebrate	Focal oculomotor changes Facial asymmetry Monoparesis or hemiparesis ↓ Cough or gag

Table 3.9	Coma: Level of Central Nervous System Involvement and Clinical Correlate		
Anatomic Site	**Pupillary Reaction**	**Breathing Pattern**	**Position**
Cerebral Hemisphere			
Forebrain	Small but reactive	Normal or brief periods of apnea, followed by voluntary deep breathing	
Deep structures, diencephalon		Cheyne-Stokes (alternating hyperpnea and apnea)	Decorticate
Brainstem			
Midbrain	Midpoint and fixed	Central hyperventilation (sustained, regular, rapid)	Decerebrate
Pons	Pinpoint	Apneustic (alternating brief pauses and end respiratory pauses)	Flaccid
Medulla		Apnea	

Further Management

- Treat underlying problem
- Treat ↑ICP (Figure 3.2) and seizures (see p. 39) if present
- Maintain homeostasis: O_2, CO_2, fluids, acid–base balance, electrolytes, and nutrition

INVESTIGATIONS

- Based on suspicion of etiology and clinical condition
- Determine need for urgent CT scan of head
  - Diffuse causes (e.g., infection, ingestion, metabolic, nonconvulsive status epilepticus): CT scan not essential immediately
  - Focal causes (e.g., head injury, intracranial hemorrhage, infection): CT scan ± contrast essential but should not delay transport to definitive care
- Other radiology: consider CXR, C-spine, abdomen; consider skeletal survey if suspect nonaccidental injury (see p. 181)
- Laboratory tests: CBC; culture; ABG; glucose, electrolytes, urea, creatinine, lactate, Ca^{2+}, Mg^{2+}, ammonium; LFTs; clotting screen; levels of ASA, acetaminophen, toxic alcohols (ethanol, methanol, ethylene glycol, isopropyl alcohol)
- Urine: urinalysis, culture, toxicology screen
- Cerebrospinal fluid (CSF): cell count, protein, glucose, Gram stain, culture, viral studies; levels of glycine, lactate; opening pressures may be useful but difficult to measure accurately in infants and young children; lumbar puncture (LP) contraindicated if comatose or if evidence of ↑ICP, hemodynamic instability, ↓ platelets, coagulopathy
- Other: ECG, EEG

3

RAISED INTRACRANIAL PRESSURE

CLINICAL FEATURES

- Early: headache, vomiting, ↓LOC, full fontanelle
- Late: Cushing triad (↓HR, ↑BP, apnea), unequal or unresponsive pupils, sunsetting eyes, papilledema; cranial nerve III, IV, VI palsies; decorticate or decerebrate posturing

MANAGEMENT

Figure 3.2 Management of Raised Intracranial Pressure

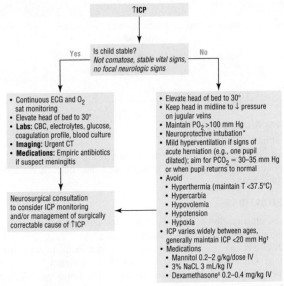

*Premedication with lidocaine may blunt ↑ICP during intubation. Select sedative agent with care (see pp. 83–84; ketamine is contraindicated in ↑ICP).
†Cerebral perfusion pressure = MAP – ICP
‡Controversial but may be of benefit if cerebral edema is secondary to space-occupying lesion (e.g., brain tumor)
© The Hospital for Sick Children, 2009. New artwork created by the Hospital for Sick Children for *The Hospital for Sick Children Handbook of Pediatrics*, 11th edition.

STATUS EPILEPTICUS

DEFINITION

- Single generalized or focal seizure lasting ≥30 min; includes any series of seizures without intervening return of consciousness, with duration >30 min

ASSESSMENT

- Common causes: fever, CNS infections, trauma, toxic ingestions, metabolic abnormalities, subtherapeutic anticonvulsant levels

INVESTIGATIONS

- Blood tests: glucose, blood gas, electrolytes, Ca^{2+}, Mg^{2+}; consider blood culture, CBC, toxicology screen, anticonvulsant levels (if indicated), metabolic workup, LFTs, urine toxicology screen
- CSF (if no contraindications to LP); metabolic workup for suspected infection or metabolic disorder
- Consider CT and EEG

MANAGEMENT

- See Figure 3.3

Figure 3.3 **Management of Status Epilepticus**

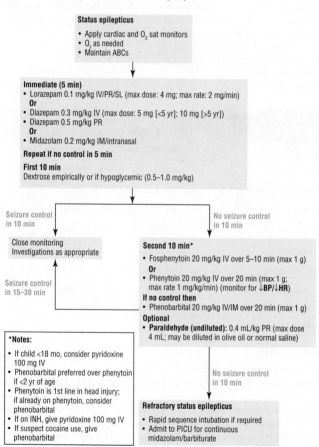

Status epilepticus
- Apply cardiac and O_2 sat monitors
- O_2 as needed
- Maintain ABCs

Immediate (5 min)
- Lorazepam 0.1 mg/kg IV/PR/SL (max dose: 4 mg; max rate: 2 mg/min)
  Or
- Diazepam 0.3 mg/kg IV (max dose: 5 mg [<5 yr]; 10 mg [>5 yr])
- Diazepam 0.5 mg/kg PR
  Or
- Midazolam 0.2 mg/kg IM/intranasal

Repeat if no control in 5 min

First 10 min
Dextrose empirically or if hypoglycemic (0.5–1.0 mg/kg)

Seizure control in 10 min → Close monitoring. Investigations as appropriate

Seizure control in 15–30 min

No seizure control in 10 min →

Second 10 min*
- Fosphenytoin 20 mg/kg IV over 5–10 min (max 1 g)
  Or
- Phenytoin 20 mg/kg IV over 20 min (max 1 g; max rate 1 mg/kg/min) (monitor for ↓BP/↓HR)

If no control then
- Phenobarbital 20 mg/kg IV/IM over 20 min (max 1 g)

Optional
- Paraldehyde (undiluted): 0.4 mL/kg PR (max dose 4 mL; may be diluted in olive oil or normal saline)

***Notes:**
- If child <18 mo, consider pyridoxine 100 mg IV
- Phenobarbital preferred over phenytoin if <2 yr of age
- Phenytoin is 1st line in head injury; if already on phenytoin, consider phenobarbital
- If on INH, give pyridoxine 100 mg IV
- If suspect cocaine use, give phenobarbital

No seizure control in 10 min →

Refractory status epilepticus
- Rapid sequence intubation if required
- Admit to PICU for continuous midazolam/barbiturate

ACUTE PSYCHOSIS

DEFINITION

- Mental state with major disturbances in thinking, relating, reality testing

DIFFERENTIAL DIAGNOSIS

- CNS lesions (e.g., tumor, abscess, hemorrhage)
- Cerebral hypoxia
- Metabolic and endocrine disturbances (e.g., electrolyte abnormalities, uremia, hepatic failure)
- Collagen-vascular diseases (e.g., SLE)
- Infections (e.g., encephalitis, malaria, HIV)
- Ingestion of toxin or medication (e.g., alcohol, barbiturates, antipsychotics, marijuana, cocaine, PCP, reserpine, opioids, heavy metals)
- Other psychiatric/developmental diagnoses
  - Pervasive developmental disorder
  - Adult-type schizophrenia
  - Manic–depressive illness
- See Table 3.10

Table 3.10	Differentiating Features of Organic and Psychiatric Psychosis	
Evaluation	Organic Cause	Psychiatric Cause
Onset	Acute	Gradual
Pathologic autonomic signs*	May be present	Absent
Vital signs	May be abnormal	Normal
Orientation	Impaired	Intact
Recent memory	Impaired	Intact
Intellectual ability	May be impaired	Intact
Hallucinations	Visual	Auditory

*↑ or ↓ in HR, RR, BP, temperature; miosis or mydriasis; skin color changes.
From Fleisher GR, Ludwig S, eds. *Textbook of Pediatric Emergency Medicine.* 5th ed. Philadelphia, Pa: Lippincott Williams & Wilkins; 2006.

MANAGEMENT

- Ensure patient and staff safety
- May require physical or chemical restraints if unable to settle the patient
- Physical restraints: apply arm, leg, torso restraints; if child/adolescent is still combative, administer chemical restraint (risk of rhabdomyolysis with continuous muscle contractions in restrained individual)

- Chemical restraints: oral administration preferred
  - First line: benzodiazepine (e.g., lorazepam); additional medications as recommended by Psychiatry
- If patient remains uncooperative or violent (threat to self or others), may require IV sedation.
  - First line: benzodiazepine (e.g., lorazepam 0.1 mg/kg SL/IM)
  - Other options: haloperidol IM, but risk of adverse reaction (e.g., acute dystonia)
- When safety of patient and staff ensured, continue with investigations, as appropriate
- Involve parent or guardian when present; ensure they understand reasons for use of physical and/or chemical restraints, when necessary

RESPIRATORY DISTRESS

DEFINITION

- Respiratory distress: $\uparrow$ work of breathing
- Respiratory failure: inability of respiratory system to provide sufficient O_2 for metabolic needs or to excrete CO_2 produced by body
- Abnormal arterial gas values:
  - Newborn PaO_2: <50 mmHg; arterial CO_2: >60 mmHg
  - Infant or older child PaO_2: <60 mmHg; $PaCO_2$: >55 mmHg
- In children, respiratory failure is a major cause of apnea/bradycardia and cardiac arrest

CLINICAL MANIFESTATIONS

- Respiratory: $\uparrow$RR, cyanosis, retractions, nasal flaring, tracheal tug, grunting; beware gasping respirations, poor effort (signs of fatigue/impending respiratory arrest)
- CVS: $\uparrow$HR, poor perfusion
- CNS: confusion, agitation, restlessness, seizures, coma

MANAGEMENT

- Early management may prevent progression to respiratory or cardiac arrest
- Maintain ABCs, including use of supplemental O_2
- ABG measurements to determine degree of hypoxia and hypercapnia
- Consider elective endotracheal intubation (see p. 17)
- Investigations and ongoing management as determined by underlying problem

FOREIGN BODY AND CHOKING

- See Figure 3.4

Figure 3.4 Management of a Choking Child

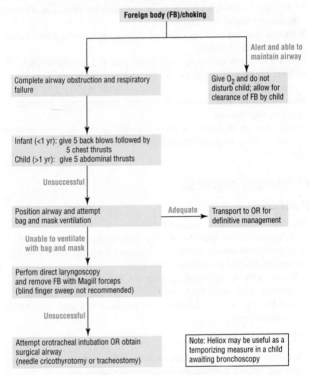

Foreign body (FB)/choking

Complete airway obstruction and respiratory failure

Alert and able to maintain airway

Give O$_2$ and do not disturb child; allow for clearance of FB by child

Infant (<1 yr): give 5 back blows followed by 5 chest thrusts
Child (>1 yr): give 5 abdominal thrusts

Unsuccessful

Position airway and attempt bag and mask ventilation → Adequate → Transport to OR for definitive management

Unable to ventilate with bag and mask

Perfom direct laryngoscopy and remove FB with Magill forceps (blind finger sweep not recommended)

Unsuccessful

Attempt orotracheal intubation OR obtain surgical airway (needle cricothyrotomy or tracheostomy)

Note: Heliox may be useful as a temporizing measure in a child awaiting bronchoscopy

Adapted from Gausche-Hill M, Fuchs S, Yamomoto L (Eds), American Academy of Pediatrics & American College of Emergency Physicians. *APLS: The Pediatric Emergency Medicine Resource* (4th ed.). Sudbury, MA: Jones & Bartlett, 2004 (pp. 64–66).

EPIGLOTTITIS AND LARYNGOTRACHEOBRONCHITIS

- See Table 3.11

STATUS ASTHMATICUS

DEFINITION

- Severe asthma exacerbation refractory to appropriate medical therapy

CLINICAL MANIFESTATIONS

- Respiratory: ↑RR, dyspnea, accessory muscle use (indrawing), prolonged expiration, diffuse expiratory wheezes; wheezing may be absent in severe exacerbations (silent chest)
- CVS: ↑HR
- CNS: altered mental status if severe

Table 3.11	Comparison of Epiglottitis and Laryngotracheobronchitis	
	Epiglottitis	**Laryngotracheobronchitis**
Definition	· Infection of epiglottis, adjacent structures · Acute febrile illness that rapidly proceeds to upper airway compromise	· Viral infection of the larynx, may involve trachea and bronchi
Clinical manifestations	· Stridor, drooling, tripod stance, very anxious child · History of fever, drooling, noisy breathing, respiratory distress, inability to swallow	· Viral prodrome · Characteristic barky cough ± stridor · Oral intake frequently affected · Nontoxic appearing · Hearing the child cough confirms diagnosis
Etiology	· *Haemophilus influenzae B, Streptococcus pneumoniae*	· Viral
Monitoring	· Assess ABCs and vital signs · ECG and O_2 saturation monitoring	· Assess ABCs and vital signs · ECG and O_2 saturation monitoring in unwell child
Management	· Obtain IV access · Cooperative child: attempt to visualize posterior pharynx with gentle use of tongue depressor · Uncooperative child: DO NOT manipulate airway, may precipitate acute airway obstruction. DO NOT attempt laryngoscopy · Severe compromise (severe stridor, hypoxia): 100% O_2, do not upset child, use gentle PPV if necessary, call for immediate anesthesia/ENT assistance · Uncertain diagnosis: lateral neck X-ray → thumbprint sign (thickness of epiglottis) · Requires intubation ideally in a controlled setting (OR)	· Severe airway compromise: give 100% O_2 and keep child calm · Provide PPV if necessary · Rarely requires intubation; anticipate need for smaller ETT · If ↑RR, ↑HR, O_2 requirement or continuous stridor, then nebulized epinephrine for symptomatic relief · If epinephrine is used, will require several hours observation or hospitalization · No evidence for use of humidifiers or water mist therapy
Medications	· Third-generation cephalosporin	· Single dose dexamethasone 0.6 mg/kg (max 20 mg) PO · Inhaled epinephrine (1:1000, 1 mg/mL solution) <5 kg: 0.5 mg/kg/dose ≥5 kg: 2.5–5 mg/dose Dilute dose to 2.5 or 3 mL in 0.9% NaCl, give via nebulizer prn to max q1h

Emergency Medicine

3

MANAGEMENT

- Assess ABCs (see pp. 5–9)
- Obtain vital signs; attach cardiac and O_2 sat monitors
- Exclude anaphylaxis based on history and physical examination (see pp. 24–26)

Medications

- Salbutamol (β_2-agonist) nebulized × 3 (0.1 mg/kg OR 0.03 mL/kg/dose of 5 mg/mL solution in 3 mL 0.9% NaCl; rough estimates: 1.25 mg for infants, 2.5 mg for younger children, 5 mg for older children)
- Ipratropium bromide (anticholinergic) nebulized × 3 (250 mcg OR 1 mL per treatment); administer concurrently with salbutamol
- Hydrocortisone 4–6 mg/kg IV q4–6h OR methylprednisolone 1–2 mg/kg IV divided q6h
- Magnesium sulfate 20–50 mg/kg IV over 20 min (monitor BP); max 2 g
- Salbutamol IV infusion for severely ill child; initial rate, 1 mcg/kg/min IV; ↑ by 1 mcg/kg/min q15min prn up to max 10 mcg/min

Intubation

- High risk in patients with status asthmaticus; avoid if possible
- When necessary, sedative drug of choice is ketamine (bronchodilator)

Complications

- Pneumothorax, hypoxia, cardiac arrest during intubation

TRANSPORT

- Safe transport crucial to patient safety; allows for needed investigations, procedures, and definitive care
- Applies to intramural (within institution) and extramural (institution to institution) movement of patient

ALL PATIENTS

Preparation

- Ensure direct physician-to-physician communication, where applicable
- Prepare equipment, including bag valve mask, medications
- STATICS: *S*cope; *T*ube; *A*irway: adequate O_2 supply, O_2 saturation monitor, oro/nasopharyngeal airway, blade; *T*ape; *I*ntroducer: stylet, Magill forceps; *C*onnector (for mask and ETT); *S*uction equipment

During Transport

- NG tube to open drainage
- Aim to maintain normothermia
- Monitor glucose for high-risk patients

RESPIRATORY PATIENT

- May need to secure definitive airway; nasal ETT preferable to oral ETT (more stable); use bite block in orally intubated patients
- Ensure adequate ventilation, oxygenation; check ETT placement (CXR)
- Insert chest tube (see p. 98) if pneumothorax and attach to Heimlich valves to avoid clamping chest tubes
- Use condenser humidifier (i.e., Swedish nose)

CARDIOVASCULAR PATIENT

- Stabilize BP and HR before transport
- Two IV cannulas or central IV access advisable; portable syringe drivers preferable to hanging fluid bags because of limited headroom

TRAUMA

- History of mechanism (blunt or penetrating) and force of trauma
- Severe injuries dictate need to search for other injuries

IMMEDIATE MANAGEMENT

- Primary survey, ABCDE: **A**irway with C-spine protection, **B**reathing and ventilation, **C**irculation, **D**isability, **E**xposure and environment control; management and assessment occur simultaneously; any change in clinical status should prompt full reassessment of primary survey (Table 3.12)
- Attach cardiac and O_2 sat monitors, catheters; initiate urgent diagnostic tests
- Secondary survey: head-to-toe examination to define presence, type, and severity of injuries; remember: "tubes and fingers in every orifice" (Table 3.13)

Table 3.12	Primary Survey of a Trauma Patient
Airway	· Maintain C-spine precautions · Clear oropharynx; have patient open mouth or perform jaw thrust, if needed · Administer O_2 to all patients initially, bag and mask ventilation, if necessary · Intubate and assist ventilation, as indicated
Breathing	· Perform inspection, palpation, percussion, auscultation of chest · Look for tension/open pneumothorax, flail chest, pulmonary contusion or hemothorax
Circulation	· Obtain IV access with two large-bore cannulas (14- or 16-gauge), preferably in upper limbs · Perform hemostasis and fluid resuscitation · Initial bolus of 20 mL/kg of crystalloid (0.9NaCl or Ringer's lactate) if signs of hypovolemic shock after trauma (even if head injury) · Continue fluid resuscitation during transport · Transfuse packed red blood cells if suspected blood loss or ongoing shock

(continued)

Table 3.12	Primary Survey of a Trauma Patient (continued)
Disability	· Perform rapid neurologic evaluation · **A**lert, response to **V**erbal stimulation, response to **P**ainful stimulation, or **U**nresponsive (AVPU) or GCS · Pupil size and reactivity · Assess movement/sensation in all 4 extremities before administration of sedation or muscle relaxant
Exposure/environment control	· Fully undress patient to enable complete examination · Prevent hypothermia: cover patient, warm IV fluids, warm environment

Table 3.13	Secondary Survey of a Trauma Patient
Head and skull	· Look for: · Scalp fractures, lacerations, hematomas · Hemorrhage from nose, mouth, ears; clear fluid (CSF) from nose or ears · Unequal/abnormally reactive pupils, abnormal extraocular movements, penetrating eye injury, visual acuity disturbances · Remove contact lenses
Maxillofacial	· Assess for midface fracture (contraindication for NG placement)
Neck	· Assume C-spine fracture until proven otherwise · Examine for C-spine tenderness, subcutaneous emphysema, laryngeal or tracheal injury (abnormal cry, stridor, subcutaneous emphysema, tracheal deviation) · Assess for blunt carotid vascular injury
Chest	· Examine for: · Flail segment or penetrating wounds · Pneumothorax or hemothorax (tracheal deviation, auscultation for reduced air entry, chest expansion) or cardiac tamponade (distended neck veins, diminished heart sounds) · Rib fractures, bruising over precordium
Abdomen	· Examine for: · Hidden penetrating wounds · Bowel sounds, guarding
Perineal	· Examine for vaginal, testicular, and penile injuries · Logroll patient to perform rectal examination for sphincter tone, blood, prostate position
Musculoskeletal/pelvis	· Assess for bruising or pelvic instability · Splint suspected pelvic fractures with circumferentially tied cloth around pelvis · Assess for compartment syndrome (see p. 718) · Examine spine during logroll (palpate for step defects and assess for point tenderness)
Neurologic examination	· Maintain full spinal immobilization · Reassess GCS or AVPU and pupil size and reactivity · Perform full motor and sensory examination of extremities

- AMPLE history: **A**llergies, **M**edications, **P**regnancy and past illnesses, **L**ast meal, **E**vents and environment
- Consider transfer to a pediatric trauma center after stabilization

Adjuncts

- Chest tube(s) in all ventilated patients with significant pneumothorax or hemothorax awaiting transport (see p. 97)
- Place NG tube (see p. 102) or orogastric tube (OG) (use OG if facial or basal skull fractures)
- Place Foley catheter (unless pelvic injury, blood visible at urethral meatus, or high-riding prostate on rectal examination) (see p. 105)
- Diagnostic studies (chest, pelvic, C-spine X-rays)
- Investigations should not delay transfer to tertiary facility

BLUNT ABDOMINAL TRAUMA

- See Figure 3.5

Figure 3.5 **Approach to Abdominal Trauma**

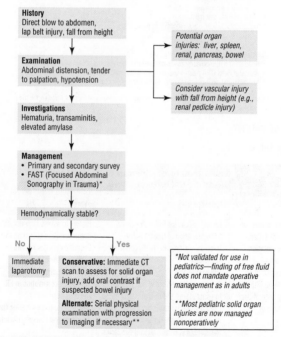

Emergency Medicine

3

HEAD INJURIES

- See Figure 3.6

Figure 3.6 **Approach to Head Injuries**

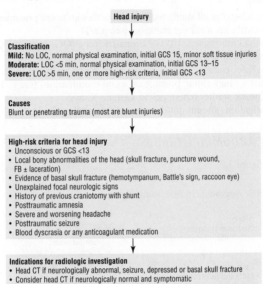

Head injury

Classification
Mild: No LOC, normal physical examination, initial GCS 15, minor soft tissue injuries
Moderate: LOC <5 min, normal physical examination, initial GCS 13–15
Severe: LOC >5 min, one or more high-risk criteria, initial GCS <13

Causes
Blunt or penetrating trauma (most are blunt injuries)

High-risk criteria for head injury
- Unconscious or GCS <13
- Local bony abnormalities of the head (skull fracture, puncture wound, FB ± laceration)
- Evidence of basal skull fracture (hemotympanum, Battle's sign, raccoon eye)
- Unexplained focal neurologic signs
- History of previous craniotomy with shunt
- Posttraumatic amnesia
- Severe and worsening headache
- Posttraumatic seizure
- Blood dyscrasia or any anticoagulant medication

Indications for radiologic investigation
- Head CT if neurologically abnormal, seizure, depressed or basal skull fracture
- Consider head CT if neurologically normal and symptomatic
- No investigation if neurologically normal and asymptomatic

© The Hospital for Sick Children, 2009. New artwork created by The Hospital for Sick Children for *The Hospital for Sick Children Handbook of Pediatrics*, 11th edition.

MANAGEMENT

- See Table 3.14

Table 3.14	Management of Children With Head Injuries Based on Severity of Injury	
Mild	**Moderate**	**Severe**
· History to rule out high-risk criteria · Documentation of trauma event · Full examination · Discharge with head injury instructions (see below)	· History to rule out high-risk criteria · Documentation of trauma event · Describe changes in child's condition since injury · Full examination · Observe in ER until child has returned to usual status and tolerates oral fluids · Discharge with head injury instructions if symptoms resolve in 2–4 h · Neurosurgical consultation if symptoms persist >4 h or abnormal neurovitals/neurologic examination	· History to assess high-risk criteria · Documentation of trauma event · Describe changes in child's condition since injury · Full examination · Monitored observation in ER · Head CT scan · Neurosurgical consultation (and hematology if bleeding disorder)

Discharge Instructions

- Patient should return to emergency department if any of the following develops:
  - Persistent or increasing headache
  - Repeated vomiting
  - Drowsiness or change in behavior
  - Weakness or clumsiness of an arm or leg
  - Stiffness of neck or complaints of pain with neck movement
  - Complaints of "seeing double"
  - Poor balance when walking
  - Seizures
  - Leakage of clear fluid from nose or ears

BURNS

BURN MAPPING

- See Figure 3.7

RESUSCITATION

- Burn patients are trauma patients: perform primary and secondary survey, obtain IV access
- For blast injuries, ensure C-spine immobilization
- Rapidly evaluate patient for symptoms of airway burns (facial burns, singed nose hairs, intraoral burns, carbonaceous sputum, signs of respiratory distress)
- If airway burns suspected, support with 100% O_2 and PPV as needed until intubation can be performed; early intubation is indicated for suspected airway burns
- 100% O_2 for all potential smoke inhalation victims; accelerates elimination of carbon monoxide
- Continuous cardiac monitoring; patients with electrical burn injuries at risk for arrhythmias
- Evaluate total burn surface area (TBSA), using diagram (see Figure 3.7) OR using child's palm (equivalent to 1% TBSA)
- Begin fluid resuscitation using the Parkland formula when TBSA ≥15%

Parkland Formula

- See Box 3.1
- Estimate of fluids required for resuscitation only; formula often underestimates needs
- Titrate fluid resuscitation to maintain urine output ≥1 mL/kg/h
- For large burns (>15% TBSA) and genitourinary burns, insert Foley catheter as soon as possible
- For large burns (>15% TBSA), insert NG tube during secondary survey

Figure 3.7 Estimation of Burn Area

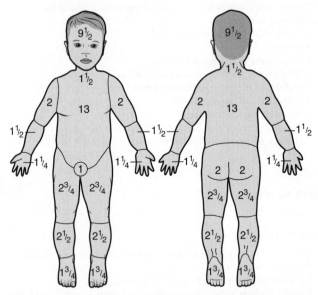

	Age in Years					
Area (%)	0	1	5	10	15	Adult
Head area	19	17	13	11	9	7
Trunk area	26	26	26	26	26	26
Arm area	7	7	7	7	7	7
Thigh area	$5^1/_2$	$6^1/_2$	$8^1/_2$	$8^1/_2$	$9^1/_2$	$9^1/_2$
Leg area	5	5	5	6	6	7

Total 3rd-degree burn _____   Total burns _____
Total 2nd-degree burn _____

Box 3.1   Parkland Formula for Fluid Resuscitation

- Resuscitation fluid = 4 mL/kg × % TBSA (second- and third-degree burns)
- 50% of IV fluids (Ringer's lactate or 0.9NaCl) over first 8 h (from time of injury)
- Remaining fluids over the next 16 h

INVESTIGATIONS

- CBC, Na^+, K^+, chloride, urea, creatinine; LFTs; amylase, blood gas, creatine kinase; urinalysis

MANAGEMENT

- Always consider possibility of abuse when evaluating a burn victim

Indications for Admission of Burn Patients

- See Box 3.2

Box 3.2	Criteria for Hospitalization of Patients With Burns

Extent:
- <2 yr: ≥6% of BSA (combination of second and third degree)
- >2 yr: ≥10% of BSA (combination of second and third degree)

Location: burns on face, neck, hands, feet, perineum

Type: chemical, electrical

Associated injuries: smoke inhalation, head injury, fractures, soft tissue trauma

Complicating medical problems: diabetes

Social situation: infants and young children, abuse, self-inflicted, psychological issues

Inpatient Management

- See p. 750

Outpatient Management

- See p. 750

DROWNING AND NEAR DROWNING

DEFINITIONS

- Drowning: a fluid submersion injury with asphyxiation leading to death within 24 h
- Near drowning: any other fluid submersion injury

MANAGEMENT

- Assess ABCs with C-spine control
- Obtain vital signs; attach cardiac and O_2 sat monitors
- Intubate if unable to protect airway or to maintain acceptable oxygenation and ventilation
- IV fluids at 50–80% of maintenance (to minimize fluid overload) unless treating shock
- NG tube, Foley catheter

- Remove wet clothing, treat hypothermia (see p. 26)
- Prevention and treatment of ↑ICP (see p. 38)
- Initial investigations: ABG, blood sugar, electrolytes, CXR
- Secondary survey: complete physical examination to rule out other injuries
- Secondary investigations: CBC; electrolytes, urea, creatinine; coagulation, ± specific drug levels, if indicated by history

FURTHER READING

Barkin RM, ed. *Pediatric Emergency Medicine: Concepts and Clinical Practice*. 2nd ed. St. Louis, Mo: Mosby Year Book; 1997.

Fleisher GR, Ludwig S, eds. *Textbook of Pediatric Emergency Medicine*. 5th ed. Philadelphia, Pa: Lippincott Williams & Wilkins; 2006.

Lalani A, Schneeweiss S, eds. *The Hospital for Sick Children Handbook of Pediatric Emergency Medicine*. Sudbury, Mass: Jones & Bartlett Publishers; 2008.

Emergency Medicine

3

Chapter 4 Poisonings and Toxicology

Nadia Luca

Margaret Thompson

Chapter 4   Poisonings and Toxicology

COMMON ABBREVIATIONS

AC	activated charcoal
ALI	acute lung injury
ABG	arterial blood gas
CBC	complete blood cell count
INR	international normalized ratio
G6PD	glucose-6-phosphate dehydrogenase
GHB	gamma hydroxybutyrate
LOC	level of consciousness
LSD	lysergic acid diethylamide
MetHb	methemoglobin
MDMA	3,4-methylenedioxymethamphetamine
MSK	musculoskeletal
PIC	poison information center
PTT	partial thromboplastin time
RR	respiratory rate
WBI	whole-bowel irrigation

APPROACH TO THE POISONED CHILD

4

INITIAL RESUSCITATION AND SUPPORT

- Ensure adequate initial resuscitation and stabilization of every potentially poisoned patient (see Chapter 1); continue to re-evaluate and provide ongoing supportive care
- Contact your local PIC

ESSENTIAL HISTORY

- Seven key questions: who (age, weight), what, when, where (route), why (intentional or accidental), how, how much
- Past medical history (medications, substances available in the home), review of systems

ESSENTIAL PHYSICAL EXAMINATION

- Eyes: pupils, extraocular movements
- Mouth: corrosive lesions, hydration of mucous membranes
- Cardiovascular: HR, BP, rhythm, perfusion
- Respiratory: RR, chest wall movement, air entry, auscultatory signs
- GI: motility and presence of bowel sounds, corrosive effects
- Neurologic/MSK: speech, reflexes, muscle tone
- Skin: color, burns, bullae
- Odors: breath, clothing

IMPORTANT LABORATORY INVESTIGATIONS

- Serum glucose/glucometer reading at bedside; urea; creatinine
- ABG to check for acid–base status
- Electrolytes (measured Na^+, K^+, Cl^-, HCO_3^-) to determine anion gap (see Chapter 16)
- Serum osmolality and calculated osmolality to determine osmolar gap (measured osmolality – calculated osmolality; increased if >10 mOsm/kg H_2O); only useful if elevated; does not rule out toxic alcohol if within normal range

$$\text{Calculated osmolality} = (2\,[Na^+] + [\text{glucose (mmol/L)}] + [\text{urea (mmol/L)}])\ \text{mOsm/kg}\ H_2O$$

OR

$$\text{Calculated osmolality} = [2(Na^+) + \text{glucose (mg/dL)}/18 + \text{urea (mg/dL)}/2.8]\ \text{mOsm/kg}\ H_2O$$

Case Dependent

- CBC, INR/PTT
- Liver transaminases (if acetaminophen detected or abdominal pain)
- Urinalysis to screen for hemoglobin, myoglobin, crystalluria
- ECG

Toxicology Screening

- See Box 4.1
- Broad-spectrum toxicology screening of urine and blood not generally recommended in emergency; treat symptoms, NOT laboratory findings: urine can be positive for days after last ingestion; many false-positive results possible
- *Communicate clinical suspicions to laboratory* for more specific testing recommendations
- Consider acetaminophen and salicylate levels in unknown overdose or decreased LOC when history is not available

APPROACH TO DECONTAMINATION

SURFACE DECONTAMINATION

Skin

- Remove contaminated clothing
- Flush exposed areas with lukewarm water or 0.9% NaCl for a minimum of 20 min
- Do not chemically neutralize unless recommended by PIC; heat generated may worsen injury

Eyes

- Remove contact lenses
- Consider use of local anaesthetic drops to facilitate irrigation

Box 4.1 Drugs Detectable in Blood and Urine

Blood

- Volatiles (ethanol, methanol, isopropanol; ethylene glycol must be specifically requested)
- Salicylates
- Acetaminophen
- Barbiturates
- Benzodiazepines (positive or negative; levels not available)
- Antidepressants (tricyclic antidepressants, many false positives and specific levels NOT helpful for acute poisonings; lithium must be specifically requested)

Urine*

- Narcotics (heroin, morphine, codeine)
- Barbiturates (specific immunoassay needed)
- Benzodiazepines (specific immunoassay needed)
- Antidepressants (amitriptyline; many false positives)
- Antipsychotics (chlorpromazine)
- Stimulants (cocaine, amphetamines)
- Hallucinogens (phencyclidine; cannabinoids require specific immunoassay)
- Cough/cold remedies
- Antihistamines (dimenhydrinate, diphenhydramine)
- Some cardiac drugs (verapamil)

*Although these substances can be detectable by some assays, few are routinely done AND none make a difference to caring for the acutely poisoned patient.

- Flush exposed eye with copious lukewarm water or 0.9% NaCl (≥1L/eye)
- If exposure to acid or base, continue irrigation until pH of tears is normal (pH 7.5–8.0)
- Careful examination of cornea, conjunctiva; refer to ophthalmologist if any abnormalities or if exposure to a base

Inhalation

- Remove from source of exposure
- Provide supplemental humidified oxygen
- Watch for worsening cardiorespiratory status (tachypnea, dyspnea, stridor, hoarse voice)

GI DECONTAMINATION

- See Table 4.1
- Evidence best for use of AC and WBI; ipecac syrup no longer recommended in any circumstance

ENHANCED ELIMINATION

- See Table 4.2

ANTIDOTES

- Given *only after* patient has been stabilized and a diagnosis has been made (exceptions: hypoglycemia, narcotic exposure)
- See Table 4.3 for a list of toxins and antidotes

Table 4.1 — Gastrointestinal (GI) Decontamination*

Treatment	Drugs	Indications	Contraindications	Dose/Administration
Single-dose AC	Most drugs; exceptions: **G**lycols **A**lcohols **M**etals (e.g., iron, lead, lithium, mercury, arsenic) **E**lectrolytes (e.g., Na+, K+) Corrosives Hydrocarbons	Within 1 h of potentially toxic ingestion; considered later depending on clinical scenario; contact local PIC	Unprotected airway, risk of aspiration, GI tract obstruction, perforation. Rarely worth fighting with patient to take	10× amount of toxin ingested OR 1 g/kg PO or by NG tube if unknown amount of toxin; adult dose = 50–100 g (comes in 25 g/250 mL or 50 g/250 mL solution; should not be further diluted)
WBI	Sustained-release/enteric-coated products Toxins poorly bound by AC (e.g., iron) Body packing of illicit drugs (e.g., cocaine, heroin)	Consider if large amounts of highly toxic sustained-release/ enteric-coated products; toxins poorly adsorbed by charcoal; body packing	GI obstruction/perforation, unprotected airway, intractable vomiting	Polyethylene glycol (PEG)-electrolyte via NG until rectal effluent clear · 9 mo–6 yr: up to 500 mL/h · 6–12 yr: up to 1000 mL/h · Adolescents/adults: up to 1500–2000 mL/h
Gastric lavage	*Not recommended for routine use for any ingestion*	Consider if recent ingestion of ++ toxic substance; contact local PIC	Unprotected airway, high aspiration potential, GI hemorrhage/perforation	Sequential instillation and aspiration of small amounts of liquid via large-bore orogastric tube; patient must be intubated

*Summary of the most current position statements of the American Academy of Clinical Toxicology and the European Association of Poison Centre and Clinical Toxicologists.

Table 4.2 Enhanced Elimination

Treatment	Drugs	Indications	Contraindications	Dose
Multidose AC	Carbamazepine, dapsone, phenobarbital, quinine, theophylline	Life-threatening ingestion of listed drugs	Unprotected airway, risk of aspiration, GI tract obstruction or perforation	10–25 g qh until clinical/laboratory variables improve; IV antiemetic to prevent vomiting
Urinary alkalinization	Salicylates, methotrexate, chlorpropamide, phenobarbital, selected other poisonings (consult local PIC)	First-line treatment in moderate-severe salicylate poisoning that does not meet criteria for hemodialysis (see pp. x) Evidence for benefit in severe methotrexate and chlorpropamide poisoning Effective in phenobarbital poisoning, BUT multidose AC superior	Renal failure, pulmonary edema, cerebral edema Caution with fluid overload if pre-existing cardiac disease	1–2 mEq/kg of 8.4% $NaHCO_3$, push Continuous infusion: 150 mEq $NaHCO_3$ in 1 L D5W at 1.5× maintenance K^+ infusion to maintain K^+ ≥4.0 q2h monitoring of urine pH (goal 7.5–8.5), output, serum pH, K^+, toxin in question Insert Foley catheter
Hemodialysis (extracorporeal removal)	Toxic alcohols (ethylene glycol, methanol), lithium, salicylates, valproic acid, theophylline, selected others	Varies according to toxin; consider in severe poisoning/poisoning refractory to initial management	Hemodynamic instability, lack of specialized equipment and expertise (e.g., dialysis capability)	

Table 4.3	Toxins and Antidotes*
Toxin	**Antidote**
Acetaminophen	*n*-Acetylcysteine (NAC)
Benzodiazepines	Flumazenil (NOT routinely recommended)[†]
β-Adrenergic antagonists	No specific antidote; consider high-dose insulin or intralipids*
Calcium channel blockers	Calcium; consider high-dose insulin infusion or intralipids*
Carbon monoxide	100% oxygen; may rarely consider hyperbaric oxygen
Cholinergic agents (pesticides)	Atropine/pralidoxime
Cyanide	Sodium nitrite/sodium thiosulfate (cyanide kit) OR hydroxycobalamin; oxygen
Digoxin	Digoxin immune Fab fragment
Heavy metals	Specific chelators
Hypoglycemics (insulin, oral hypoglycemics)	Glucose (D25W in children); consider octreotide if oral hypoglycemic ingestion
Iron	Deferoxamine
Methanol/ethylene glycol	Fomepizole OR ethanol (if fomepizole unavailable)
Methemoglobin	Methylene blue (contraindicated in G6PD deficiency)
Opiates	Naloxone

*Consult your PIC for dosing and appropriate use.
[†]Can precipitate seizures or arrhythmias.

TIPS FOR IDENTIFYING UNKNOWN POISONS

- Presenting signs/symptoms may conform to a particular toxic syndrome; may help identify class of drug/toxin ingested (Table 4.4)
- If ↑ anion gap, differential diagnosis suggested by mnemonic MUDPILE CATS (Box 4.2)
- If ↑ osmolar gap, causes suggested by mnemonic ME DIE (see Box 4.2)

SELECTED POISONINGS

- See Table 4.5
- See Figure 4.1

Table 4.4	Common Toxic Syndromes	
Toxic Syndrome	**Clinical Signs**	**Common Causes**
Anticholinergic syndrome	Tachycardia; hypertension; skin flushed, hot, dry; dilated pupils; urinary retention; ↓ bowel sounds; delirium, hallucinations, mumbling speech; ± hyperthermia; ± myoclonic jerking; ± seizures	Antidepressants (tricyclic agents); antihistamines (diphenhydramine); antipsychotic agents; atropine; scopolamine; antiparkinsonism medications (amantadine, benztropine); plants (e.g., Jimson weed)
Sympathomimetic syndrome	Tachycardia; hypertension; hyperthermia; diaphoresis; dilated pupils; hyperreflexia; delusions, paranoia	Amphetamines; methamphetamines and derivatives (e.g., MDMA [Ecstasy]); cocaine; decongestants (ephedrine); caffeine; theophylline; withdrawal from sedatives/hypnotics; may be mimicked by ASA toxicity or hypoglycemia
Cholinergic syndrome	Mnemonic DUMBELS: **D**iaphoresis, diarrhea; **U**rinary incontinence; **M**iosis; **B**ronchospasm, bronchorrhea, bradycardia; **E**mesis; **L**acrimation; **S**alivation	Organophosphate pesticides, carbamate pesticides, physostigmine, edrophonium, mushrooms (some), nerve gases
Sympatholytic/ sedative/hypnotic syndrome	Bradycardia, hypotension, pinpoint/ small pupils, hypothermia, ↓GI peristalsis, respiratory depression, coma, hyporeflexia	Clonidine, methyldopa, narcotics, barbiturates (phenobarbital), benzodiazepines and other sedatives, hypnotics, ethanol

Box 4.2	Differential Diagnosis of Increased Anion and Osmolar Gaps

Increased Anion Gap
- **M**ethanol
- **U**remia
- **D**iabetic ketoacidosis (also starvation and alcoholic ketoacidosis)
- **P**araldehyde, phenformin (also metformin)
- **I**ron, isoniazid
- **L**actic acidosis (anything that causes hypotension, seizures)
- **E**thylene glycol
- **C**yanide, CO
- **A**cetylsalicylic acid
- **T**oluene
- **S**olvents

Increased Osmolar Gap
- **M**ethanol
- **E**thylene glycol
- **D**iuretics (mannitol, sorbitol, glycerin)
- **I**sopropyl alcohol
- **E**thanol

Table 4.5 — Presentation and Management of Common Poisonings

Toxin/Exposure	Clinical Presentation	Key Investigations	Management

Acetaminophen
Toxic dose: >200 mg/kg in children, >7.5 g in large children and adults
	Stage I: 0.5–24 h
	Nausea, vomiting, lethargy, pallor, diaphoresis, malaise; rarely change in LOC
	Stage II: 24–72 h
	Initial symptoms resolve; RUQ pain, liver enlargement/tenderness; ↑AST/ALT, bilirubin, INR; oliguria, renal function abnormalities
	Stage III: 72–96 h
	Stage I symptoms reappear; jaundice, encephalopathy; peak elevation of AST/ALT, coagulation defects, lactic acidosis, hypoglycemia; acute renal failure; death
	Stage IV: 4 d–2 wk
	Symptoms resolve, liver/renal functions normalize
		- Obtain 4 h postingestion acetaminophen level, plot on Rumack-Matthew nomogram (Figure 4.1)
		- Baseline electrolytes, glucose, urea, creatinine, liver transaminases, INR
		- Repeat acetaminophen level, liver transaminases, INR after NAC treatment
			1. Administer AC
			2. NAC:
			  · Indications:
			   a) A 4 h or greater level above the possible hepatotoxic line when plotted on nomogram (see Figure 4.1)
			   b) History of ingestion of >200 mg/kg and no level available within 8–10 h of ingestion
			   c) Presentation >24 h postingestion with detectable acetaminophen level and evidence of hepatotoxicity
			  · Administration:
			   - Various IV/oral protocols; contact local PIC* (see sample at end of table)
			   - Outcome excellent if NAC started within 8–10 h of ingestion; treatment initiated >8 h postingestion beneficial, but effectiveness diminishes with time

Barbiturates and anticonvulsants	· CNS depression: lethargy, ataxia, slurred speech, nystagmus · Respiratory depression (apnea, hypoxia), hypotension · Other: delirium, bullous skin lesions, hypothermia	Stat and serial anticonvulsant levels if testing available; peak often delayed by 24–48 h in overdose	1. Support ventilation, circulation; watch for seizures, arrhythmias 2. Consider AC 3. Consider multidose AC for phenobarbital, carbamazepine (see Table 4.2) 4. Consider urinary alkalinization (see p. 58); effective for phenobarbital intoxication 5. Consider dialysis for carbamazepine, valproic acid, phenobarbital

(continued)

Table 4.5 Presentation and Management of Common Poisonings *(continued)*

Toxin/Exposure	Clinical Presentation	Key Investigations	Management

Calcium channel blockers	· Hypotension, bradycardia, dysrhythmias, noncardiogenic pulmonary edema, coma, seizures (severe)
	· Hyperglycemia, metabolic acidosis
		· ECG, continuous cardiorespiratory monitoring
		· Electrolytes (especially K⁺, Ca²⁺), glucose, urea, creatinine, ABG
			1. GI decontamination:
			  a) AC is preferred method
			  b) Consider WBI for large ingestions of sustained-release preparations (See Table 4.1)
			2. IV fluid resuscitation (20 mL/kg 0.9%NaCl)
			3. Specific drugs and antidotes (see Table 4.3)
			  a) 10% CaCl 0.1 mL/kg IV OR 10% calcium gluconate 0.3 mL/kg IV slow push for symptomatic hypotension/bradycardia
			  b) If response to Ca²⁺, repeat bolus or continuous infusion
			  c) Vasopressors if hypotension unresponsive to fluids and calcium
			  d) High-dose regular insulin (0.5–1.0 units/kg IV bolus followed by 0.5–1.0 units/kg/h infusion, titrating as necessary) if inadequate response to above measures (frequent glucose checks)
			  e) Consider intralipid 20% bolus 1.5 mL/kg over 5 min followed by infusion. Consult PIC
			  f) Aminnone or milrinone: for hypotension unresponsive to fluids, Ca²⁺, vasopressors, insulin
			  g) Other inotropes, as hemodynamic monitoring dictates

(continued)

Table 4.5 Presentation and Management of Common Poisonings *(continued)*

Toxin / Exposure	Clinical Presentation	Key Investigations	Management
Insecticides (organophosphates)	Cholinergic signs (muscarinic: mnemonic DUMBELS, see Table 4.4; nicotinic: weakness, muscle fasciculations), CNS signs (coma, convulsions), respiratory insufficiency		1. Airway management: suction ± assisted ventilation 2. AC once airway secured 3. If dermal exposure: remove clothes, irrigate skin 4. Atropine 0.05 mg/kg IV (max 2 mg); double dose q5min until bronchial secretions dry, wheezing stops 5. Pralidoxime chloride 20–40 mg/kg (max 8 g) IV slowly; repeat dose and/or continuous infusions may be necessary 6. Benzodiazepines for seizures

Iron
· Elemental iron: 33% in ferrous fumarate; 20% in ferrous sulfate; 12% in ferrous gluconate
· Potentially toxic dose: 20–60 mg/kg elemental iron
· Highly toxic dose: >60 mg/kg
· Lethal dose: 200–300 mg/kg
	· *Gastrointestinal phase* (30 min–6 h): direct injury to GI mucosa; vomiting, bloody diarrhea, abdominal pain, hypotension, shock, metabolic acidosis
	· *Quiescent phase* (6–24 h): resolution of GI symptoms; may not be seen in severe poisoning
	· *Delayed phase* (4 h–4 d): abrupt relapse with multiple organ failure; shock; profound metabolic acidosis, coagulopathy, hepatic dysfunction, renal failure, pulmonary failure, CNS dysfunction
	· *Hepatotoxicity* (within 2 d): coma, coagulopathy, jaundice
	· *Bowel obstruction* (2–4 wk); GI scarring ± obstruction, classically at gastric outlet
		· Serum iron concentration at 4–6 h
		· CBC, electrolytes, urea, creatinine, blood gas, liver enzymes, glucose, INR, type and crossmatch
		· Abdominal X-ray (looking for radio-opaque pills)
			1. Supportive care for nausea, vomiting, diarrhea, fluid loss
			2. GI decontamination: WBI if tablets seen on X-ray (see Table 4.1)
			3. If asymptomatic, normal laboratory values, and ingested <20 mg/kg, may discharge home; otherwise, observe for at least 8 h
			4. Deferoxamine indicated if any of the following:
			  a) Severe symptoms: altered mental status, hemodynamic instability, persistent vomiting and/or diarrhea
			  b) Serum iron level >90 µmol/L (>500 mcg/dL); NB: brief chelation may be necessary if level 63–90 µmol/L (300–500 mcg/dL) and symptomatic
			  c) Iron level not available and >60 mg/kg elemental iron ingested and symptomatic
			  d) Anion gap metabolic acidosis

(continued)

Table 4.5 Presentation and Management of Common Poisonings (continued)

Toxin/Exposure	Clinical Presentation	Key Investigations	Management
Opiates and opioids (narcotics) (e.g. morphine, heroin, codeine, hydrocodone, fentanyl, meperidine, methadone, dextromethorphan)	· Mild to moderate: sedation, miosis, hypotension, bradycardia, flushing, nausea · Severe: respiratory depression, apnea, coma, ALI · Seizures: rare, but may occur with meperidine and dextromethorphan ingestions	· Positive response to naloxone (may consider qualitative urine screen for verification and to identify co-ingestions)	1. Airway/ventilatory support 2. AC 3. Naloxone 0.1 mg/kg/dose IV/ETT (max 2 mg/dose); repeat prn to maintain reversal; contact PIC for continuous naloxone infusion 4. After naloxone therapy, must be in constant care setting, discharged only when fully awake and ≥3 h have elapsed; symptomatic methadone intoxication must be observed ≥24 h and ≥6 h after naloxone infusion discontinued
Salicylates · Sources include ASA, salicylic acid, bismuth salicylate, methyl salicylate (oil of wintergreen) · Toxic dose of ASA: >150 mg/kg: lethal dose: >500 mg/kg · Oil of wintergreen: 1 mL = 1.4 g ASA	· Common symptoms: tachypnea, nausea, vomiting, diaphoresis, tinnitus - Severe cases: hyperthermia, hyperventilation, tachycardia, lethargy, confusion · May progress to convulsions, coma, ALI, and death	· Serum salicylate level on presentation and q2h until peak and declining ×2 · ABG: initially mixed picture of respiratory alkalosis and metabolic acidosis (infants/young children tend to be acidemic, whereas older children/adults tend to be alkalemic); as become more ill, respiratory and metabolic acidosis with acidemia · Glucose usually low, INR elevated (clinical bleeding unusual), lactate elevated · CBC, electrolytes, urea, creatinine, Ca²⁺, acetaminophen level · Urine for ketones, blood pH q1h while alkalinization therapy in progress	1. AC 10 g per gram drug ingested 2. Supplemental glucose 3. Volume resuscitation; add KCl once voided 4. Airway intervention (if required) followed by hyperventilation (iatrogenic respiratory acidosis) → decreases brain salicylate levels, cerebral edema 5. Urinary akalinization (see p. 58) 6. Indicated if any of the following: a) Symptomatic ingestion (other than tinnitus) if level not available b) Acute ingestion and a salicylate level of >3.5 mmol/L c) Metabolic acidosis 6. Hemodialysis indicated if any of the following: a) Sick patient and contraindications to alkalinization (ALI, cerebral edema, renal failure)

(continued)

Table 4.5   Presentation and Management of Common Poisonings (continued)

Toxin/Exposure	Clinical Presentation	Key Investigations	Management
			b) Sick patient and failure to alkalinize after 2 h of aggressive bicarbonate therapy c) Clinical deterioration (including refractory acidosis) despite appropriate supportive care d) High levels (>7.2 mmol/L acute; >5.0 mmol/L chronic)

Toxic alcohols	*Methanol:* retinal injury, visual disturbances (blurring, central scotomata), blindness, abdominal pain and vomiting, metabolic acidosis
	Ethylene glycol: flank pain, hematuria, oliguria, renal failure, metabolic acidosis
	Both: inebriation, hyperventilation (Kussmaul's), seizures, coma, death
		· Stat serum ethylene glycol, methanol, ethanol levels
		· Electrolytes, blood gas, glucose, urea, creatinine, amylase, serum osmolality, Ca²⁺, urinalysis
		· Anion gap (latent period up to 40 h for methanol, 4–24 h for ethylene glycol)
		· Osmolar gap (increased early, disappears as toxic alcohol is metabolized)
			1. Consider gastric lavage if early
			2. Fomepizole (15 mg/kg loading dose): specific antagonist of ADH; optimum antidote but not always available
			3. Ethanol infusion (second line): consult local PIC for loading and maintenance infusion doses
			4. Folic acid: enhances elimination of formic acid (1 mg/kg in children up to 50 mg IV q4h) until methanol undetectable
			5. Pyridoxine and thiamine: involved in minor elimination pathways of ethylene glycol to nontoxic products
			6. Hemodialysis indicated if any of the following:
			  a) Evidence of end-organ damage (any degree of visual impairment, renal failure, or metabolic acidosis)
			  b) Methanol level >15 mmol/L (early) (exact level debated)
			  c) Ethylene glycol level >8 mmol/L (early)

(continued)

Table 4.5 Presentation and Management of Common Poisonings (continued)

Toxin / Exposure	Clinical Presentation	Key Investigations	Management
Tricyclic antidepressants (e.g., amitriptyline, imipramine)	Narrow therapeutic index; three major toxic syndromes: · Anticholinergic (see Table 4.4) · CNS: confusion, delirium, hallucinations, hyperreflexia; late—seizures, obtundation, coma · Cardiovascular: hypotension, sinus tachycardia, QRS prolongation (may predict risk of seizure, arrhythmia), ventricular arrhythmias; hallmark ECG pattern: deep S wave in I, aV_R and tall R wave in aV_L	Cardiac monitor × 24 h, and hourly ECGs until 6h after ingestion	1. Administer AC 2. Treat hypotension with fluid boluses 3. Inotropes as necessary: norepinephrine bitartrate first choice (theoretical due to TCA depletion of norepinephrine) 4. If QRS >100 ms or arrhythmia: $NaHCO_3$ 1–2 mEq/kg IV boluses, repeated as necessary; keep pH 7.45–7.55 5. If QRS prolongation or arrhythmia refractory, consider lidocaine or phenytoin 6. Treat seizures with benzodiazepines, and/or phenobarbital 7. Consider intralipids; contact local PIC for dosing

*Sample NAC protocol:
· 150 mg NAC/kg over 15 min (usually given over 60 min to avoid adverse reactions)
· 50 mg NAC/kg over 4 h
· 100 mg NAC/kg over 16 h
· Total = 300 mg NAC/kg over 21 h; Note: total fluids must be adjusted for children less than 35 kg to avoid fluid overload.

Figure 4.1 Semilogarithmic Plot of Plasma Acetaminophen Levels Versus Time

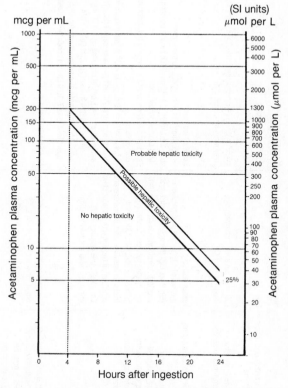

Adapted from Rumack BH, Matthew H. Acetaminophen poisoning and toxicity. *Pediatrics.* 1975;55:871–876. Modified form presented here is used with the permission of Micromedix, Inc., Englewood, Colorado.

ENVIRONMENTAL CONTAMINANTS

- See Table 4.6

RECREATIONAL DRUGS

- See Table 4.7
- See pp. 123–124 for tips on dealing with stable adolescents in the emergency setting who are using drugs

Table 4.6   Common Environmental Contaminants

Substance	Route of Exposure	Symptoms/Signs	Investigations	Management
Asbestos	Still found in old buildings	Long-term exposure linked to lung cancer, malignant mesothelioma	CXR	No known treatment
Carbon monoxide	Smoke inhalation from fires, combustion, appliances, car exhaust	*Minor:* headache, nausea, vomiting *Major:* chest pain, arrhythmia, confusion, loss of consciousness	ECG in all patients; carboxyhemoglobin level	100% oxygen via nonrebreather mask; hyperbaric oxygen may rarely be considered
Lead	Paint, gasoline, folk remedies, cosmetics, pottery glaze, ceramic food containers, leaded pipes, soil; rare in developed countries	Headache, abdominal pain, constipation, poor appetite *Severe:* loss of milestones, poor coordination, hearing loss, renal insufficiency; lead encephalopathy–ataxia, persistent vomiting, lethargy, stupor, coma, seizures	Venous lead level • If elevated: erythrocyte protoporphyrin (EP) level, CBC (hypochromic, microcytic anemia), reticulocyte count, serum iron, iron binding capacity, ferritin, urea, creatinine; abdominal XR ("lead flecks" in intestinal tract indicate recent ingestion); if treating with chelator, check Ca^{2+}, Mg^{2+}, liver enzymes, G6PD, urinalysis, renal and liver function	Based on lead level: • <0.5 μmol/L (<10 mcg/dL): no treatment • 0.5–2.1 μmol/L (10–45 mcg/dL): remove environmental lead sources, follow level • >2.1 μmol/L (>45 mcg/dL): consider treatment with oral chelator • >3.4 μmol/L (>70 mcg/dL) and/or lead encephalopathy: consult with local PIC and give dimercaprol (British antilewisite* [BAL], dithiol chelating agent) 75 mg/m² IM q4h × 3–5 d; 4 h after BAL, start CaNa₂ EDTA 1000–1500 mg/m²/d as continuous infusion for 5 d; repeat lead level 7–10 d later to check for rebound
Organic mercury	Marine fish (e.g. swordfish, tuna), fish from polluted fresh waters (e.g., pike, bass)	Paresthesia, malaise, ataxia, visual field defects, deafness; teratogenic to fetal brain; FDA recommends pregnant women limit weekly consumption	May measure mercury levels in whole blood (however, normal levels do not exclude mercury poisoning)	No known treatment

(continued)

Table 4.6   Common Environmental Contaminants (continued)

Substance	Route of Exposure	Symptoms/Signs	Investigations	Management
Inorganic mercury	Dental amalgams, thermometers, batteries, fluorescent bulbs, mercury mines	Interstitial pneumonitis, intention tremor, inflamed gums, excess salivation, psychiatric symptoms (anxiety, insomnia); renal accumulation–nephrotic syndrome, renal tubular dysfunction	Urinary excretion of mercury	Chelating agents considered for symptomatic patients with confirmed poisoning

*Note: Suspended in peanut oil: check for allergy; also, may cause hemolysis in patients with G6PD deficiency.

Table 4.7	Common Substances of Abuse	
Substance	**Clinical Presentation**	**Management**
Amphetamines ("speed," "crystal meth," Ritalin, ephedrine)	Tachycardia, hypertension, arrhythmias, hyperthermia, hallucinations, tremors, hyperacute sensorium, rhabdomyolysis, seizures, coma	AC Benzodiazepines for agitation, seizures, hypertension Aggressive cooling Short-acting IV antihypertensives for refractory hypertension Avoid β-blockers
Cocaine	Hypertension, tachycardia, cardiac ischemia, hyperthermia, respiratory distress, intestinal infarction, rhabdomyolysis, mydriasis, psychomotor agitation, coma, seizures, cerebrovascular accident	Judicious use of benzodiazepines for seizures, hypertension, and/or agitation Aggressive cooling Short-acting IV antihypertensives for refractory hypertension Serial ECGs and cardiac enzymes, if chest pain Avoid β-blockers and succinylcholine
Ecstasy (MDMA, "E," "love drug," "rave drug")	Euphoria, increased alertness, hyperthermia, nausea, mydriasis, ataxia, tachycardia, hypertension, hyponatremia, rhabdomyolysis, cerebrovascular accident, seizure	Single-dose AC if recent ingestion Benzodiazepines for hyperthermia, agitation, hypertension, and/or seizures Aggressive cooling Avoid β-blockers
Ethanol (a child not used to exposure may get serious toxic effects with as little as 10–15 mL/kg beer, 4–6 mL/kg wine, 1–2 mL/kg 80-proof liquor)	*Mild:* sedation, impaired judgment, slurred speech, ataxia *Moderate:* hypotension, ↓K⁺, hypoglycemia, hypothermia, respiratory distress, coma *Severe:* death in 50%	Laboratory tests: electrolytes, glucose, ethanol level, osmolar gap Consider AC if suspect drug co-ingestion Treat hypoglycemia, hypokalemia Consider hemodialysis if ethanol level >110 mmol/L (>500 mg/dL)
GHB	Miosis, nystagmus, ataxia, bradycardia, hypotension, respiratory depression, coma	Supportive care; attention to airway, oxygenation
Heroin	See p. 64	
Ketamine ("special K")	Dissociative anesthetic, nystagmus, analgesia, amnesia, hallucinations, tachycardia, mild hypertension, emesis, rhabdomyolysis	Laboratory tests: electrolytes, creatinine Can discharge home once at baseline mental status Benzodiazepines for agitation

(continued)

Table 4.7	Common Substances of Abuse *(continued)*	
Substance	Clinical Presentation	Management
LSD	Psychosis with hyperalertness, delusions, hallucinations, visual perception distortion, paresthesias, dizziness, hyperthermia, seizures	Laboratory tests: CPK, creatinine, liver enzymes Benzodiazepines for seizures and/or anxiety Otherwise treat as per sympathomimetics
Marijuana	Tachycardia, miosis, euphoria, delusions, paranoia, dry mouth, ↑ appetite	Benzodiazepines for psychotic reactions/ acute delirium Observation: general improvement in 4–6 h

METHEMOGLOBINEMIA

- Form of hemoglobin in which Fe^{2+} is oxidized to Fe^{3+}, which cannot bind oxygen
- Oxygen affinity of remaining ferrous (Fe^{2+}) heme increased, thus Hb-dissociation curve is left-shifted and oxygen delivery to tissues impaired
- Causal exogenous agents: metoclopramide, nitrites, sulfonamides, local anesthetic agents (benzocaine, lidocaine)

CLINICAL PRESENTATION

- 30–50% MetHb: headache, fatigue, dyspnea, lethargy, cyanosis
- >50% MetHb: respiratory depression, altered consciousness, shock, seizures, death

MANAGEMENT

- Measure saturation gap: O_2 saturation by pulse oximetry vs. ABG
- Laboratory test: Evelyn-Malloy method: expresses MetHb as % of total Hb
- Consider blood transfusion or exchange transfusion if patient in shock

Methylene Blue

- Indications: patient symptomatic or MetHb >30%
- Dose: 1–2 mg/kg IV over 5 min; may repeat q30–60min (max 7 mg/kg)
- Contraindication: G6PD deficiency (try ascorbic acid or exchange transfusion)

Dart RC, Caravati EM, McGuigan MA, Whyte IM, Dawson AH, Seifert SA, Schonwald S, Yip L, Keyes DC, Hurlbut KM, Erdman AR, eds. *Medical Toxicology*. 3rd ed. Philadelphia, Pa: Lippincott Williams & Wilkins; 2004.

Ford M, Delaney KA, Ling L, Erikson T. *Clinical Toxicology*. Philadelphia, Pa: WB Saunders; 2001.

Goldfrank LR, Flomenbaum N, Hoffman RS, Howland MA, Lewin N, Nelson LS, eds. *Goldfrank's Toxicologic Emergencies*. 8th ed. New York, NY: McGraw-Hill; 2006.

Klaasen CD, ed. *Casarett and Doull's Toxicology: The Basic Science of Poisons*. 6th ed. New York, NY: McGraw-Hill; 2001.

Olson KR, ed. *Poisoning & Drug Overdose*. 5th ed. New York, NY: Lange Medical Books/McGraw-Hill; 2007.

USEFUL WEB SITES

Agency for Toxic Substances and Disease Registry. Available at: http://www.atsdr.cdc.gov.

American Academy of Clinical Toxicology. Available at: http://www.clintox.org.

Toxic plant index. Available at: http://chppm-www.apgea.army.mil/ento/plntndx.htm.

TOXNET—National Library of Medicine Specialist Information Services. Available at: http://toxnet.nlm.nih.gov.

The Vaults of Erowid (information about psychoactive plants and chemicals). Available at: http://www.erowid.org.

Poisonings and Toxicology

4

Chapter 5 Pain and Sedation

Mark O. Tessaro

Basem Naser

Chapter 5   Pain and Sedation

COMMON ABBREVIATIONS

ABC   airway, breathing, and circulation
PCA   patient-controlled analgesia
ETT   endotracheal tube

PAIN MANAGEMENT IN CHILDREN

- Age-related differences exist in behavioral responses to pain
- No evidence that sensitivity to pain differs between pediatric and adult patients
- Analgesia is frequently underused in children
- Providers of analgesic drugs should be familiar with their side effects and their potential interactions; opioid pharmacokinetics and pharmacodynamics differ between neonates and older infants and children
- Neonatal dosing may differ from guidelines presented herein

GENERAL PRINCIPLES OF PAIN ASSESSMENT

- See Figure 5.1
- Obtain pain history from child and/or parents
- Assess children based on developmental level and situation
- Assess pain routinely and regularly to tailor therapy; tools and results must be charted

VITAL SIGNS

- Physiologic measures (e.g., HR, RR, BP) can be used as adjuncts to self-reported and behavioral observations but are NOT sensitive or specific indicators of chronic pain

SELF-REPORT

- Self-report tools are more convenient and should be used whenever possible: children ≥4 yr can self-report and children ≥7 or 8 yr can use numeric scales
- Behavioral observation tools (e.g., vocalization, verbalization, facial expression, motor response, body posture, activity, appearance) can be used with preverbal/nonverbal children and as adjuncts to older children's self-report
- Verbal numeric self-reported scale (for school-aged and adolescent patients) rates pain on a scale of 0 (no pain) to 10 (worst pain)

Figure 5.1 Pain Assessment and Management of the Child

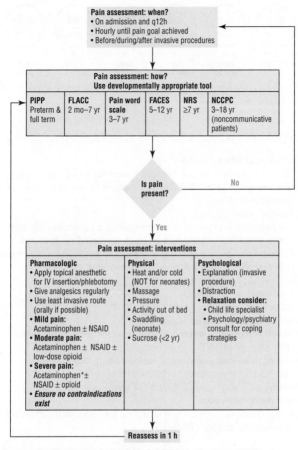

Pain assessment: when?
- On admission and q12h
- Hourly until pain goal achieved
- Before/during/after invasive procedures

Pain assessment: how?
Use developmentally appropriate tool

PIPP	FLACC	Pain word scale	FACES	NRS	NCCPC
Preterm & full term	2 mo–7 yr	3–7 yr	5–12 yr	≥7 yr	3–18 yr (noncommunicative patients)

Is pain present? → No

Yes

Pain assessment: interventions

Pharmacologic	Physical	Psychological
• Apply topical anesthetic for IV insertion/phlebotomy • Give analgesics regularly • Use least invasive route (orally if possible) • **Mild pain:** Acetaminophen ± NSAID • **Moderate pain:** Acetaminophen ± NSAID ± low-dose opioid • **Severe pain:** Acetaminophen*± NSAID ± opioid • ***Ensure no contraindications exist***	• Heat and/or cold (NOT for neonates) • Massage • Pressure • Activity out of bed • Swaddling (neonate) • Sucrose (<2 yr)	• Explanation (invasive procedure) • Distraction • **Relaxation consider:** • Child life specialist • Psychology/psychiatry consult for coping strategies

Reassess in 1 h

Algorithm based on the Hospital for Sick Children's pain assessment policy and pain management clinical practice guideline.

Adapted from The Hospital for Sick Children Clinical Practice Guideline on Pain Management.
PIPP, Premature Infant Pain Profile; *FLACC*, Faces Legs Activity Cry Consolability; *NRS*, Numenic Rating Scale; *NCCPC*, Noncommunicating children's pain checklist.

PAIN SCALES

- Many different scales are available (see Figure 5.1)
- FACES commonly used (Figure 5.2)

Figure 5.2 **FACES Scale**

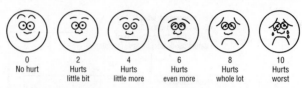

0	2	4	6	8	10
No hurt	Hurts little bit	Hurts little more	Hurts even more	Hurts whole lot	Hurts worst

Reprinted with permission from Hockenberry MJ, Wilson D, Winkelstein ML. *Wong's Essentials of Pediatric Nursing.* 7th ed. St. Louis, Mo: Mosby; 2005:1259.

GENERAL PRINCIPLES OF PAIN MANAGEMENT

- Prevent pain when possible
  - Better to prevent than treat; requirements for analgesics are lower if children wake up comfortable after surgery or are pretreated before painful procedures
- Give analgesics regularly
  - For pain that is expected to be constant (e.g., postsurgical), analgesics should be ordered and given as scheduled medications ("around the clock"); prn dosing should be used for breakthrough pain only (i.e., preambulation, preprocedures)
- Use the least invasive route
  - Oral route, when possible
  - IM is least acceptable
- Use the analgesic ladder (Figure 5.3)
  - Match analgesia to severity of pain (e.g., for severe pain, begin with nonopioid AND opioid analgesics)
  - Use of more than one class of analgesic (e.g., acetaminophen and NSAIDs); promotes better pain relief
- Treating pain with opioids does NOT lead to psychological dependence/addiction
- Use equianalgesic doses when changing routes or switching from one opioid to another (Table 5.1)

PHARMACOLOGIC METHODS OF PAIN CONTROL

- See Tables 5.2, 5.3, and 5.4

Figure 5.3 Analgesic Ladder

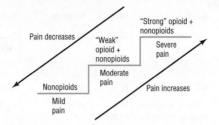

© The Hospital for Sick Children Clinical Practice Guideline on Pain Management.

Table 5.1	Equianalgesic Dosing*		
Drug	**Potency (Relative to Morphine)**	**IV Loading Dose (mg/kg)**	**PO Equivalent**
Meperidine	0.1	0.5–1.0	1.5–2 × IV dose
Morphine	1	0.05–0.10	3–5 × IV dose
Hydromorphone	5	0.015	1.3–6.7 × IV dose
Fentanyl IV	100	0.0005–0.001	N/A
Fentanyl patch	100	N/A; 25-mcg patch delivers 25 mcg/h; absorption continues for 12–24 h after removal; change patch q72h	

*Based on a single dose.
From Yaster M, Krane EJ, Kaplan RF, Coté CJ, Lappe DG. *Pediatric Pain Management and Sedation Handbook*. St. Louis, Mo: Mosby; 1997:40.

5

ADJUVANT THERAPY

- Adjuvant drugs (e.g., anticonvulsants [gabapentin], tricyclic antidepressants [amitriptyline], ketamine, and clonidine) may be important in treatment of neuropathic pain
- Benzodiazepines may be helpful for treatment of painful muscle spasms
- Oral sucrose reduces procedural pain in neonates and young infants

Table 5.2 — Pediatric Systemic Dosage Guidelines

Medication	Dosage	Route	Frequency	Maximum dose
Acetaminophen	10–15 mg/kg/dose	PO/PR	q4–6h	75 mg/kg/d or 4 g/d, whichever is less
NSAIDs*				
Ibuprofen	5–10 mg/kg/dose	PO	q6–8h	40 mg/kg/d
Naproxen	<25 kg: 7 mg/kg/dose 25–49 kg: 250 mg/dose >50 kg: 500 mg/dose	PO PO/PR PO/PR	q12h	1 g/d
Diclofenac	1 mg/kg/dose	PO/PR	q8–12h	3 mg/kg/d
Ketorolac	0.5 mg/kg/dose	IV	q6h for only 48 h	15 mg/dose
Opioids†				
Codeine‡	1.0–1.5 mg/kg/dose	PO	q4h	3–6 mg/kg/d
Morphine§	0.15–0.3 mg/kg/dose 0.05–0.1 mg/kg/dose 0.01–0.04 mg/kg/dose	PO/PR IV IV infusion	q3–4h q2–4h Continuous infusion ‖	
Meperidine#	0.5–1.0 mg/kg/dose 1–2 mg/kg/dose	IV PO	q3–4h q3–4h	100 mg/dose 150 mg/dose

*Use of NSAIDs may decrease opioid usage by 30–50%; ensure adequate hydration and renal function with NSAID use (follow urea and creatinine levels).

†For nonintubated infants <3 mo, initial opioid dose should be reduced to one third to one fourth of dose recommended above.

‡Codeine is metabolized into morphine; however, 10% of the population lacks the enzyme, and in them, codeine has no analgesic effect.

§Dosages recommended are initial doses: IV dose may be repeated q10min until child is comfortable, then administer q3–4h; for breakthrough pain: 0.02–0.05 mg/kg IV q2–4h; prn should be prescribed when around-the-clock or continuous morphine is ordered.

‖Morphine infusion; 0.5 × body weight (kg) = no. of mg morphine; dilute to 50 mL in syringe; therefore, 1 mL/h = 0.01 mg/kg/h.

#Avoid use in severe renal impairment: metabolite may cause seizures.

© The Hospital for Sick Children, 2009. New artwork created by The Hospital for Sick Children for *The Hospital for Sick Children Handbook of Pediatrics*, 11th edition.

Table 5.3 — Neonatal Opioid Infusion Guidelines

Population	Pain Severity	Morphine (mcg/kg/h)	Fentanyl (mcg/kg/h)
Preterm neonate	Mild	0–2	0.5
	Moderate	2–5	0.5
	Severe	5–10	1
Term neonate	Mild	0–5	0–0.5
	Moderate	5–10	0.5–1
	Severe	10–20	1–2

From Yaster M, Krane EJ, Kaplan RF, Coté CJ, Lappe DG. *Pediatric Pain Management and Sedation Handbook.* St. Louis, Mo: Mosby; 1997:199.

Table 5.4	Adverse Effects of Opioid Analgesics*
Adverse Effect	**Management**
Nausea/vomiting	· Antihistamine (e.g., dimenhydrinate)[†] 1 mg/kg q6h prn IV/PO · Serotonin receptor antagonist (e.g., ondansetron) 0.1 mg/kg/dose q8h prn IV/PO (up to 4 mg max)
Constipation	· Stool softeners (e.g., docusate sodium 5 mg/kg/d q6-8h)
Pruritus	· Antihistamine (e.g., diphenhydramine[†] 1 mg/kg q6h IV/PO)
Somnolence	· Reduce dose of opioid · Consider naloxone (start low to avoid reversal of analgesia; see Opioid Reversal in text)
Respiratory depression	· Stop opioid · Mild: stimulation and oxygen · Severe: respiratory support · Naloxone: see Opioid Reversal in text

*Routine close monitoring of all patients taking opioids permits early recognition and management of any adverse effect. All opioids may produce nausea, constipation, biliary tract spasms, sedation, and respiratory depression. These adverse effects are variable among patients.

[†]When dimenhydrinate and diphenhydramine are used in combination, reduce the dose of each to 0.5 mg/kg/dose to avoid sedation.

© The Hospital for Sick Children, 2009. New artwork created by The Hospital for Sick Children for *The Hospital for Sick Children Handbook of Pediatrics*, 11th edition.

MANAGEMENT OF PATIENTS TAKING OPIOIDS

MONITORING

- Monitor all patients taking medications with potential cardiorespiratory compromising effects; see institution-specific guidelines for details

OPIOID REVERSAL

- Naloxone (opioid antagonist) should be available for reversal of adverse opioid effects (Table 5.5)
- In patients with significant opiate exposure, use lowest naloxone dose possible and titrate carefully to avoid rebound hypertension, tachycardia, arrhythmias, and pulmonary edema

OPIOID TAPERING

- Consider tapering for any patient who has received opioids >5 d
  - Switch to PO (providing PO route is acceptable)
  - Weaning dose: for PO or intermittent IV, decrease daily dose by 10–20% *of initial daily dose* every day
- Consider IV morphine boluses for breakthrough pain

Table 5.5	Naloxone Administration
Step	**Comment**
Discontinue opioids and other sedation	
Evaluate ABCs	See pp. 5-9
Administer naloxone IV over 2 min	· Respiratory depression: · 1-2 mcg/kg · Respiratory arrest: · 0.1 mg/kg to a maximum of 2 mg · Use lowest effective dose to reverse respiratory effects and not analgesia
Observe for response	· Patient should open eyes and respond within 2 min
Titrate naloxone	· If no response within 2 min, repeat dose · If no effect after 10 mcg/kg has been given, consider nonopioid causes of unresponsiveness
Discontinue naloxone	· When patient responds
Observation	· Monitor for at least 2 h · Naloxone duration is less than that of most opioids, and repeated doses may be necessary · Consider use of naloxone infusion
Replacement analgesia	· Use nonopioids during observation

Adapted from McCaffery M, Pasero C. *Pain: Clinical Manual.* St. Louis, Mo: Mosby; 1999; and from Yaster M, Krane EJ, Kaplan RF, Coté CJ, Lappe DG. *Pediatric Pain Management and Sedation Handbook.* St. Louis, Mo: Mosby; 1997:48–49.

PATIENT-CONTROLLED ANALGESIA

- Device that provides basal opioid infusion with patient-administered supplemental boluses for breakthrough pain
- Common indications: postoperative pain, sickle cell pain crises, posttrauma, burns, cancer pain, before dressing changes
- In the absence of contraindications, initiate PCA using morphine; hydromorphone or fentanyl may be used in cases of morphine intolerance (nausea, vomiting) or renal impairment (Table 5.6)

LOCAL ANESTHETICS

- See Table 5.7
- Local anesthetics should be considered for all venipunctures and IV starts

SURGICAL PAIN MANAGEMENT

- See Table 5.8

Table 5.6   PCA Initiation in Opioid-Naïve Patients

Drug	Basal Rate (mcg/kg/h)	Bolus Dose (mcg/kg)	Lockout Period (min)	Maximum Dose
Morphine	10–30	10–30	6	Set max dose/2-h period as 80% of total dose in 2 h if all boluses were used
Hydromorphone	3–5	3–5	6	
Fentanyl	0.15–1	0.2–0.5	6	

From Yaster M, Krane EJ, Kaplan RF, Coté CJ, Lappe DG. *Pediatric Pain Management and Sedation Handbook.* St. Louis, Mo: Mosby; 1997:100.

Table 5.7   Local Anesthetic Dosage Guidelines

Medication	Maximum Dose	Duration After Infiltration	Route
Lidocaine plain 1% or 2%	5 mg/kg	60–120 min	SC
Lidocaine with epinephrine 1/200,000	7 mg/kg	120–360 min	SC
Bupivacaine 0.25% or 0.5% (± epinephrine 1/200,000)	2–3 mg/kg	240–480 min	SC
Topical Anesthesia			
TAC (lacerated skin): tetracaine 0.5%, adrenaline 0.05%, cocaine 11.8%	3 mL	60–360 min	Not for mucous membranes; avoid over areas of end-arterial perfusion*–risk of ischemia
EMLA (intact skin): 1-g patch contains lidocaine 25 mg, prilocaine 25 mg	2.5 g	1–2 h	Under occlusive dressing for 60 min; not for abraded skin, mucous membranes; risk of methemoglobinemia in infants and neonates
LET (lacerated skin): 1 mL contains lidocaine 40 mg, epinephrine HCl 0.5 mg, tetracaine 5 mg	3 mL	60–360 min	Not for mucous membranes; avoid over areas of end-arterial perfusion*–risk of ischemia
Tetracaine HCl (Ametop) 4% gel (intact skin)		4–6 h	Not for abraded skin; not for mucous membranes; under occlusive dressing for 30–40 min

*Areas of end-arterial perfusion: pinna, tip of nose, fingers, toes, penis.
From Yaster M, Krane EJ, Kaplan RF, Coté CJ, Lappe DG. *Pediatric Pain Management and Sedation Handbook.* St. Louis, Mo: Mosby; 1997:59–69; and from Schechter NL, Berde CB, Yaster M. *Pain in Infants, Children, and Adolescents.* Philadelphia, Pa: Lippincott Williams & Wilkins; 2002:243.

Pain and Sedation

5

Table 5.8 An Approach to Surgical Pain Management

Preoperative/Intraoperative	Postoperative Day 1-2	Transition Postoperative Day 3-4	Discharge Home
Preoperative **<4 yr:** Acetaminophen 30–40 mg/kg PR under GA (max dose 75 mg/kg/d) **>4 yr:** 1 h preoperative/on call to operating room: 1. Lidocaine (Maxilene) to back of both hands 2. Acetaminophen 15 mg/kg PO (max dose 75 mg/kg/d) **Intraoperative** For children > 2 yr: ketorolac 0.5 mg/kg IV (max 15 mg bolus) upon skin closure	**1. Acetaminophen** PO = 10–15 mg/kg q6h PR = 20 mg/kg q6h (max dose 75 mg/kg/d) + **2. Ketorolac** IV = 0.5 mg/kg q6–8h (max dose 15 mg/dose 2 mg/kg/d) + **3. IV opioid boluses** q2–4h prn **a) Morphine** 50 mcg/kg bolus (max 3 mg bolus) OR **b) Hydromorphone** 15–20 mcg/kg bolus (max 1 mg/kg bolus)	**1. Acetaminophen** + **2a. Diclofenac** PO/PR = 1 mg/kg q8–12h (max 50 mg/dose, 3 mg/kg/d) OR **2b. Ibuprofen** PO = 5–10 mg/kg q6–8h (max 40 mg/kg/d or 2400 mg) + **3. Oral opioid boluses** q3–4h Around-the-clock for first day of transition, then prn **a) Morphine** 0.15–0.3 mg/kg/dose (max 15 mg/dose) OR **b) Hydromorphone** 40–80 mcg/kg/dose OR **c) Oxycodone** 0.1–0.2 mg/kg q4–6h (max 10 mg/dose) ± **4.** IV opioid bolus as above, q2h for breakthrough or poorly controlled pain	**1. Acetaminophen** + **2a. Diclofenac** OR **2b. Ibuprofen** + **3. Oral opioid** q4–6h prn; give 1–3 weeks' supply **a) Morphine** OR **b) Hydromorphone** OR **c) Oxycodone** OR **d) Codeine** (ineffective in 10% of patients) PO = 1 mg/kg ± **4. Oral diazepam*** q6h prn; give 2–4 days' supply

Additional column notes: **b) Hydromorphone** 2–4 mg/dose if patient > 50 kg (max 4 mg/dose); **c) Oxycodone** available as Percocet (oxycodone 15 mg + acetaminophen 325 mg) NB: not to exceed acetaminophen max dose

*For muscle spasm in patients with cerebral palsy following orthopedic procedures.

© The Hospital for Sick Children, 2009. New artwork created by The Hospital for Sick Children for *The Hospital for Sick Children Handbook of Pediatrics*, 11th edition.

SEDATION

DEFINITIONS

- Minimal sedation: anxiolysis with maintenance of consciousness; often obtained from a single drug, given once, at a low dose
- Moderate sedation (formerly, *conscious sedation*): medically controlled depressed consciousness in which the patient maintains protective reflexes (swallowing, coughing, gagging), an independently patent airway, and the ability to respond appropriately to stimulation or command. Usually achieved with a combination of sedative and analgesic drugs
- Deep sedation: medically controlled depressed consciousness in which the patient *may not* maintain protective reflexes, an independent airway, or the ability to respond
- Note: Sedation is a continuum in which patients can easily progress into deeper levels of sedation

PREPARATION

- History: allergies, airway issues, medications, previous adverse reactions to anesthesia, last oral intake
- NPO: see p. 21
- Continuous saturation and cardiac monitoring
- Equipment for airway management and resuscitation: bag valve mask, ETT, O_2, suction, laryngoscope, intubation medications (see p. 16)
- Personnel: at least two qualified individuals trained in the sedation, procedure, and monitoring being used
- See Table 5.9

DISCHARGE CRITERIA

- Independent patent airway and stable cardiovascular function
- Intact protective reflexes (swallowing, coughing, gagging) and easy arousability
- Able to talk and sit unaided, if developmentally appropriate
- Adequate hydration

Table 5.9	Sedation Drugs*			
Drug	Indication	Route	Dosage	Side Effects
Chloral hydrate[†]	Sedation, immobility for nonpainful procedures, hypnosis	PO/PR	· Pediatric/infants: 80–100 mg/kg PO/PR; administer 20–45 min before procedure; may repeat with 40 mg/kg in 1 h (max 2 g/dose)	· Respiratory depression, residual sedation, paradoxical excitement, headache, GI upset, acute intermittent porphyria · Avoid in gastritis

(continued)

Table 5.9	Sedation Drugs* (continued)			
Drug	**Indication**	**Route**	**Dosage**	**Side Effects**
Barbiturates				
Pentobarbital[†]	Sedation, sleep induction, immobility for nonpainful procedures	IV	· Pediatric/infants: 2.5 mg/kg IV over 1 min (max 50 mg); if needed wait 1 min then 1.25 mg/kg IV over 30 s (max 25 mg); wait 1 min again then 1.25 mg/kg IV over 30 s (max 25 mg); wait 1 min more then give additional 1 mg/kg (max 20 mg) if required (max total dose, 4–6 mg/kg IV or 200 mg IV, whichever is less)	· Respiratory depression, hypotension, laryngospasm, paradoxical excitement, apnea *Note:* give slowly to avoid side effects
		IM/PR	· <15 kg: 6 mg/kg; >15 kg: 5 mg/kg · Administer 20–30 min before procedure (max dose IM/PR 200 mg/dose)	
Benzodiazepines[†]				
Midazolam	Sedation, anxiolytic amnesia, hypnosis, relief of muscle spasm	IV	· Pediatric/infant/neonate: 0.05 mg/kg IV; may be repeated × 1 prn (max total dose 0.15 mg/kg dose IV)	· Respiratory depression, laryngospasm, apnea, hypotension
		PO	· Pediatric/infant: <20 kg: 0.5–0.75 mg/kg PO >20 kg: 0.3–0.5 mg/kg PO · Administer 15–30 before procedure (max dose 20 mg)	
Diazepam	Relief of muscle spasm, sedation	IV	· 0.1 mg/kg; may be repeated × 1 prn (max total dose 20 mg IV)	· Ataxia, respiratory depression, laryngospasm, hypotension, blurred vision, diplopia, paradoxical excitement
		PO	· 0.2 mg/kg (max dose 20 mg) · Administer 45–60 min before procedure	

(continued)

Table 5.9 — Sedation Drugs* (continued)

Drug	Indication	Route	Dosage	Side Effects
Lorazepam[†]	Anxiolytic, sedation, hypnosis, mild amnesia	SL	· 0.05 mg/kg 30–60 min before procedure (max dose 4 mg)	· Same as diazepam
		IV	· 0.03–0.05 mg/kg (max dose 4 mg)	

*Sedation drugs may precipitate attack of acute intermittent porphyria.
†Administer cautiously in patients with hepatic, renal, or pulmonary disease.

© The Hospital for Sick Children, 2009. New artwork created by The Hospital for Sick Children for *The Hospital for Sick Children Handbook of Pediatrics*, 11th edition.

FURTHER READING

American Academy of Pediatrics Committee on Fetus and Newborn, Committee on Drugs, Section on Anesthesiology, Section on Surgery, and Canadian Paediatric Society, Fetus and Newborn Committee: Prevention and management of pain and stress in the neonate. *Pediatrics*. 2000;105:454–461.

Berde CB, Sethna NF. Analgesics for the treatment of pain in children. *N Engl J Med*. 2002;347:1094–1103.

Golianu B, Krane EJ, Galloway KS, Yaster M. Pediatric acute pain management. *Pediatr Clin North Am*. 2000;47:589–599.

USEFUL WEB SITES

Pediatric Pain Letter. Available at: http://pediatric-pain.ca/ppl/.

Position statement. Acetaminophen and ibuprofen in the management of fever and mild to moderate pain in children. Available at: www.cps.ca/english/statements/DT/dt98-01.htm.

Prevention and management of pain and stress in the neonate. Available at: http://www.cps.ca/english/statements/FN/fn07-01.htm.

Pain and Sedation

5

Chapter 6 Procedures

Clare Hutchinson
Jonathan Pirie

Chapter 6   Procedures

COMMON ABBREVIATIONS

ASIS	anterior superior iliac spine
AXR	abdominal X-ray
CSF	cerebrospinal fluid
F	French
IO	intraosseous
IVC	inferior vena cava
NG	nasogastric
LET	lidocaine, epinephrine, tetracaine
SCM	sternocleidomastoid muscle
SVC	superior vena cava
UAC	umbilical artery catheter
UVC	umbilical venous catheter

PAIN CONTROL AND ANTISEPTIC TECHNIQUE

PAIN CONTROL

* Appropriate pain control is an essential part of every procedure
* Topical anesthetic appropriate for intact skin procedures, when time allows
* 1% lidocaine SC may be used for more invasive procedures (e.g., central line placement, chest tube insertion, LP)
* Depending on invasiveness of procedure, moderate to deep sedation may be required
* Physicians must have the requisite knowledge and skills to administer more potent IV analgesics and anxiolytics

ANTISEPTIC TECHNIQUE

* Antiseptic swabs may suffice for peripheral catheter insertion, pneumothorax aspiration
* Povidone–iodine (Betadine) or other antiseptic solutions are appropriate for most procedures; sterile gown, draping, and mask may be required for more invasive procedures

VASCULAR PROCEDURES

PERIPHERAL IV CATHETERIZATION

Equipment

* Tourniquet, tape
* 16–24-gauge angiocatheter
* IV fluid setup

6

Method

- Use cephalic, median basilic, median antecubital, fifth interdigital, saphenous veins; dorsal arch of foot (Figure 6.1)
- Restrain extremity and prepare with antiseptic solution
- Apply tourniquet and squeeze limb above the site to distend veins
- Puncture skin 0.5–1 cm distal to desired site of entry to vein at an angle of 15–45°
- When blood returns, advance further by 1–2 mm; thread plastic cannula into vein while keeping needle steady
- Release tourniquet, remove needle, tape cannula into place, and attach line tubing

Figure 6.1 Sites for Peripheral Intravenous Access

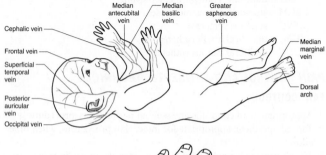

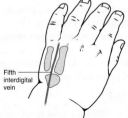

From Baldwin GA. *Handbook of Pediatric Emergencies*. 3rd ed. Philadelphia, Pa: Lippincott Williams & Wilkins; 2001:19. Reprinted by permission of Lippincot Williams and Wilkins. Available at http://lww.com

Complications

- Bleeding, infection, extravasation

SCALP IV CATHETERIZATION

Equipment

- Razor, tape
- Rubber band tourniquet
- 25–27-gauge butterfly needle
- 2-mL syringe with sterile 0.9% NaCl

Method

- Use frontal, superficial temporal, posterior auricular, occipital veins (see Figure 6.1)
- Shave selected area and cleanse with antiseptic; may apply rubber band around scalp to facilitate venous filling
- Attach syringe with 0.9% NaCl to butterfly needle and flush
- Puncture skin directly over vein at a 30° angle until blood returns, then lower angle and advance needle into vein
- Release rubber band and test patency with 0.9% NaCl infusion; tape securely

Complications

- Bleeding, infection, extravasation

INTRAOSSEOUS ACCESS

Equipment

- 18- or 20-gauge IO infusion needle, bone marrow aspiration needle, or 20-gauge spinal needle

Method

- Hold needle with stylet firmly and insert 2 cm inferior and 1 cm medial to the tibial tuberosity (Figure 6.2A)
- Insert needle at 90° angle to bony surface or angled slightly away from joint space, using "screwing" motion until through cortex (felt with a "give")
- Can also insert in lower third of femur in the midline, 1–2 cm above the external condyle (Figure 6.2B)
- Remove stylet and check access with aspiration of marrow and 0.9% NaCl flush

Complications

- Bleeding, infection, extravasation
- Risk of dislodging easily (if not fixed securely) with resulting subcutaneous infusion
- Osteomyelitis and subcutaneous abscess; epiphyseal damage; fat embolism

EXTERNAL JUGULAR CATHETERIZATION

Equipment

- Central line kit or angiocatheter setup, 0.9% NaCl
- IV line and fluid
- 2-0 suture, sterile dressing

Figure 6.2 Intraosseous Infusion

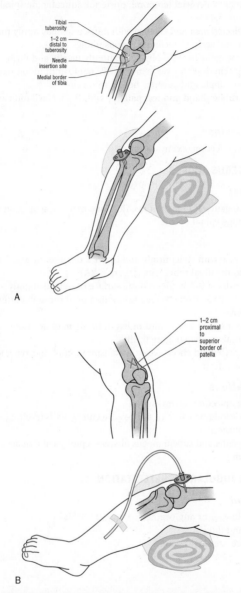

Tibial tuberosity

1–2 cm distal to tuberosity

Needle insertion site

Medial border of tibia

A

1–2 cm proximal to superior border of patella

B

Adapted from Henretig FM, King C, eds. *Textbook of Pediatric Emergency Procedures*. Baltimore, Md: Williams & Wilkins; 1997:292, 294. Reprinted by permission of Lippincot Williams and Wilkins. Available at http://lww.com

Method

- Place patient in 15–30° Trendelenburg position (roll under shoulder helpful)
- Insert needle caudally (toward the feet) in vein over SCM (Figure 6.3)
- When blood returns to hub, advance cannula, remove needle, and attach infusion
- Secure cannula with suture; apply sterile dressing

Complications

- Bleeding, infection, extravasation
- Pleural puncture

INTERNAL JUGULAR CATHETERIZATION

Equipment

- Central line kit (3–5F Cook catheter, metal needle, blade, guidewire, infusion catheter)
- 5-mL syringe, IV line and fluid
- 2-0 suture, sterile dressing

Method (Seldinger)

- Sterile preparation; roll under shoulder, head to left
- Right side is preferred because course of SVC is straight, left dome of lung is higher, thoracic duct is on the left

Figure 6.3 Internal and External Jugular Vein Cannulation

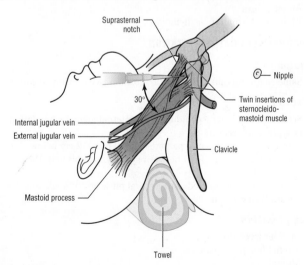

Suprasternal notch

Nipple

30°

Twin insertions of sternocleido-mastoid muscle

Internal jugular vein

External jugular vein

Clavicle

Mastoid process

Towel

Adapted from Levin DL, Morris FC, eds. *Essentials of Pediatric Intensive Care*. St. Louis, Mo: Quality Medical Publishing; 1990:807–809.

Procedures

6

- Imagine straight line between mastoid process and suprasternal notch; insert needle at midpoint of this line, aimed toward the ipsilateral nipple (see Figure 6.3)
- In older children, a triangle is formed by middle third of the clavicle and the two bellies of SCM; vein lies under lateral border of medial belly of SCM
- Insert needle at 30° angle toward ipsilateral nipple while aspirating with attached syringe
- When blood returns, advance 1–2 mm farther; steady needle with one hand; expect venous flow; cover hub with finger to prevent blood loss
- Insert guidewire through needle several centimeters past needle tip; if it does not advance easily, remove wire, resite needle to ensure flow, then replace wire
- Remove needle while ensuring guidewire is in place; keep pressure on vein to limit blood loss
- Use blade to make a small nick at entry site, then thread dilator over wire, puncture skin, and remove dilator
- Thread flushed catheter over wire in a twisting motion and remove wire
- Check for adequate flow through catheter lumen; attach infusion setup
- Secure cannula with suture; apply sterile dressing

Complications

- Venous laceration
- Arterial line placement
- Pneumothorax, hemothorax
- Air embolism
- Right atrial irritation, arrhythmias

FEMORAL VEIN CATHETERIZATION

Equipment

- Same as for internal jugular catheterization (see previous section)

Method

- Setup and Seldinger technique as per internal jugular cannulation (see previous section)
- Externally rotate hips and palpate femoral pulse, 2 cm below inguinal ligament, halfway between symphysis pubis and ASIS (Figure 6.4)
- Insert needle 0.5 cm medial to femoral pulse at 30° angle directed toward the umbilicus

Complications

- Vascular laceration
- Arterial line placement
- Air embolism

Figure 6.4 **Femoral Vein Cannulation**

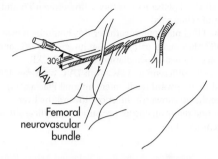

NAV, nerve, artery, vein.
Adapted from Levin DL, Morris FC, eds. *Essentials of Pediatric Intensive Care*. St. Louis, Mo: Quality Medical Publishing; 1990:809.

- Bowel perforation
- Infection (including osteomyelitis)
- Avascular necrosis of hip

UV AND UA CATHETERIZATION

Equipment

- 5F UVC, 3.5F UAC, insertion kit, 3-way stopcock, 0.9% NaCl
- Smaller-size catheters may be required for premature infants (see p. 105)

Method

- Tie a loose knot with umbilical tie at base of stump, for hemostasis
- Cut stump with clean stroke of scalpel to within 2 cm of stump base (Figure 6.5A)
- Evert edges of stump with mosquito forceps (Figure 6.5B)
- Identify two arteries and one thin-walled larger vein
- Gently use dilator to open vessels if needed, especially arteries (see Figure 6.5B)
- Attach catheter and 5-mL syringe to 3-way stopcock; prime setup with 0.9% NaCl
- Use "shoulder-umbilical" graph to estimate catheter insertion length (Figures 6.6 and 6.7)
- Use forceps to gently put traction on cord, and insert catheter into vessel to desired distance
- If catheter does not insert easily, suspect false tract and check for blood flow by aspirating
- Once easy blood return is confirmed at the desired insertion depth, secure the catheter with suture to cord, and secure with "bridge-tape" support (Figure 6.5C)

Procedures

6

- Confirm position with two views CXR and AXR
  - High UAC placement: catheter tip between T6 and T9 (above origin of celiac axis)
  - Low UAC placement: catheter tip should be between L3 and L5
  - UVC placement: catheter tip at junction of IVC and right atrium, projecting just above diaphragm on AP CXR
  - Note: To differentiate UAC from UVC on X-ray: UAC turns down and then upward (as it enters internal iliac artery); UVC takes only a cephalad (upward) direction, toward the liver
- With line removal, ensure pressure at umbilical site for 3–5 min to prevent bleeding

Figure 6.5 Insertion of Umbilical Vein and Artery Catheters

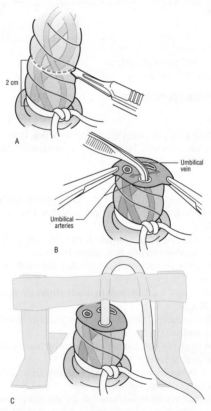

Adapted from Fleisher GR, Ludwig S, eds. *Textbook of Pediatric Emergency Medicine*. Philadelphia, Pa: Lippincott Williams & Wilkins; 2000:1804. Reprinted by permission of Lippincot Williams and Wilkins. Available at http://lww.com

Figure 6.6 Umbilical Vein Catheter Insertion Length

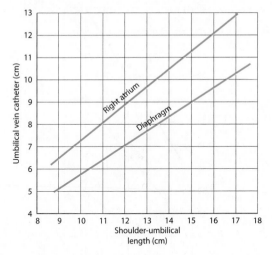

Adapted from Dunn PM. Localization of the umbilical catheter by post-mortem measurement. *Arch Dis Child.* 1966;41:70–71; adapted and reproduced with permission from the BMJ Publishing Group.

Complications

* Infection
* Thrombosis
* Ischemia of lower limbs with arterial spasm or stenosis
* Necrotizing enterocolitis
* Air embolus
* Massive bleeding with dislodgement

RADIAL ARTERY ACCESS

Equipment

* 20–24-gauge angiocatheter
* 23–25-gauge butterfly needle with 1–3-mL syringe for single sampling
* Heparinized infusion setup, if indwelling catheter

Method

* Feel for pulse at radial, dorsalis pedis, or posterior tibial arteries
* For radial insertion, hyperextend and immobilize the wrist
* If radial placement, ensure ulnar flow with Allen test:
    * Elevate fisted hand for 30 s, apply pressure to occlude both radial and ulnar arteries, open hand, release ulnar pressure, color should return within 7 s

Figure 6.7 Umbilical Artery Catheter Insertion Length

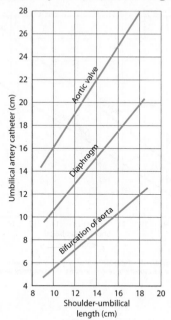

Adapted from Dunn PM. Localization of the umbilical catheter by post-mortem measurement. *Arch Dis Child.* 1966;41:72–73; adapted and reproduced with permission from the BMJ Publishing Group.

- Clean area, and insert needle at 30° angle, bevel up
- With blood return, advance 1–2 mm
- If blood return ceases or slows, distal wall of the artery may have been punctured (Figure 6.8A)
- If this occurs, pull back very slowly until flashback is seen again (Figure 6.8B)
- Advance catheter with twisting motion; remove needle and ensure arterial flow
- Attach heparinized infusion; secure with tape or operation-site dressing
- For sampling only, may use butterfly needle, aspirating syringe to assist blood return
- Ensure compression of vessel for 3–5 min after removal

Complications

- Infection, bleeding
- Arterial spasm
- Distal ischemia

Figure 6.8 Insertion of a Radial Arterial Catheter

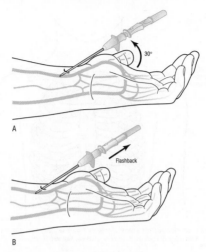

Adapted from Fleisher GR, Ludwig S, eds. *Textbook of Pediatric Emergency Medicine*. Philadelphia, Pa: Lippincott Williams & Wilkins; 2000:1806. Reprinted by permission of Lippincot Williams and Wilkins. Available at http://lww.com

CARDIORESPIRATORY PROCEDURES

NEEDLE ASPIRATION OF PNEUMOTHORAX

Equipment
- 14–16-gauge angiocatheter
- 3-way stopcock; 5–10-mL syringe

Method
- In emergent tension pneumothorax, insert angiocatheter in midclavicular line at second intercostal space (Figure 6.9)
- Remove stylet; should be rush of air
- Can attach 3-way stopcock to syringe to keep closed system until chest tube inserted, but watch for signs of reaccumulation of air
- CXR to look for resolution of pneumothorax

Complications
- Pneumomediastinum
- Bleeding

THORACENTESIS

Equipment
- 18-gauge needle, 3-way stopcock, 20-mL syringe

Figure 6.9 Needle Aspiration of Tension Pneumothorax

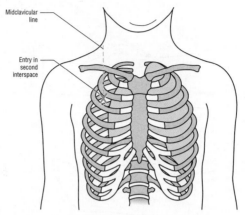

From Henretig FM, King C, eds. *Textbook of Pediatric Emergency Procedures.* Baltimore, Md: Williams & Wilkins; 1997:395. Reprinted by permission of Lippincot Williams and Wilkins. Available at http://lww.com

Method
- Patient should be placed in sitting position, back toward the person performing the procedure, head and neck supported (Figure 6.10A)
- Insert needle along posterior axillary line at sixth or seventh rib interspace, following superior aspect of rib (Figure 6.10B)
- Aspirate small aliquots of fluid (up to 50 mL) slowly to prevent cardiovascular decompensation
- CXR postprocedure to look for iatrogenic pneumothorax, remaining fluid

Complications
- Bleeding
- Pneumothorax
- Infection

CHEST TUBE INSERTION

Equipment
- Chest tube insertion kit, chest tube (Table 6.1)
- Scalpel, hemostat, Kelly forceps, 2-0 suture, Pleur-evac (underwater seal)

Method
- Landmark fifth interspace between the anterior and midaxillary line; site adjusted according to intrapleural fluid level (Figure 6.11)
- Infiltrate skin with lidocaine; make 1–2-cm incision through skin with scalpel

Figure 6.10 Thoracentesis

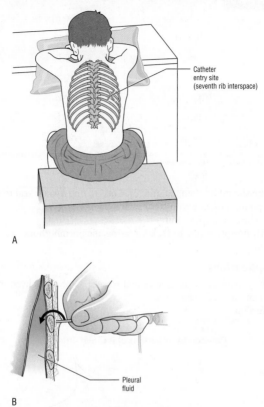

Catheter entry site (seventh rib interspace)

A

Pleural fluid

B

- Dissect underlying tissue and intercostal muscle bluntly with curved forceps along superior aspect of rib until penetration of pleura
- Use forceps to grip distal tip of chest tube and guide through pleural opening
- Alternately, can use Seldinger technique with needle insertion along superior edge of rib until release of pleural fluid; thread guidewire through lumen and remove needle, use dilator over guidewire to widen opening and remove, then thread chest drain over guidewire into chest and remove wire
- Advance tube 4–10 cm, depending on size of child or until fluid/ condensation appears in tube

Procedures

6

Table 6.1	Chest Tube Sizes by Age	
Age	**Size (F)**	
Newborn	10–12	
6 mo	10–12	
1 yr	16–20	
4 yr	20–28	
10 yr	28–32	
>14 yr	28–32	

From Fleisher GR, Ludwig S, eds. *Textbook of Pediatric Emergency Medicine*. Philadelphia, Pa: Lippincott Williams & Wilkins; 2000:1839. Reproduced with permission.

- Tube should be clamped until attached to underwater seal to prevent inspiration of air into pleural cavity
- Fix chest tube with suture
- CXR postprocedure to look for iatrogenic pneumothorax, remaining fluid

Complications

- Injury to lungs, heart, mediastinal vessels, diaphragm, liver, spleen
- Pneumothorax, hemothorax
- Infection

6

Figure 6.11 Position for Insertion of a Chest Tube

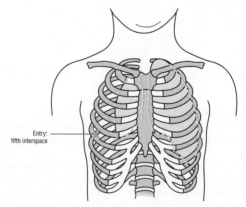

Entry:
fifth interspace

Adapted from Fleisher GR, Ludwig S, eds. *Textbook of Pediatric Emergency Medicine*. Philadelphia, Pa: Lippincott Williams & Wilkins; 2000:1838. Reprinted by permission of Lippincot Williams and Wilkins. Available at http://lww.com

PERICARDIOCENTESIS

Equipment
- Continuous ECG monitoring
- 20-gauge 2.5-inch spinal needle
- 3-way stopcock with 50-mL syringe

Method
- Patient should be supine; head of the bed elevated to 30–45°
- Localize area just below xiphoid process; sterilize and place sterile drapes
- Anesthetize area with topical anesthetic and injection of local anesthetic
- Insert spinal needle at angle of 60–70° relative to abdomen, pointing toward the left shoulder (Figure 6.12)
- Advance slowly, aspirating gently
- A "pop" may be felt on entry of the pericardial sack
- If epicardium is touched, may cause dysrhythmias on ECG monitoring
- Once fluid is drained, remove needle, and apply sterile dressing
- CXR postprocedure to look for iatrogenic pneumothorax, hemothorax

Figure 6.12 **Pericardiocentesis**

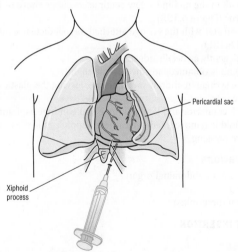

Xiphoid process

Pericardial sac

Adapted from Fleisher GR, Ludwig S, eds. *Textbook of Pediatric Emergency Medicine*. Philadelphia, Pa: Lippincott Williams & Wilkins; 2000:1844. Reprinted by permission of Lippincot Williams and Wilkins. Available at http://lww.com

Procedures

6

Complications

- Arrhythmia
- Cardiac trauma (injury to coronary arteries, puncture of cardiac chambers)
- Pneumothorax
- Hemothorax
- Diaphragmatic perforation

GASTROINTESTINAL PROCEDURES

PERITONEAL TAP

Equipment

- 18–22-gauge over-the-needle catheter
- 20-mL syringe; 50–100-mL syringe; T connector

Method

- Patient should be placed either sitting or in a lateral decubitus position (Figure 6.13A and C)
- Sterilize the area and place sterile drapes
- Anesthetize area with topical anesthetic and injection of local anesthetic
- Landmark in the midline, a few centimeters either above or below umbilicus (Figure 6.13B)
- Insert catheter with the syringe attached, perpendicular to abdomen (Figure 6.13D)
- Aspirate gently as needle advances
- Once fluid is obtained, advance needle slightly
- Remove syringe; withdraw metal needle, leaving the plastic catheter in place
- Attach T connector and larger syringe and continue aspirating fluid
- Once fluid is removed, remove catheter; apply sterile dressing and pressure dressing

Complications

- Perforation of abdominal organ
- Bleeding
- Infection (peritonitis)

NG TUBE INSERTION

Equipment

- 8–12F NG tube, lubricant

Method

- Estimate length of insertion by measuring distance from nose to ear to stomach, and mark on tube
- Lubricate tip and insert through either nostril; use oral route if suspicion of facial injury, skull fracture, or dysmorphic facies

Figure 6.13 Peritoneal Tap

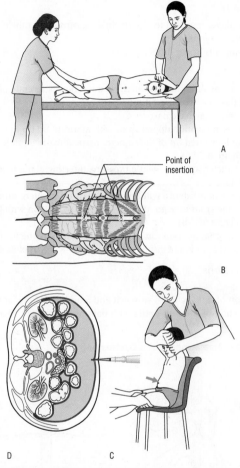

Point of insertion

A

B

D   C

From Fleisher GR, Ludwig S, eds. *Textbook of Pediatric Emergency Medicine*. Philadelphia, Pa: Lippincott Williams & Wilkins; 2000:1848. Reprinted by permission of Lippincot Williams and Wilkins. Available at http://lww.com

- Watch for coiling in pharynx; if older, ask patient to swallow during insertion
- While listening with stethoscope over stomach, rapidly instill 5 mL of air through tube; should hear "pop" if adequate insertion into stomach

Complications

- Intracranial, esophageal, or bronchial insertion
- Perforation, bleeding

REPLACEMENT OF A GASTROSTOMY TUBE

Equipment

- Foley catheter matched to size of child's gastrostomy tube (G-tube)
- 0.9% NaCl, syringes
- Lubricant, absorbent dressing, tape

Method

- Replacement should not be attempted if tube has recently been placed (last few weeks) or if tube has been out of place for more than 4–6 h (tract may have narrowed)
- Gently insert a cotton-tipped swab with lubricant on tip to assess tract
- Position lubricated tip of the catheter perpendicular to abdominal wall (Figure 6.14A)
- Insert catheter, applying gentle pressure, directing along previously assessed tract
- A decrease in resistance will be felt once catheter enters stomach
- Insert catheter far enough to allow inflation of balloon with 0.9% NaCl (Figure 6.14B)
- Ensure appropriate position by aspirating stomach contents through catheter, with option of instilling 30 mL of 0.9% NaCl before aspirating

Complications

- Bleeding
- Insertion of tube between stomach and anterior abdominal wall
- Obstruction of stomach outlet with balloon of newly replaced tube

Figure 6.14 Replacement of a Gastrostomy Tube

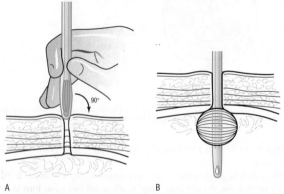

A   B

Adapted from Fleisher GR, Ludwig S, eds. *Textbook of Pediatric Emergency Medicine*. Philadelphia, Pa: Lippincott Williams & Wilkins; 2000:1852. Reprinted by permission of Lippincot Williams and Wilkins. Available at http://lww.com

GENITOURINARY PROCEDURES

BLADDER CATHETERIZATION

Equipment
- Sterile Foley catheter set (Table 6.2)
- Lubricant, sterile water
- For intermittent catheterization, use a feeding tube of appropriate diameter up to the age of 7 yr; after 7 yr, use a disposable urinary catheter of appropriate diameter

Table 6.2	Urinary Catheter Sizes	
Age (yr)	Intermittent Catheterization	Indwelling Catheters
0-5	3.5-5F feeding tube	3.5-5F feeding tube
5-7	5F feeding tube	5F feeding tube
7-10	8-10F Foley disposable urinary catheter	8-10F Foley (Silastic)
10-14	10F Foley disposable urinary catheter	10F Foley (Silastic)
>14	12-14F Foley disposable urinary catheter	10-14F Foley (Silastic)

Method
- Separate labia to visualize urethra under clitoral hood in females (Figure 6.15A); extend penis in males
- Swab area with antiseptic; drape sterile towel above and below
- Lubricate catheter, apply traction to surrounding skin, and introduce catheter into urethral meatus (Figure 6.15B)
- Advance until urine returns; inflate balloon with 3–5 mL of sterile water, pull back gently to ensure that inflated balloon stays in bladder (Figure 6.15C)
- Attach outlet to sterile closed system or remove if not indwelling

Complications
- Trauma, bleeding, perforation
- Infection
- Urethral stenosis

SUPRAPUBIC BLADDER ASPIRATION

Equipment
- 23–25-gauge butterfly or needle (2–3 cm)
- 3–5-mL syringe

Figure 6.15 Insertion of a Foley Catheter

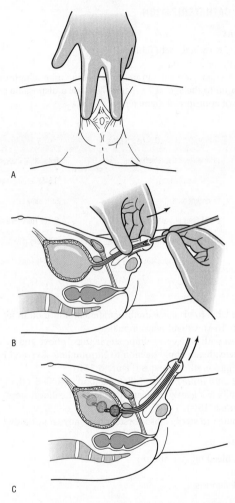

A

B

C

Adapted from Fleisher GR, Ludwig S, eds. *Textbook of Pediatric Emergency Medicine*. Philadelphia, Pa: Lippincott Williams & Wilkins; 2000:1856. Reprinted by permission of Lippincot Williams and Wilkins. Available at http://lww.com

Method

- Most appropriate in children < 2 yr
- Place infant in frogleg position (Figure 6.16A) and clean area 1–2 cm (1 finger's breadth) above symphysis pubis in midline where a transverse abdominal crease is usually present

- Advance needle at 10–20° angle from perpendicular to abdominal wall, aiming toward the head while gently aspirating (Figure 6.16B)
- Stop advancing needle once urine returns; attach syringe and aspirate

Complications
- Bleeding
- Infection
- Bowel penetration

Figure 6.16 **Suprapubic Bladder Aspiration**

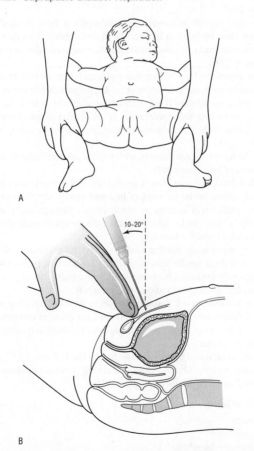

A

10–20°

B

Procedures

6

CENTRAL NERVOUS SYSTEM PROCEDURES

LUMBAR PUNCTURE

Equipment

- Infant (22–24-gauge short) or child (22-gauge long) LP kit including needle with stylet, CSF specimen tubes
- Manometer, 3-way stopcock

Method

- Ensure no head injury or evidence of raised intracranial pressure (see p. 38)
- Place child on side in lateral decubitus position; have assistant restrain child by holding feet and head and curving the spine to achieve maximum flexion; ensure back is perpendicular to bed (Figure 6.17A)
- Locate superior edges of both iliac crests and draw an imaginary line between them to intersect spine at L_4–L_5; palpate this or the next intervertebral space upward (L_3–L_4); insertion of needle in L_3–L_4 or L_4–L_5 disk space ensures that needle entry is below level of spinal cord
- With sterile technique, cleanse skin with antiseptic solution; use sterile drapes
- Anesthetize area appropriately with topical anesthetic patch and injection of local anesthetic
- Confirm landmarks and insert needle and stylet slowly with bevel up, angled perpendicular to plane of bed and toward direction of umbilicus; resistance will increase as needle passes through fascia; will then be a slight "pop" and a "give" when needle passes through dura (not always felt in small infants)
- Remove stylet while holding needle steady and check for CSF; if none, withdraw needle slowly, checking for fluid, or reinsert stylet and advance further; if hit bone, withdraw needle carefully to just below skin surface and redirect angle slightly
- Attach 3-way stopcock and manometer to measure opening pressure
- Let CSF drain into sterile tubes and send for relevant investigations (e.g., Gram stain/culture, protein/glucose, virology, cell count—usually last tube)
- Remove needle and apply pressure to site for 1–2 min
- May also perform LP with child in a sitting position; landmarks are same as just described (Figure 6.17B)

Complications

- Headache
- Epidermal cyst
- CSF leakage; bleeding
- Infection
- Brainstem herniation

Figure 6.17 **Lumbar Puncture**

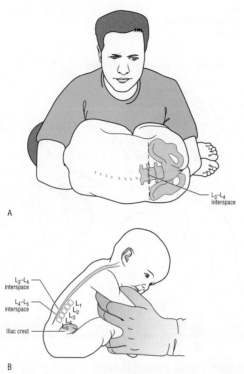

A

B

Adapted from King C, Henretig FM. *Pocket Atlas of Pediatric Emergency Procedures.* Philadelphia, Pa: Lippincott Williams & Wilkins; 2000:125. Reprinted by permission of Lippincot Williams and Wilkins. Available at http://lww.com

VENTRICULOPERITONEAL SHUNT TAP

Equipment

- 23–25-gauge butterfly needle
- Sterile collection tubes
- Manometer, 3-way stopcock
- Razor blade

Method

- Locate shunt reservoir on child's head (Figure 6.18A)
- Shave hair around reservoir and pump
- Insert butterfly needle into reservoir (Figure 6.18B)
- Brisk flow of CSF may indicate distal blockage of shunt; use sterile collection tubes
- Attach manometer, if pressure measurement indicated

Complications

- Bleeding
- Introduction of infection
- CSF leakage

Figure 6.18 **Ventriculoperitoneal Shunt Tap**

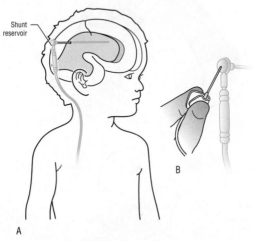

Adapted from Fleisher GR, Ludwig S, eds. *Textbook of Pediatric Emergency Medicine*. Philadelphia, Pa: Lippincott Williams & Wilkins; 2000:1816. Reprinted by permission of Lippincot Williams and Wilkins. Available at http://lww.com

MUSCULOSKELETAL PROCEDURES

ARTHROCENTESIS

Equipment

- 20-gauge needle with 10-mL syringe
- EDTA tube for cell count; sterile tube for Gram stain/culture; plain blood tube for protein, glucose

Method

- Clean area and anesthetize with topical anesthetic and injection of local anesthetic
- Restrain child if necessary and have assistant hold joint stable
- Insert 20-gauge needle and aspirate fluid
- Knee: aspirate from lateral side by flexing knee slightly and directing needle downward at a 10–20° angle beneath middle of patella (Figure 6.19A)

- Elbow: aspirate from lateral side by flexing elbow at 90° angle and directing needle into triangle formed by head of radius, lateral epicondyle, and olecranon
- Ankle: aspirate from anteromedial aspect, with ankle at 90°; direct needle between anterior tibialis tendon and medial malleolus (Figure 6.19B)
- Shoulder: aspirate from anterolateral aspect with arm hanging externally rotated, and direct needle below and lateral to coracoid process
- Assess for yellow/red color, cloudy disposition; place in designated tubes

Figure 6.19 Arthrocentesis of the Knee and Ankle

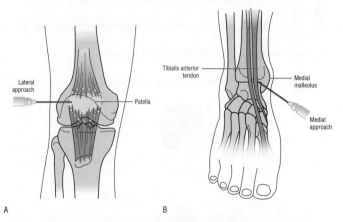

A   B

Adapted from Fleisher GR, Ludwig S, eds. *Textbook of Pediatric Emergency Medicine*. Philadelphia, Pa: Lippincott Williams & Wilkins; 2000:1872. Reprinted by permission of Lippincot Williams and Wilkins. Available at http://lww.com

Complications
- Infection
- Bleeding
- Epiphyseal damage

SPLINTING

Equipment
- Bucket of water at room temperature; stocking, cotton padding, gauze, "cling" or flannel wrap
- Sedation and analgesia preparations, as needed (see Chapter 5)

Method

- Determine type of splint:
  1. "Long arm posterior splint" for elbow, forearm (Figure 6.20A)
  2. "Posterior ankle splint" for distal fibula, ankle, foot (Figure 6.20B)
- Measure and cut plaster to appropriate length, ensuring coverage of joints above and below injury while maintaining mobility of fingers or toes
- Upper extremity splints require 8–10 layers; lower extremity splints require 12–15 layers
- Use stockinette that will extend slightly farther than splint so that it can fold back over ends of plaster
- Wrap circumferentially with cotton; overlap each turn by 50%, adding extra padding at bony prominences
- Keep joints in neutral positions (e.g., elbow at 90°, wrist in slight dorsiflexion)
- Immerse plaster, squeeze out extra water, and mold slab into place, avoiding wrinkles
- Wrap with cling or flannel wrap to hold in place

Figure 6.20 Long Arm Posterior Splint and Posterior Ankle Splint

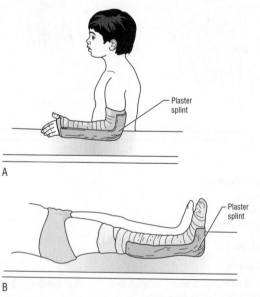

Adapted from Fleisher GR, Ludwig S, eds. *Textbook of Pediatric Emergency Medicine*. Philadelphia, Pa: Lippincott Williams & Wilkins; 2000:1886. Reprinted by permission of Lippincot Williams and Wilkins. Available at http://lww.com

Complications
- Pressure sores, dermatitis
- Neurovascular compromise

SIMPLE LACERATION REPAIR

GLUING

Equipment
- Tissue adhesive (e.g., 2-octylcyanoacrylate [Dermabond])
- Topical anesthetic (e.g., lidocaine eutectic mixture [LET])

Method
- Indications
  - For repair of superficial lacerations <4 cm length and <0.5 cm width
  - Should only be used in clean wound in which edges can easily be approximated
  - Should not be used in wounds in which dehiscence is likely to occur (near a joint), on scalp, eyebrow, eyelid, or crossing mucocutaneous junctions
- After cleaning, wound should be dried and hemostasis attained
- LET topical anesthetic may be used for pain control; will also aid in vascular constriction and hemostasis; apply 20–30 min before procedure (see Table 5.7, p. 81)
- Appose wound edges with slight eversion, using forceps or fingers
- Apply thin layer of tissue adhesive over wound edges, holding wound in apposition for 30-60 s to allow polymerization
- Repeat this maneuver 2–3 times to allow optimal wound closure, holding wound in apposition for 2–3 min after final application

Complications
- Wound dehiscence
- Adhesion of materials used for preprocedure cleaning (e.g., gauze) to glued wound

SUTURING

Equipment
- Nonabsorbable suture for superficial laceration repair; size depends on location of repair
- Absorbable synthetic suture for deeper repair
- Needle, depending on operator preference and depth of wound
- Sterile gauze dressing
- Antibiotic ointment

Method

- Preparation of wound should include cleansing area with povidone–iodine solution, irrigation of wound with 0.9NaCl
- Ensure edges of wound can be approximated with good alignment
- Edges should be everted to avoid depressed scar once healed
- Simple interrupted stitches may be used to repair superficial skin wounds, with knots placed to side to avoid irritation and inflammation of wound
- Other techniques such as vertical and horizontal mattress stitches are used for deeper, more complex wounds and should be reserved for those with adequate training and experience
- Simple skin lacerations should be dressed with sterile gauze and anti-bacterial ointment
- Tetanus prophylaxis, as appropriate
- Removal of nonabsorbable sutures is dependent on location of wound (Table 6.3)

Complications

- Wound infection
- Wound dehiscence

Table 6.3	Timely Suture Removal
Wound Location	**Time of Removal (days)**
Neck	3–4
Face, scalp	5
Upper extremities, trunk	7–10
Lower extremities	8–10
Joint surface	10–14

From Fleisher GR, Ludwig S, eds. *Textbook of Pediatric Emergency Medicine.* Philadelphia, Pa: Lippincott Williams & Wilkins; 2000:1490. Reprinted by permission of Lippincot Williams and Wilkins. Available at http://lww.com

INCISION AND DRAINAGE

ABSCESS

Equipment

- Scalpel, No. 15 blade, mosquito clamp, syringe with 18-gauge needle
- 0.9% NaCl, packing/gauze

Method

- Should not be attempted for very large abscesses, deep abscesses in sensitive areas (e.g., perirectal), or abscesses in nasolabial folds or palmar or deep plantar spaces
- Anesthetize area with application of topical anesthetic and injection of local anesthetic
- Define area of maximum fluctuation; can try aspirating with 18-gauge needle
- Make crosslike incision with scalpel to make diamond-shaped opening
- With mosquito clamp, dissect loculations to release fluid
- Irrigate with 0.9% NaCl and pack with soaked gauze

Complications

- Bleeding
- Scarring
- Nerve or vessel damage

FURTHER READING

King C, Henretig FM. *Pocket Atlas of Pediatric Emergency Procedures.* Philadelphia, Pa: Lippincott Williams & Wilkins; 2000.
Roberts JR, Hedges JR. *Clinical Procedures in Emergency Medicine.* 3rd ed. Philadelphia, Pa: WB Saunders; 1998.

Procedures

6

Section II Subspecialty Pediatrics

Chapter 7 Adolescent Medicine

Ellie Vyver
Miriam Kaufman

Chapter 7   Adolescent Medicine

COMMON ABBREVIATIONS

AN	anorexia nervosa
BMI	body mass index
BN	bulimia nervosa
CBC	complete blood cell count
CVS	cardiovascular system
ED-NOS	eating disorder not otherwise specified
ESR	erythrocyte sedimentation rate
FSH	follicle-stimulating hormone
FTT	failure to thrive
LFT	liver function test
LH	luteinizing hormone
T_4	thyroxine
TSH	thyroid-stimulating hormone

INTERVIEWING THE ADOLESCENT

* HEADS framework for interviewing (Table 7.1)
* Take usual medical and detailed psychosocial history
* Interview alone; quiet and private setting, if possible
* Nonjudgmental and nonlabeling approach; avoid assumptions
* Ensure confidentiality but state limits up front (e.g., will not keep confidential information about suicidal intent, major self-harm, plan to harm others; if younger than 16 yr, abuse is reportable)
* Check one's own feelings, attitudes, and potential biases

EATING DISORDERS

* Often do not fall into traditional classification → high index of suspicion
* Incidence and prevalence increasing among adolescents and children <12 yr
* Differential diagnosis: AN, BN, ED-NOS, food avoidant emotional disorder, organic causes of weight loss, other psychiatric disorders
* High morbidity: all body systems affected; consequences on brain development, bone acquisition, growth may be irreversible
* Higher mortality than other psychiatric illnesses; death in up to 20% from suicide or medical complications (e.g., adverse cardiac event, renal failure)
* Impaired quality of life: social isolation, comorbid anxiety and mood disorders, failure to complete postsecondary education, unemployment
* Early intervention is key to a favorable prognosis

Table 7.1		HEADS Interview
H	Home	Living situation, relationships with parents, siblings, family support, stresses and responsibilities, independence
E	Education/employment	Present, past, and changes in school performance, career goals, likes/dislikes, connectedness to school, details of employment, including safety, number of h/wk
	Eating	Attitudes about body size and shape, changes in weight, dieting, views on "healthy eating," exercise, weight control strategies
A	Activities	Hobbies/interests, friends, sports, clubs or other groups
	Adherence/compliance	With medications, treatments, therapies
D	Drugs	Smoking, alcohol, caffeine, over-the-counter, prescription, herbal and street drugs; ask about friends, family use first, then ask about the teen's use; if history is positive for use, consider CRAFFT screen (see Table 7.3)
S	Sexuality	Sexual activity, birth control, condom use, sexually transmitted infections, sexual orientation; ask about friends first, then about the teen; elicit what adolescent means by sexual activity
	Suicide/depression	Mood, "boredom," appetite, sleep, loss of interest, thoughts/attempts of suicide/self-harm
	Safety	Home and school violence, bullying, sexual abuse/date rape, seat belts, safety equipment for sports or activities

AN

- Refusal to maintain body weight consistent with health for gender, age, and height (i.e., maintenance of body weight <85% of expected)
- In children and adolescents: failure to gain expected weight and/or height
- Intense fear of gaining weight or becoming fat
- Distorted body image
- Postmenarchal amenorrhea (absence of at least three consecutive menstrual periods or occurring only after hormone administration [e.g., estrogen, birth control pill])
- Restricting subtype (no regular binge eating or purging behavior) or binge/purge subtype

BN

- Recurrent episodes of binge eating: consuming large amount in short period of time; feeling out of control during episodes
- Recurrent inappropriate compensatory behavior to prevent weight gain (e.g., self-induced vomiting; misuse of laxatives, diuretics, enemas, or other medications; fasting; excessive exercise)
- Overly influenced by body weight and shape; weight often within normal limits

APPROACH TO EATING DISORDERS

- See Table 7.2 for comparison of clinical and laboratory findings in AN and BN

Table 7.2	Comparison of Typical Clinical Features and Laboratory Findings in Anorexia Nervosa and Bulimia Nervosa	
Features	**Anorexia Nervosa**	**Bulimia Nervosa**
General examination	Hypothermia and cold extremities, dry skin, lanugo, carotenemia, alopecia	Eroded tooth enamel (posterior aspect upper teeth), Russell's sign (callus on knuckles), subconjunctival hemorrhages, parotid enlargement
GI	Slowed gastric emptying, constipation, hyper-cholesterolemia, increased liver enzymes	Esophagitis, gastric dilatation, rarely rupture, Mallory-Weiss tears, vocal cord dysfunction
CVS	Sinus bradycardia, arrhythmias, hypotension, low-voltage ECG with flattened or inverted T waves, prolonged Q-Tc interval, pericardial effusion, poor peripheral perfusion, edema, cardiac muscle atrophy, mitral valve prolapse	Cardiomyopathy (suspect ipecac poisoning), prolonged Q-Tc interval, edema
Endocrine	Amenorrhea, growth delay/failure, delayed puberty, hypercortisolemia, sick euthyroid syndrome, partial DI, failure to acquire peak bone mass	Irregular menses
Metabolic	Dehydration with $\uparrow Na^+$, $\downarrow Na^+$ from $\uparrow H_2O$ intake, tubular necrosis, $\downarrow$ renal function, hypophosphatemia, $\downarrow K^+$, hypoglycemia, $\downarrow Ca^{2+}$, $\downarrow Mg^{2+}$	Hypochloremic hypokalemic metabolic alkalosis if vomiting; hyperchloremic metabolic acidosis if laxative abuse; $\uparrow$ amylase; $\uparrow Na^+$ secondary to dehydration
Hematologic	B_{12} and folate deficiency, vitamin K deficiency, coagulopathy, pancytopenia, $\downarrow$ ESR	
Neurologic	Structural brain changes, atrophy in severe cases, seizure, syncope, poor concentration	

Note: Features of AN and BN often overlap.

Adolescent Medicine

7

History

- Is weight loss a result of decreased intake vs. output? Has it been voluntary?
- Weight history—highest and lowest weights, time of greatest weight loss, social environment just before and at start of weight loss, attitudes about size and shape

- Plot weight and height on growth curve; previous weight curve is most predictive of ideal body weight; BMI and weight for height are less useful
- Dietary history: food choices and portion size; history of uncontrolled eating, purging, and exercise (types and frequency); diet aids, laxative use, smoking/drug use
- Menstrual history: age at menarche, regularity of menstruation, weight at time of last normal menstrual period
- Review of systems: fever, night sweats, arthralgia, rashes, abdominal pain, hematemesis, chest pain, dyspnea, palpitations, alopecia, cold intolerance, constipation
- Psychiatric and social/family history

Physical Examination

- Vital signs: orthostatic changes in HR and BP (taken after lying down for 2 min followed by standing for 2 min), temperature
- Complete physical examination, paying particular attention to features in Table 7.2

Initial Workup

- CBC and differential, electrolytes, bicarbonate, Ca^{2+}, Mg^{2+}, PO_4^-, glucose, urea, creatinine, amylase, albumin, liver enzymes, coagulation profile, bilirubin, ESR
- TSH and free T_4, FSH, LH, estradiol, prolactin
- 12-lead ECG
- Urinalysis, particularly for specific gravity, hematuria/proteinuria
- Consider other investigations to rule out organic causes of weight loss

Indications for Hospitalization

- Significant bradycardia (daytime HR <50; nighttime HR <45) or hypotension
- Significant orthostatic changes ($\downarrow$ in systolic BP >20 mm Hg, $\uparrow$ in HR >35 beats/min)
- Arrhythmias, including prolonged Q-Tc interval
- Dehydration
- Electrolyte or acid–base abnormalities
- Absolute weight <75–80% ideal body weight
- Arrested growth and development
- Acute food refusal
- Suicidal ideation

Initial Management of Inpatients

- Bed rest
- Monitoring of vital signs, including orthostatic changes in BP, HR
- Cardiac monitoring for severe bradycardia, other arrhythmias
- Judicious use of fluids: avoid large amounts of IV fluids unless patient is in shock; if IV fluids are warranted, avoid high-glucose solution because it may cause refeeding syndrome

- Initial caloric intake should approximate intake before hospitalization; slowly increase by 250-kcal/d increments until seeing weight increases of approximately 1 kg/wk (initial weight loss may be due to inadequate caloric intake, shifts in extracellular and intracellular fluids, "water loading" before hospitalization; rapid weight gain may be due to edema)
- Monitor Na^+, K^+, Cl^-, glucose, Ca^{2+}, Mg^{2+}, and PO_4^- daily for 5 d after initiation of feeding (oral or nasogastric); nadir in PO_4^- typically day 4 of refeeding; supplement PO_4^-, Ca^{2+}, Mg^{2+}, and K^+, as necessary
- Team approach optimal (e.g., pediatrician, dietitian, psychiatrist or psychologist, social worker, family)

Refeeding Syndrome

- Cardiovascular collapse and death can occur in malnourished patients aggressively renourished with parenteral or enteral nutrition; be extremely cautious with patients hospitalized at body weight <70%; risk is greatest during first week of refeeding and is associated with intracellular shifts in PO_{4-}
- $\downarrow K^+$ and $\downarrow Mg^{2+}$ can lead to cardiac arrhythmias
- Increased metabolic demand can lead to increased cardiac workload, heart failure
- Delirium can occur during or after second week of refeeding

SUBSTANCE USE

- See Table 4.5 for overdose management

TIPS FOR INTERVENING IN THE EMERGENCY SETTING

- See Tables 7.3 and 7.4 for tips for interviewing the adolescent about substance use
- Disclose drug screening tests
- Give results without parents present

Table 7.3	CRAFFT Screen for Problematic Substance Use
C	Have you ever driven a *CAR* or driven with someone else while high or drunk?
R	Do you ever drink or use drugs to *RELAX*, feel better, or fit in?
A	Do you ever drink or get high *ALONE*?
F	Do you ever *FORGET* things while drinking or using drugs?
F	Do your *FAMILY* or *FRIENDS* ever tell you to cut down on drinking or drug use?
T	Has your alcohol or drug use ever gotten you in *TROUBLE*?

Note: Two or more positive answers suggest problematic use and need for further assessment.

Table 7.4		**DARES Approach to Motivational Interviewing**
D	Develop discrepancy	Between present state and how adolescent wants to be; explore decisional balance (pros and cons of current behavior vs. change); compare times before problem began and present situation; envision a changed vs. unchanged future
A	Avoid arguments	Ambivalence to change is normal; arguing causes a normal reflex reaction in the opposite direction
R	Roll with resistance	Adolescents expect a predictable and authoritative encounter; assume a different role that focuses on their values and concerns; shift attention away from stumbling blocks to a more workable issue (harm reduction)
E	Express empathy	Confrontation = increased resistance Support and empathy = decreased resistance
S	Support self-efficacy	Adolescent as the expert; avoid imposing change; affirm strengths and support belief in the possibility of change; emphasize personal choice and control; provide resources

ADOLESCENT PARENTING

- See Table 7.5 for health issues common to teen parents and their infants

Table 7.5	**Health Supervision for Teen Parents and Their Infants**
Mother	**Infant**
· Less likely to graduate; encourage progression toward educational goals · Higher risk of unemployment, poverty; help find social supports · ↑ risk of relationship instability; monitor for domestic violence · High risk of subsequent pregnancy within 2 yr of first pregnancy; contraception counseling postpartum · Monitor for postpartum depression and substance use	· Growth → increased risk of low birth weight and prematurity if poor prenatal care; ↑ risk of FTT · ↑ risk of poor nutrition; promote breastfeeding; monitor for iron deficiency anemia · Development → earlier motor development but ↑ risk of speech and language delay; ↑ risk of behavioral/emotional difficulties · ↑ risk of accidental injury; safety counseling

FURTHER READING

American Academy of Pediatrics, Committee on Adolescence and Committee on Early Childhood, Adoption, and Dependent Care. Care of adolescent parents and their children. *Pediatrics.* 2001;107:429–434.

Goldenring JM, Rosen DS. Getting into adolescent heads: an essential update. *Contemp Pediatr.* 2004;21:64–90.

Kaufman M. *Easy for You to Say: Q&As for Teens Living with Chronic Illness or Disability.* Buffalo, NY: Firefly Books; 2005.

Neinstein LS, ed. *Adolescent Health Care: A Practical Guide.* Philadelphia, Pa: Lippincott, Williams & Wilkins; 2007.

Society of Adolescent Medicine. Eating disorders in adolescents: position paper of the Society for Adolescent Medicine. *J Adolesc Health.* 2003;33:496–503.

USEFUL WEB SITES

Adolescent Health Working Group—Adolescent Provider Toolkit. Available at: www.ahwg.net/resources/toolkit.htm.

Canadian Paediatric Society. Adolescent Health section. Available at: www.cps.ca/english/publications/AdolesHealth.htm.

Guidelines for Adolescent Depression Toolkit. Available at: www.glad-pc.org/documents/GLAD-PCToolkit.pdf.

The Society of Adolescent Medicine (SAM). Available at: www.adolescenthealth.org.

The Society of Obstetrics and Gynaecology of Canada. Available at: www.sexualityandu.ca.

Chapter 8 Allergy and Immunology

Vy Hong-Diep Kim
Adelle R. Atkinson

Chapter 8   Allergy and Immunology

COMMON ABBREVIATIONS

AD	autosomal dominant
ADA	adenosine deaminase
AR	autosomal recessive
CMV	cytomegalovirus
CVID	common variable immunodeficiency
EBV	Epstein-Barr virus
G6PD	glucose-6-phosphate dehydrogenase
NOBI	neutrophil oxidative burst index
PEG	polyethylene glycol
PID	primary immunodeficiency
PNP	purine nucleoside phosphorylase
RAST	radioallergosorbent test
SCID	severe combined immunodeficiency
SLE	systemic lupus erythematosus
SPT	skin prick test
XL	X-linked

ALLERGY

ANAPHYLAXIS

- See p. 24 for emergent management of anaphylaxis

IMMUNE RESPONSES

- See Table 8.1
- See Box 8.1

ALLERGIC RHINITIS

- Comorbidities: asthma, sinusitis, otitis media, eczema, lymphoid hypertrophy/obstructive sleep apnea, allergic conjunctivitis, nasal polyps, food allergy
- Characteristic signs: horizontal nasal crease ("allergic salute"); allergic shiners (dark circles beneath eyes); Dennie-Morgan folds (creases on lower eyelid parallel to lower lid margin); pale, bluish, edematous nasal turbinates; tearing, scleral or conjunctival injection, periorbital swelling; eczema; wheezing
- See p. 133 for treatment options

Table 8.1	Classification of Hypersensitivity Immune Responses	
Type of Hypersensitivity	Pathologic Immune Mechanisms	Examples
I: Anaphylactic or immediate hypersensitivity reactions	IgE antibody	Anaphylaxis, allergic rhinitis, allergic asthma, acute urticaria
II: Cytotoxic reactions	IgM, IgG antibodies against antigens bound to cell membrane structures	Immune hemolytic anemia, Rh hemolytic disease in newborn, autoimmune hyperthyroidism, myasthenia gravis, Goodpasture syndrome, penicillin-induced hemolytic anemia
III: Immune-complex mediated	Complexes of circulating antigens and IgM or IgG antibodies	Serum sickness (fever, skin rash, arthralgia/arthritis, glomerulonephritis); some adverse reactions to cephalosporins, sulfonamides, penicillins, may take a week to manifest; poststreptococcal glomerulonephritis
IV: Delayed hypersensitivity	T lymphocytes	Tuberculin skin test reactions, contact dermatitis

© The Hospital for Sick Children, 2009. New artwork created by The Hospital for Sick Children for *The Hospital for Sick Children Handbook of Pediatrics*, 11th edition.

FOOD ALLERGY

- Adverse immune response to food proteins; must distinguish between immune-mediated (allergic) and non–immune-mediated (intolerance or toxic reactions)
- Symptoms: gastrointestinal (vomiting, diarrhea, abdominal pain, cramping), skin eruptions (urticaria, angioedema, dermatitis), respiratory (rhinoconjunctivitis, bronchospasm), anaphylaxis; usually occur within 2 h of ingestion

Box 8.1	Common Investigations for Allergy

Skin Prick Testing (SPT)
- Most specific screening method to detect IgE antibodies if history of reaction to allergen
- Positive reaction: wheal ≥3 mm larger than negative saline control; read 15 min after application of reagents; positive histamine control ensures reliable testing
- Antihistamines withheld 1 wk before skin testing

CAP-RAST (Radioallergosorbent Test)
- Quantifies in vitro specific IgE to particular allergen (e.g., to follow food-specific IgE antibody concentrations)
- Useful when SPT not possible; not as sensitive or specific as standardized SPT

Provocation Testing
- Gold standard in diagnosis of IgE-mediated hypersensitivity
- Only in controlled setting equipped to deal with anaphylaxis

© The Hospital for Sick Children, 2009. New artwork created by The Hospital for Sick Children for *The Hospital for Sick Children Handbook of Pediatrics*, 11th edition.

- Most common food allergens: cow's milk, egg, peanuts, tree nuts (almonds, cashew nuts, walnuts, pistachios), wheat, soy, fish, shell-fish, sesame seeds
- Peanuts are leading cause of food-induced anaphylaxis
- Early childhood allergies to milk, egg, soy, wheat usually resolve by school age (80%)
- Peanut, tree nut and seafood allergies generally considered lifelong; 20% of peanut allergy may resolve by age 5 yr (recurrence possible)
- Egg allergy is not a contraindication to MMR immunization
- Influenza and yellow fever vaccines still contraindicated in children with egg allergy (see p. 482)
- Pollen–food allergy syndrome (oral allergy syndrome)—form of contact urticaria with pruritus, tingling ± angioedema of lips, tongue, palate, oropharynx; rarely systemic symptoms; most commonly associated with ingestion of fresh fruits, raw vegetables, certain nuts in pollen-sensitized individuals

Other Food Reactions
- Food protein–induced enterocolitis: onset in early infancy with recurrent emesis, bloody diarrhea, hypoalbuminemia, abdominal distension; cow's milk and soy proteins implicated most often; usually resolves by age 2–3 yr

Specific Interventions
- Strict elimination of food identified as allergen; avoid generalized elimination diets: risk of malnutrition, eating disorders
- "Allergy-aware" or "allergy-safe" classroom: do not trade/share foods; hand washing before and after eating; no food allowed in activities; scrutinize ingredient labels
- Medical alert bracelet (MedicAlert®) identification
- Prescribe autoinjectable epinephrine (EpiPen® or Twinject®) if history of life-threatening food allergy

ADVERSE DRUG REACTIONS

Drug-Related Reactions

Nonimmunologic
- Intolerance: lowered threshold to normal pharmacologic action of drugs in susceptible persons (e.g., salicylates causing tinnitus)
- Idiosyncratic reactions: qualitative abnormal response in genetically susceptible persons (e.g., hemolytic anemia with exposure to oxidant drugs in G6PD-deficient patients)
- Pseudoallergic reactions: resemble allergic reactions but no immunologic mechanism involved (e.g., skin rash with radiocontrast material)

Immunologic
- 6–15% of all adverse drug reactions; penicillin, cephalosporins most frequent offenders

Evaluation for Suspected Drug Allergy

- Detailed history: timing; all prescription, nonprescription, biologic (e.g., monoclonal antibodies, IVIG) drugs; characterization of reaction, similar past reactions
- Skin testing to evaluate IgE-mediated reactions (if available for particular drug); negative SPT confirmed with intradermal testing, then oral challenge as gold standard

Latex Allergy

- Risk factors: contact with latex articles (multiple surgical procedures [e.g., spina bifida, genitourinary anomalies, repeated catheterizations, contact with health care workers]); atopy
- Management: avoidance (especially stretchable latex [e.g.,balloons, gloves]), latex-free surgery, autoinjectable epinephrine if risk of anaphylaxis

Penicillin Allergy

- About 90% of persons deemed penicillin allergic based on history are not truly allergic; confirm with skin testing and oral challenge
- If negative SPT to major and minor determinants of penicillin (the major breakdown products of penicillin), then 1% chance of having allergic reaction

Cephalosporin Allergy

- Cross-reactivity with penicillins decreases with increasing generation of cephalosporins (first generation: 5–16%; second: 4%; third or fourth: 1–3%); avoid in proven penicillin sensitivity (for those with significant β-lactam allergy, consider macrolides or clindamycin)
- If required in penicillin-sensitive patient, graded challenge may be done

Sulfonamide Allergy

- Skin rashes common
- Urticaria: develops 1–2 d after onset of treatment; resolves 1–2 d after treatment ends
- Idiosyncratic reactions: less common, occur later (10–12 d) into therapy (e.g., erythema multiforme, Stevens-Johnson syndrome, toxic epidermal necrolysis; see p. 205)

Management

- Discontinue suspected medication immediately; rarely, suppressive therapy (with antihistamines ± corticosteroids) with continuation of offending drug may be appropriate if no alternative therapy and mild reaction
- Symptomatic relief as necessary with epinephrine, antihistamines, corticosteroids (see p. 133)
- Educate to avoid future exposure; consider cross-reactivity with other drugs

- Desensitization for IgE-mediated life-threatening drug allergy may be performed in controlled hospital setting if offending drug is only treatment of choice; consult allergist
- Non–IgE-mediated adverse drug reactions that are contraindicated for in vivo challenge or desensitization: Stevens-Johnson syndrome, toxic epidermal necrolysis, chemical hepatitis, drug-induced nephritis, bone marrow suppression, hemolytic anemia, serum sickness
- If history is unclear as to cause and effect, consult allergist to determine whether graded challenge appropriate
- Medical alert bracelet (MedicAlert®) identification for all with potentially life-threatening allergies

INSECT STING ALLERGY

- Prevalence: 1–3% of general population
- Most commonly Hymenoptera order: honeybee, yellow jacket, yellow hornet, white-faced hornet, paper wasp

Clinical Reactions

- See Table 8.2

Investigations

- SPT with Hymenoptera venom is standard method of identifying specific causative insect
- Severe systemic reactions may decrease venom-specific IgE to undetectable level; false-negative result may occur if SPT done within 2–4 wk of reaction

Management of Acute Reactions

- Local reactions: resolve spontaneously; symptomatic treatment with cold compresses, oral analgesics, antihistamines
- Large local reactions: cold compresses, elevation of affected limb, analgesia, antihistamines; if extensive and disabling, consider oral steroids (2–4 d)
- Systemic reactions: treat anaphylaxis (see p. 24); intermittent application of a tourniquet (for 1 min q3–5min) proximal to site (if sting is on extremity) may delay the systemic absorption of venom
- If stinger is visible, should be removed carefully to avoid further venom injection

Prophylactic Management

- Avoidance measures (e.g., long sleeves, no bare feet, use straw when drinking from can), specific venom immunotherapy

MANAGEMENT OF ALLERGIES

Pharmacologic

- See Table 8.3

8

Table 8.2   Types of Reactions to Insect Stings

Type	Immediate			Delayed
	Local Reactions	Large Local Reactions	Systemic Reactions	
Timing	Within minutes up to about 4 h after sting			Develop days after the sting
Clinical	Swelling, erythema, burning sensation at site	Cover two large joints or involve an entire limb	Urticaria, pruritus, angioedema, vomiting, dyspnea, wheezing, hypotension	Rare; serum sickness, vasculitis, glomerulonephritis, Guillain-Barré syndrome, encephalitis, or myocarditis
Course	Resolve within hours or few days	Swelling may increase over 24–48 h, resolves in 5–10 d	IgE mediated; mild symptoms to severe life threatening	
Risk with subsequent sting	Not predictive of systemic reactions to subsequent stings	5% risk of anaphylaxis to subsequent stings	60–70% recurrence of anaphylaxis with subsequent sting	

© The Hospital for Sick Children, 2009. New artwork created by The Hospital for Sick Children for The Hospital for Sick Children Handbook of Pediatrics, 11th edition.

Table 8.3 — Pharmacologic Management of Allergic Disorders

Disorder and Treatment	Comments
Allergic rhinitis	
First-Generation Oral Antihistamines **Diphenhydramine** (5 mg/kg/d PO/IV/IM ÷ q6h) **Hydroxyzine** (2 mg/kg/d PO ÷ tid or qid)	Effective but cause somnolence, central nervous system depression
Second-Generation Oral Antihistamines **Cetirizine** (2–6 yr: 5 mg PO od or ÷ bid; >6 yr: 5–10 mg PO od or ÷ bid) **Loratadine** (2–9 yr and/or <30 kg: 5 mg PO daily; ≥10 yr and/or >30 kg: 10 mg PO od) **Fexofenadine** (>12 yr: 60 mg PO q12h) **Desloratadine** (>12 yr: 5 mg PO od)	Fewer side effects (nonsedating), preferred as first-line therapy; may be given once daily (cetirizine, loratadine); cetirizine and loratadine can be used in patients as young as 2 yr
Intranasal Corticosteroids **Fluticasone propionate** (4–11 yr: 1–2 sprays [50 mcg each] in each nostril od; ≥12 yr: 2 sprays in each nostril od) **Budesonide** (starting dose: >6 yr: 2 sprays [each 64 mcg] in each nostril od or 1 spray in each nostril bid [total daily dose, 256 mcg]) **Mometasone** (≥12 yr: 2 sprays [each 50 mcg] in each nostril od)	Effective in relieving all symptoms of allergic and nonallergic rhinitis, especially congestion
Urticaria	
Diphenhydramine (see above) **Hydroxyzine** (see above) **Ketotifen fumarate** (6 mo–3 yr: 0.05 mg/kg PO bid; >3 yr: 1 mg PO bid) **Cetirizine** (see above) **Loratadine** (see above)	
Allergic conjunctivitis	
Sodium cromoglycate (>5 yr: 2 drops in each eye qid) **Olopatadine hydrochloride** (1–2 drops in each affected eye bid) **Levocabastine hydrochloride** (≥12 yr: 1 drop in each eye bid)	Topical medications

© The Hospital for Sick Children, 2009. New artwork created by The Hospital for Sick Children for *The Hospital for Sick Children Handbook of Pediatrics*, 11th edition.

Immunotherapy

- Recommended for those ≤16 yr with history of IgE-mediated systemic reactions to Hymenoptera stings or for adults with cutaneous systemic reactions (e.g., urticaria, angioedema)
- Consider as third-line therapy (first-line: allergen avoidance; second-line: pharmacotherapy) for patients with history of IgE-mediated allergic rhinitis or asthma (controversial) exacerbated by environmental allergens
- Standardized allergens used in increasing concentrations over months with maintenance therapy for 4–5 yr; consult allergist
- Contraindications: non–IgE-mediated allergy, IgE-mediated food allergies, severe uncontrolled asthma, comorbid autoimmune disease, age <5 yr, symptoms consisting only of atopic dermatitis, previous failed trial of immunotherapy, no symptom reduction after 2 yr of therapy

IMMUNOLOGY

- See Box 8.2 for clinical "red flags" suggestive of an immune disorder

Box 8.2	"Red Flags" for Immunodeficiencies

- Recurrent pyogenic infections in different sites or more than one severe pyogenic infection (e.g., meningitis, pneumonia, sepsis, osteomyelitis)
- Frequent or chronic sinusitis or otitis media, skin infections or abscesses, furunculosis, organ abscesses, lymphadenitis, severe course with varicella-zoster infection
- Prolonged infection with poor response to antibiotics
- Infections with unusual organisms or opportunistic infections (e.g., *Pneumocystis jiroveci, Aspergillus, Mycobacterium avium-intracellulare*)
- Illness after live viral vaccination (e.g., MMR, varicella, yellow fever)
- Adverse transfusion reaction
- Poor wound healing; delayed separation of umbilical cord (>3 weeks)
- Chronic diarrhea, often with malabsorption; failure to thrive
- Persistent thrush
- Skin rashes (e.g., intractable atopic dermatitis)
- Family history of unexplained early infant deaths, increased susceptibility to infection, consanguinity, multiple autoimmune or rheumatic diseases
- Absence of lymph nodes and tonsils

© The Hospital for Sick Children, 2009. New artwork created by The Hospital for Sick Children for *The Hospital for Sick Children Handbook of Pediatrics*, 11th edition.

APPROACH TO IMMUNODEFICIENCIES

- See Boxes 8.3 and 8.4

PRIMARY IMMUNODEFICIENCIES

- See Tables 8.4 and 8.5

SECONDARY IMMUNODEFICIENCIES

- See Box 8.5

Box 8.3 Screening Tests for Primary Immunodeficiencies

- CBC with WBC differential (for lymphopenia, neutropenia, thrombocytopenia, anemia)
- Quantitative immunoglobulins: IgG, IgA, IgM
- Antibody titers to protein vaccines if previously immunized (e.g., diphtheria, tetanus, polio, measles, mumps, rubella)
- Delayed-type hypersensitivity skin test (intradermal skin test with 0.1 mL heat-killed *Candida* 1:100 dilution)
- CXR: thymic shadow

© The Hospital for Sick Children, 2009. New artwork created by The Hospital for Sick Children for *The Hospital for Sick Children Handbook of Pediatrics*, 11th edition.

Box 8.4 Specific Tests for Suspected Immunodeficiencies

Tests of B-Lymphocyte Function
- Quantitative immunoglobulins: IgG (consider subclasses), IgA, IgM
- B-lymphocyte quantitation by flow cytometry
- Antibody response to protein vaccines (tetanus, diphtheria, polio, measles, mumps, rubella antibody titers)
- Antibody response to polysaccharide vaccine (pneumococcal polysaccharide vaccine)
- Isohemagglutinins (only if child >1 yr; assesses IgM response to carbohydrate antigen)

Tests of T-Lymphocyte Function
- Total lymphocyte count
- T-cell and subset quantitation by flow cytometry (CD3/total T-cell, CD4/T-helper, CD8/T-suppressor/cytotoxic counts)
- CXR for thymic shadow
- Delayed-type hypersensitivity skin test (intradermal skin test with 0.1 mL heat-killed *Candida* 1:100 dilution)
- In vitro T-cell proliferative responses to mitogens, antigens, or allogenic cells (day 3 and day 6 proliferations)
- Thymic biopsy

Tests of Phagocytic Cell Function
- Neutrophil count and morphology
- NOBI by flow cytometry
- Adhesion antigen (CD11/CD18) by flow cytometry
- Chemotaxis assays

Tests of Complement System Function
- Total hemolytic complement (CH50), C3, C4

Other Tests
- HIV testing
- ADA and PNP levels
- Molecular cytogenic studies

© The Hospital for Sick Children, 2009. New artwork created by The Hospital for Sick Children for *The Hospital for Sick Children Handbook of Pediatrics*, 11th edition.

Table 8.4   Typical Features of Primary Immunodeficiencies

Features	T-Cell Defect	B-Cell Defect	Phagocytic Cell Defect	Complement Defect
Onset of infections	First year of life to late childhood	Later childhood to adulthood	Early onset	First decade of life, most commonly 5–6 yr
Pathogens involved	Bacteria: streptococci, Pseudomonas Viruses: CMV, EBV, varicella, parainfluenza, enteric viruses Fungi and parasites: *Candida* organisms; opportunistic infections; *Pneumocystis jiroveci* pneumonia (PJP)	Bacteria: streptococci, *Haemophilus* organisms, mycoplasmas Viruses: echovirus,* polio Parasites: *Giardia* organisms	Bacteria: staphylococci, pseudomonads, *Serratia* and *Klebsiella* organisms Fungi: *Candida* and *Aspergillus* organisms	Bacteria: *Neisseria* organisms, pneumococci
Clinical	Failure to thrive, protracted diarrhea, persistent oral candidiasis, viral or PJP pneumonitis	Recurrent sinopulmonary infections, chronic GI symptoms, malabsorption, mycoplasma arthritis, enteroviral meningoencephalitis	Skin: dermatitis, impetigo, cellulitis Lymph nodes: suppurative adenitis Oral cavity: periodontitis, ulcers Internal organs: abscesses, osteomyelitis	Infections: meningitis, arthritis, septicemia, recurrent sinopulmonary infections
Special	Lymphopenia, severe erythroderma	Autoimmunity, increased risk of lymphoma	Delayed separation of umbilical cord (>3 wk), poor wound healing	Rheumatoid disorders: SLE, vasculitis, dermatomyositis, scleroderma, glomerulonephritis, angioedema

*Most commonly in X-linked agammaglobulinemia.
Adapted from Report of an IUIS Scientific Group: Primary immunodeficiency diseases. *Clin Exp Immunol.* 1999;118:S1–S28; and from Woroniecka M, Ballow M. Office evaluation of children with recurrent infection. *Pediatr Clin North Am.* 2000;47:1211–1224.

Table 8.5 Selected Primary Immunodeficiency Disorders

Disorder	Serum Ig	B Cells	T Cells	Inheritance	Associated Features
Predominantly Antibody Deficiencies (50%)					
X-linked agammaglobulinemia	All ↓	↓↓↓	Normal	XL	Severe bacterial infections
CVID	↓IgG and usually IgA ± IgM	Normal or ↓	Normal or ↓	Variable	Presents in second–fourth decades, ↑ risk of lymphoreticular and GI malignancies, malabsorption and autoimmune disorders
Transient hypogammaglobulinemia of infancy	↓IgG and IgA	Normal	Normal	Unknown	Recurrent moderate bacterial infections
Dysgammaglobulinemia	Normal	Normal	Normal	Variable	Inability to make antibodies to specific antigens
Disorders of Cell-Mediated Immunity (10%)					
DiGeorge syndrome	Normal or ↓	Normal	↓ or normal	De novo defect or AD	Hypoparathyroidism, conotruncal malformation, abnormal facies
Chronic mucocutaneous candidiasis	Normal	Normal	Normal	AD, AR, sporadic	Chronic mucocutaneous candidiasis
Disorders of Combined Humoral and Cellular Immunity (20%)					
T-B+ SCID:					
Common γ chain deficiency	↓	Normal or ↑	↓↓↓	XL	Hemophagocytic lymphohistiocytosis
T-B- SCID:					
RAG1/2 deficiency	↓ →	↓↓↓	↓↓↓	AR	Defective gene recombination
ADA deficiency	→	Progressive ↓	Progressive ↓	AR	Costochondral junction flaring
T+B- SCID:					
Omenn syndrome	↓; ↑IgE	Normal or ↓	Present	AR	Erythroderma, eosinophilia, adenopathy, hepatosplenomegaly

(continued)

Table 8.5 Selected Primary Immunodeficiency Disorders (continued)

Disorder	Serum Ig	B Cells	T Cells	Inheritance	Associated Features
Disorders of Combined Humoral and Cellular Immunity (20%)					
Other:					
Wiskott-Aldrich syndrome	↓IgM; often ↑ IgA and IgE	Normal	Progressive ↓	XL	Thrombocytopenia, small platelets, eczema, lymphomas, autoimmune disease, bacterial infections
Ataxia-telangiectasia	Often ↓IgA, IgE, and IgG subclasses; ↑IgM	Normal	↓	AR	Ataxia, telangiectasia, increased alpha fetoprotein, lymphoreticular and other malignancies, increased X-ray sensitivity
Phagocytic Cell Defects (18%)					
Chronic granulomatous disease	Normal	Normal	Normal	XL (mostly) or AR	Neutrophils and monocytes/macrophages affected
Complement Deficiencies (2%)					
Early classic pathway components (C1, C2, C4); associated with collagen vascular disease					
Late complement components (C5, C6, C7, C8, C9); associated with recurrent *Neisseria* infections					
C3 (shares characteristics of early and late component deficiencies)					

Adapted from Notarangelo L, Casanova J-L, Conley ME, et al, for the IUISPID Classification Committee. Primary immunodeficiency diseases: an update from the International Union of Immunological Societies Primary Immunodeficiency Diseases Classification Committee Meeting in Budapest, 2005. *J Allergy Clin Immunol.* 2006;117:883–896.

- Infections (e.g., HIV, EBV)
- Nutritional deficiencies (e.g., protein, calorie, vitamin, or mineral malnutrition)
- Protein-losing states (e.g., nephrotic syndrome, protein-losing enteropathy, intestinal lymphangiectasia)
- Malignancy (e.g., leukemia, lymphoma)
- Immunosuppressive agents (e.g., antineoplastic drugs, corticosteroids, radiation)
- Adverse drug reactions (e.g., myelosuppression from sulfonamides, anticonvulsants)
- Hematologic disorders (e.g., sickle cell disease)
- Metabolic disorders (e.g., severe uremia, galactosemia)
- Systemic inflammatory disease (e.g., sarcoidosis)
- Splenectomy
- Prematurity

MANAGEMENT OF IMMUNODEFICIENCIES

- Family studies, genetic counseling; prenatal diagnosis available for some PIDs
- Prompt recognition and aggressive treatment of infection
- Prophylactic antibiotics—see Chapter 23
- No live attenuated vaccines for diagnosed or suspected immune deficiencies and some secondary immunodeficiencies (generalized malignant disease, immunosuppressive agents, high-dose corticosteroids); may cause vaccine-induced infection; give inactivated polio vaccine to patient and MMR and/or varicella vaccine to family
- Active management of varicella exposure (chickenpox)—see p. 488
- Selective IgA deficiency: washed red cell concentrate to avoid anaphylaxis, and use IVIG with caution
- If blood transfusion required in patients with T-cell defects, use only irradiated leukocyte-poor CMV-negative products to avoid graft-versus-host disease and CMV infection
- Gamma globulin replacement monthly for B-cell defects
- Bone marrow transplantation for T-cell and combined defects, if appropriate
- Enzyme replacement (e.g., PEG-conjugated ADA for specific enzyme deciency)

FURTHER READING

Fleisher TA, Ballow M. Primary immune deficiencies: presentation, diagnosis, and management. *Pediatr Clin North Am.* 2000;47:1197–1354.

Middleton E, Reed CE, Ellis EF, et al. *Allergy Principles and Practice.* 5th ed. St. Louis, Mo: Mosby-Year Book; 1998.

Ochs HD, Smith CIE, Puck JM. *Primary Immunodeficiency Diseases—A Molecular and Cellular Approach.* 2nd ed. New York, NY: Oxford University Press; 2006.

Shearer WT, Leung DYM, eds. Mini-primer on allergic and immunologic diseases. *J Allergy Clin Immunol.* 2006;117(suppl 2):S429–S494.

Stiehm ER. *Immunologic Disorders in Infants and Children.* 5th ed. Philadelphia, Pa: WB Saunders; 2004.

USEFUL WEB SITES

American Academy of Allergy, Asthma and Immunology. Available at: http://www.aaaai.org.

American College of Allergy, Asthma and Immunology online. Available at: http://www.acaai.org.

Canadian Society of Allergy and Clinical Immunology. Available at: http://www.csaci.medical.org.

Canadian immunization guide. Available at: http://www.naci.gc.ca.

The Jeffrey Modell Foundation. Available at: http://www.jmfworld.com.

Chapter 9 Cardiology

Andrea Wan
Derek Wong
Fraser Golding

Chapter 9   Cardiology

COMMON ABBREVIATIONS

A-fib	atrial fibrillation
A-flutter	atrial flutter
ABC	airway, breathing, circulation
ACE	angiotensin-converting enzyme
AoV	aortic valve
AS	aortic stenosis
ASD	atrial septal defect
AV	atrioventricular
AVSD	atrioventricular septal defect
BT	Blalock-Taussig
CBC	complete blood cell count
CHD	congenital heart disease
CHF	congestive heart failure
CMV	cytomegalovirus
CoA	coarctation of the aorta
CRP	C-reactive protein
DCM	dilated cardiomyopathy
EBV	Epstein-Barr virus
ESR	erythrocyte sedimentation rate
GAS	group A streptococcal
GXT	graded exercise test
HCM	hypertrophic cardiomyopathy
HLHS	hypoplastic left heart syndrome
IE	infective endocarditis
IVC	inferior vena cava
JVP	jugular venous pressure
LA	left atrium
LAD	left axis deviation
LAE	left atrial enlargement
LBBB	left bundle branch block
LLSB	left lower sternal border
LPA	left pulmonary artery
LQTS	long QT syndrome
LUSB	left upper sternal border
LV	left ventricle
LVE	left ventricular enlargement
LVH	left ventricular hypertrophy
LVOTO	left ventricular outflow tract obstruction
MAPCA	multiple aortopulmonary collateral arteries

MV	mitral valve
PA	pulmonary artery
PAC	premature atrial contraction
PDA	patent ductus arteriosus
PGE/PGE$_1$	prostaglandin E/prostaglandin E$_1$
PPHN	persistent pulmonary hypertension of the newborn
PPS	peripheral pulmonary stenosis
PS	pulmonary stenosis
PVC	premature ventricular contraction
PVR	pulmonary vascular resistance
RA	right atrium
RAD	right axis deviation
RAE	right atrial enlargement
RBBB	right bundle branch block
RCM	restrictive cardiomyopathy
RPA	right pulmonary artery
RR	respiratory rate
RUSB	right upper sternal border
RV	right ventricle
RVH	right ventricular hypertrophy
RVOTO	right ventricular outflow tract obstruction
SEM	systolic ejection murmur
SVC	superior vena cava
SVR	systemic vascular resistance
SVT	supraventricular tachycardia
TAPVD	total anomalous pulmonary venous drainage
TGA	transposition of the great arteries
TOF	tetralogy of Fallot
TR	tricuspid regurgitation
TSH	thyroid-stimulating hormone
TV	tricuspid valve
V-fib	ventricular fibrillation
VSD	ventricular septal defect
VT	ventricular tachycardia
WPW	Wolff-Parkinson-White

FOCUSED CARDIOLOGY EXAMINATION

HISTORY

- Presenting illness: failure to thrive, dyspnea, orthopnea, tachypnea, palpitations, syncope, exercise intolerance, difficulty feeding, cyanosis, lethargy, chest pain
- Family history: sudden death, CHD, unexplained deaths (possible familial arrhythmia), pacemakers, premature (age < 55 yr) myocardial infarction/stroke

PHYSICAL EXAMINATION

- General examination: dysmorphic features, growth parameters
- Vital signs: RR, HR, four-limb BP, preductal/postductal saturations
- Head/neck: JVP, cyanosis, bruits (carotid, cranial)
- Cardiac: RV heave, LV apex location, S_1/S_2 (normal splitting), S_3, S_4, murmurs, thrills, perfusion, peripheral pulses, peripheral edema
- Respiratory: crackles, respiratory distress
- Abdominal: hepatomegaly, splenomegaly, bruits

INVESTIGATIONS

- ECG: arrhythmias, chamber enlargement
- Holter: correlate symptoms with rhythm disturbance, response to medication; assess pacemaker function
- GXT: response to exercise (i.e., HR, BP, O_2 consumption, ECG changes, cardiac output), quantitative functional assessment
- CXR: visceral situs, cardiac size/shape/location, pulmonary vascularity, position of aortic arch
- Echocardiography: real-time two-dimensional images of cardiac anatomy, function, and hemodynamics
- CT scan: cardiac, vascular and airway anatomy, pericardial abnormalities, lung parenchyma
- Cardiac MRI: cardiac anatomy and function, vascular and airway anatomy, lung parenchyma, quantitative measures of blood flow

CARDIAC MURMURS

- Timing, location, radiation, pitch, intensity, additional heart sounds (e.g., clicks, thrills, gallop)
- See Table 9.1 and Box 9.1

Table 9.1	Characteristics of Innocent and Pathologic Murmurs	
Characteristics	**Innocent**	**Pathologic**
Timing	Systolic	Systolic or diastolic
Intensity	Grade 1–2	Grade 3–6
Associated sounds	None	Clicks, thrills, gallop rhythm
Response to inspiration	Louder after inspiration	No change
Response to change in position	Quieter when upright compared with supine	No change

Cardiology

Box 9.1	Murmur Intensity Grading

Grade 1: soft, barely audible
Grade 2: same intensity as heart sounds
Grade 3: greater intensity than heart sounds
Grade 4: grade 3 + thrill
Grade 5: heard with diaphragm of stethoscope at 45° to chest wall, + thrill
Grade 6: heard with diaphragm of stethoscope completely off chest wall

INNOCENT MURMURS

- Still's: musical vibratory systolic murmur along left sternal border (young children)
- Pulmonary flow: soft blowing murmur at upper left sternal border (older children)
- PPS: same as pulmonary flow but radiates to back (resolves by 3–6 mo)
- Carotid bruit: 2/6 intensity systolic murmur above clavicles, along carotids (all ages)
- Venous hum: continuous murmur above or below clavicles; intensity changes with rotation of head and compression of jugular vein; disappears when supine (young children)

PEDIATRIC ECG

- See Table 9.2 for summary of normal ECG values

HEART RATE

- 300 divided by number of "large" squares on the ECG (assuming the paper speed is 25 mm/s) (Figure 9.1)

Figure 9.1 **How to Count Heart Rate Based on ECG**

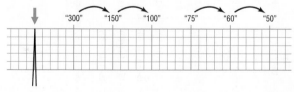

From Dubin D. *Rapid Interpretation of EKGs*. St Louis, Mo: Mosby; 1991. Revised and updated 4th ed. Tampa, Fl: Cover Publishing Company, 1991:60. Courtesy of Dale Dubin.

RHYTHM

- Regular vs. irregular, narrow complex vs. wide complex QRS, sinus rhythm vs. other
- Criteria for sinus rhythm: P wave for every QRS complex, QRS complex for every P wave; normal P wave axis (upright P wave in II and usually I and aV$_F$)

Table 9.2　Normal ECG Values for Age

Age	Heart Rate Minimum–Maximum*	Mean Frontal Plane QRS Axis*	PR Interval*	QRS Duration*	R Wave Amplitude*	Lead V_1 S Wave Amplitude*	R/S Ratio*	R Wave Amplitude*	Lead V_6 S Wave Amplitude*	R/S Ratio*
0-1 mo	100-180 (120)	+75-+180 (+120)	0.08-0.12 (0.10)	0.04-0.08 (0.06)	4-25 (15)	1-20 (10)	0.5-∞ (1.5)	1-21 (6)	0-12 (4)	0.1-∞ (2)
2-3 mo	110-180 (120)	+35-+135 (+100)	0.08-0.12 (0.10)	0.04-0.08 (0.06)	2-20 (11)	1-18 (7)	0.3-10.0 (1.5)	3-20 (10)	0-6 (2)	1.5-∞ (4)
4-12 mo	100-180 (150)	+30-+135 (+160)	0.09-0.13 (0.12)	0.04-0.08 (0.06)	3-20 (10)	1-16 (8)	0.3-4.0 (1.2)	6-20 (13)	0-4 (2)	2.0-∞ (6)
1-3 yr	100-180 (130)	0-+110 (+60)	0.10-0.14 (0.12)	0.04-0.08 (0.06)	1-18 (9)	1-27 (13)	0.5-1.5 (0.8)	3-24 (12)	0-4 (2)	3.0-∞ (20)
4-5 yr	60-150 (100)	0-+110 (+60)	0.11-0.15 (0.13)	0.05-0.09 (0.07)	1-18 (7)	1-30 (14)	0.1-1.5 (0.7)	4-24 (13)	0-4 (1)	2.0-∞ (20)
6-8 yr	60-130 (100)	-15-+110 (+60)	0.12-0.16 (0.14)	0.05-0.09 (0.07)	1-18 (7)	1-30 (14)	0.1-1.5 (0.7)	4-24 (13)	0-4 (1)	2.0-∞ (20)
9-11 yr	50-110 (80)	-15-+110 (+60)	0.12-0.17 (0.14)	0.05-0.09 (0.07)	1-16 (6)	1-26 (16)	0.1-1.0 (0.5)	4-24 (14)	0-4 (1)	4.0-∞ (20)
12-16 yr	50-100 (75)	-15-+110 (+60)	0.12-0.17 (0.15)	0.05-0.09 (0.07)	1-16 (5)	1-23 (14)	0.0-1.0 (0.3)	4-22 (14)	0-5 (1)	2.0-∞ (9)
>16 yr	50-90 (70)	-15-+110 (+60)	0.12-0.20 (0.15)	0.05-1.0 (0.08)	1-14 (3)	1-23 (10)	0.0-1.0 (0.3)	4-21 (10)	0-6 (1)	2.0-∞ (9)

*Mean values are noted in brackets.
From the Texas Children's Hospital. In: Carson A, Gilette PC, McNamara DB, eds. A Guide to Cardiac Dysrhythmias in Children. New York, NY: Grune and Stratton; 1980.

AXIS

- Look at limb leads (I, II, III, aV$_R$, aV$_L$, aV$_F$) to determine cardiac axis (Figure 9.2)
- At birth, mean QRS axis between +60° and +160°; by 1 yr, between +10° and +100°

Figure 9.2 **Determining Cardiac Axis**

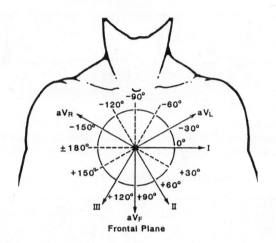

Frontal Plane

INTERVALS AND WAVES

P Wave

- Represents atrial activation
- Tall P wave (>3 mV in height): RAE
- Wide (>0.12 ms in width) or bifid P wave: LAE

PR Interval

- Represents physiologic delay in AV node

First-Degree AV Block

- PR interval >120 ms (Figure 9.3)

Figure 9.3 **First-Degree Atrioventricular Block**

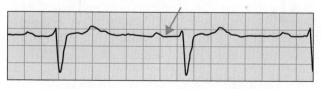

Second-Degree AV Block

Mobitz Type I (Wenckebach)
- Progressive prolongation of PR interval with eventual nonconducted P wave followed by conducted sinus beat with shorter PR interval (Figure 9.4)

Figure 9.4 **Mobitz Type I Atrioventricular Block (Wenckebach)**

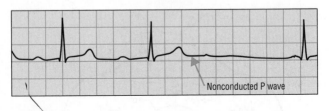

Nonconducted P wave

Mobitz Type II
- Nonconducted P waves that occur outside ventricular refractory period, without progressive prolongation of PR interval (Figure 9.5)

Figure 9.5 **Mobitz Type II Atrioventricular Block**

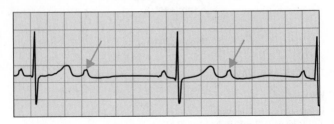

Third-Degree Block (Complete Heart Block)
- No relationship between P waves and QRS complexes (Figure 9.6)

Figure 9.6 **Complete Heart Block**

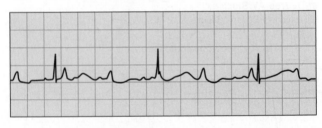

QRS Complex

- Q waves should be seen in leads II, III, aV_F, V_5–V_6; are usually narrow, low voltage
- QRS complex duration should be <60 ms in infants <1 yr, <80 ms in children/adolescents
- RBBB: right axis, rSR' in leads V_4R, V_1, V_2; wide slurred S in I, V_5, V_6
- LBBB: left axis, wide slurred R in leads I, aV_L, V_5, V_6; wide S in V_1, V_2

QT Interval

- Corrected for HR using formula

$$QTc = \frac{QT}{\sqrt{RR\ interval}}$$

- QTc ≤440 ms in children (>6 m old) and adults
- Causes of QTc prolongation: hypothermia, ↓K^+, ↓Ca^{2+}, drugs, cerebral brain injury, congenital

ST Segments

- Normal ST segments may be ↑ up to 1 mm
- Diffuse ST segment elevation: pericarditis, myocarditis, or pericardial effusion
- Local ST segment elevation: coronary ischemia

T Waves

- From birth to 7 d, T wave may be upright in V_1
- From 7 d to approximately 7 yr, T wave in V_1 should be inverted
- In adolescents, T wave should be upright in V_1

VENTRICULAR HYPERTROPHY

- See Table 9.3

Table 9.3	ECG Findings Suggestive of Hypertrophy
RVH	**LVH**
· RAD · rSR' pattern with R' > R in V_1, V_3R, V_4R · Q waves in V_3R, V_4R · Monophasic R wave in V_1, V_3R, V_4R · Abnormal T wave orientation in V_1 · R wave in V_1 > 95th percentile for age · S wave in V_6 > 95th percentile for age	· S wave in V_1 > 95th percentile for age · R wave in V_6 > 95th percentile for age · Deep Q waves in V_5-V_7 · ST depression or T wave inversion in V_5-V_7

ECG FINDINGS IN CONGENITAL HEART DISEASE AND K ABNORMALITIES

- See Table 9.4

Table 9.4	Characteristic ECG Changes in Selected Disorders
Abnormality	**ECG Findings**
AVSD	Left or northwest axis deviation
ASD	RBBB pattern in V_1 and inferior leads
HLHS	Low-amplitude QRS voltages in lateral leads
Anomalous left coronary artery from the pulmonary artery (ALCAPA)	Deep Q waves in I, aV_L, V_6; ST segment and T wave abnormalities in inferolateral leads
Hyperkalemia	Peaked T waves
Hypokalemia	Flat T waves or U waves

© The Hospital for Sick Children, 2009. New artwork created by The Hospital for Sick Children for *The Hospital for Sick Children Handbook of Pediatrics*, 11th edition.

CARDIAC APPROACH TO CXR

- See Table 9.5

Table 9.5	Cardiac Characteristics on Pediatric CXR
Characteristics	**CXR Findings**
Situs	· Normal left-sided structures: heart, stomach bubble · Normal right-sided structures: liver, minor fissure of right middle lobe of lung
Cardiac position	· Levocardia: apex of heart directed to left · Dextrocardia: apex of heart directed to right
Cardiothoracic ratio	· Ratio of diameter of cardiac silhouette to diameter of thoracic cage · Newborn < 0.6; outside newborn period < 0.5
Aortic arch sidedness	· Left- or right-sided aortic arch (relative to trachea)
Pulmonary markings	· Normal, ↑ or ↓

© The Hospital for Sick Children, 2009. New artwork created by The Hospital for Sick Children for *The Hospital for Sick Children Handbook of Pediatrics*, 11th edition.

ARRHYTHMIAS

TACHYARRHYTHMIAS

- See Figure 9.7

Supraventricular Tachycardia

- See Table 9.6 and Figure 9.8

Figure 9.7 An Approach to Tachyarrhythmias

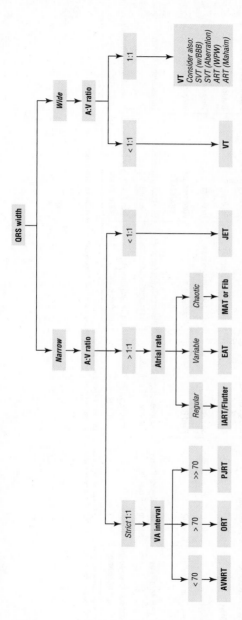

ART, antidromic re-entrant tachycardia; AVNRT, AV node re-entrant tachycardia; EAT, ectopic atrial tachycardia; IART, intra-atrial re-entrant tachycar-
dia; ORT, orthodromic re-entrant tachycardia; PJRT, paroxysmal junctional re-entrant tachycardia; JET, junctional ectopic tachycardia; MAT, multifocal atrial tachycardia.
From Walsh EP Saul JP, Triedman JK. *Cardiac Arrhythmias in Children and Young Adults with Congenital Heart Disease.* Philadelphia, Pa: Lippincott Williams & Wilkins; 2001. Reprinted by permission of Lippincot
Williams and Wilkins. Available at http://lww.com

Table 9.6 Different Types of SVT and Their Differentiating Characteristics

Characteristics	AVNRT	AVRT	AET	A-Flutter	A-Fib
Frequency	15% of SVT	70% of SVT	Uncommon	Rare	Rare
Population at risk	Older children	Younger children		Postoperative CHD	Postoperative CHD, WPW
Onset	Sudden	Sudden	Warm up (slow increase)	Sudden	Sudden
Offset	Sudden	Sudden	Cool down (slow decrease)	Incessant	Incessant
Heart rate variability	Fixed HR	Fixed HR	Variable HR	Fixed atrial rate with variable QRS	Irregularly irregular
P wave morphology	May have retrograde P wave close to QRS complex	May have retrograde P wave close to QRS complex	P waves different compared with normal sinus rhythm	Saw-tooth pattern (best seen in II, V₂)	No discernible P waves
Response to adenosine or vagal maneuvers	Terminates	Terminates	Blocks temporarily but resumes quickly	Blocks at AV node; flutter waves persist	Blocks at AV node, but A-fib continues

AET, atrial ectopic tachycardia; AVNRT, AV node re-entrant tachycardia; AVRT, AV re-entrant tachycardia.
© The Hospital for Sick Children, 2009. New artwork created by The Hospital for Sick Children for *The Hospital for Sick Children Handbook of Pediatrics*, 11th edition.

Figure 9.8 Supraventricular Tachycardia

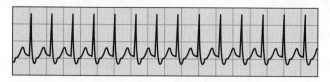

Management of SVT

- Acute management if unstable: see Figure 1.4
- Acute management if stable: attempt vagal maneuvers, adenosine 0.15–0.25 mg/kg IV bolus
- Long-term management: beta blockade for short term, medium and long term; electrophysiologic study and ablation for definitive diagnosis and management for recurrent and symptomatic SVT or if nonresponsive to medical management

VT

- Definition: greater than 3 sequential ventricular beats at rate above upper limit of normal for age
- Causes: electrolyte abnormalities ($\uparrow K^+$, $\downarrow Mg^{2+}$), CHD, LQTS, idiopathic VT, arrhythmogenic RV dysplasia
- ECG characteristics: wide complex tachycardia, AV dissociation, ventricular rate faster than atrial rate (Figure 9.9)

Figure 9.9 Ventricular Tachycardia

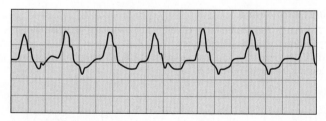

Management of VT

- Acute management for unstable patients (see p. 10)
- Acute management for stable patients: amiodarone loading dose 5 mg/kg IV over 1 h then 5–15 mcg/kg/min as a continuous infusion or lidocaine 20–50 mcg/kg/min as a continuous infusion
- Long-term management: amiodarone, automated implantable cardiac defibrillator, electrophysiologic study for intracardiac mapping for possible ablation

ECTOPIC BEATS

- See Table 9.7

Table 9.7	Premature Ectopic Beats	
Characteristics	**PACs**	**PVCs**
Epidemiology	Common in children with normal hearts	50-70% of children with normal hearts (with Holter)
Causes	Stimulants, caffeine, hypoxia hyperthyroidism, digoxin, amphetamines	Hypoxia, inflammation, cardiomyopathy, electrolyte abnormalities, cardiac tumors
ECG characteristics	P wave with different morphology than normal sinus rhythm P wave, followed by narrow QRS complex; P wave may not be conducted if ventricle is refractory	Wide QRS complex with no preceding P wave; appears earlier than anticipated with change in T wave morphology
Management	No treatment required; treat reversible underlying causes	No treatment required; treat reversible underlying causes

© The Hospital for Sick Children, 2009. New artwork created by the Hospital for Sick Children for *The Hospital for Sick Children Handbook of Pediatrics*, 11th edition.

Benign Versus Worrisome PVCs

- Benign PVCs: monomorphic (i.e., QRS morphology same for each one), disappear, or become less frequent with exercise
- Worrisome PVCs: underlying CHD, polymorphic PVCs, personal or family history of sudden death or syncope, incessant or very frequent PVCs

BRADYCARDIAS

Sinus Arrhythmia

- Normal finding, common in children, not associated with pathologic condition, requires no treatment
- ECG characteristics: normal variation of HR with respiration (slower during expiration) (Figure 9.10)

Figure 9.10 Sinus Arrhythmia

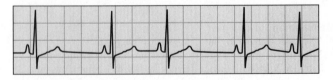

Sinus Bradycardia

- Definition: HR less than lower limit of normal for age
- Causes: hypothermia, hypothryroidism, anorexia nervosa, malnutrition, hypokalemia, hypoxia, CNS injury, atrial cardiac surgery
- Management: treat underlying reversible cause if present; consider atropine, isoproterenol, or pacing if symptomatic

AV BLOCK

- Epidemiology: most caused by damage to AV node (e.g., inflammation, postsurgical)
- Causes of AV block: maternal lupus (congenital heart block), rheumatic fever, IE, myocarditis, Lyme disease, diphtheria, cardiomyopathies, ASD, Ebstein anomaly, AVSD, congenitally corrected TGA, cardiac surgery, digoxin toxicity
- Types of AV block: see pp. 147–148
- Pathophysiology: no conduction of electrical signal from atria to ventricles; resultant ventricular escape rate may be too slow to maintain adequate cardiac output
- Acute management: ABCs (see pp. 5–9), isoproterenol infusion, or transcutaneous pacing to ↑HR and cardiac output
- Long-term management:
  - No treatment required for first-degree or type I second-degree heart block (Wenckebach)
  - Permanent pacemaker for high-risk type II second-degree (Mobitz) or complete heart block

ECG SYNDROMES

- See Table 9.8

Table 9.8	Characteristics of Selected ECG Syndromes	
Characteristics	**WPW**	**LQTS**
Incidence	1/1000–3/1000 of general population	1/5000 of general population
Associated abnormalities	Ebstein anomaly	Deafness (Jervell and Lange-Nielson syndrome)
Inheritance pattern	Not inherited	AD or AR (6 subtypes)
Baseline ECG findings	Short PR interval, delta wave	QTc >upper limit of normal
Risk of sudden death	1/1000 patient-years	⅔ higher risk of death than general population
Commonly associated arrhythmias	A-fib with rapid AV conduction degenerating to V-fib	Torsades de pointes
Management	Beta blockade, catheter ablation	Beta blockade, implantable defibrillator
Additional information	Risk factors for sudden death: family history of sudden death, A-fib, delta wave at high HRs	30% can have normal baseline QTc with LQTS apparent with provocation testing; only 75% are gene positive

© The Hospital for Sick Children, 2009. New artwork created by the Hospital for Sick Children for *The Hospital for Sick Children Handbook of Pediatrics*, 11th edition.

APPROACH TO THE CHILD WITH CONGENITAL HEART DISEASE

APPROACH TO THE CYANOTIC CHILD

- History, physical examination, ECG, CXR, hyperoxic test
- Hyperoxic test: place infant in 100% FIO_2, measure preductal PaO_2; preductal $PaO_2 < 150$ mm Hg suggests cyanotic CHD
- See Figure 9.11 and Table 9.9
- Noncardiac causes of cyanosis: PPHN, sepsis, fever, lung disease, hypoglycemia
- Acute management of cyanotic CHD:
  - PGE_1 for any suspected cyanotic heart lesion (0.01–0.1 mcg/kg/min); potential side effects include apnea, fever, ↓BP (secondary to vasodilation)
  - Accept saturations of >70% acutely; if intubated, aim for CO_2 ~ 45 mm Hg
  - Transfer child emergently to pediatric cardiologist for evaluation and management

Figure 9.11 Approach to the Cyanotic Newborn

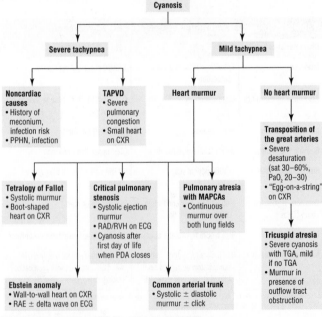

© The Hospital for Sick Children, 2009. New artwork created by TØ158
he Hospital for Sick Children for *The Hospital for Sick Children Handbook of Pediatrics*, 11th edition.

9

Table 9.9 Congenital Cyanotic Heart Lesions

Characteristics	TGA	TOF	Common Arterial Trunk	TAPVD	Tricuspid Atresia
Epidemiology	· Most common cyanotic lesion in neonates	· Most common cyanotic lesion in children · Associated with DiGeorge syndrome	· Associated with DiGeorge syndrome	· Supracardiac (50%) · Cardiac (20%) · Infracardiac (20%) · Mixed types (10%)	
Structural abnormalities	· Aorta arises from RV, PA arises from LV · See Figure 9.12	· Large unrestrictive VSD · RVOTO · RVH · Overriding aorta · See Figure 9.13	· Systemic and pulmonary vessels from single great vessel · Large VSD · See Figure 9.14	· Pulmonary veins drain to site other than LA · See Figure 9.16	· No connection between RA and RV · See Figure 9.15
Pathophysiology	· Systemic venous blood returns to RV and out aorta · Pulmonary venous blood returns to LV and out PA · Mixing occurs at PFO/ASD	· RVOTO limits pulmonary blood flow · R→L shunting across VSD · "Pink Tets" have mild RVOTO and CHF rather than cyanosis	· Ratio of SVR:PVR determines symptoms · Lower PVR results in more pulmonary blood flow, higher saturations, heart failure ± coronary ischemia	· Pulmonary blood drains to other venous structure · ASD with R→L shunt causing cyanosis · Infracardiac TAPVD always obstructed	· Mixing between desaturated blood from RA and fully saturated blood from pulmonary veins in LA
Associated lesions	· ASD · VSD · PS · AS · PDA	· Right aortic arch in 25%	· Truncal valve stenosis or insufficiency · Arch interruption · Coronary abnormalities	· VSD · ASD · Right atrial isomerism	· Pulmonary atresia · PS/AS · CoA · TGA

(continued)

Table 9.9 Congenital Cyanotic Heart Lesions (*continued*)

Characteristics	TGA	TOF	Common Arterial Trunk	TAPVD	Tricuspid Atresia
Clinical features	· Single loud S_2 ± soft SEM · Degree of cyanosis depends on mixing of blood across ASD	· Single loud S_2, 2–3/6 SEM (due to RVOTO) · Degree of cyanosis depends on RVOTO	· Cyanosis, CHF · 3/6 SEM, ± click, diastolic murmur (truncal valve insufficiency)	· Severe obstruction: severe tachypnea, cyanosis · Mild obstruction: CHF, cyanosis	· Cyanosis, normal S1, single S2 · 2–3/6 systolic murmur at LLSB
CXR findings	· "Egg on a string"	· "Boot-shaped" heart	· Cardiomegaly · ↑ pulmonary flow · Right aortic arch (25%)	· ↑ pulmonary markings · Bilateral white-out if obstructed · "Snowman sign" in supracardiac TAPVD	· Normal cardiac silhouette · Enlarged RA, ↓ pulmonary vascularity
ECG findings	· RAD · RVH	· RAD · RVH	· RAD · RVH · LVH · ST depression	· RVH · RAE	· LAD · RAE · LVH · ↓ voltages in V_1-V_3
Treatment	· PGEs ± balloon septostomy · Arterial switch operation in newborn period	· Repair at 4–6 mo	· Definitive surgical treatment within 2–4 wk	· If obstructed, emergent surgery · If unobstructed, elective repair	· PGEs and surgery · See p. 162
Long-term complications	· Aortic/PA dilation · Coronary artery abnormalities · AI · PI	· Residual RVOTO · PI · RV dilation · Poor RV function · Ventricular arrhythmias	· Truncal valve insufficiency · RVOTO · Ventricular arrhythmias	· Residual or recurrent pulmonary vein stenosis · Atrial arrhythmia	See pp. 162-164

CYANOTIC HEART LESIONS

- See Figures 9.12 through 9.16

Figure 9.12 **Transposition of the Great Arteries**

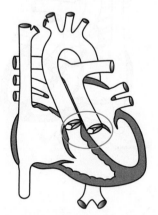

© The Hospital for Sick Children, 2003. Courtesy of *The Hospital for Sick Children Handbook of Pediatrics*, 10th edition, Fig 4.16, p. 100. (Original modified/created by SickKids using Mullins and Mayer software).

Figure 9.13 **Tetralogy of Fallot**

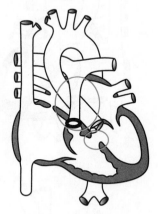

© The Hospital for Sick Children, 2003. Courtesy of *The Hospital for Sick Children Handbook of Pediatrics*, 10th edition, Fig 4.25, p. 103. (Original modified/created by SickKids using Mullins and Mayer software).

Figure 9.14 **Common Arterial Trunk**

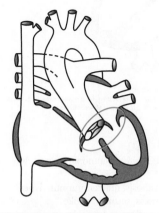

© The Hospital for Sick Children, 2003. Courtesy of *The Hospital for Sick Children Handbook of Pediatrics*, 10th edition, Fig 4.27, p. 105. (Original modified/created by SickKids using Mullins and Mayer software).

Figure 9.15 **Tricuspid Atresia**

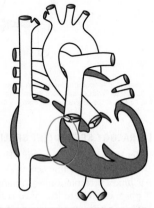

© The Hospital for Sick Children, 2003. Courtesy of *The Hospital for Sick Children Handbook of Pediatrics*, 10th edition, Fig 4.22 to 4.24, p. 102. (Original modified/created by SickKids using Mullins and Mayer software).

Figure 9.16 Types of Total Anomalous Pulmonary Venous Return

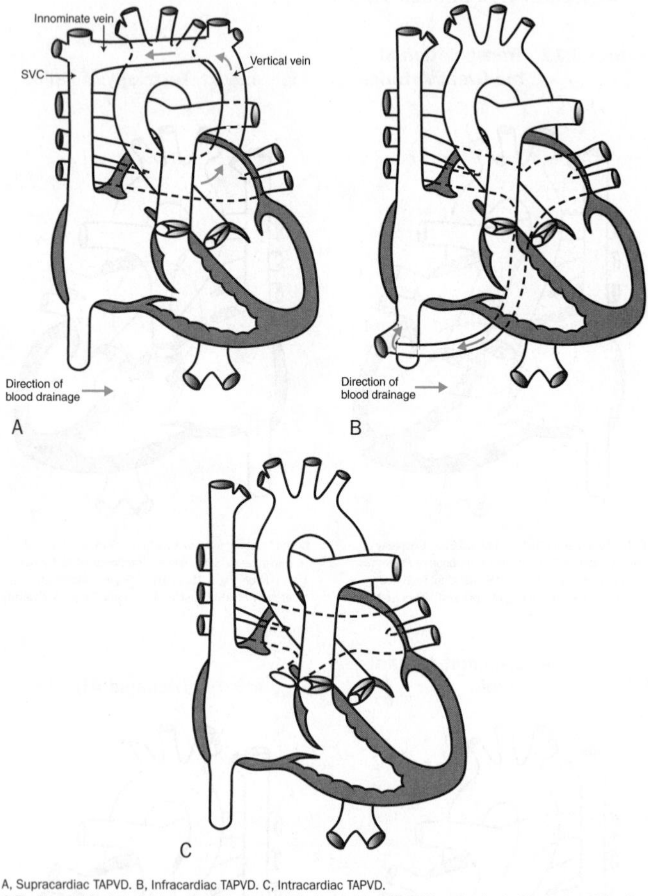

A, Supracardiac TAPVD. B, Infracardiac TAPVD. C, Intracardiac TAPVD.
© The Hospital for Sick Children, 2003. Courtesy of *The Hospital for Sick Children Handbook of Pediatrics*, 10th edition, Fig 4.26, p. 105. (Original modified/created by SickKids using Mullins and Mayer software).

TETRALOGY SPELLS (TET SPELLS)

- Tet spells: due to worsening RVOTO with ↓ pulmonary blood flow, more R→L shunting across VSD
- Clinical presentation: worsening cyanosis, quieter murmur, hyperpnea; can lead to loss of consciousness, seizures, stroke
- Should be recognized immediately and treated quickly

Acute Management of Tet Spells

1. ABCs and supplemental O_2 (see pp. 5–9)
2. Knee to chest position: ↑SVR, promotes L→R shunting across VSD
3. Morphine: ↓ hyperpnea and agitation
4. Propranolol or esmolol: ↓ dynamic subpulmonary stenosis
5. Phenylephrine or ketamine: ↑SVR, promotes L→R shunting across VSD and ↑ pulmonary blood flow
6. When no response to medical therapy, emergent intervention includes transcatheter stenting of outflow tract/PDA or surgical placement of shunt

EBSTEIN ANOMALY

Pathophysiology

* TV displaced downward into RV, with septal leaflet adherent to interventricular septum and portion of RV being "atrialized" (Figure 9.17)
* TV has variable degree of regurgitation
* May be anatomic or functional pulmonary stenosis/atresia
* ASD may shunt R→L

Figure 9.17 Ebstein Anomaly

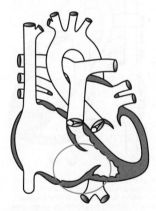

© The Hospital for Sick Children, 2003. Courtesy of
The Hospital for Sick Children Handbook of Pediatrics,
10th edition, Fig 4.17, p. 100. (Original modified/
created by SickKids using Mullins and Mayer software).

Clinical Findings

* Physical examination: cyanosis at birth (high PVR); as PVR drops, ↑ pulmonary flow, ↓ cyanosis, normal S_1, widely split S_2, 2/6–3/6 pansystolic murmur at LLSB (TR), S_3/S_4
* CXR: wall-to-wall heart due to dilated RA and severe TR
* ECG: RAE, RBBB, first-degree AV block (40%), WPW in 20% of patients with Ebstein

Acute Management

- PGEs (0.01–0.1 mcg/kg/min) if severely cyanotic at birth
- With adequate pulmonary blood flow, patients may be weaned from PGEs
- Mild cases may require no intervention
- Surgical intervention on TV is technically challenging with suboptimal results

CONGENITAL HEART DISEASE PRESENTING WITH CARDIOGENIC SHOCK

- Cardiogenic shock typically caused by obstructive lesions on left side of heart (Table 9.10 and Figure 9.18)

Figure 9.18 **Hypoplastic Left Heart Syndrome**

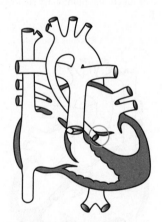

© The Hospital for Sick Children, 2003. Courtesy of
The Hospital for Sick Children Handbook of Pediatrics,
10th edition, Fig 4.18, p. 101. (Original modified/
created by SickKids using Mullins and Mayer software).

SINGLE VENTRICLE PALLIATION

Step 1

- Norwood procedure (see Cardiac Surgical Procedures, p. 176) goal is to establish reliable but restricted pulmonary blood flow, systemic cardiac output, unrestricted systemic–venous and pulmonary–venous mixing
- Saturations: 75–85%

Table 9.10 Congenital Left Heart Obstructive Lesions

Characteristics	CoA	Aortic Stenosis	HLHS
Epidemiology	Turner syndrome: 30% have CoA	Valvular (70%), subvalvular (25%), supravalvular (5%)	
Structural abnormalities	Discrete narrowing of aortic arch at level of PDA	· Valvular AS due to thickened, dysplastic AoV · Subvalvular AS due to muscle or membrane	· MV, LV, AoV are small; functions like single ventricle physiology · AoV or MV can be stenotic or atretic · Aortic arch is hypoplastic (see Figure 9.18)
Pathophysiology	Pressure load on LV; if severe can lead to LV dysfunction; descending aorta may be supplied via PDA; as PDA closes—cardiogenic shock	Pressure load on LV; if severe can lead to LV dysfunction; in neonatal critical AS, systemic blood flow supplied via PDA; as PDA closes—cardiogenic shock	Fully saturated blood from LA mixes with venous blood from RA, is ejected out RV to PA, and through PDA to body; as PDA closes, ↓ systemic perfusion
Associated lesions	Hypoplasia of transverse arch, VSD, bicuspid AoV (85%)	Supravalvular AS may be associated with Williams syndrome	MV or AoV stenosis or atresia, hypoplastic aortic arch
Clinical features	Gradient between upper and lower extremities; systolic murmur at LUSB border radiating to back; weak/absent femoral pulses; gallop rhythm if CHF	Can be asymptomatic; exercise intolerance, normal S_1, narrow S_2, 2/6–4/6 SEM at RUSB ± thrill that radiates to carotids, CHF if severe and ↓ heart function	Normal S_1, single loud S_2, usually no murmur, poor perfusion, weak pulses
CXR findings	Cardiomegaly, rib notching (in older children), "3 sign" (indentation in aorta)	Dilated aorta, cardiomegaly, pulmonary edema if severe CHF	Moderate cardiomegaly, ↑ pulmonary vascular markings
ECG findings	RVH in neonates (can be normal); older children may have LVH	LVH ± strain, coronary ischemia if obstruction severe and function poor	RAD, RVH, poor left-sided forces (i.e., no Q wave in V_6, small QRS voltages in lateral precordial leads)
Treatment	If in shock, ABCs, resuscitation; in neonates, can use PGEs to keep PDA open; surgery in neonates or balloon dilation ± stents in older children	If cardiogenic shock, ABCs, resuscitation; in neonates, PGEs; AoV balloon dilation or surgical repair/replacement	ABCs, resuscitation, PGE infusion, single ventricle palliation
Long-term complications	Recurrent/residual CoA, hypertension, aortic aneurysms	If severe LVOTO, risk of sudden death; recurrent stenosis or insufficiency	See Single Ventricle Palliation, p. 162–164

© The Hospital for Sick Children, 2009. New artwork created by The Hospital for Sick Children for *The Hospital for Sick Children Handbook of Pediatrics*, 11th edition.

Cardiology

9

163

Step 2

- Bidirectional cavopulmonary shunt (Glenn procedure) (see Cardiac Surgical Procedures, p. 176) and ligation of BT shunt; done at 4–6 mo
- Saturations: 80–85%
- If bilateral SVCs, left SVC anastomosed to LPA—increased risk of thrombus formation in pulmonary artery segment between the two SVCs

Step 3

- Fontan procedure (see Cardiac Surgical Procedures, p. 176); done at 2–4 yr
- Saturations: >90%
- Long-term complications: rhythm disturbances, thromboembolic complications, ↓ cardiac function, valve regurgitation, protein-losing enteropathy

CONGENITAL HEART DISEASE PRESENTING WITH CONGESTIVE HEART FAILURE

- See Table 9.11 and Figures 9.19 through 9.23

Figure 9.19 Atrial Septal Defect

Figure 9.20 Ventricular Septal Defect

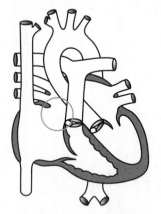

© The Hospital for Sick Children, 2003. Courtesy of *The Hospital for Sick Children Handbook of Pediatrics*, 10th edition, Fig 4.11, p. 97. (Original modified/created by SickKids using Mullins and Mayer software).

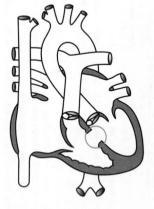

© The Hospital for Sick Children, 2003. Courtesy of *The Hospital for Sick Children Handbook of Pediatrics*, 10th edition, Fig 4.13, p. 97. (Original modified/created by SickKids using Mullins and Mayer software).

Table 9.11

Congenital Lesions Causing Congestive Heart Failure

Characteristics	ASD (see Figures 9.19, 9.22)	VSD (see Figure 9.20)	AVSD (see Figure 9.21)	PDA (see Figure 9.23)
Epidemiology		Most common CHD	25% of T21 have AVSD	
Structural abnormalities	· Secundum (50–70%) · Primum (15%) · Sinus venosus (10%)	· Perimembranous (70%) · Outlet (5%) · Inlet (5%) · Muscular (5–20%)	· Complete: single "common" AV valve · Partial: 2 separate orifices	· Arterial duct between descending aorta and LPA (most common)
Pathophysiology	· Secundum: defect near PFO · Sinus venosus: defect in upper atrial septum · Primum: defect in inferior atrial septum · L→R shunt causing RV volume overload	· L→R shunting between ventricles · Degree of shunt depends on size of VSD · Volume overload to left-sided structures and pulmonary vasculature	· L→R shunting between atria or ventricles; often large ASD and VSD · Primum ASD along spectrum of AVSD · Causes volume overload · Leads to pulmonary hypertension	· L→R shunting; degree of shunting depends on size of PDA and pressure difference between aorta and PA
Associated lesions	· Sinus venosus ASD associated with anomalous pulmonary veins · VSD		· TOF · DORV · Right or left isomerism	

Clinical features	· Asymptomatic
	· Soft SEM at upper left sternal border
	· Widely fixed split S_2
		· Depends on size
		· Small: pansystolic murmur ± thrill
		· Moderate/large
		  · CHF
		  · Cyanosis
		  · Pulmonary hypertension
			· Signs of CHF
			· Pansystolic murmur (due to VSD or valvular regurgitation)
				· Bounding pulses
				· Wide pulse pressure
				· Normal S_1
				· Loud S_2
				· Systolic murmur in neonates
				· Continuous murmur in older children, if small-moderate

(continued)

Cardiology

9

Table 9.11 Congenital Lesions Causing Congestive Heart Failure (continued)

Characteristics	ASD (see Figures 9.19, 9.22)	VSD (see Figure 9.20)	AVSD (see Figure 9.21)	PDA (see Figure 9.23)
CXR findings	· Can be normal · Mild cardiomegaly · Enlarged RA and RV · Increased pulmonary blood flow	· Cardiomegaly · Increased pulmonary blood flow	· Cardiomegaly · Increased pulmonary blood flow	· Mild cardiomegaly · Increased pulmonary blood flow
ECG findings	· Incomplete RBBB in V_1, II, III, aVF, RVH, RAD	· Can be normal · LAE · LVH	· Superior QRS axis · Long PR interval · RVH/LVH	· Normal · With larger PDA: can have LAE, LVH, RVH
Treatment	· If no CHF, follow for closure · Small-moderate: can have closure in cath lab · Large or sinus venosus ASDs: need surgery	· 40% perimembranous and 80% muscular VSDs close by 2 yr · Treat CHF · Surgical/device closure at 4–6 mo, earlier if refractory CHF	· Treat CHF · Should be repaired by 6 mo	· Treat CHF · Follow for closure · If small/moderate: transcatheter device closure · If large or symptomatic in neonates: surgical ligation
Long-term complications	· Atrial arrhythmia · Pulmonary hypertension (occurring at age 20–30s)	· Residual VSD · Postoperative heart block	· Pulmonary hypertension · Valvular regurgitation or stenosis	· Pulmonary hypertension if very large

© The Hospital for Sick Children, 2009. New artwork created by The Hospital for Sick Children for *The Hospital for Sick Children Handbook of Pediatrics*, 11th edition.

Figure 9.21 **Atrioventricular Septal Defect**

Figure 9.22 **Sinus Venosus Atrial Septal Defect**

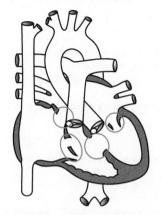

© The Hospital for Sick Children, 2003. Courtesy of
The Hospital for Sick Children Handbook of Pediatrics,
10th edition, Fig 4.14, p. 97. (Original modified/
created by SickKids using Mullins and Mayer software).

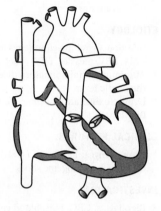

© The Hospital for Sick Children, 2003. Courtesy of
The Hospital for Sick Children Handbook of Pediatrics,
10th edition, Fig 4.12, p. 97. (Original modified/
created by SickKids using Mullins and Mayer software).

Figure 9.23 **Patent Ductus Arteriosus**

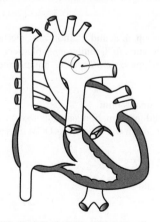

© The Hospital for Sick Children, 2003. Courtesy of
The Hospital for Sick Children Handbook of Pediatrics,
10th edition, Fig 4.15, p. 98. (Original modified/
created by SickKids using Mullins and Mayer software).

MYOCARDITIS

- Characterized by inflammatory changes in myocardium and necrosis of adjacent myocytes

ETIOLOGY

- Infectious: viral infection (coxsackievirus, adenovirus, echovirus, CMV, EBV, measles, HIV); bacterial, fungal, protozoal
- Autoimmune/inflammatory diseases: lupus, Kawasaki disease, rheumatic fever
- Drugs/toxins: anthracylines, lead, allergic drug hypersensitivity reaction

CLINICAL FEATURES

- Fever, tachycardia, signs of CHF, exercise intolerance, palpitations, chest pain, cardiogenic shock

INVESTIGATION

- Blood tests: CBC, ESR, blood culture, troponins, CK-MB, viral studies
- ECG: tachycardia, low QRS voltage, ST-T wave changes, heart block, arrhythmias
- CXR: cardiomegaly, ↑ pulmonary vascular markings
- Echocardiogram: decreased cardiac function, chamber enlargement, AV valve regurgitation, thrombus, pericardial effusion
- Endomyocardial biopsy: used in some centers to direct treatment

MANAGEMENT

- Acute: ABCs (see pp. 5, 8, and 9), inotropes, mechanical support
- Intermediate: diuretics, ACE inhibitors, β-blockers
- Controversial therapies: steroids, IVIG, immunotherapy

PROGNOSIS

- Outcomes for neonates poor
- Patients with mild inflammation generally recover completely
- One third to one fourth will progress to DCM requiring transplantation

CARDIOMYOPATHIES

- See Tables 9.12 and 9.13

Table 9.12	Cardiomyopathies in Children		
Characteristics	HCM	DCM	RCM
Epidemiology	AD (30–60%); mutations in muscle proteins; can be due to metabolic diseases or infant of diabetic mother	60% idiopathic, 30% familial; secondary to myocarditis, toxins, myopathy, arrhythmia, autoimmune diseases, myopathies (see Table 9.13)	Rare in children; can be idiopathic or secondary to systemic disease (e.g., scleroderma, sarcoidosis, metabolic diseases, radiation)
Structural abnormalities	Hypertrophied ventricular septum leading to LVOTO	Dilated, poorly contractile ventricle	Dilated atrium
Pathophysiology	Stiff hypertrophied ventricle that does not fill well; LVOTO due to subAS; subendocardial ischemia due to severe hypertrophy	Dilated, poorly contractile ventricle leads to congestion and poor systemic perfusion	Noncompliant ventricle results in poor filling
Associated lesions	LVOTO, mitral insufficiency		
Clinical features	Sudden death can be initial presentation; exercise intolerance, syncope, chest pain, or dyspnea on exertion, SEM at left sternal border	Dyspnea, orthopnea, poor exercise tolerance, 90% present with CHF, gallop, hepatomegaly	Dyspnea, orthopnea, poor exercise tolerance, CHF, gallop, sudden death, arrhythmia
CXR findings	LVE	Cardiomegaly, ↑ pulmonary blood flow	Dilated atria, ↑ pulmonary vascular markings
ECG findings	LVH, ST-T wave changes, abnormal Q waves	Sinus tachycardia, nonspecific ST changes, low voltage, LVH	RAE/LAE, arrhythmia
Treatment	Activity restriction; β-blockers; myectomy for severe LVOTO, implantable defibrillator	Management of CHF (diuretics, β-blockers, ACE inhibitors), transplantation if end-stage	Manage CHF, arrhythmia; transplantation if end-stage
Long-term complications	Sudden death, worsening LVOTO	Arrhythmia, sudden death	Arrhythmia, sudden death

© The Hospital for Sick Children, 2009. New artwork created by The Hospital for Sick Children for *The Hospital for Sick Children Handbook of Pediatrics*, 11th edition.

Table 9.13	Causes of Dilated Cardiomyopathy
Infectious	Viral: coxsackievirus, adenovirus, echovirus, EBV, CMV, HIV Bacterial: diphtheria, *Mycoplasma*, meningococcus Fungal: histoplasmosis, coccidioidomycosis Parasites: Chagas disease, toxoplasmosis
Metabolic	Lysosomal storage disease, mitochondrial disease
Endocrine	Hyperthyroidism, pheochromocytoma
Autoimmune	Lupus, scleroderma, rheumatic fever
Neuromuscular/myopathic	Muscular/myotonic dystrophy, Friedreich ataxia
Hematologic	Anemia, sickle cell anemia, beta thalassemia
Toxin induced	Anthracyclines, radiation, cyclophosphamide, chloroquine, hemosiderosis
Other	Chronic tachyarrhythmia, coronary artery abnormality/chronic ischemia

Adapted from Allen HD, Adams FH, Moss AJ. *Moss and Adams' Heart Disease in Infants, Children and Adolescents: Including the Fetus and Young Adults.* 6th ed. Philadelphia, Pa: Lippincott Williams and Wilkins; 2001; and from Behrman RE, Kliegman RM, Jenson HB. *Nelson Textbook of Pediatrics.* 17th ed. Philadelphia, Pa: Saunders; 2004:1572–1576.

INITIAL INVESTIGATIONS

- Echocardiogram: functional or structural abnormalities, hemodynamic parameters
- ECG: ischemia, hypertrophy, chamber enlargement
- Holter: arrhythmias, ischemia
- GXT: arrhythmias, ischemia, functional capacity
- Blood tests: CBC, troponins, CK-MB, blood gas, TSH, carnitine, amino acids, lactate, trace metals, organic acids, as indicated
- Endomyocardial biopsy/skeletal muscle biopsy may be considered
- For treatment options, see Table 9.12

INFECTIVE ENDOCARDITIS

ETIOLOGY

- Usually occurs in association with structural heart disease
- Risk factors: indwelling lines, IV drug use, immunocompromised patients
- Organisms: viridans streptococci (most common), *Staphylococcus*, HACEK (*Haemophilus* species, *Actinobacillus actinomycetemcomitans, Cardiobacterium hominis, Eikenella corrodens, Kingella* species); gram-negative organisms and fungi uncommon unless neonate, immunocompromised, or IV drug user

CLINICAL FEATURES

- Symptoms: fever, myalgia, arthralgia, malaise
- Signs: new heart murmur or change in murmur, CHF, embolic phenomena (petechiae, hepatosplenomegaly, splinter hemorrhages, Janeway lesions, Osler nodes, pulmonary emboli)

INVESTIGATIONS

- Blood tests: three successive separate blood cultures, CBC, ESR, CRP, creatinine, urea
- Echocardiogram: underlying structural disease, vegetations, cardiac function; transthoracic echocardiogram adequate in children and may not need transesophageal echocardiogram; negative findings on echocardiogram do *not* rule out endocarditis

DIAGNOSIS

- Duke criteria (Box 9.2)

Box 9.2   Modified Duke Criteria for the Diagnosis of Infective Endocarditis

Major Criteria
- Blood culture positive for microorganism typical for IE from two separate cultures, or single culture positive for *Coxiella burnetii,* or antiphase 1 IgG antibody titer >1:800
- Evidence of endocardial involvement on echocardiogram

Minor Criteria
- Predisposing heart condition or IV drug use
- Fever
- Vascular phenomenon: major arterial emboli, septic pulmonary infarcts, mycotic aneurysm, intracranial hemorrhage, conjunctival hemorrhage, Janeway lesion
- Immunologic phenomenon: glomerulonephritis, Osler nodes, Roth spots, rheumatoid factor
- Microbiologic evidence: positive blood culture that does not meet major criteria or serologic evidence of active infection with organism consistent with IE

Definite IE

Pathologic Criteria
- Microorganisms demonstrated by culture or histologic examination of vegetation, vegetation that has embolized, or intracardiac abscess

OR
- Pathologic lesions; vegetation or intracardiac abscess confirmed by histologic examination showing active IE

Clinical Criteria
- 2 major criteria, OR
- 1 major and 3 minor criteria, OR
- 5 minor criteria

Possible IE
- 1 major and 1 minor criterion, OR
- 3 minor criteria

Rejected
- Firm alternative diagnosis, OR
- Resolution of symptoms with antibiotic therapy for <4 d, OR
- No pathologic evidence of IE at surgery or autopsy with antibiotic therapy for <4 d, OR
- Does not meet criteria for possible IE

With permission from the American Heart Association.

MANAGEMENT

- Acute management: antibiotics, treatment of CHF, cardiac surgery if severe valvular regurgitation, aortic root abscess, large vegetation, or embolic phenomena
- Long-term management: management of residual lesions or sequelae
- For antibiotic prophylaxis guidelines for bacterial endocarditis, see p. 989

ACUTE RHEUMATIC FEVER

- Due to autoimmune sequelae of GAS pharyngitis
- Diagnosis based on Jones criteria (Table 9.14)

Table 9.14	Revised Jones Criteria
Major manifestations	Carditis, polyarthritis, chorea, erythema marginatum, subcutaneous nodules
Minor manifestations	Arthralgia, fever, elevated ESR or CRP, prolonged PR interval on ECG
Evidence of antecedent GAS infection	Positive throat culture or rapid antigen test for GAS, raised or rising streptococcal antibody titer
2 major OR 1 major and 2 minor manifestations must be present, plus evidence of antecedent GAS infection	
Recurrent episodes require only 1 major OR several minor manifestations, plus evidence of antecedent GAS infection	

From Special Writing Group of the Committee on Rheumatic Fever, Endocarditis, and Kawasaki Disease of the Council on Cardiovascular Disease in the Young of the American Heart Association. Guidelines for the diagnosis of rheumatic fever, Jones Criteria, 1992 update. *JAMA.* 1992;268:2070.

INVESTIGATIONS

- Blood tests: CBC, ESR, antistreptolysin O titer
- ECG: prolonged PR interval
- Echocardiogram: function, pericardial effusion, valvular regurgitation

MANAGEMENT

- Acute (see Table 9.15)
- Long-term (see Table 9.16)

SYNCOPE

- Common in childhood, usually benign
- See Tables 9.17 and 9.18 for classification and etiology

Table 9.15   Management of Acute Rheumatic Fever

General	· Bed rest and monitor for carditis · If carditis, gradual ambulation over period of at least 4 wk
Immediate treatment of pharyngitis	· Penicillin VK 125–300 mg PO tid–qid for 10 d · Erythromycin 30–50 mg/kg/d ÷qid for 10 days (if penicillin allergy)
Continued antibiotic prophylaxis	· Penicillin G IM every 4 wk (not available in Canada) · Penicillin VK 125–300 mg PO bid · Erythromycin 30–50 mg/kg/d ÷qid (if penicillin allergy)
Anti-inflammatory therapy	· ASA 100 mg/kg/d ÷qid for 2 wk, then 60–70 mg/kg/d for 3–6 wk · Prednisone 1–2 mg/kg/d for 2–3 wk followed by taper if carditis present
Heart failure therapy	· Diuretics and/or ACE inhibitors in patients with severe symptoms · May need valve repair or replacement if severe/chronic rheumatic valve disease
Chorea	· Consider neuroleptics, benzodiazepines, antiepileptics if severe · Usually considered self-limiting and benign

© The Hospital for Sick Children, 2009. New artwork created by The Hospital for Sick Children for *The Hospital for Sick Children Handbook of Pediatrics*, 11th edition.

Table 9.16   Duration of Prophylaxis for People Who Have Had Acute Rheumatic Fever: Recommendations of the American Heart Association

Category	Duration
Rheumatic fever without carditis	5 yr or until 21 yr of age, whichever is longer
Rheumatic fever with carditis but without residual heart disease	10 yr or well into adulthood, whichever is longer
Rheumatic fever with carditis and residual heart disease	At least 10 yr since last episode and at least until 40 yr of age, sometimes lifelong

From Dajani A, Taubert K, Ferrieri P, Peter G, Shulman S, and Committee on Rheumatic Fever, Endocarditis and Kawasaki Disease of the Council on Cardiovascular Disease in the Young, and American Heart Association. Treatment of acute streptococcal pharyngitis and prevention of rheumatic fever: a statement for health professionals. *Pediatrics*. 1995;96:758–764.

Table 9.17   Classification of Syncope

Neurally Mediated	Vasovagal, Orthostatic
Cardiovascular	Arrhythmia (LQTS, extreme tachycardia/bradycardia), obstructive (severe AS, PS, HOCM, pulmonary HTN), myocardial dysfunction (infarction, Kawasaki disease, coronary anomalies)
Noncardiovascular	Seizure, metabolic (hypoglycemia, electrolyte abnormality), psychogenic (hyperventilation)

From Mcleod KA. Syncope in childhood. *Arch Dis Child*. 2003;88:350–353. Adapted and reproduced with permission from the BMJ Publishing Group.

Table 9.18   Syncope in Childhood

	Vasovagal	Orthostatic	Cardiac
History	· Associated with fright, pain, heat, prolonged standing, crowding · Prodrome of dizziness, pallor, diaphoresis, hyperventilation · Loss of consciousness usually <1 min, with gradual awakening	· Usually occurs on changing position · May have history of prolonged bed rest, dehydration, medications (e.g., antihypertensives, vasodilators)	· Exercise induced · Syncope when supine · Associated chest pain · Family history of sudden death · History of structural heart disease
Physical findings	· Normal	· Orthostatic BP and HR (record BP and HR when supine, and again after standing for 5–10 min) · 10–15 mm Hg drop is abnormal, especially if HR does not increase	Focused cardiac examination (see pp. 143–144)
Investigations to consider	· No investigations necessary	· Electrolytes, fasting blood glucose · Orthostatic BP and HR · EEG if suspect seizure	ECG, GXT, 24-h Holter monitor, cardiac event recorder, echocardiogram
Management	· Reassurance · Cross legs if prodromal signs · Encourage fluids · Frequent severe episodes despite simple measures, consider medication (β-blocker, fludrocortisone)	· Stand up slowly · Encourage fluids, ↑ salt in diet	Etiology specific

CHROMOSOMAL ABNORMALITIES AND SYNDROMES ASSOCIATED WITH CARDIAC DISEASE

- See Tables 9.19 and 9.20

Table 9.19	Chromosomal Abnormalities Associated With Congenital Heart Disease	
Chromosomal Abnormality	**% Risk of Heart Disease**	**Associated Lesion(s)**
Trisomy 13	90	VSD, ASD, PDA
Trisomy 18	95	VSD, DORV, PDA
Trisomy 21	40	AVSD, VSD, ASD, TOF
Tetrasomy 22 (cat-eye)	40	TAPVR, TOF, VSD
Deletion 4p	50	ASD, VSD, PDA
Deletion 5p (cri du chat syndrome)	30	VSD, ASD, PDA
Deletion 22q (various)	85	Conotruncal anomalies
45 XO (Turner syndrome)	15	CoA
47 XXY (Klinefelter syndrome)	50	VSD, PDA, MVP, TOF
Fragile X	50–75	MVP (in older patients)

Adapted from Freedom RM, Benson LN, Smallhorn JF, eds. *Neonatal Heart Disease*. New York, NY: Springer-Verlag; 1992:8. With kind permission of Springer Science and Business Media.

Table 9.20	Syndromes Associated With Congenital Heart Disease	
Syndrome	**% Risk of Heart Disease**	**Associated Lesion(s)**
Alagille	–	Peripheral PS
Apert	10	VSD, TOF
Asplenia/polysplenia	Almost 100	AVSD, TGA, TAPVR
CHARGE	60–70	TOF, AVSD, DORV, VSD
Crouzon disease	–	PDA, CoA
Cutis laxa	–	PS, pulmonary hypertension
DiGeorge (deletion 22q)	85	Conotruncal anomalies
Ehlers-Danlos (some types)	50	MVP, dilated aortic root
Ellis-van Creveld	50–60	Common atrium, ASD
Goldenhar	15	TOF, VSD

(continued)

Table 9.20	Syndromes Associated With Congenital Heart Disease *(continued)*	
Syndrome	**% Risk of Heart Disease**	**Associated Lesion(s)**
Holt-Oram	100	ASD, VSD, AV block
Hurler/Hunter/other MPS	–	Valvular insufficiency
Kartagener	100	Dextrocardia
LEOPARD	50	PS
Marfan	60–80	MVP, AI, dilated aortic root
Noonan	50	PS
Osteogenesis imperfecta	5–10	Aortic incompetence
Rubinstein-Taybi	–	VSD
Smith-Lemli-Opitz	–	VSD, PDA
TAR	20	TOF, ASD
Tuberous sclerosis	30	Cardiac rhabdomyoma
VATER/VACTERL	>50	VSD, TOF, ASD, PDA
Williams (deletion 7q)	90–100	AS, PS, renal stenosis

Adapted from Freedom RM, Benson LN, Smallhorn JF, eds. *Neonatal Heart Disease*. New York, NY: Springer-Verlag; 1992:8. With kind permission of Springer Science and Business Media.

9

CARDIAC SURGICAL PROCEDURES

- Staged surgical palliation for single ventricle physiology:
  - Norwood (Stage 1): aortic arch reconstruction, atrial septectomy, and shunt to the disconnected PAs (Figure 9.24)
  - Hybrid (alternative Stage 1): bilateral pulmonary artery bands and ductal stenting
  - Bidirectional cavopulmonary connection (Glenn anastomosis; Stage 2): SVC to PA connection (Figure 9.25)
  - Fontan (Stage 3): IVC-to-PA connection (RA to PA anastomosis, extracardiac conduit or lateral tunnel) ± fenestration (Figure 9.26)
- Blalock-Hanlon: surgical atrial septectomy
- BT shunt (modified): polyethylene terephthalate (Dacron) shunt from innominate artery to PA
- Damus-Kaye-Stansel: MPA transection near bifurcation with end-to-side proximal MPA anastomosis to aorta (part of Norwood stage I)
- Jatene: arterial switch for correction of complete TGA
- Konno: aortic root enlargement
- Mustard: atrial baffle of systemic veins for palliation of complete TGA; replaced by Jatene arterial switch

Figure 9.24 **Norwood Procedure**

Figure 9.25 **Bidirectional Cavopulmonary Connection**

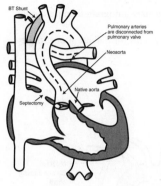

© The Hospital for Sick Children, 2003. Courtesy of *The Hospital for Sick Children Handbook of Pediatrics*, 10th edition, Fig 4.20, p. 101. (Original modified/ created by SickKids using Mullins and Mayer software).

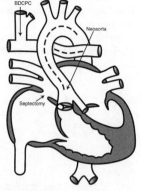

© The Hospital for Sick Children, 2003. Courtesy of *The Hospital for Sick Children Handbook of Pediatrics*, 10th edition, Fig 4.21, p. 101. (Original modified/ created by SickKids using Mullins and Mayer software).

Figure 9.26 **Fontan Procedure**

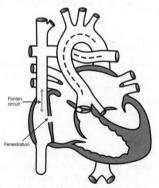

© The Hospital for Sick Children, 2003. Courtesy of *The Hospital for Sick Children Handbook of Pediatrics*, 10th edition, Fig 4.19, p. 101. (Original modified/ created by SickKids using Mullins and Mayer software).

Cardiology

9

- Rashkind: transcatheter balloon atrial septostomy
- Rastelli operation: placement of valved conduit-graft between RV and PA and intraventricular tunnel to direct LV blood to the aorta via VSD (for TGA with VSD and PS)
- Ross: AoV replacement with pulmonary autograft, then pulmonary homograft
- Senning: atrial baffle of pulmonary veins for palliation of complete TGA; replaced by Jatene switch
- See Figure 9.27 for shunts

Figure 9.27 Cardiac Shunts

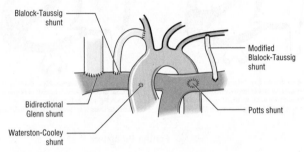

From The Johns Hopkins Hospital. In: Robertson J, Shilkofski N, eds. *The Harriet Lane Handbook.* 17th ed. Philadelphia, Pa: Mosby; 2005:195.

FURTHER READING

Allen HD, Adams FH, Moss AJ. *Moss & Adams' Heart Disease in Infants, Children and Adolescents: Including the Fetus and Young Adults.* 6th ed. Philadelphia, Pa: Lippincott Williams and Wilkins; 2001.

Park MK. *Pediatric Cardiology for Practitioners.* 4th ed. St. Louis, Mo: Mosby; 2002.

USEFUL WEB SITES

American College of Cardiology. Available at: www.acc.org.
American Heart Association. Available at: www.americanheart.org.
Canadian Cardiovascular Society. Available at: www.ccs.ca.
Heart and Stroke Foundation Canada. Available at: www.heartandstroke.ca.
The Nevil Thomas Adult Congenital Heart Library. Available at: www.achd-library.com.
Pediheart. Available at: www.pediheart.org.

Chapter 10 Child Maltreatment

Sharon Naymark
Emma Cory

Chapter 10 Child Maltreatment

COMMON ABBREVIATIONS

CBC	complete blood cell count
INR	international normalized ratio
NAI	nonaccidental injury
PTT	partial thromboplastin time
STI	sexually transmitted infection

BACKGROUND

INDICATORS/RED FLAGS

- Consider child maltreatment whenever red flags are present:
  - Injury not consistent with history provided and/or age/developmental stage of child
  - Inconsistent or changing history
  - Delay in seeking medical attention
  - Multiple injuries or injuries of different ages
  - Evidence of neglect or failure to thrive

REPORTING

- Any person who has reason to suspect child abuse or neglect has a legal obligation to report this information to the local child welfare agency
- Reports should be made directly and should not be delegated to another individual
- Child welfare agency will determine need for police involvement
- Individuals have ongoing duty to report to child welfare agency if new concerns become apparent

DOCUMENTATION

- Chart can be used for legal purposes; write legibly, include time and date
- Include drawings, measurements, body diagrams; consider photographs (consent required)

PHYSICAL ABUSE

HISTORY

- Thorough history of events leading to injury (location, time, response of child/caregiver, progression of symptoms), developmental stage of child
- Family or personal history of bleeding disorders or predisposition to fractures

PHYSICAL EXAMINATION

- Growth variables (weight, height, head circumference) and percentiles
- Thorough examination with focus on skin (completely undress), neurologic features (fontanelle, fundi), mouth (frenulum), abdomen, and musculoskeletal (palpation for tenderness, swelling)

MEDICAL EVALUATION

- Laboratory investigations: CBC, INR/PTT for bruising; consider extended coagulation workup and urine for organic acids (to rule out glutaric aciduria) for intracranial hemorrhage/retinal hemorrhages
- Skeletal survey (see p. 242) for all children <2 yr with concerns of abuse; children >2 yr based on clinical suspicion; *no* role for babygram (1–2 views of entire body)
- Ophthalmology: dilated fundoscopic examination to assess for retinal hemorrhages
- Neuroimaging: CT and/or MRI
- Consider bone scan if equivocal findings on initial skeletal survey or if strong suspicion of skeletal injury with normal skeletal survey
- Consider follow-up skeletal survey after 10–14 d in certain high-risk cases

INJURY PATTERNS

Bruising

- Areas with underlying bone bruise more easily (e.g., forehead, shins), unlike areas with more soft tissue (e.g., cheeks, buttocks)
- Age/development level: bruising in nonambulatory children unusual
- Location: less common in well-cushioned areas (cheeks, buttocks, back) and ears
- Pattern: object outlines usually indicate inflicted injury (loop marks, handprints)
- Dating of bruises: age of bruises cannot be reliably estimated based on color

Fractures

- Correlate fracture with mechanism of injury (e.g., spiral fractures imply a twisting mechanism, transverse fractures imply a bending force or direct impact)
- Age/development level: fractures in nonambulatory children unusual
- Location: metaphysis, rib, vertebra, scapula, sternum highly suspicious for NAI (Figures 10.1 and 10.2)
- Pattern: multiple, complex skull fractures may suggest NAI
- Age of injury: fractures of different ages and delay in seeking treatment raise concerns
- Rib fractures: subtle in the acute form; more obvious with healing; typical mechanism is anterior–posterior compression of rib cage during forceful squeezing or shaking (see Figure 10.1)

- Metaphyseal fractures: also known as classic metaphyseal lesion, corner fracture, bucket-handle fracture; subtle in the acute form; more obvious with healing; caused by shearing of new bone formation from ends of long bones; typical mechanism is forceful tug or twist of a limb or flailing of limbs during shaking of infant (see Figure 10.2)

Figure 10.1 Mechanism and Location of Rib Fractures

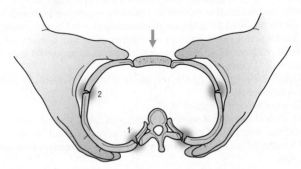

Often identified posteriorly (1) or laterally (2).

Figure 10.2 Mechanism of Metaphyseal Fractures

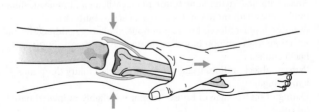

Shaken Baby Syndrome
- Forceful shaking results in rapid acceleration and deceleration of the head with associated flailing of the limbs and compression of the rib cage
- Presentation: variable and often nonspecific symptoms—irritability, lethargy, crying, vomiting, poor feeding, breathing problems, respiratory arrest, seizures, death; most often no or few external signs of trauma
- Diagnosis: brain injury, intracranial hemorrhages, retinal hemorrhages, rib/skull/metaphyseal fractures

Burns

- Injury depends on temperature, mechanism, duration of exposure, presence of clothing, first aid applied (see Chapter 33)
- Age/developmental level: contact burns unusual in nonmobile infants
- Location: buttocks or feet in stocking distribution may indicate forced immersion
- Pattern: concerns should be raised when the pattern of burn(s) does not fit with the history provided

SEXUAL ABUSE

HISTORY

- Time/date of abuse, description of events, known information about perpetrator, vaginal or anal bleeding/pain, discharge, past history (medical, gynecologic), psychological (current suicidal thoughts or behavioral changes)
- Forensic interview should be done by trained professional—in nonacute asymptomatic cases, examination can often be deferred until interviews completed by child welfare agency; acute assault or pain/bleeding/discharge requires immediate evaluation

PHYSICAL EXAMINATION

- General examination plus Tanner stage, external genital and anal examinations, hymen (configuration, rim, edges, injuries), other skin injuries

INVESTIGATIONS

- Consider swabs for STIs (gonorrhea, *Chlamydia, Trichomonas*): vaginal swabs in symptomatic prepubertal females vs. cervical swabs in any adolescent; vaginal swabs technically difficult; referral to experienced practitioner recommended; no role for speculum examination in prepubertal child
- Offer pregnancy test
- Consider HIV, hepatitis B, VDRL serologic tests
- Sexual assault evidence kit requires patient consent and police involvement; should be done within 72 h of assault

CLASSIFICATION OF GENITAL EXAMINATION FINDINGS

- Most examination findings are normal or nonspecific; this does not rule out abuse
- Findings seen in newborns or commonly seen in nonabused children:
  - Neither confirm nor discount a child's clear disclosure of abuse
  - Examples: genital redness, labial adhesions, hymenal bumps/notches, anal fissures or skin tags

- Indeterminate findings:
  - May be supportive of a child's clear disclosure of sexual abuse but should be interpreted with caution if child has not made a disclosure
  - Examples: genital herpes, genital warts
  - Often require referral to a child welfare agency for further evaluation
- Findings diagnostic of trauma and/or sexual contact:
  - Support a child's disclosure of abuse and are highly suggestive of abuse, even in the absence of a disclosure
  - Examples: acute laceration of the hymen, healed hymenal laceration, gonorrhea and *Chlamydia* outside the neonatal period, presence of sperm
  - Refer to child welfare agency

MANAGEMENT

- Discourage repeated questioning/examination of child
- STI prophylaxis (can be given in acute cases without swabs)
- Emergency contraception
- Consider hepatitis B immunization and immunoglobulin
- Consider HIV prophylaxis for high-risk cases: requires expert consultation, repeated HIV test in 3–6 mo

FURTHER READING

Adams J. Guidelines for medical care of children who may have been sexually abused. *J Pediatr Adolesc Gynecol.* 2007;20:163–172.

Dubowitz H. Preventing child neglect and physical abuse: a role for pediatricians. *Pediatr Rev.* 2002;23:191–196.

Canadian Paediatric Society. Joint statement on shaken baby syndrome. *Paediatrics Child Health* 2001;6:663-667. Reaffirmed 2005.

Kleinman PK. *Diagnostic Imaging of Child Abuse.* St. Louis, Mo: Mosby, Inc; 1998.

10

Chapter 11 Dentistry

Ereny Bassilious
Teresa D. Berger
Shonna L. Masse

Chapter 11 Dentistry

EARLY CHILDHOOD CARIES AND DENTAL CARE

EARLY CHILDHOOD CARIES

- Typically begins on maxillary incisors and first primary molars
- May appear as chalky white spots to brown or black holes in enamel
- Parents may not be aware of caries until tooth begins to discolor or enamel begins to "chip" away
- Risk factors: bottle feeding with any liquid other than water while being put to sleep, use of bottle as pacifier, breastfeeding on demand, not brushing teeth after feedings

RECOMMENDATIONS FOR DENTAL CARE

- Infants should not be put to sleep with bottle containing liquid with fermentable carbohydrates
- Encourage infants to drink from cup by first birthday
- Damp washcloth to wipe gums from birth until first tooth erupts, then use soft-bristled toothbrush 3 times/d
- First dental visit by first tooth eruption or first birthday
- Use pacifier for children who have need for nonnutritive sucking (easier to wean than thumb)
- Characteristics of appropriate pacifier: single piece plastic, vent holes on outside surface, appropriate size for age

TEETHING

- See Table 11.1
- See Figure 11.1
- Symptoms (e.g., irritability, drooling)
- Symptomatic treatment: cold teething rings, acetaminophen or ibuprofen as analgesic, if necessary
- Avoid teething gels because of risk of overdose, aspiration, methemoglobinemia

ODONTOGENIC INFECTIONS

- Most common is dental abscess: raised, soft, fluctuant, intraoral or extraoral swelling
- Risk of spreading and systemic involvement if untreated
- Immediate referral to dentist
- Consider admission and/or IV antibiotics (clindamycin) if:
  1. Periorbital or submandibular cellulitis
  2. Rapid progression of facial cellulitis
  3. Unwell child

Table 11.1	Chronology of Human Dentition			
Teeth	Eruption		Exfoliation	
	Maxillary	**Mandibular**	**Maxillary**	**Mandibular**
Primary teeth				
Central incisors	6–8 mo	5–7 mo	7–8 yr	6–7 yr
Lateral incisors	8–11 mo	7–10 mo	8–9 yr	7–8 yr
Canines	16–20 mo	16–20 mo	11–12 yr	9–11 yr
First molars	10–16 mo	10–16 mo	10–12 yr	10–12 yr
Second molars	20–30 mo	20–30 mo	10–12 yr	11–13 yr
Permanent teeth				
Central incisors	7–8 yr	6–7 yr		
Lateral incisors	8–9 yr	7–8 yr		
Canines	11–12 yr	9–11 yr		
First premolars	10–11 yr	10–12 yr		
Second premolars	10–12 yr	11–13 yr		
First molars	6–7 yr	6–7 yr		
Second molars	12–13 yr	12–13 yr		
Third molars	17–22 yr	17–22 yr		

Copyright © 2007 Elsevier. From Kliegman RM, Behrman RE, Jenson HB, Stanton BF, eds. *Nelson Textbook of Pediatrics*. 18th ed. Philadelphia, Pa: WB Saunders; 2007:47.

Figure 11.1 **Identification System for Primary and Permanent Teeth**

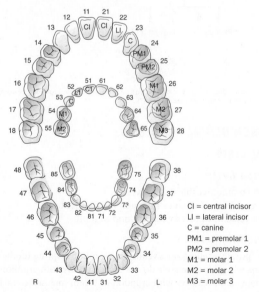

CI = central incisor
LI = lateral incisor
C = canine
PM1 = premolar 1
PM2 = premolar 2
M1 = molar 1
M2 = molar 2
M3 = molar 3

Adapted from the *Ontario Dental Association Fee Guide 2003–2007*, by permission of the Ontario Dental Association.

TREATMENT

- Antibiotics are effective at containing and reducing spreading of infection before definitive treatment (Figure 11.2)
- Tooth extraction is often treatment of choice after 1 dose of IV antibiotics or 2 doses of oral antibiotics

Figure 11.2 **Algorithm for Selecting Antimicrobial Therapy for Odontogenic Infections**

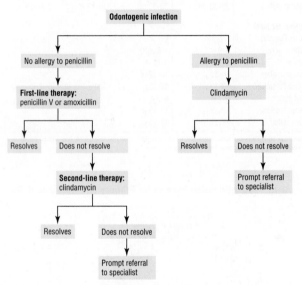

Adapted from Sandor GKB, Low DE, Judd PL, Davidson RJ. Antimicrobial treatment options in the management of odontogenic infections. *J Can Dent Assoc.* 1998;64(7).

COMMON DENTAL PROBLEMS

DENTAL CYSTS

Eruption Cyst

- Most common visible dental cyst
- Out-pouching of alveolus in region of erupting tooth
- Management: resolves with eruption of tooth

Eruption Hematoma

- Blue/purple swelling on alveolus in region of erupting tooth
- Forms when blood vessels do not recede upon tooth eruption
- Management: resolves with eruption of tooth; may see some bleeding with eruption

Mucocele

- *Small* fluid-filled vesicle; overlying mucosa is normal in color
- Occurs on lower lip, palate, or floor of mouth
- Due to severance/blockage of salivary duct and gland
- Management: surgical excision and removal of involved salivary gland

Ranula

- *Large*, soft, dome-shaped mucous-filled swelling on floor of mouth
- Due to severance/blockage of salivary gland duct
- Management: excision or marsupialization

ULCERS

Aphthous Ulcers

- Also known as canker sores
- Well-circumscribed, ulcerative lesions with white, necrotic base surrounded by red halo
- Occur on "unbound" mucosa (inside of cheeks, inside of lips)
- Etiology unclear; may be infectious
- Management: self-limiting, lesions heal within 10–14 d without scarring; symptomatic treatment: topical anesthetics such as mouth wash with lidocaine may help decrease pain

Acute Herpetic Gingivostomatitis

- Caused by HSV type 1
- Intraoral vesicular lesions on *any* mucosal surface
- Vesicles rupture, leaving painful ulcers
- Fiery red gingiva
- Symptoms: fever, cervical lymphadenopathy, malaise; headaches precede intraoral signs by 3–4 d

Management

- Self-limiting disease lasting 10–14 d
- Symptomatic treatment: soft, bland diet with extra fluids; acetaminophen for fever, pain
- Good oral hygiene imperative for healing
- Antibiotics contraindicated
- Consider antivirals only if patient is immunocompromised

Recurrent Herpes Labialis

- Painful recurrent vesicles on lips
- Triggers: stress, sunlight, trauma
- Management: symptomatic treatment

Traumatic Ulcers

- Due to accidental intraoral trauma, cheek biting, or after dental local anesthesia
- Management: symptomatic treatment; resolves in 10–14 d

Tight Frenulum (Tongue Tie)

- Can affect feeding and speech articulation but not language development
- Management: typically does not require treatment; surgical release of frenulum if feeding affected

Teeth Discoloration

- See Table 11.2

Table 11.2	Differential Diagnosis of Tooth Discoloration
Cause	**Description**
Decay/caries	Brown/black
Plaque accumulation	Yellow
Foods (tea/coffee, curry, berries, wine)	According to substance
Previous trauma	Yellow, gray, or brown
Exfoliation of teeth	Reddish (due to entrapment of vessels)
Liquid iron supplement	Black stain
Fluorosis	Porous, chalky white, brown
Illness, malnutrition, prematurity, birth trauma (forceps)	May cause hypocalcification—opaque white patches or horizontal lines
Tetracycline (during pregnancy or as infant—4 mo in utero until 7 yr)	Brown/yellow
Chromogenic bacteria	Black line stain around gingival margin of teeth
Neonatal hyperbilirubinemia	Blue to black discoloration of primary teeth
Kidney failure	Mottled enamel
Cystic fibrosis (staining due to meds)	Mottled enamel

DENTAL TRAUMA

- See Table 11.3

THE MEDICALLY COMPROMISED DENTAL PATIENT

IMMUNOCOMPROMISED PATIENTS

- Any immunocompromised child should be referred to dentist for complete oral examination as soon as possible after diagnosis
- Definitive dental treatment for any oral diseases (including dental caries and periodontal disease) should be completed before receiving

Table 11.3	Description and Management of Dental Trauma	
Type of Injury	**Description**	**Management of Dental Trauma**
Crown fractures	No pulpal exposure (enamel and dentin only)	Permanent and primary teeth: referral to dentist within 24 h
	With pulpal exposure (enamel, dentin, pulp)	Permanent and primary teeth: immediate referral to dentist
Nondisplacement injuries	Concussion: injury to tooth/supporting structures; NO abnormal loosening/ displacement	Permanent and primary teeth: referral to dentist within 24 h
	Subluxation: injury to tooth/supporting structures; abnormal loosening but NO displacement	Permanent teeth: immediate referral to dentist Primary teeth: if significantly loose: immediate referral; if minimally loose: referral within 24 h
Displacement injuries	Extrusion: partial displacement of tooth from socket	Permanent and primary teeth: immediate referral to dentist
	Luxation: displacement of tooth in a direction other than axially	Permanent and primary teeth: immediate referral to dentist
	Intrusion: displacement of tooth axially into alveolus	Permanent and primary teeth: immediate referral to dentist
Avulsion	Complete displacement of tooth from socket	Permanent teeth: *immediate reimplantation within 5 min*; if not possible, store and transport tooth in chilled milk or patient's saliva Primary teeth: immediate referral if caregivers cannot locate avulsed tooth (rule out intrusion); avulsed primary teeth are not replanted (risk of ankylosis, infection)

immunosuppression, if possible (e.g., organ transplantation); this will eliminate potentially life-threatening sites of infection
- Regular dental follow-up required; cyclosporine can cause gingival enlargement; excellent oral hygiene practices required for prevention; surgical removal of excessive gingival tissue may be required

CARDIAC PATIENTS

- See endocarditis prophylaxis guidelines, p. 989
- Definitive dental treatment for any oral diseases (including dental caries and periodontal disease) should be completed before elective open-heart surgery, if possible
- Regular dental follow-up required

FURTHER READING

Nowak AJ, Casamassimo PS. *The Handbook of Pediatric Dentistry.* 3rd ed. The American Academy of Pediatric Dentistry; 2007.

Pinkham JR, Casamassimo PS, Fields HW, McTigue DJ, Nowak AJ. *Pediatric Dentistry: Infancy Through Adolescence.* 4th ed. St. Louis, Mo: Mosby; 2005.

USEFUL WEB SITES

American Academy of Pediatric Dentistry. Available at: **www.aapd.org**.

Dentistry

11

Chapter 12 Dermatology

Marissa O. Joseph
Elena Pope

Chapter 12 Dermatology

COMMON ABBREVIATIONS

ABC	airway, breathing, circulation
BP	benzoyl peroxide
BSA	body surface area
β-HCG	beta-human chorionic gonadotropin
CBC	complete blood cell count
CN V1	cranial nerve 5, first branch
EB	epidermolysis bullosa
EM	erythema multiforme
GABHS	group A β-hemolytic streptococcus
H&E	hematoxylin and eosin stain
HPV	human papilloma virus
HSP	Henoch-Schönlein purpura
HSV	herpes simplex virus
KOH	potassium hydroxide
5% LCD	5% liquor carbonis detergens
LFT	liver function test
NF	neurofibromatosis
NICH	noninvoluting congenital hemangioma
RICH	rapidly involuting congenital hemangioma
SA	salicylic acid
SBE	subacute bacterial endocarditis
SJS	Stevens-Johnson syndrome
SLE	systemic lupus erythematosus
SPF	sun protection factor
SSSS	staphylococcal scalded skin syndrome
TEN	toxic epidermal necrolysis
UVA	ultraviolet A
UVB	ultraviolet B

MORPHOLOGY

- See Table 12.1

NEONATAL ERUPTIONS

VESICULOPUSTULAR DISEASE

Differential Diagnosis

- Neonatal HSV (grouped vesicles on erythematous base)
- Neonatal varicella (macules, papules, evolving vesicles that crust over; presents within 5 d of birth)

Table 12.1

Table 12.1	**Quick-Glance Differential Diagnosis by Lesion Morphology**
Morphology	**Diagnosis (Representative Examples)**
Vesiculobullous	Infectious: impetigo, HSV, varicella, SSSS, hand-foot-and-mouth disease Autoimmune: linear IgA dermatosis, pemphigus vulgaris, bullous lupus Congenital: EB, incontinentia pigmenti, aplasia cutis congenita Physical/mechanical: burns, sucking blister, friction blister, sunburn Other: contact dermatitis, miliaria, lymphangioma, EM, SJS, TEN
Pustular	Neonates: erythema toxicum, transient neonatal pustular melanosis, acne, *Candida* infection, folliculitis Children: varicella, acne, folliculitis, meningococcemia, pustular psoriasis, drug eruption
Papulosquamous	Psoriasis, tinea corporis, SLE, lichen planus, pityriasis rosea, seborrheic dermatitis, drug reaction, chronic dermatitis, cutaneous T-cell lymphoma
Dermatitic	Diaper, atopic, seborrheic, contact dermatitis; nummular eczema, immuno-deficiencies, Langerhans cell histiocytosis, scabies, Wiskott-Aldrich syndrome, candidiasis, tinea corporis, acrodermatitis enteropathica
Vascular	Mottling, hemangioma, urticaria, port-wine stain, livedo reticularis, spider angioma, erythema infectiosum, vascular malformations, pyogenic granuloma
Purpuric	Thrombocytopenia, HSP and other vasculitides, congenital infection, coagulopathy, SLE, Kasabach-Merritt syndrome, meningococcemia, SBE
White	Flat: vitiligo, ash-leaf macule, postinflammatory hypopigmentation, pityriasis alba, tinea versicolor, morphea, Waardenburg syndrome, lichen sclerosus Raised: milia, closed comedones, molluscum contagiosum, keratosis pilaris, scar
Brown	Flat: mongolian spot, café au lait spot, junctional nevus, ephelid (freckle), postinflammatory hyperpigmentation, transient neonatal hypermelanosis, incontinentia pigmenti, tinea versicolor, Addison disease, Becker nevus Raised: congenital melanocytic nevus, dermal nevus, dermatofibroma, melanoma, mastocytoma
Yellow	Carotenemia, sebaceous gland hyperplasia, jaundice, xanthoma, nevus sebaceous, juvenile xanthogranuloma

© The Hospital for Sick Children, 2009. New artwork created by The Hospital for Sick Children for *The Hospital for Sick Children Handbook of Pediatrics*, 11th edition.

Dermatology

12

- Neonatal pustulosis (benign "baby acne"; presents in first month of life)
- Infantile acne (associated with scarring and virilizing tumors; presents at 3–6 mo)
- Acropustulosis of infancy (pustules/vesicles on palms and soles; presents/recurs birth–3 yr)
- Erythema toxicum (discrete vesicles, papules, pustules on erythematous base; spares palms and soles; new lesions up to 10 d)
- Transient neonatal pustular melanosis (pustules/pigmented macules; more common in black infants; presents at birth)
- Miliaria (blockage of eccrine ducts, associated with excess heat/humidity)

- Sucking blisters (solitary ovoid blister or erosion on noninflamed skin)
- Impetigo neonatorum (flaccid, well-demarcated bullae; leaves erosions, crust, collarette of scale)
- Congenital candidiasis (usually "sick"; generalized erythematous papules, vesicles, pustules, erythroderma; presents on first day of life)
- Infantile scabies (papules, vesicles, pustules, burrows in axillae, neck, web spaces, palms, soles)

Investigations

- Vesicular or pustular fluid
  - Gram stain, C&S (*Staphylococcus aureus* on culture of orifices in impetigo), viral culture
  - Electron microscopy (eosinophils on Giemsa or Wright stain of contents of pustule in HSV)
  - HSV/VZV polymerase chain reaction (PCR)
- Lesion scraping
  - Tzanck smear (multinucleated giant cells in HSV)
  - KOH preparation (fungal hyphae in *Candida*)
  - Burrow (isolation of *Sarcoptes scabiei* mite, eggs, or feces)
- Skin biopsy
  - H&E, immunofluorescence
- Serology
  - TORCH (toxoplasmosis, rubella, CMV, herpes) workup, VDRL

MACULAR

- Café au lait macule (well-demarcated light brown macules; associated with neurofibromatosis, McCune-Albright and Russell-Silver syndrome)
- Ash-leaf spot (irregular hypopigmented macule; associated with tuberous sclerosis)
- Congenital pigmented nevi (darkly pigmented brown-black lesions, may be >20 cm)
- Nevus simplex (stork bite/angel's kiss)
- Nevus flammeus (port-wine stain)

NODULAR

Subcutaneous Fat Necrosis

- Erythematous plaques/nodules over cheeks, arms, trunk, buttocks, legs
- Starts in first few weeks of life if hypoxia/hypothermia/trauma at birth; benign, self-limited
- Associated with hypercalcemia

VASCULAR

- See Table 12.2

| **Table 12.2** | **Differential Diagnosis of Common Vascular Lesions** |

Diagnosis	Classification	Clinical Features	Investigations/ Management
Lymphangioma	Vascular malformation	· Present at birth, gradually enlarge over years · Large flesh-colored or bluish mass, or hemorrhagic vesicles	· Surgery · Recurrence common
Nevus flammeus (port-wine stain)	Vascular malformation	· Present at birth, grows proportionately with child · Associated with Sturge-Weber syndrome in 10% of CN V1 distribution · Klippel-Trénaunay syndrome: associated asymmetry (soft tissue overgrowth)	· CN V1 distribution, involvement of large areas on head: requires MRI head · Some respond to pulsed dye laser
Pyogenic granuloma	Tumor	· Solitary red firm nodule; 5-6 mm · Bleeds easily with trauma · Common sites: umbilicus, hands, feet	· Silver nitrate · Curettage and electro-dessication of base is curative
Infantile hemangioma	Tumor	· Benign tumor of endothelial cells · May be present at birth, usually begins at 4 wk-3 mo · Often starts as macule, grows disproportionately · Rapid growth phase until 6-9 mo, then spontaneous regression · Superficial (bright red, papular), deep (bluish, nodular), and mixed	· Majority self-resolve: 30% by 3 yr, 50% by 5 yr, 90% by 9 yr · Neuroimaging (CNS/spine) for periorbital lesions, large segmental lesions · Evaluation of airway for lesions in "beard distribution" · Indications for systemic steroids: airway, ocular obstruction, cardiac failure, ulceration, significant cosmetic disability (prednisone 2 mg/kg/d with gradual taper) · Ophthalmology and ENT referral, when appropriate · May need systemic antibiotics for ulceration and secondary infection
Congenital hemangioma	Tumor	· Present at birth · 2 types: RICH; NICH	· For NICH with congestive heart failure: systemic steroids, ± embolization

Dermatology

12

FEBRILE CHILD WITH A RASH

- See Table 12.3

Table 12.3	Febrile Child With a Rash
Conditions	**Clinical Features**
Viral exanthem	· Morbilliform red eruption, usually nonpruritic · Associated with measles, rubella, roseola, enteroviruses, mononucleosis
Juvenile idiopathic arthritis	· Polymorphous rash
Scarlet fever (group A streptococci)	· Flesh-colored papular "sandpaper" rash, strawberry tongue, Pastia sign (lines of petechiae in skinfolds)
Rheumatic fever (group A streptococci)	· Erythema marginatum, subcutaneous nodules
Acute SLE	· Malar rash, photosensitivity, oral/nasal ulcers
Kawasaki disease	· Polymorphous rash, palmoplantar desquamation or erythema, oral changes
HSP	· Palpable petechiae and purpura, commonly on buttocks and lower legs
Hand-foot-and-mouth disease (coxsackievirus A16, enterovirus 71)	· Red macules, vesicles on buccal mucosa, palate, tongue, dorsum of hands and feet after viral prodrome
Acute dermatomyositis	· Heliotrope rash (periorbital violaceous), Gottron papules, nail fold changes, shawl sign (rash over anterior chest, neck), malar rash
Lyme disease (Borrelia burgdorferi)	· Erythema migrans (large erythematous annular lesion)
Subacute bacterial endocarditis	· Splinter hemorrhages (red lines in nails), Osler nodes
Acute hepatitis	· Jaundice, purpuric rash over lower limbs
Meningococcemia, gonococcemia	· Petechiae and purpura
Drug hypersensitivity syndrome	· Erythroderma; morbilliform, papulosquamous, urticarial, or bullous lesions
Typhoid fever (Salmonella typhi)	· Rose spots: sparse salmon-colored, blanching, maculopapular rash over the trunk

© The Hospital for Sick Children, 2009. New artwork created by The Hospital for Sick Children for *The Hospital for Sick Children Handbook of Pediatrics,* 11th edition.

DERMATITIS

Diaper Dermatitis

- See Table 12.4

Dermatology

12

Table 12.4	Differential Diagnosis of Diaper Dermatitis		
Disease	**Lesions**	**Sites**	**Management**
Irritant contact dermatitis (due to urine, feces)	· Shiny red macules, patches, ulcerations, erosions	· No flexural involvement	· Disposable diapers · Frequent diaper changes · Liberal use of emollients (e.g., petrolatum) and barrier creams (e.g., zinc oxide) · 1% hydrocortisone cream tid
Seborrheic dermatitis ("cradle cap")	· Yellow, greasy plaques on erythematous base	· Scalp, axillae, trunk, flexural areas	· 1% hydrocortisone cream tid
Candida	· Beefy red patches with peripheral scale; "satellite lesions"	· Flexural areas, oral thrush	· 1% hydrocortisone powder in clotrimazole cream tid
Psoriasis	· Well-demarcated papules/plaques with thick scale	· Trunk, extremities, nails, scalp, flexural areas	· Medium-potency topical corticosteroid (see Topical Corticosteroids section)
Bullous impetigo	· Bullae on red base, erosions, crusts	· Any, including flexural	· Antistaphylococcal systemic antibiotics
Langerhans cell histiocytosis	· Hemorrhagic papules/plaques with scale, purpura, erosions, crust	· Scalp, axillae, trunk, flexural areas	· For skin disease: moderate to potent topical steroids, psoralen + UVA (PUVA)
Acrodermatitis enteropathica	· AR, zinc deficiency · Presents at 4–10 wk or when weaning off breast · Triad: dermatitis alopecia, diarrhea	· Scalp, perioral (perlèche), anogenital, fingers, alopecia, red discoloration of hair (zebra hair)	· 1–3 mg/kg/d zinc sulfate · Side effects: GI upset, emesis, microcytic anemia

© The Hospital for Sick Children, 2009. New artwork created by The Hospital for Sick Children for *The Hospital for Sick Children Handbook of Pediatrics*, 11th edition.

Dermatology

12

Atopic Dermatitis

- Acute: pruritus, erythema, vesicles, exudate, crust
- Chronic: xerosis, scaling, lichenification, Dennie-Morgan folds under eyes
- Personal/family history of atopy
- Clinical diagnosis: relapsing, itchy, dry, skin rash; 65% onset before 1 yr (90% before 5 yr)
- Distribution:
  - Infant: cheeks, forehead, scalp, extensor surfaces
  - Child: antecubital and popliteal fossae, wrists, ankles (i.e., flexural surfaces)
- Aggravating factors: sweating, contact sensitivity, secondary infection
- Complications: impetigo, cellulitis, eczema herpeticum, molluscum contagiosum
- If difficult to treat, consider immunodeficiency, Langerhans cell histiocytosis

Management

- See Table 12.5

<table>
<tr><td colspan="2">Table 12.5   Management of Atopic Dermatitis</td></tr>
</table>

Behavioral Measures	Medical Management
· Cotton clothing, keep room cool, humidifier · Avoid irritants: mild soaps, detergents; double rinse · Avoid bleaches, fabric softeners, wool or synthetic fibers · Daily to tid bath with capful of oil (e.g., Aveeno, Alpha Keri oil) · Leave skin damp and apply emollient · No good evidence for food triggers, if aggravated by certain foods can avoid or apply petrolatum (e.g., Vaseline) around mouth before meal · Avoid elimination diets (do not help, and compromise nutrition)	· Moisturizers: prefer emollients such as petrolatum (e.g., Vaseline, Glaxal Base) · Topical steroids: 1% hydrocortisone ointment to face and folds, betamethasone valerate 0.05% ointment tid to affected body areas · Topical immunomodulators: tacrolimus 0.03% ointment bid for >2 yr age; pimecrolimus ointment bid; may experience burning first several days · UVB light, calcineurin inhibitors (cyclosporine/tacrolimus), or mycophenolate mofetil: for recalcitrant and severe cases · Antipruritic: essential, especially if sleep disturbance; hydroxyzine 3–5 mg/kg/d divided tid-qid or diphenhydramine 5 mg/kg/d divided q6h · Antibiotics: topical if mild secondary infection (e.g., fusidic acid ointment); if more severe, then PO antistaphylococcal coverage (e.g., cephalexin, cloxacillin) for 10–14 d; if septic, use IV treatment · Acyclovir: if eczema herpeticum, route and duration dependent on clinical status

© The Hospital for Sick Children, 2009. New artwork created by The Hospital for Sick Children for *The Hospital for Sick Children Handbook of Pediatrics*, 11th edition.

Poison Ivy Contact Dermatitis

- Very pruritic vesicular dermatitis often in a linear distribution
- Obtain exposure history; beware indirect exposure via pets, clothing; airborne contact possible (e.g., burning of leaves), may be severe
- Treat with potent topical steroid (e.g., betamethasone valerate 0.1% tid, or stronger; see Topical Corticosteroids section)
- If extensive, prednisone 1 mg/kg/d (max 40–60 mg/d) tapered slowly over 2–3 wk

ACNE VULGARIS

- Noninflammatory lesions: open (blackheads) or closed (whiteheads) comedones
- Inflammatory lesions: papules, pustules, cysts (not true cysts), nodules
- Etiologic agent: *Propionibacterium acnes*

Topical Agents

- See Table 12.6

Systemic Treatment

- Used when moderate to severe, not responding to topical agents, or multiple sites involved (e.g., face, chest, back)

Table 12.6	Topical Acne Treatments
BP gel and cream (2.5–20%)	· Anti-inflammatory properties (inhibits *P. acnes*), mild comedolytic · Start qhs to bid, 5% strength and increase to 10% prn · Side effects include drying, peeling
Topical antibiotics	· 2% clindamycin solution, 2% erythromycin solution/gel · Anti-inflammatory properties, best used in combination with other treatments
Topical retinoids	· Tretinoin 0.01%, 0.025%, 0.05% cream/gel; adapalene: decreases comedones · Side effects include photosensitivity (need sunscreen SPF ≥ 30), redness, peeling, hypopigmentation · Start qhs or on alternate days with 0.01% cream (if dry) or gel (if oily skin), gradually increase strength and frequency as tolerated
Combination treatments	· Contains BP, retinoid, and antibiotic in one preparation (e.g., Clindoxyl gel: 1% clindamycin + 5% BP or Stievamycin gel: various strengths of retinoids + 4% erythromycin)

© The Hospital for Sick Children, 2009. New artwork created by The Hospital for Sick Children for *The Hospital for Sick Children Handbook of Pediatrics*, 11th edition.

Systemic Antibiotics

- Tetracycline: contraindicated if <8 yr or pregnant; 250 mg tid × 3 wk, then bid tapered to effect
- Minocycline: 100 mg bid × 1 wk, then daily
- Erythromycin: 250 mg tid × 3 wk, then bid

Isotretinoin (Accutane)

- Useful in nodulocystic acne to prevent scarring; best used in consultation with dermatologist
- 20-wk course of 1 mg/kg/d
- Tests needed before initiation and monthly: LFTs, urinalysis, CBC, cholesterol, triglycerides, β-HCG
- Highly teratogenic, avoid conception during and 1 mo posttreatment; need two forms of contraception
- Side effects: cheilitis, xerostomia, xerophthalmia, conjunctivitis, myalgia, headache, teratogenicity, hepatitis, hypercholesterolemia, hypertriglyceridemia, pseudotumor cerebri

PAPULOSQUAMOUS DISORDERS

Psoriasis

- Autoimmune inflammatory disorder often with positive family history
- Lesions: well-demarcated erythematous plaques with adherent silvery scale ± itch + Koebner phenomenon (trauma induces new lesions)
- Distribution: extensor surfaces, scalp, flexures/folds (inverse psoriasis); nails (pitting, onycholysis, thickening, oil drop sign)
- Variants: palmar-plantar, pustular, guttate (may follow GABHS)
- Associations: psoriatic arthritis

Management

- Goal: limit inflammation and minimize scale; no cure presently
- See Table 12.7
- Systemic:
  - No systemic corticosteroids (cause erythroderma on withdrawal)
  - Methotrexate, biologic immunomodulatory therapies (e.g., infliximab [Remicade])
  - Guttate psoriasis: throat/perianal swab for *Streptococcus*, treat appropriately
  - UVA, UVB light therapy: needs referral by dermatologist

TINEA INFECTIONS

- See Table 12.8

Table 12.7	Topical Treatments for Psoriasis	
	First Line	**Second Line**
Skin	· Midpotency steroids · Face: hydrocortisone-17-valerate bid · Body: betamethasone valerate ointment/cream bid	· Betamethasone valerate qam · Calcipotriene (Dovonex) qhs
Excessive scale	Add 3% SA and 5% LCD to steroid	N/A
Scalp	· Tar shampoo + midpotency steroid lotion qam · 10% SA in mineral oil qhs	N/A

© The Hospital for Sick Children, 2009. New artwork created by The Hospital for Sick Children for *The Hospital for Sick Children Handbook of Pediatrics*, 11th edition.

Table 12.8	Tinea Infections	
Diagnosis	**Clinical Features**	**Management**
Capitis (head)	· Causes: *Trichophyton tonsurans* or *Microsporum canis* (rare; fluoresces with Wood lamp) · Very contagious · 5 clinical patterns: 1) diffuse scaling, 2) circumscribed alopecia with scale, 3) black dot (broken hairs), 4) kerion (boggy mass), 5) pustular	· Scraping for KOH and fungal culture · Systemic treatment only · Terbinafine PO for 4 weeks (<20 kg, 62.5 mg daily; 20–40 kg, 125 mg daily; >40 kg, 250 mg daily)
Corporis (body)	· *M. canis*, *T. mentagrophytes*, *T. tonsurans*, *T. rubrum*	· Systemic treatment rarely needed · Topical terbinafine, ciclopirox, clotrimazole, ketoconazole all efficacious applied bid · May take up to 4 wk
Pedis (feet)	· *T. tonsurans*, *T. rubrum* · Vesicles, erosions, maceration between toes, scaling	
Faciei (face)	· *M. canis*, *T. verrucosum*	
Cruris (groin)	· *T. mentagrophytes*, *Epidermophyton floccosum* · Inner thighs and inguinal folds	

© The Hospital for Sick Children, 2009. New artwork created by The Hospital for Sick Children for *The Hospital for Sick Children Handbook of Pediatrics*, 11th edition.

ALOPECIA

- General approach: examine skin, hair, nails, mucous membranes; fungal scrapings (culture, KOH), hair shaft microscopy, biopsy rarely
- See Table 12.9

INFESTATIONS

- See Table 12.10

Table 12.9	Common Causes of Alopecia			
Disease	**Description**	**Associations**	**Management**	**Prognosis**
Alopecia areata	· Nonscarring · Scalp normal · Totalis: >90% scalp · Universalis: all areas	· Autoimmune disease (e.g., thyroid, adrenals) · Atopic dermatitis	· High-potency (see Topical Corticosteroids section) or intralesional steroids	· 95% regrow in 1 yr (except totalis and universalis) · 30% recurrence
Trichotillomania	· Circumscribed with irregular borders · Varied lengths	· Traumatic events · Excoriations	· Referral to psychiatrist	
Telogen effluvium	· Diffuse loss	· Precipitated by stressful events (illness, crash diet, medications)	· Diagnosis by microscopic examination for telogen root	· Complete regrowth

© The Hospital for Sick Children, 2009. New artwork created by The Hospital for Sick Children for *The Hospital for Sick Children Handbook of Pediatrics*, 11th edition.

Table 12.10	Clinical Features and Management of Infestations	
Diagnosis	**Clinical Features**	**Investigations/Treatment**
Scabies (infantile, see Neonatal Eruptions, p. 194)	· *S. scabiei hominis* · Incubation period 3–6 wk · Pruritic papules/burrows in web spaces, can progress to nodules, dermatitis · Abdomen, dorsa of hands, genitalia, skin folds · Few (6–10) mites; reaction mainly due to allergy to mites · Nodules can persist for months · Return to school once treated	· Clinical diagnosis + isolation of *S. scabiei* mite, eggs, or feces from burrow · Treat all contacts · 5% permethrin cream/lotion, from neck down for 8–14 h, on 2 occasions 1 wk apart · Alternatively, ivermectin 200 mcg/kg/dose PO × 1 dose (>15 kg, or >5 yr) · Wash bedding/clothing in hot water · Treat pruritus with antihistamines, topical mid-potency steroids (see Topical Corticosteroids section)
Pediculosis (lice)	· Louse 3–4 mm long, eggs 1 mm, firmly adherent to hair shaft · Capitis (head louse): postauricular and occipital regions common, also excoriated papules/pustules when on body · Pubis (crab louse): smaller lice, affects eyelashes and pubic hair, transmitted via sexual contact	· Wash and towel-dry hair; apply permethrin 1% for 10 min and rinse; repeat in 7 d · Vinegar-and-water (1:1) soaks and fine-tooth comb · If eyelash involvement, apply petrolatum bid-tid for 10 d · Soak combs, hair accessories in permethrin shampoo or boil for 10 min; wash clothing/bedding in hot water

© The Hospital for Sick Children, 2009. New artwork created by The Hospital for Sick Children for *The Hospital for Sick Children Handbook of Pediatrics*, 11th edition.

BACTERIAL INFECTIONS

- See Table 12.11

VIRAL INFECTIONS

- See Table 12.12

Table 12.11	Clinical Features of Cutaneous Bacterial Infections	
Diagnosis	**Clinical Features**	**Management**
Cellulitis	· Poorly demarcated erythema, warmth, induration ± tenderness	· Systemic antibiotics (see Chapter 24)
Impetigo	· Caused by *S. aureus* and GABHS · Moist, honey-colored crusts overlying erosions, may see fragile vesicles/ bullae (bullous impetigo)	· Swab lesion, send for culture · If localized, use topical antibiotics · Systemic treatment against *S. aureus* and GABHS (e.g., cephalexin) for 10–14 d
SSSS	· *S. aureus* exfoliative toxin A causes skin exfoliation at granular layer · Tender erythematous eruption of central face, neck, axillae, groin, torso · Bullae, generalized desquamation; typically normal conjunctivae and mucous membranes	· Usually benign self-limited course, mortality <1% · Minimize handling · Bland emollient during desquamation (e.g., petrolatum) · Cloxacillin for 7–10 d

© The Hospital for Sick Children, 2009. New artwork created by The Hospital for Sick Children for *The Hospital for Sick Children Handbook of Pediatrics*, 11th edition.

Table 12.12	Clinical Features of Selected Cutaneous Viral Infections	
Diagnosis	**Clinical Features**	**Investigations/Management**
Molluscum contagiosum	· Caused by poxvirus · Flesh-colored umbilicated papules anywhere on skin	· Clinical diagnosis, can express curdlike material · Spontaneous regression after 2 yr; majority require no treatment · Curettage (uncomfortable), cantharidin (Cantharone) (blisters)
Verrucae (warts)	· Caused by HPV · Vulgaris (anywhere on body), plantar (palms and soles), accuminata (genitals), and flat (sites of trauma, face, or extremities)	· Untreated: mean lifespan 2 yr · Vulgaris and plantar: 60% SA with bandage for 1 wk, debride and continue with weaker over-the-counter preparations · Liquid nitrogen in older children/adolescents · Accuminata: topical imiquimod 5 times/wk until resolution or 25% podophyllin left on 4–6 h, repeated weekly; suspect child abuse
Varicella (chickenpox)	· Hallmark: lesions in varying stages; abrupt onset; very pruritic erythematous macules, papules, and vesicles that crust and leave erosions	See Chapter 24

© The Hospital for Sick Children, 2009. New artwork created by The Hospital for Sick Children for *The Hospital for Sick Children Handbook of Pediatrics*, 11th edition.

URTICARIA

- Acute <6 wk; chronic >6 wk
- Usually idiopathic, history of inciting agent (often not found)
- Careful airway/respiratory assessment, particularly if angioedema present
- No routine investigations; if chronic, refer to dermatologist
- Acute treatment: maintain ABCs (see pp. 5–9), antihistamine × 10 d if persistent; short-course systemic steroids, depending on severity (see p. 133)

EM, SJS, AND TEN

- See Table 12.13

Table 12.13	Clinical Features and Management of Erythema Multiforme (EM), Stevens-Johnson Syndrome (SJS), and Toxic Epidermal Necrolysis (TEN)		
	EM	**SJS**	**TEN**
Etiology	HSV, mycoplasma, EBV	Drugs*	Drugs*
Prodrome	1–3 d	1–3 d; fever, occasionally flulike symptoms	Fever and tender red skin
Clinical features	· Target lesions, typically on acral areas; all lesions appear within 72 h · Central bullae in cases of mycoplasma-induced EM · Koebner phenomenon[†] · 1–3 mucosal surfaces involved	· Diffuse petechial patches with blister formation progressing to epidermal necrolysis over 1–2 d · ≥2 mucosal surfaces · <10% BSA involved	· Blisters that progress in hours to skin necrosis · Nikolsky sign[‡] · ≥2 mucosal surfaces · >30% BSA involvement
Clinical course	· Resolves within 2–4 wk · Low mortality	· Resolves in 1 wk · Low mortality	· High mortality · Eye complications · Bronchiolitis obliterans
Management	· Supportive · Systemic steroids controversial (may benefit severe mucosal involvement) · Acyclovir prophylaxis for recurrent HSV	· Supportive · Stop offending drug · IVIG 3 g/kg divided over 2 d · No systemic steroids	· Supportive · Stop offending drug · IVIG 3 g/kg divided over 2 d · Burn unit care (wound care)

*Drugs include NSAIDs, penicillin, sulfa antibiotics, and anticonvulsants.
[†]Trauma to skin induces similar lesions.
[†]Lateral pressure to skin leads to separation of epidermis.

Dermatology

12

INHERITED DERMATOSES

Ichthyoses

- Heterogeneous group of dermatoses affecting cornified layer of epidermis resulting in excessive scaling of skin; treatment with emollients, topical retinoids

EB

- See Table 12.14
- Group of heterogeneous mechanobullous diseases characterized by development of blisters after trauma to skin
- Usually present at birth or in infancy
- Treatment: education, symptomatic management, support; special attention to temperature control, airway involvement, fluid balance, infection with extensive blistering (particularly in neonates)

Table 12.14	Classification and Features of Epidermolysis Bullosa (EB)
EB simplex	Generally more benign, nonscarring; fewer complications
Junctional EB	More severe; generalized forms often fatal or can heal with atrophy, may present with severe airway involvement and granulation tissue around nails and orifices
Dystrophic EB	More severe scarring and atrophy; multisystem involvement

© The Hospital for Sick Children, 2009. New artwork created by The Hospital for Sick Children for *The Hospital for Sick Children Handbook of Pediatrics*, 11th edition.

NF

- See Box 12.1

Box 12.1	Diagnostic Criteria for Neurofibromatosis-1 (NF-1)*

- 6 or more café au lait macules >5 mm before puberty, >15 mm after puberty
- Axillary or inguinal freckling
- 2 or more neurofibromas, or 1 plexiform neurofibroma
- Optic glioma
- Lisch nodules (iris hamartomas)
- Characteristic bony lesions (sphenoid dysplasia, thinning of bony cortex ± pseudoarthrosis)
- First-degree relative(s) with NF-1

*Requires 2/7 criteria for diagnosis.
© The Hospital for Sick Children, 2009. New artwork created by The Hospital for Sick Children for *The Hospital for Sick Children Handbook of Pediatrics*, 11th edition.

Tuberous Sclerosis

- AD inheritance
- Cutaneous findings: adenoma sebaceum, periungual fibroma, fibrous plaque of forehead, shagreen patch, dental pits, gum hypertrophy

TOPICAL CORTICOSTEROIDS

POTENCIES

- Very low (e.g., 1% hydrocortisone)
- Low (e.g., betamethasone valerate 0.05%, hydrocortisone-17-valerate)
- Moderate (e.g., betamethasone valerate 0.1%, mometasone furoate)
- High (e.g., betamethasone dipropionate, fluocinonide 0.05%)
- Very high (e.g., clobetasol-17-propionate)

SIDE EFFECTS

- Increase with potency and duration; atrophy, striae, hypertrichosis, perioral dermatitis, delayed wound healing, exacerbation of skin infections

PRESCRIPTION CONSIDERATIONS

- Ointment most potent, greasy, and hydrating; use on thick dry skin, avoid on hairy areas or face
- Creams less potent than ointment, avoid on hairy areas, can be used on face
- Lotions and gels more drying, much less potent, good in hairy areas, avoid on dry skin
- Quantities: bid application for 1 wk (30–60 g); bid application for 1 mo (120–240 g)

FURTHER READING

Hurwitz S. *Clinical Pediatric Dermatology: A Textbook of Skin Disorders of Childhood and Adolescence*. 3rd ed. Philadelphia, Pa: WB Saunders; 2005.
Schachner LA, Hansen RC. *Pediatric Dermatology*. 3rd ed. Philadelphia, Pa: Churchill Livingstone; 2003.
Weston WL, Morelli JG, Lane AT. *Color Textbook of Pediatric Dermatology*. 4th ed. St. Louis, Mo: Mosby; 2007.

USEFUL WEB SITES

Dermatologic Image Database. Available at: www.dermnet.org.nz.
Dermatology image atlas—Johns Hopkins University. Available at: http://dermatlas.med.jhmi.edu/derm.
Emedicine—dermatology. Available at: www.emedicine.com/derm.

Dermatology

12

Chapter 13 / Development

Joelene F. Huber

Elizabeth A. Jimenez

Chapter 13 Development

COMMON ABBREVIATIONS

ABA	applied behavioral analysis
ADHD	attention deficit/hyperactivity disorder
ADI-R	Autism Diagnostic Interview—Revised
ADL	activities of daily living
ADOS	Autism Diagnostic Observation Schedule
ARND	alcohol-related neurodevelopmental disorder
ASD	autism spectrum disorder
CARS	Childhood Autism Rating Scale
CP	cerebral palsy
DSM-IV-TR	*Diagnostic and Statistical Manual of Mental Disorders*, 4th ed - *Text Revision*
FAS	fetal alcohol syndrome
FASD	fetal alcohol spectrum disorder
GMFCS	Gross Motor Function Classification System
MR	mental retardation
PDD NOS	pervasive developmental disorder not otherwise specified

APPROACH TO PEDIATRIC DEVELOPMENT

DEVELOPMENTAL HISTORY

* A complete pediatric medical history is required
  * Prenatal, delivery, and neonatal histories are very important
  * Sleep and diet
* For each of the following areas of development, determine when major milestones were first reached, current level of function, and presence of any regression:
  * Gross motor (e.g., timing of sitting, walking, running, stairs, tricycle)
  * Fine motor (e.g., pincer grasp, buttons, zippers, use of scissors, utensils, cups)
  * Language
    – Vocabulary (e.g., timing of first words, number of words)
    – Expressive language (e.g., use of language: syntax, point of view, ability to tell a narrative, use of jargon, echolalia, perseveration)
    – Receptive language (e.g., understanding, following commands with and without context)
    – Articulation
    – Fluency (e.g., stuttering)
    – Languages exposed to (e.g., home, school, community)
    – Reading (e.g., phonologic abilities, hyperlexia)

- Social: eye contact, interest in peers, nonverbal communication, responds to name
- Behavior and temperament: discuss any aggressive, maladaptive, self-injurious, or repetitive behaviors and whether redirection is possible
- Play: in parallel or along with other children, appropriate use of toys, with similar- or different-aged children, imaginative play
- ADL: toileting, dressing, feeding, sleeping, money skills, telephone, safety
- Academics: school program, school performance, special services at school
- Family history: three-generation pedigree, paying attention to presence of ASDs; developmental delays; learning disabilities; seizures; genetic, metabolic, and psychiatric conditions; substance abuse; consanguinity
- Social history: home environment, school/day care program, rehabilitation services, special services, funding resources, respite, social supports
- Complete review of systems
- Additional corroborative history, with parental permission, may be taken from therapists, teachers, or other caregivers

DEVELOPMENTAL PHYSICAL EXAMINATON

- Growth parameters: percentiles for height, weight, and head circumference
- Complete general physical examination and neurologic examination; note dysmorphic features
- Important to look for stigmata of neurocutaneous syndromes
- Set up room with items such as toys, blocks, books, paper, crayons, and child scissors; observe/elicit skills in each domain to corroborate with history

DIAGNOSTIC TESTS

Genetics

- Chromosomal analysis for all patients with global developmental delay or ASDs
- DNA analysis for fragile X syndrome in all patients with unexplained MR, global delay, and/or ASD
- Testing for other genetic syndromes based on clinical suspicion (e.g., 22q deletion syndrome, Rett syndrome)
- Genetics consultation if dysmorphic features and no etiology identified

Neuroimaging

- MRI preferable to CT scan except when craniosynostosis or intracranial calcifications (congenital infection, tuberous sclerosis) suspected
- Indicated in patients with microcephaly or macrocephaly, seizures, loss of psychomotor skills, neurologic signs, or history of perinatal injury
- Role in patients with normocephaly and no focal neurologic signs is unclear

Metabolic Testing

- Focused metabolic workup when clinically indicated (e.g., consanguinity, neonatal hypotonia, coarse facial features, developmental regression, lethargy, early seizures, recurrent vomiting, food intolerances, odors)
- Extremely low yield in absence of above clinical suspicion

Other Tests

- Audiometry and vision assessments for all patients with developmental or behavior concerns
- EEG if any clinical suspicion of seizures (including staring spells)
- Psychometric testing

NORMAL PATTERNS OF GROWTH AND DEVELOPMENT

- See Table 13.1

DEVELOPMENTAL RED FLAGS

- See Box 13.1

Box 13.1 | **Developmental Red Flags**

Warrant further investigation and treatment:
- Not walking by 18 mo of age
- No single words by 18 mo of age
- Not putting two words together by 2 yr of age
- Not responding to name by 12 mo of age
- Not pointing to show by 15 mo of age
- Regression of developmental milestones

Development

13

Table 13.1 Emerging Developmental Milestones From Birth to 5 Years

Age	Gross Motor	Fine Motor	Social	Language	Self-Help
Birth	Kicks legs and thrashes arms; Moro, stepping, placing, and grasp reflexes present	Looks at objects or faces	Responds positively to feeding and comforting	Cries; startled by loud sudden sounds	Alert; interested in sights and sounds
1 mo	Raises head and chest when lying on stomach	Follows moving objects with eyes	Social smile; becomes active when sees human face	Cries in distinct way when hungry	Responds to voices; turns head toward voice
2 mo	Ventral suspension: head sustained in plane of body; pull to sitting: head lags; holds head steady when held sitting	Holds objects put in hand; hand regard; follows moving object 180°	Recognizes mother/primary caregiver; listens to voice and coos	Makes sounds: "ah," "eh," "ugh"; laughs	Reacts to sight of bottle or breast
3 mo	Ventral suspension: lifts head and chest, arms extended; tonic neck posture predominant; pull to sitting: head lag partially compensated; early head control with bobbing motion; back rounded	Shakes rattle; reaches toward and misses objects; waves at toy	Recognizes most familiar adults	Says "ahh," "ngah"	Increases activity when shown toy

(continued)

Table 13.1 Emerging Developmental Milestones From Birth to 5 Years (continued)

Age	Gross Motor	Fine Motor	Social	Language	Self-Help
4 mo	Turns around when lying on stomach; in prone position, lifts head and chest—head in approximate vertical axis, legs extended; pull to sitting: no head lag; head steady, held forward; sitting with full truncal support; when held in standing/erect position, pushes with feet	Puts toys or other objects in mouth	Interested in own image in mirror—smiles, playful; laughs out loud; may show displeasure if social contact is broken; excited at sight of food	Squeals, "ah-goo" sounds	Reaches for larger objects; sees small objects but makes no move to them
5 mo	Rolls from stomach to back	Picks up objects with one hand	Reacts differently to strangers (stranger anxiety)	Makes razzing sounds–gives "raspberries"	
6 mo	Rolls from back to stomach	Transfers objects from one hand to another	Reaches for familiar persons	Babbles; turns to own name	Looks for object after it disappears from sight
7 mo	Sits without support; may support most of weight when standing; bounces actively	Holds two objects (one in each hand) at same time; grasps using radial palm; rakes at small object	Gets upset and afraid if left alone	Makes sounds such as "da," "ba," "ga," "ka," "ma"	Anticipates being lifted by raising arms
8 mo	Crawls on hands and knees	Uses forefinger to poke, push, or roll small objects	Plays "peek-a-boo"	Makes sounds like "ma-ma," "da-da," "ba-ba" (two-syllable babbling)	Feeds self cracker or cookie

(continued)

Table 13.1 Emerging Developmental Milestones From Birth to 5 Years *(continued)*

Age	Gross Motor	Fine Motor	Social	Language	Self-Help
9 mo	Pulls self to standing position	Picks up small objects using only finger and thumb (pincer grasp)	Resists having toy taken away	Imitates speech sounds	
10 mo	Sidesteps/walks around furniture while holding on	Picks up two small objects in one hand	Plays "pat-a-cake"		
11 mo	Stands alone well	Puts small objects in cup or other container	Shows or offers toy to adult	Uses "Mama" or "Dada" specifically for parent	Picks up spoon by handle
12 mo	Climbs up on chairs or other furniture; walks with one hand held; "cruises"	Turns pages of books a few at a time	Imitates simple acts such as hugging or loving doll; plays simple ball game; makes postural adjustment to dressing	Says one word clearly; points in response to word	Removes socks
13 mo	Walks without help	Builds tower of two or more blocks	Plays with other children	Shakes head to express "no"; hands object to you when asked	Lifts cup to mouth and drinks
14 mo	Stoops and recovers	Marks with pencil or crayon	Gives kisses	Asks for food or drink with sounds or words	Insists on feeding self
15 mo	Runs	Scribbles with pencil or crayon	Greets people with "hi" or similar; hugs parents	Says two words besides "Mama" or "Dada"; makes sounds in sequences that sound like sentences	Feeds self with spoon

(continued)

Table 13.1 Emerging Developmental Milestones From Birth to 5 Years (continued)

Age	Gross Motor	Fine Motor	Social	Language	Self-Help
18 mo	Sits on small chair; walks up stairs with one hand held; kicks a ball—good balance and coordination; moves toys into and out of container	Builds tower of four or more cubes; imitates vertical strokes; dumps small object from bottle	Sometimes says "no" when interfered with; kisses parent with puckering of lips; exhibits shared attention (points to share interesting observation with another)	Uses five or more words as names of things (i.e., water, cookie, clock); follows a few simple instructions; understands phrases such as "Give me that" when gestures are used; recognizes names of common objects; identifies one or more parts of body	Feeds self; eats with a fork; seeks help when in trouble; may complain when wet or soiled; knows use of toothbrush and comb
24 mo	Runs well; walks up and down stairs, one step at a time; opens doors; climbs on furniture; throws and kicks ball	Builds tower of six cubes; performs circular scribbling; imitates horizontal stroke; folds paper once imitatively	Tells immediate experiences; listens to stories with pictures	Puts two to three words together; knows "I"; points to appropriate picture when someone says "Show me the dog"; has expressive vocabulary of 50–250 words	Handles spoon well; helps to undress
30 mo	Jumps	Builds tower of eight cubes; makes horizontal and vertical strokes but generally will not join them to make a cross; imitates circular stroke, forming closed figure	Pretends in play	Refers to self by pronoun "I"; knows full name	Helps put things away

(continued)

Development

13

215

Table 13.1 Emerging Developmental Milestones From Birth to 5 Years (continued)

Age	Gross Motor	Fine Motor	Social	Language	Self-Help
36 mo	Goes up stairs alternating feet; rides tricycle; stands momentarily on one foot	Builds tower of nine cubes; imitates construction of "bridge" of three cubes; copies circle; imitates cross	Plays simple games (in "parallel" with other children)	Knows age and sex, counts three objects correctly; repeats three numbers or sentence of six syllables; expressive vocabulary of over 1000 words; remembers some recent past events	Toilet trained; helps in dressing (unbuttons clothing, puts on shoes); washes hands
48 mo	Hops on one foot; throws ball overhand; uses scissors to cut out pictures; climbs well	Imitates construction of "gate" of five cubes; copies cross and square; draws person with two or four parts besides head; can name longer of two lines	Plays with several children—beginning of social interaction and role-playing	Counts four pennies accurately; tells story; asks many questions; uses four- to five-word sentences; uses plurals; can repeat three or four numbers; knows four colors	Uses toilet alone
60 mo	Skips	Copies triangle; can name heavier of two weights	Asks questions about meaning of words; participates in domestic role-playing	Repeats sentence of 10 syllables; counts 10 pennies correctly; follows three-part instructions; can name penny, nickel, and dime; uses pronouns properly	Dresses and undresses

Adapted from Parker S, Zuckerman B, eds. *Behavioral and Developmental Pediatrics: A Handbook for Primary Care.* Boston, Mass: Little, Brown; 1995:420–421.

GLOBAL DEVELOPMENTAL DISABILITY/INTELLECTUAL DISABILITY (COGNITIVE-ADAPTIVE DISORDERS)

- American Association on Intellectual and Developmental Disabilities definition: "a disability characterized by significant limitations both in intellectual functioning and in adaptive behavior as expressed in conceptual, social, and practical adaptive skills. This disability originates before the age of 18"
- *DSM-IV-TR* Mental Retardation Severity classification based on IQ level: Mild, 50–55 to approximately 70; Moderate, 35–40 to 50–55; Severe, 20–25 to 35–40; Profound, <20 or 25
- Etiology identified in 40–60% of patients
- Presents most often as developmental delay in >2 areas during infancy or preschool years
- Described as global developmental delay until after age 5 yr, when diagnosis is more certain
- Diagnosis: evaluations should occur serially over time to identify evolving phenotypes
- Rule out underlying genetic or metabolic causes; see Diagnostic Tests section
- Management: family and educational support, routine health evaluations; anticipate and plan for future independent functioning level, and refer for genetic counseling if appropriate

AUTISM SPECTRUM DISORDERS

- Heterogeneous group of disorders characterized by severe and pervasive impairments in several developmental areas: reciprocal social interaction, language and communication skills, and presence of stereotyped behaviors, restricted interests, and activities (*DSM-IV-TR*)
- ASD includes autistic disorder, Asperger's disorder, and PDD NOS
- Prevalence: 6/1000 children
- 2:1 to 6.5:1 male predominance
- Recurrence rate in siblings: 2–8%

APPROACH TO ASD

Diagnostic Criteria

AUTISM

- See Box 13.2
- Autism red flags: combined language and social delays, regression in language and social milestones in second or third year of life (occurs in approximately one third)
- Best predictors in 18-mo-old: lack of response to name and pointing for interest

Box 13.2 Diagnostic Criteria for Autistic Disorder

DSM-IV-TR Criteria

A. A total of at least six items from (1), (2), and (3), with at least two from (1), and one each from (2) and (3):

1. Qualitative impairment in social interaction, as manifested by at least two of the following:
   a. Marked impairment in the use of multiple nonverbal behaviors, such as eye-to-eye gaze, facial expression, body postures, and gestures to regulate social interaction
   b. Failure to develop peer relationships appropriate to developmental level
   c. Lack of spontaneous seeking to share enjoyment, interests, or achievements with other people (e.g., by a lack of showing, bringing, or pointing out objects of interest)
   d. Lack of social or emotional reciprocity

2. Qualitative impairment in communication, as manifested by at least one of the following:
   a. Delay in, or total lack of, the development of spoken language (not accompanied by an attempt to compensate through alternative modes of communication such as gesture or mime)
   b. In individuals with adequate speech, marked impairment in the ability to initiate or sustain a conversation with others
   c. Stereotyped and repetitive use of language or idiosyncratic language
   d. Lack of varied spontaneous make-believe play or social imitative play appropriate to developmental level

3. Restricted, repetitive, and stereotyped patterns of behavior, interests, and activities, as manifested by at least one of the following:
   a. Encompassing preoccupation with one or more stereotyped and restricted patterns of interest that is abnormal either in intensity or focus
   b. Apparently inflexible adherence to specific, nonfunctional routines or rituals
   c. Stereotyped and repetitive motor mannerisms (e.g., hand or finger flapping or twisting or complex whole-body movements)
   d. Persistent preoccupation with parts of objects

B. Delays or abnormal functioning in at least one of the following areas, with onset before age 3 yr:
   1. Social interaction
   2. Language as used in social communication
   3. Symbolic or imaginative play

C. Not better accounted for by Rett disorder or childhood disintegrative disorder

Reprinted with permission from the *DSM-IV-TR: Diagnostic and Statistical Manual of Mental Disorders. Text Revision*, Fourth Edition, copyright 2000. American Psychiatric Association.

ASPERGER'S DISORDER

- See Box 13.3

Diagnostic Evaluation

- Detailed developmental history (may use ADI-R)
- Clinical observation (ADOS is gold standard)
- CARS

Box 13.3   Diagnostic Criteria for Asperger's Disorder

DSM-IV-TR Criteria

A. Qualitative impairment in social interaction, as manifested by at least two of the following:
1. Marked impairment in the use of multiple nonverbal behaviors such as eye-to-eye gaze, facial expression, body postures, and gestures to regulate social interaction
2. Failure to develop peer relationships appropriate to developmental level
3. A lack of spontaneous seeking to share enjoyment, interests, or achievements with other people (e.g., by a lack of showing, bringing, or pointing out objects of interest to other people)
4. Lack of social or emotional reciprocity

B. Restricted repetitive and stereotyped patterns of behavior, interests, and activities, as manifested by at least one of the following:
1. Encompassing preoccupation with one or more stereotyped and restricted patterns of interest that is abnormal either in intensity or focus
2. Apparently inflexible adherence to specific, nonfunctional routines or rituals
3. Stereotyped and repetitive motor mannerisms (e.g., hand or finger flapping or twisting, or complex whole-body movements)
4. Persistent preoccupation with parts of objects

C. The disturbance causes clinically significant impairment in social, occupational, or other important areas of functioning.

D. There is no clinically significant general delay in language (e.g., single words used by 2 yr old, communicative phrases used by 3 yr old).

E. There is no clinically significant delay in cognitive development or in the development of age-appropriate self-help skills, adaptive behavior (other than in social interaction), and curiosity about the environment in childhood.

F. Criteria are not met for another specific pervasive developmental disorder or schizophrenia.

Reprinted with permission from the *DSM-IV-TR: Diagnostic and Statistical Manual of Mental Disorders. Text Revision*, Fourth Edition, copyright 2000. American Psychiatric Association.

Development

13

Additional Testing

- Formal evaluation of cognitive function and adaptive skills by psychologist
- Speech, language and communication assessment by speech language pathologist

Medical Evaluation

- See Developmental History and Developmental Physical Examination sections, above

Strategies for Management

- Early intervention: behavioral therapy (ABA); speech and language therapy
- Medication to treat specific symptoms and behaviors
- Family and educational support

DIAGNOSIS

- See Box 13.4

Box 13.4   Diagnostic Criteria for Attention Deficit/ Hyperactivity Disorder

A. Either 1 or 2:

1. Six (or more) of the following symptoms of **inattention** have persisted for at least 6 mo to a degree that is maladaptive and inconsistent with developmental level:
   a. Often fails to give close attention to details or makes careless mistakes in schoolwork, work, or other activities
   b. Often has difficulty sustaining attention in tasks or play activities
   c. Often does not seem to listen when spoken to directly
   d. Often does not follow through on instructions and fails to finish schoolwork, chores, or duties in workplace (not caused by oppositional behavior or failure to understand instructions)
   e. Often has difficulty organizing tasks and activities
   f. Often avoids, dislikes, or is reluctant to engage in tasks that require sustained effort (such as schoolwork or homework)
   g. Often loses things necessary for tasks or activities (e.g., toys, school assignments, pencils, books, or tools)
   h. Is often easily distracted by extraneous stimuli
   i. Is often forgetful in daily activities

2. Six (or more) of the following symptoms of **hyperactivity-impulsivity** have persisted for at least 6 mo to a degree that is maladaptive and inconsistent with developmental level:
   Hyperactivity
   a. Often fidgets with hands or feet or squirms in seat
   b. Often leaves seat in classroom or in other situations in which remaining seated is expected
   c. Often runs about or climbs excessively in situations in which it is inappropriate (in adolescents or adults, may be limited to subjective feelings of restlessness)
   d. Often has difficulty playing or engaging in leisure activities quietly
   e. Is often "on the go" or often acts as if "driven by motor"
   f. Often talks excessively
   Impulsivity
   g. Often blurts out answers before questions have been completed
   h. Often has difficulty awaiting turn
   i. Often interrupts or intrudes on others (e.g., butts into conversations or games)

B. Some hyperactive-impulsive or inattentive symptoms that caused impairment were present before age 7 yr

C. Some impairment from symptoms is present in two or more settings (e.g., at school and at home)

D. There must be clear evidence of clinically significant impairment in social, academic, or occupational functioning

E. Symptoms do not occur exclusively during course of pervasive developmental disorder, schizophrenia, or other psychotic disorder and are not better accounted for by another mental disorder (e.g., mood disorder, anxiety disorder, dissociative disorder, or personality disorder)

Reprinted with permission from the *DSM-IV-TR: Diagnostic and Statistical Manual of Mental Disorders. Text Revision*, Fourth Edition, copyright 2000. American Psychiatric Association.

Development

13

TREATMENT

- Behavioral management strategies
- Medications shown to be effective in treating children with ADHD
  - Stimulants are first line; available in short, intermediate, and extended-release forms
  - Methylphenidate (e.g., Ritalin, Concerta)
    - Common side effects include decreased appetite, weight loss, sleep disruption, growth suppression, tachycardia, hypertension, hypotension, palpitations, nervousness, irritability, emotional lability, dizziness, crying, tics (do not administer to patients with motor tics or Tourette syndrome)
  - Amphetamines (e.g., Dexedrine, Adderall)
    - Common side effects include decreased appetite, sleep disruption, weight loss, irritability, hypertension, tachycardia, palpitations; do not administer to children with structural heart abnormalities

CEREBRAL PALSY

- Permanent but nonprogressive disorder characterized by impaired motor control, including coordination and balance dysfunction, and/or abnormal movements
- Caused by injury to the developing brain
- Prevalence: 2/1000–5/1000 live births
- Etiology may not be found in >50%
- Risk factors: echogenicities in periventricular white matter (strongest predictive factor); very low birth weight (<1500 g) (15–20% risk); intraventricular hemorrhage; kernicterus (bilirubin encephalopathy); delays in greater than four motor milestones; Apgar score of <3 at 10 min (poor predictor)

DIAGNOSIS AND MANAGEMENT

- Should not diagnose before 6 mo of age
- Serial evaluations over time are necessary
- Classification of CP may not be clearly identifiable until 18 to 36 mo of age (Table 13.2)
- Physical examination: special attention to motor abilities, tone, asymmetry or persistence of primitive reflexes, deep tendon reflexes; examine for contractures
- Audiometry (high-frequency and sensorineural hearing loss common in athetoid CP), vision and cognitive testing
- Management goals: improve motor function and mobility, facilitate communication, improve independence in activities of daily living, provide educational support, prevent musculoskeletal complications (e.g., contractures)
- Treatment may include physical, occupational, and speech therapy, assistive devices (e.g., walkers, augmentative communication, orthotic

bracing), antispasticity medications (e.g., baclofen), botulinum toxin A injections, and orthopedic surgery
- Classification and prognostic information defined in the Gross Motor Function Classification System for Cerebral Palsy (available in *Dev Med Child Neurol*, 1997;39:214-223)

Table 13.2	Clinical Classification of Cerebral Palsy
Type	Frequency (%)
Spastic 　Hemiparesis 　Monoparesis 　Diplegia* 　Quadriparesis	70–80
Dyskinetic 　Athetoid 　Dystonic 　Chorea 　Ballismus 　Tremor	10–15
Rigid	5
Ataxic	1
Mixed	10–15

Reprinted from Taft LT. Cerebral palsy. *Pediatrics in Review*. 1995;16:411–418.

FETAL ALCOHOL SPECTRUM DISORDER

- FASD is a clinical spectrum caused by prenatal alcohol exposure (FAS and ARND)
- Specific timing and amount of fetal alcohol exposure leading to FASD are unclear; however, the syndrome was described only in children of problem drinking mothers
- Incidence of FASD: 9.1/1000
  - Higher rates in subpopulations (e.g., 190/1000 in some North American First Nations populations)
- Diagnosis
  - Known or suspected maternal alcohol use during pregnancy with features from three areas:
    1. Craniofacial anomalies: short palpebral fissures, ptosis, hypoplasia of midface, upturned nose, smooth philtrum, thin upper lip
       – Plot palpebral fissure length (≥ 2 SD below mean is significant)
       – Philtrum length should be one third of the lower one third of the face

– Examine lip and philtrum and rank according to lip philtrum
  guide (rank of 4 or 5 is significant)
– See Further Reading section (Koren and Nulman, 2006)
2. Growth impairment: small for gestational age, postnatal growth
   retardation (low weight compared with height)
3. Neurodevelopmental features: microcephaly; corpus callosum
   agenesis; cerebellar hypoplasia; attention deficit hyperactivity;
   language and learning difficulties; cognitive, memory, and
   abstract reasoning impairment; fine and gross motor deficits;
   tremors; sociopathy; maladaptive behavior; not learning from
   experience; delinquency; and rule breaking
   • For suspected fetal alcohol exposure, with lack of a confirmed his-
     tory of maternal alcohol intake, neonatal meconium testing for fatty
     acid ethyl esters (FAEE) is very specific to fetal exposure to alcohol
 • Associated birth defects: congenital heart defects, cleft lip and/or
   palate, sensorineural hearing loss, skeletal and limb deformities, renal
   anomalies, ophthalmologic abnormalities
 • Management: developmental assessment; speech, occupational, and
   physical therapy, as needed; cognitive testing; educational support;
   medical and/or surgical management of birth defects; routine health
   evaluation, including growth monitoring

FURTHER READING

American Academy of Pediatrics, Committee on Quality Improvement,
   Subcommittee on Attention-Deficit/Hyperactivity Disorder. Clinical practice
   guideline: diagnosis and evaluation of the child with attention-
   deficit/hyperactivity disorder. *Pediatrics.* 2000;105:1158–1170.
Johnson CP, Myers SM, and the Council on Children with Disabilities.
   Identification and evaluation of children with autism spectrum disorders.
   Pediatrics. 2007;120:1183–1215.
Myers SM, Johnson CP, and the Council on Children with Disabilities.
   Management of children with autism spectrum disorders. *Pediatrics.*
   2007;120:1162–1182.
Koren G, Nulman I. *The Motherisk Guide to Diagnosing Fetal Alcohol Spectrum
   Disorder (FASD).* 2nd ed. Toronto, Ontario, Canada: The Hospital for Sick
   Children; 2006.
Thackray H, Tifft C. Fetal alcohol syndrome. *Pediatr Rev.* 2001;22:47–55.
Walker WO Jr, Johnson CP. Mental retardation: overview and diagnosis. *Pediatr
   Rev.* 2006;27:204–212.

USEFUL WEB SITES

National Institute of Mental Health information. Available at: http://www.nimh.nih.gov
Pediatric Development and Behavior information. Available at: http://www.dbpeds.org
Centers for Disease Control and Prevention – Department of Health and Human
   Services; Child Development section. Available at: http://www.cdc.gov/ncbddd/
   child/default.htm

Development

13

Chapter 14 Diagnostic Imaging and Interventional Radiology

Arif Manji

Ganesh Krishnamurthy

Bairbre Connolly

Chapter 14 Diagnostic Imaging and
Interventional Radiology

COMMON ABBREVIATIONS

AF	air–fluid
AP	anterior to posterior
AXR	abdominal X-ray
BA	biliary atresia
C+ CT	contrast-enhanced computed tomography
C– CT	nonenhanced computed tomography
C+ MRI	contrast-enhanced magnetic resonance imaging
C tube	cecostomy tube
CBD	common bile duct
CVL	central venous line
CXR	chest X-ray
DDH	developmental dysplasia of the hip
DMSA	dimercaptosuccinic acid
DTPA	diethylenetriamine pentaacetic acid
ESSB	esophagus, stomach, and small bowel (fluoroscopy study)
GA	general anesthesia
GB	gallbladder
GE	gastroesophageal
G tube	gastrostomy feeding tube
GJ tube	gastrojejunostomy feeding tube
GU	genitourinary
HCl	hydrochloric acid
IBD	inflammatory bowel disease
IGT	image-guided therapy
J tube	jejunostomy tube
Lat	lateral
LGI	lower gastrointestinal (contrast study)
MAG3	mercapto acetyl triglycine
MRCP	magnetic resonance cholangiopancreatography
NEC	necrotizing enterocolitis
NJ tube	nasojejunal tube
PA	posterior to anterior
PICC	peripherally inserted central catheter
RLQ	right lower quadrant
RUQ	right upper quadrant
SCFE	slipped capital femoral epiphysis
SMA	superior mesenteric artery
SMV	superior mesenteric vein
SVC	superior vena cava
SXR	skull X-ray

UGI	upper gastrointestinal (series)
UPJ	ureteropelvic junction
US	ultrasonography
VCUG	voiding cystourethrogram
VP	ventriculoperitoneal
VUR	vesicoureteral reflux

GENERAL PRINCIPLES

IMAGING MODALITIES
- See Table 14.1

CONTRAST AGENTS
- See Table 14.2
- Used to examine structures without inherent contrast differences relative to surroundings
- Administration: oral, rectal, or IV injection before imaging

BRAIN
- See Table 14.3

HEAD AND NECK
- See Tables 14.4 and 14.5 and Figure 14.1

Table 14.1 Imaging Modalities

Modality	Advantages	Disadvantages	Contraindications
Plain film XR	Inexpensive, noninvasive, readily available	Radiation exposure, generally poor at distinguishing soft tissues	Pregnancy (relative)
CT	Excellent delineation of bones and soft tissues; spiral CT fast data acquisition; may allow 3D reconstruction; CT angiography less invasive than conventional angiography	High radiation exposure; sedation/GA may be needed; patient anxiety; relatively high cost; caution with contrast in renal failure/allergy; metal causes artifact	Pregnancy (relative); contraindication to contrast agents
MRI	No radiation involved; excellent soft tissue resolution and discrimination; MR angiography and venography offer noninvasive assessment of vessels and flow	Claustrophobia; sedation/GA may be needed; metal causes artifact; may be less readily available	Ferromagnetic metal foreign bodies, cardiac pacemaker
US	Low cost, noninvasive, no radiation, determines cystic vs. solid; real-time imaging useful for interventions	Highly operator dependent; air in bowel may prevent imaging of midline abdominal structures	
Nuclear medicine	Functional imaging data	Radioactive substance injected, ingested, or inhaled; frequently needs IV ± sedation; urine and body fluids radioactive	
PET-CT	Excellent tumor detection	IV needed; high radiation dose; ± sedation/GA	Pregnancy
Fluoroscopy (GI/GU)	Real time; rarely requires sedation	Radiation involved; bladder catheterization for VCUG	Pregnancy

Diagnostic Imaging and Interventional Radiology

14

227

Table 14.2 Types and Uses of Contrast in Imaging

Modality	Agent	Routes and Study Type	Contraindications
XR	Barium	PO/PR–routine GI studies	Perforation, toxic megacolon
	Iodinated contrast	PO/PR–suspected perforation in GI/GU studies	Allergy (relative)
	Iodinated contrast	Via urinary catheter–GU studies	Allergy (relative)
CT	Iodinated contrast	IV–highlights vessels, inflammation PO/PR–bowel opacification	Renal failure
MRI	Gadolinium	IV–highlights vessels, inflammation	Renal failure

Table 14.3 Brain Imaging

Pathology	Modality
Congenital anomalies	· Antenatal US or MRI helpful · Postnatal MRI confirms diagnosis, assesses gray/white matter differentiation and maturation; useful in follow-up
Germinal matrix hemorrhage	· US best for evaluation of IVH and its sequelae
Hypoxic-ischemic encephalopathy	· MRI, diffusion-weighted imaging, and MR spectroscopy
Congenital infections	· CT optimal (e.g., shows intracranial calcifications of TORCH infections) · For congenital herpes infection, consider MRI
Metabolic disease	· MRI with MR spectroscopy
Trauma	· SXRs of limited value; use C– CT for initial evaluation of head trauma (accidental and nonaccidental), intracranial hemorrhages, and fractures; perform C+ CT if see fracture adjacent to the dural venous sinuses; diffuse axonal injury is best evaluated using MRI
Tumors	· CT frequently performed initially · C+ MRI best for tumor evaluation (diagnosis and follow-up)
Stroke and vasculitis	· MRI, MR angiography, and diffusion-weight imaging · <6 hr: immediately active acute stroke program
VP shunt malfunction	· Shunt series (AP/Lat SXR, AP CXR, AP AXR) show the course and integrity of the shunt tubing (kinks, breaks) · Head C– CT assesses ventricular size

Table 14.4	Head and Neck Imaging
Pathology	**Modality**
Orbital cellulitis	· C+ CT of the orbits determines if infection is preseptal or postseptal and identifies cavernous sinus thromboses
Sinusitis	· Sinus AP/Lat XR useful only if >6 yr of age · C– CT (occasionally C+ CT) evaluates complications of sinusitis
Thyroid disease	· US is initial modality to assess size, symmetry, and focal lesions
Neck and upper airway disease	· See Table 14.5 and Figure 14.1 for Lat neck XR findings

Table 14.5	Lateral Neck X-Ray in Neck and Upper Airway Disease
Diagnosis	**Findings on Lateral Neck X-Ray**
Croup	*Steeple sign:* subglottic narrowing
Epiglottitis	*Thumbprint sign:* enlarged, indistinct epiglottis
Retropharyngeal abscess	Soft tissue, air, or enlargement of prevertebral soft tissues · Anterior to C2: >7 mm or > ½ vertebral body width · Anterior to C6: >14 mm or >1 full vertebral body width · Loss of normal "step-off" at ~C4 False positives: neck flexed and end-expiration Further evaluation and confirmation with C+ CT

Figure 14.1 **Lateral Neck X-Ray for Evaluating Retropharyngeal Abscess**

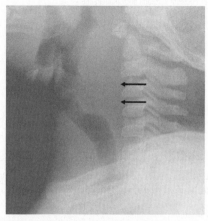

Increased prevertebral soft tissue shadow (*arrows*) displacing the hypopharynx suggests retropharyngeal abscess.

CONGENITAL ANOMALIES

- Antenatal US helpful; postnatal confirmation with spine and brain MRI (to assess for associated anomalies)
- Spine US is the screening investigation of choice; simple sacral dimples are innocuous and do not require workup unless they are large, located farther away from the anus, or in association with other cutaneous stigmata

TRAUMA (SPINE AND CORD INJURY)

- Start with AP/Lat XR for cervical spine injury; request odontoid views if suspect atlanto-occipital instability
- If AP/Lat XR findings normal, flexion/extension views unlikely to be abnormal
- If AP/Lat XR findings equivocal/abnormal, flexion/extension views still unlikely to be abnormal but may help rule out injury in an alert child with no neurologic signs complaining of neck pain/tenderness
- See Table 14.6 and Figure 14.2
- C– CT with multiplanar reconstruction is best for detecting vertebral fractures; additional C+ CT useful when associated vascular injury suspected
- If neurologic deficit present, perform spine MRI to assess spinal cord and root/nerve integrity

Table 14.6	ABCDS for Reading C-Spine Films
Alignment	Look for continuous lines with smooth contour and no step-offs · Anterior vertebral body (spinal) line · Posterior vertebral body (spinal) line · Facet line · Spinolaminar line · Spinous process line
Bones	Chips or fractures
Count	Must visualize all 7 cervical vertebral bodies in entirety
Disk spaces	Look for consistent distance between each vertebral body
Soft tissue	Look for swelling, especially prevertebral

SCOLIOSIS

- Standard AP (3-foot XR) and Lat spinal XR
- PA view can be used in girls to reduce breast radiation

Figure 14.2 Normal Lateral X-Ray of C-Spine

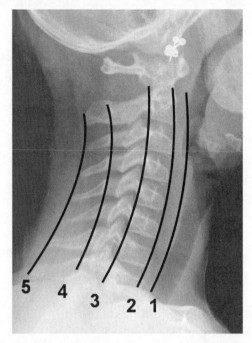

Line 1, Prevertebral soft tissue line: runs along the posterior border of airway through the first four or five vertebral bodies, then widens around laryngeal cartilage and parallels the remaining cervical vertebrae. Line 2, Anterior spinal line: demarcates anterior border of cervical vertebral bodies. Line 3, Posterior spinal line: demarcates posterior border of cervical vertebral bodies. Line 4, Spinolaminar line: connects junction of lamina and spinous process. Line 5, Spinous process line: joins the tips of spinous processes. These lines should run smooth and parallel, with no abrupt step-offs.

CHEST

APPROACH TO CXR

- See Table 14.7 and Figures 14.3A and B on p. 233
- Initial imaging study for all suspected thoracic disease
- Standard views: upright PA and left Lat
- Supplemental views: oblique, lordotic, left or right Lat decubitus
- May require portable AP depending on acuity

Table 14.7	Basic Approach to CXR
Identification	Date, Name, Indications
Exposure	Thoracic disk spaces should be just visible through heart
Rotation	Medial ends of clavicles should be equidistant from spinous process
Inspiration	Poor inspiration—poor aeration, vascular crowding, compressed and widened central shadow Older children: 6 anterior and 8 posterior ribs normally seen (general rule) Hyperinflation—lucent lungs, flattened diaphragm, small heart
Soft tissues	Look for air in the soft tissues Note presence of thymus (normally seen up to age 10 yr)
Abdomen	Look for free air under diaphragm in upright CXR
Bones	Check cervical and thoracic spine, shoulder girdle, ribs, sternum
Mediastinum	Trachea, heart, great vessels, spine Look for mediastinal or tracheal shift, widened mediastinum
Hila	Pulmonary vessels, mainstem and segmental bronchi, lymphadenopathy
Lungs	Lung parenchyma, pleura, diaphragm

INFILTRATE

- See Table 14.8 on p. 234
- Cells or fluid (blood, pus, edema) involving the bronchoalveolar airspace or peribronchial interstitial space; need to consider volume loss, seen as a density or opacity on a CXR

ATELECTASIS

- Loss of lung aeration ranging from subsegmental to entire lung collapse, with volume loss
- Appears radio-opaque; differentiated from infiltrate based on linear or wedge pattern (subsegmental) or associated volume loss (lobar or entire lung collapse)
- Indirect signs: hilar/mediastinal shift toward collapse, ± hemidiaphragm elevation

Figure 14.3A Posteroanterior CXR

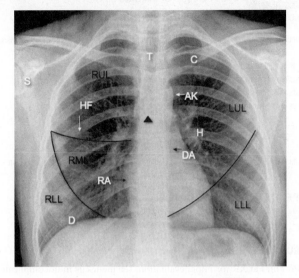

Figure 14.3B Lateral CXR

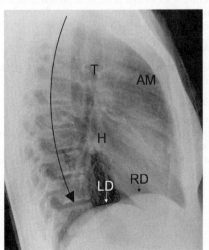

A, Anterior mediastinum (AM), aortic knuckle (AK), clavicle (C), descending aorta (DA), dome of diaphragm (D), hilum (H), horizontal fissure (HF), left dome of diaphragm (LD), left lower lobe (LLL), left upper lobe (LUL), right atrium (RA), right dome of diaphragm (RD), right lower lobe (RLL), right middle lobe (RML), right upper lobe (RUL), scapula (S), trachea (T), tracheal bifurcation (*arrowhead*). B, (*Long curved arrow*) Radiolucency normally increases from superior to inferior region, along the thoracic vertebrae.

Table 14.8	Specific Signs of Infiltrate on CXR
Sign	**Pathology**
Silhouette sign	Lobar consolidation/infiltrate (may also represent atelectasis or mass)
· Loss of right heart border	· Right middle lobe
· Loss of right hemidiaphragm	· Right lower lobe
· Loss of left heart border	· Lingula
· Loss of left hemidiaphragm	· Left lower lobe
Air bronchograms	Radiolucent branching bronchi visible through opacified airspace disease
Peribronchial cuffing	Interstitial infiltrate, edema, and/or bronchial inflammation

PARENCHYMAL ABNORMALITIES

- C– CT for mets, diffuse lung disease (HRCT)
- C+ CT best (e.g., for lung abscess, pneumatocele or contusion)

PLEURAL EFFUSIONS

- PA and Lat XR for initial evaluation; see meniscus in uncomplicated effusion; Lat XR more sensitive (initial posterior pooling)
- Lat decubitus film shows layering dependently, unless effusion loculated
- US most sensitive for detecting minimal pleural fluid, extent, loculations, septations, and pleural thickening
- C+ CT occasionally helpful as adjunct

MEDIASTINAL MASS

- CT or MRI determine location, mass effect on airway and vessels, and can help determine etiology

PNEUMOTHORAX

- Most obvious on expiratory upright CXR
- Shows visceral pleura paralleling the chest wall, separating partially collapsed lung from pleural air
- Mediastinal shift and diaphragmatic inversion indicate tension pneumothorax

ABDOMEN

OBSTRUCTION

- See Table 14.9

Table 14.9	Imaging of Abdominal Obstruction		
Diagnosis	Modality	Utility	Findings
Bowel obstruction: general approach	AXR (supine and upright)	Initial modality of choice	· Dilated bowel loops, AF levels, distal paucity of gas · Small or large bowel pattern
	AXR (Lat decubitus or cross-table Lat)	Adjunct	Detects free air or AF levels when difficult to obtain upright film, or for confirmation
	Contrast studies	Adjunct	ESSB for proximal small bowel, contrast enema for distal small bowel and large bowel
Pyloric stenosis	US	Modality of choice	Pylorus length >17 mm Thickness ≥15 mm
	UGI	Rarely used	String or double-track sign, delayed gastric emptying, etc.
Esophageal atresia ± tracheoesophageal fistula	CXR	Initial modality	Attempt NG tube insertion: coiled tube in a dilated proximal esophageal pouch
	UGI: air, rarely contrast	Caution with contrast	Outlines upper pouch Gap length measurement
Duodenal atresia/ stenosis/obstruction	AXR	Initial modality	"Double bubble" sign: marked distension of stomach and proximal duodenum No distal air beyond second portion of duodenum
	UGI	Diagnostic	Can distinguish different causes of duodenal obstruction

14

(continued)

Table 14.9	Imaging of Abdominal Obstruction *(continued)*		
Diagnosis	**Modality**	**Utility**	**Findings**
Malrotation (with midgut volvulus is surgical emergency)	UGI	Modality of choice	1. Abnormal position of duodenojejunal junction (ligament of Treitz): below and right of normal (normal is to the left of the spine at or above level of pylorus) 2. Complete duodenal obstruction or "corkscrew" filling pattern down right spine in volvulus
	LGI	Adjunct	Cecum high and more midline, not in RLQ
	US	Adjunct	Inverted SMA and SMV relationship (normally vein is to the right of artery at level of the head of the pancreas)
	AXR	Initial test but not diagnostic	Cecum not in RLQ Not indicative of volvulus
Intussusception	US	Modality of choice	Ideally done when symptomatic Telescoping of bowel seen
	Pneumatic reduction	Treatment of choice for ileocolic intussusception	Air enema reduction under fluoroscopic guidance: contraindicated in suspected perforation
Hirschsprung disease	AXR	Initial	Distal bowel obstruction: dilated loops with AF levels on upright (nonspecific)
	Barium enema	Suggestive	Small-caliber rectum Colonic dilatation proximal to narrowed (aganglionic) segment (colon diameter > rectum)

INFLAMMATION

- See Table 14.10

HEPATOBILIARY DISEASE

- See Table 14.11

Table 14.10 **Imaging of Abdominal Inflammatory Conditions**

Diagnosis	Modality	Utility	Findings
Neonatal NEC	AXR	Modality of choice	· Multiple static dilated bowel loops · Pneumatosis intestinalis: intramural gas in bowel wall · Late signs: portal venous gas and pneumoperitoneum · Serial AXRs q4–6h initially · Cross-table Lat and/or decubitus help detect free air
	US + Doppler	Adjunct	· Bowel perfusion and free air
Appendicitis	US	Modality of choice	· High specificity and sensitivity · Visualization of normal appendix required to rule out appendicitis
	AXR	Adjunct, poor	· Radio-opaque fecalith in 5–10%
	C+ CT abdomen/pelvis	Complex cases or if excess bowel gas present	· Inflammation of appendix and peritoneum; associated abscesses/complications
IBD	AXR	Initial modality for sequelae	· Nonspecific findings, perforation · Toxic megacolon: >5.5–6 cm transverse colon
	ESSB contrast study	Crohn's diagnosis and sequelae	· Indirect visualization of small bowel segments not accessible by endoscopy · Strictures
	LGI	Ulcerative colitis	· Ulceration, lead-pipe colon
	US	Sequelae	· Abscess, bowel wall thickening
	C+ CT (IV + PO) abdomen/pelvis	Sequelae	· Bowel wall thickening, abscess, fistula, megacolon
	MRI abdomen/pelvis	Adjunct	· Fistula: higher sensitivity than CT

14

Table 14.11   Imaging of Hepatobiliary Disease

Diagnosis	Modality	Utility	Findings
Cholelithiasis/ choledocholithiasis	US	Modality of choice	· Location of stone (better sensitivity for detection in GB than CBD) · Intrahepatic biliary dilatation seen with CBD stone *If associated cholecystitis:* · GB wall thickening · Pericholecystic fluid · Sonographic Murphy sign (RUQ tenderness by US probe)
	MRCP	Adjunct	· Entire biliary tree seen
BA	US	Initial modality	In a *fasting* infant: · Rule out choledochal cyst · Absent or deformed GB, length <2 cm · No ductal dilatation · Irregular GB wall
	Nuclear medicine Biliary scan (Chotetec)	Modality of choice	Following 5 d phenobarbital
	Cholangiogram (percutaneous/ intraoperative)	Adjunct	Patency of biliary tree excludes BA
Liver disease	US with Doppler	Initial modality	· Focal/diffuse parenchymal abnormalities · Abnormalities of biliary tree · Patency of blood vessels and direction of flow with color-flow Doppler · Confirmation of ascites
	C+ CT abdomen	Adjunct	Good for focal parenchymal disease, biliary tract disease
	MRI, MRCP	Adjunct	Good for parenchymal and vascular abnormalities; occasionally for intra- and extrahepatic biliary pathology

OTHER ABDOMINAL CONDITIONS

- See Table 14.12 and Figure 14.4

Table 14.12	Imaging of Other Abdominal Conditions		
Diagnosis	Modality	Utility	Findings
Meckel diverticulum	US	Poor	· Nonspecific · May show intussusception
	Meckel scan: Tc-pertechnetate scintigraphy	Modality of choice	· Uptake by ectopic gastric mucosa · >1 dose ranitidine before scan inhibits gastric secretion, thus increasing increasing its visualization
Abdominal mass	US	Initial modality	Size, nature, organ of origin
	C+ CT abdomen and pelvis	Adjunct	Aids diagnosis, location, other involved structures, lymphadenopathy; follow-up; best for calcifications
	MRI abdomen	Adjunct	Soft tissue characteristics
Abdominal trauma	C+ CT abdomen and pelvis	Modality of choice	Solid and hollow viscus injuries; fluid

**Figure 14.4 Pneumatosis Intestinalis Seen in Patient
With Necrotizing Enterocolitis**

14

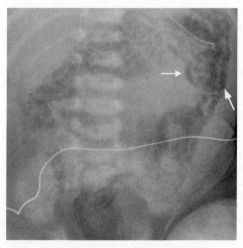

AXR: Linear lucencies (*arrows*) represent extraluminal air (air in the wall of the bowel) suggestive of pneumatosis in NEC.

CONGENITAL ANOMALIES

- US for detection and follow-up (e.g., dysplastic kidneys, hydronephrosis, horseshoe kidney, UPJ obstruction, cysts)

URINARY TRACT INFECTION

- See Table 14.13

Table 14.13	Imaging in Urinary Tract Infections	
Modality	**Indication**	**Findings**
Renal US	First episode of pyelonephritis <6 yr of age	Renal size/position, hydronephrosis, structural architecture, corticomedullary differentiation, and lower urinary tract
VCUG	First episode of pyelonephritis <6 yr of age	Presence/grade of VUR, bladder and urethral abnormalities (e.g., ureterocele, posterior urethral valve), postvoid residual urine (not precise)
DMSA scan	To look for scarring, differential function (e.g., postpyelonephritis)	Binds to cortical tubular cells; absent uptake correlated with scars, infarcts, masses; assesses each kidney's contribution to global renal function
MAG3 Lasix washout study	Obstructed kidney	Assess excretion/drainage from kidney

TESTICULAR TORSION

- US with color Doppler

UTERINE AND OVARIAN PATHOLOGY

- US most useful in diagnosing ovarian torsion and pelvic pathology
- MRI used for congenital malformations such as cloacal abnormality

MUSCULOSKELETAL SYSTEM

TRAUMA

- AP and Lat XR for fractures; occasionally need comparison film of contralateral side
- Oblique views may help (e.g., scaphoid fracture)
- Appearance of ossification centers key in differentiating normal from Salter-Harris epiphyseal injuries (see Chapter 31)
- Certain fractures (e.g., pelvic) may require CT for treatment planning
- MRI useful in evaluating bone, cartilage, soft tissue, and ligamentous changes

OSTEOMYELITIS

- Mainly involves metaphysis
- Bone scan and MRI show early changes; XR does not show changes until after approximately 10 d

HIP DISORDERS

- See Table 14.14 and Figure 14.5

Table 14.14	Imaging of the Hip	
Pathology	**Modality**	**Findings**
DDH	US—screening modality of choice	Shallow acetabulum, ± subluxation of head
	XR: AP and frog-leg view	Displaced and small femoral head
Legg-Calvé-Perthes disease	XR: AP and frog-leg view	Small epiphysis → widened articular space → subchondral fracture → resorption
SCFE	XR: AP and frog-leg view	Femoral head height loss, slipped medially and posteriorly; widened physis; *Klein's line:* line along superior border of femoral metaphysis misses the head (see Figure 14.5)
Hip effusion	US	Fluid in joint space

Figure 14.5 **Approximating Klein's Line for Slipped Capital Femoral Epiphysis on Frog-Leg X-Ray**

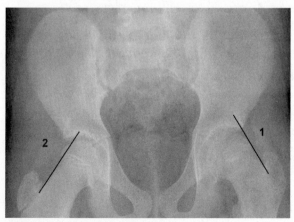

Left SCFE. Klein's line—drawn along the superior aspect of the femoral neck—should intersect portion of the femoral head (*line 2*). *Line 1* on left does not intersect femoral head, consistent with SCFE.

BONE AGE

- Bone age: AP XR of *left* wrist (± additional views of knee)

SKELETAL SURVEY

- Skeletal survey: 12 views (skull, spine, chest, abdomen, extremities)
- Mainly performed in skeletal dysplasias, metabolic disorders, histio-cytosis, and child abuse (latter may require additional imaging [e.g., head CT])

BONE TUMORS

- AP and Lat XR best for initial diagnosis
- MRI best for extent of involvement (especially joint/soft tissue), metastases

CATHETERS AND TUBES

CENTRAL LINES

- On CXR, look for catheter tip at junction of SVC and right atrium, below right mainstem bronchus
- Some extension into right atrium acceptable, but if noted to be low in the right atrium and curving to the left on PA film, may be in right ventricle

UMBILICAL ARTERIAL AND VENOUS CATHETERS

- See Chapter 6

ENDOTRACHEAL TUBES

- On CXR, ETT tip should be approximately midway between thoracic inlet and carina; watch for atelectasis if ETT too far down one bronchus, usually the right

GASTROSTOMY AND GASTROJEJUNOSTOMY TUBES

GENERAL PRINCIPLES

- See Figure 14.6 and Table 14.15

TECHNIQUES OF G AND GJ TUBE PLACEMENT

- Technique of choice depends on local expertise or institutional preferences
  - Surgical
  - Laparoscopic
  - Percutaneous endoscopic gastrostomy
  - Image guided

Figure 14.6 Algorithm for Selecting Feeding Tube

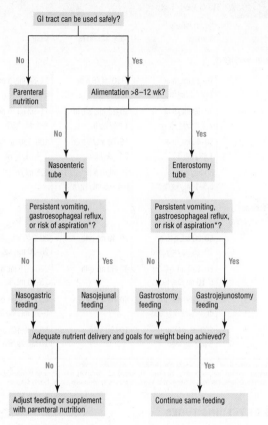

14

*Despite treatment with prokinetic and acid inhibitory agents.
© The Hospital for Sick Children, 2003. Courtesy of *The Hospital for Sick Children Handbook of Pediatrics*, 10th edition, Fig. 25.3. p. 597.

Table 14.15	Guidelines for Initiating and Progressing Tube Feedings		
Age (yr)	Initial Hourly Infusion	Daily Increases	Goal
Continuous Feedings			
0-1	10-20 mL/h or 1-2 mL/kg/h	5-10 mL/8 h or 1 mL/kg/h	21-54 mL/h or 6 mL/kg/h
1-6	20-30 mL/h or 2-3 mL/kg/h	10-15 mL/8 h or 1 mL/kg/h	71-92 mL/h or 4-5 mL/kg/h
6-14	30-40 mL/h or 1 mL/kg/h	15-20 mL/8 h or 0.5 mL/kg/h	108-130 mL/h or 3-4 mL/kg/h
>14	50 mL/h or 0.5-1 mL/kg/h	25 mL/8 h or 0.4-0.5 mL/kg/h	125 mL/h
Bolus Feedings (Not for GJ Tubes)			
0-1	60-80 mL q4h or 10-15 mL/kg/feed	20-40 mL q4h	80-240 mL q4h or 20-30 mL/kg/feed
1-6	80-120 mL q4h or 5-10 mL/kg/feed	40-60 mL q4h	280-375 mL q4h or 15-20 mL/kg/feed
6-14	120-160 mL q4h or 3-5 mL/kg/feed	60-80 mL q4h	430-520 mL q4h or 0-20 mL/kg/feed
>14	200 mL q4h or 3 mL/kg/feed	100 mL q4h	500 mL q4h or 10 mL/kg/feed

Note: Rates expressed per kg body weight are useful for small-for-age patients.
From Wilson SE. Pediatric enteral feeding. In: Grand RJ, Sutphen JL, Dietz WH, eds. *Pediatric Nutrition, Theory and Practice.* Toronto, Ontario, Canada: Butterworths; 1987. Reprinted by permission of Dr. James Sutphen.

TYPES OF FEEDING TUBES

- Pigtail catheters (e.g., Dawson-Mueller): loop at distal end with locking device proximally
- Balloon-style G tube
- Foley catheter (temporary replacement catheter)
- Low-profile devices: Bard button (mushroom-shaped dome tip); MIC-KEY devices (silicone balloon tip inflatable with saline)
- See Figure 14.7

Figure 14.7 Types of Feeding Tubes

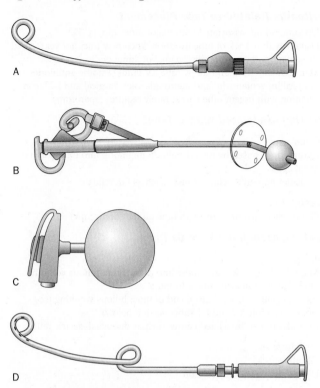

A

B

C

D

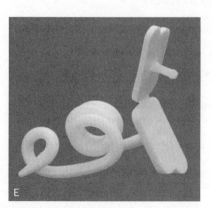

E

A, Mac-Loc G tube. B, balloon-style G
tube. C, Mickey button tube. D, GJ tube.
E, Chait Trapdoor cecostomy tube.
© The Hospital for Sick Children, 2003.
Courtesy of *The Hospital for Sick Children
Handbook of Pediatrics*, 10th edition,
Fig. 20.1. p. 464.

COMPLICATIONS ASSOCIATED WITH G AND GJ TUBES

Peritonitis Related to Tube Placement
- Uncommon but associated with major morbidity (1.5%)
- Usually within 1 wk of tube insertion when new tract not yet formed
- Presentation: fever, irritability, pain, vomiting; peritoneal signs
- Management: NPO and nil by tube, IV fluids, empiric antibiotics (ampicillin, gentamicin, and metronidazole), surgical and IGT consultation with urgent tube check; rarely requires laparotomy

Vomiting Associated With G Tube

Causes
- Obstruction caused by pigtail/balloon migration into duodenum or esophagus
- Consider non–tube-related causes such as GE reflux

Investigation
- G-tube check (contrast through tube under fluoroscopy)

Vomiting Associated With GJ Tube

Causes
- Migration of gastric coil of tube into duodenum: bilious vomiting
- Tube leak in stomach: vomits formula
- Intussusception around distal end of tube: bilious vomiting (see Intussusception Around GJ Tubes section below)
- Consider non–tube-related causes such as duodenal–gastric reflux

Investigations
- GJ-tube check
- US to rule out intussusception

Intussusception Around GJ Tubes
- Highest risk: <1 to 2 yr of age
- Presentation: typically bilious vomiting, irritability; may be asymptomatic
- Rarely irreducible or ischemic
- Diagnosis: US, fluoroscopy

Management
- Refer for tube revision: exchange tube over wire, cut distal pigtail, shorten tube, or change tube type; US confirms intussusception reduced
- If severe symptoms: hold feeding ± temporary replacement of GJ with G tube
- If recurrent intussusception: consider further shortening of GJ to GD tube, continuous G-tube feeding or fundoplication

Blocked G or GJ Tube

- Blockage usually from failure to flush tube after use or after administration of medications (PPIs, commonly crushed tablets)
- Flush with saline in 5- or 10-mL syringe using forceful pressure
- Try carbonated beverage or cranberry juice; specific alkaline/acid solution may be indicated depending on medication

Dislodged G or GJ Tube

- Gently insert Foley catheter of same size or smaller into stomach and secure with tape
- Within 8 wk of initial insertion: Foley catheter position must be confirmed by contrast fluoroscopy before feeding started (increased risk of peritoneal placement when tract is not completely formed)
- >8 wk after insertion: Foley catheter or new tube position confirmed by withdrawing gastric juice via syringe before feeding
- If safe for gastric feeding, may run feeds and medications through Foley until new tube is placed; if not safe, keep Foley in situ to maintain tract patency
- If GJ partly dislodged, secure with tape until evaluated; often can still be used

Tube Site Infections

Granulation Tissue
- Pinkish red, moist with clear/cloudy exudates, may bleed
- Consider frequent saline soaks, hydrogen peroxide, or silver nitrate

Skin Irritation With Leakage
- Daily skin care: clean peristomal area, keep dry, apply skin barriers
- Gastric acid suppression for G and GJ tubes

Skin Inflammation (Not Definite Cellulitis)
- Clean daily with saline soaks; dry and apply barrier cream
- Trial of topical antimicrobial ointment

Cellulitis
- Topical antibiotics initially
- Candidal infection: local antifungal ± oral if oral candidiasis present
- Subcutaneous abscess (rare): drainage + systemic antibiotics

CECOSTOMY TUBES

GENERAL PRINCIPLES

- Indicated in patients with problematic fecal incontinence (e.g., spina bifida, imperforate anus)
- Pigtail catheter is inserted into cecum under image guidance, replaced by low-profile Chait tube after 6–8 wk
- Antegrade enemas through tube to wash out and empty colon through rectum and prevent accidental soiling

COMPLICATIONS

- Similar to G/GJ tubes (see Complications Associated With G and GJ Tubes section on p. 246)

Peritonitis

- Early postinsertion
- Beware of ascending infection along VP shunt: give empiric antibiotics (ampicillin, gentamicin, metronidazole), IV fluids, ± neurosurgical and general surgical consultation

Blocked C Tube

- Attempt unblocking, as with G/GJ tube
- If unsuccessful, will require unblocking/exchange to be performed under fluoroscopy

Dislodged C Tube

- Temporary Foley replacement or tape partially dislodged tube, as with G/GJ
- Requires reinsertion under fluoroscopy

Tube Site Infections

- See Gastrostomy and Gastrojejunostomy Tubes section (p. 242)

VASCULAR ACCESS

- Central venous access devices inserted by image guidance; include tunneled and nontunneled CVLs, implantable devices (subcutaneous ports), and PICCs

INDICATIONS

- See Box 14.1

Box 14.1	Indications for Central Venous Line Insertion

- Hemodialysis, plasmapheresis
- Total parenteral nutrition
- Chemotherapy, vesicant drugs
- Poor IV access
- IV therapy >2 wk
- Hyperosmolar infusions
- Frequent blood sampling
- Unstable medical condition requiring inotropic support and/or multiple continuous infusions

PREPROCEDURAL EVALUATION

- Age, medical condition, catheter type, and developmental stage affect whether GA, sedation, or local anesthetic is appropriate
- Consider preprocedural Hb, PLT, INR, and PTT for all central access (generally not required if PICC requested)

COMPLICATIONS

- See Table 14.16 for recommendations regarding line removal

Table 14.16	Suggested Removal Priority for Central Venous Lines		
	Removal Priority		
Reason for Removal	**A**	**B**	**C**
Line insertion site/tunnel			
Infection at insertion site			X
Tunnel infection	X		
Positive blood culture*			
Only peripheral			X
Only CVL		X	
Both		X	
Condition of patient			
Too unstable to remove†			
Septic shock		X	
Fever, not systemically unwell			X
No clinical response in 48–72 h	X		
Complications			
Endocarditis	X		
Endovasculitis	X		
Septic emboli	X		
Blood culture positive at 48–72 h of treatment	X		
Organism			
Coagulase-negative *Staphylococcus*			X
S. aureus	X		
Streptococcus group			X
Gram-negative bacilli			X
Bacillus spp.	X		
Fungus	X		
Polymicrobial		X	
Mycobacterium	X		

A, recommend immediate removal; B, recommend removal, depending on venous access and CVL dependence;
C, recommend trial of treating with line in place.
*See specific organism for removal priority.
†Use clinical judgment.
© The Hospital for Sick Children, 2003. Courtesy of *The Hospital for Sick Children Handbook of Pediatrics*, 10th edition.

Infection

- Exit-site skin infection: local discharge/redness at site
- Tunnel infection: tracking of redness, swelling, tenderness along subcutaneous course
- Catheter-related bacteremia: positive culture from catheter *and* from peripheral venous sample with either
  1. greater quantitative culture from catheter, or
  2. catheter culture positive earlier than peripheral culture

Occlusion

- CXR to check for line position and for breakage
- Blood related: treat with alteplase (tPA) instillation for 2–4 h; see pp. 470–472
- Chemical occlusions can be unblocked with instillation of 0.1 mol/L HCl for 2–4 h
- If unblocking unsuccessful or if occlusion recurs, consider venous thrombosis as cause
- Avoid high pressure or excessive force using small syringes (≤ 5 mL), as line may rupture
- May require unblocking or rewiring by interventional radiologist

Thrombosis

- US: sensitive for detecting vessel clots (including jugular vein)
- Lineogram: contrast study of catheter may detect tip clot and fibrin sheath formation
- Venography: gold standard—for catheter-related clots within vein (excluding jugular vein)
- Management: see pp. 470–472

Migration/Dislodgement

- CXR and contrast study of catheter (lineogram) to confirm line position

Fracture

- External breakage: repair kits available (requires experienced personnel)
- Internal breakage: exchange/retrieval (requires experienced personnel)

CHEST TUBES

IMAGE-GUIDED INSERTION

- Locking pigtail catheters routinely used; no sutures or large incision required
- Pigtails softer, more flexible, less painful than standard tubes but more likely to block

DECREASED DRAINAGE: ETIOLOGY AND MANAGEMENT

- All pleural fluid drained (confirm with CXR or US)
- Failure in system (check all seals) or inadequate suction
- Tube blocked: flush catheter through stopcock with Luer-Lok saline syringe; never let chest tube be open to air
- Loculated collection: confirm with US or CT chest; fibrinolytics (tPA) beneficial in loculated collections
- Tube malposition or kink: confirm by CXR or rarely CT chest; may require tube manipulation under fluoroscopy

Removal of Pigtail Chest Tube

- Should be done by experienced personnel
- Prerequisites: gauze with petrolatum (Vaseline) for airtight dressing, clamp, scissors, gloves
- Two ways to remove tube:
  1. Clamp tube. Cut the distal end of the tube to release tension on internal thread, thereby unlocking distal pigtail. Keep cut end of tube covered with finger to avoid air entry. Release clamp. Pull out tube, placing petrolatum dressing on site in same motion. Dress with gauze.
  2. Clamp tube. Release lock on tube by turning anticlockwise. Ensure thread not caught in stopcock. Ensure system closed to air, then release clamp. Pull out tube, placing petrolatum dressing on site in same motion. Dress with gauze.

FURTHER READING

Carty H. *Imaging Children*. London, England: Churchill Livingstone; 2004.

Donnelly L, Jones B, O'Hara S, et al. *Diagnostic Imaging: Pediatrics*. Salt Lake City, Utah: Amirsys; 2005.

Stringer DA. *Pediatric Gastrointestinal Imaging & Intervention*. Hamilton, Ontario, Canada: BC Decker Inc; 2000.

Diagnostic Imaging and Interventional Radiology

14

USEFUL WEB SITES

Introduction to pediatric radiology. Available at: **www.med-ed.virginia.edu/ courses/rad/peds** (interactive systems-based Web site of general pediatric radiology, with excellent images and teaching text in a quiz format)

Oregon Health & Science University. Available at: **www.ohsu.edu/radiology/teach/ kojima/** (comprehensive list of normal values and measurements for organs in pediatrics)

Pediatric Imaging Teaching Files. Available at: **www.uhrad.com/pedsarc.htm** (case based, with over 80 cases, each with clinical history, images, brief differential diagnoses, and teaching points)

Pediatric radiology. Available at: **www.cchs.net/pediatricradiology** (Web-based teaching curriculum of pediatric radiology aimed primarily for radiology residents, with questions, answers, and results)

Radiology articles. Available at: **www.emedicine.com/radio** (section covering pediatric radiology, divided by disease entity and easy to search)

Virtual Pediatric Hospital. Available at: **www.virtualpediatrichospital.org** (case-based problems, directs the reader to different resources)

Chapter 15 Endocrinology

Caroline McLaughlin
Rayzel M. Shulman
Kusiel Perlman

Chapter 15 Endocrinology

COMMON ABBREVIATIONS

ACTH	adrenocorticotropic hormone
ADH	antidiuretic hormone
BG	blood glucose
CAH	congenital adrenal hyperplasia
CHO	carbohydrate
DHEAS	dehydroepiandrosterone sulfate
DHT	dihydrotestosterone
DKA	diabetic ketoacidosis
DM1	type 1 diabetes mellitus
DM2	type 2 diabetes mellitus
DSD	disorders of sexual development
ECF	extracellular fluid
FFA	free fatty acids
FSH	follicle-stimulating hormone
GH	growth hormone
hCG	human chorionic gonadotropin
HHS	hyperglycemic hyperosmolar state
HPA	hypothalamic–pituitary axis
IAI	intermediate-acting insulin
LAI	long-acting insulin
LHRH	luteinizing hormone–releasing hormone
OGTT	oral glucose tolerance test
PTH	parathyroid hormone
RAI	rapid-acting insulin
SIADH	syndrome of inappropriate antidiuretic hormone
SG	specific gravity
T_3	triiodothyronine
T_4	thyroxine
TSH	thyroid-stimulating hormone
TSI	thyroid-stimulating immunoglobulin (TSH receptor–stimulating antibodies)
VSD	ventricular septal defect

Endocrinology

15

DIABETES MELLITUS

TYPE 1

Diagnostic Criteria

- One random BG >11 mmol/L or two fasting plasma BG >6.9 mmol/L, glycosuria ± ketonuria, and symptoms of hyperglycemia

Clinical Features

- Polyuria, polydipsia, polyphagia, weight loss
- Approximately 25% present with DKA

Epidemiology

- Incidence varies; 0.1–45 per 100,000 children <18 yr worldwide, 15–17 per 100,000 in the United States; 9–25 per 100,000 in Canada

Genetic Susceptibility

- Risk increases with family history of DM1 (5% for first-degree relatives)

Management of Stable, Newly Diagnosed Diabetes (No DKA)

- Initiation of diabetes education can be achieved on outpatient basis
- Admission to hospital indicated only to correct ketoacidosis or other factors making ambulatory care difficult (e.g., distance, language, psychosocial)

Insulin

- See Table 15.1
- Initial daily insulin dose: 0.4–0.6 units/kg/d divided ⅔ before breakfast and ⅓ before supper
- Each dose divided ⅔ IAI, ⅓ RAI
  - For example, for a child who weighs 30 kg, the total initial daily insulin dose based on 0.5 units/kg/d would be 15 units; 10 units total given before breakfast, divided as 7 units IAI and 3 units RAI; 5 units total before dinner, divided as 3 units IAI and 2 units RAI
- For most children, especially if >5 yr, nighttime dose split as RAI before supper and IAI at bedtime
- If starting on a basal/bolus regimen, total daily dose is divided into 50% LAI and 50% RAI
- Monitor BG levels before meals, before bed, and as indicated
- Younger patients and during initial education period, target BG is 6–12 mmol/L; for patients >6 yr when patient and family comfortable with management, BG target decreased to 4–10 mmol/L
- Anticipate decrease in insulin requirements in first few weeks with increased activity and honeymoon period
- Comprehensive outpatient educational program and ongoing communication with diabetes team essential in long-term management

Table 15.1	Onset, Peak, and Duration of Action of Insulin Preparations		
Insulin	Onset	Peak	Duration
Rapid-acting: Lispro (Humalog) Aspart (Novolog/Novorapid)	5-10 min	0.5-2.5 h	3-4 h
Intermediate-acting: Humulin N Novolin NPH	1-4 h	6-12 h	18-24 h
Long-acting: Glargine (Lantus) Detemir (Levemir)	1-2 h 1-2 h	Peakless Mild peak	18-28 h 12-24 h

Outpatient Management of Intercurrent Illness

- Check BG and urine ketones every 4 h around the clock
- Do not stop insulin
- The dose of RAI may need to be adjusted, but insulin is always required (Table 15.2)
- Ensure fluid intake
- May provide carbohydrates as fluid
- Treat the underlying illness
- If the child vomits ≥2 times in 6–8 h OR refuses to take fluids, should be seen urgently in the emergency department (Figure 15.1)

Table 15.2	Insulin Adjustment During Intercurrent Illness				
BG (mmol/L)	<6	6-13	13-17	>11	>17
Urine ketones	-ve or +ve	-ve or +1	-ve	+2 to +3	-ve or +ve
Action	Decrease daily insulin by 20% per day until BG 6-11	Wait and monitor, give usual insulin	Give usual insulin at usual time AND at same time, add 10% of total daily dose as RAI	Give usual insulin at usual time AND add 20% of total daily insulin dose as RAI q4h until ketones negative and BG <11	

DKA

- See Figure 15.2 for management

Figure 15.1 Emergency Room Management of Intercurrent Illness

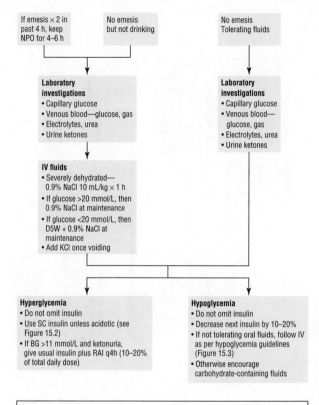

If emesis × 2 in past 4 h, keep NPO for 4–6 h

No emesis but not drinking

No emesis Tolerating fluids

Laboratory investigations
- Capillary glucose
- Venous blood—glucose, gas
- Electrolytes, urea
- Urine ketones

Laboratory investigations
- Capillary glucose
- Venous blood— glucose, gas
- Electrolytes, urea
- Urine ketones

IV fluids
- Severely dehydrated— 0.9% NaCl 10 mL/kg × 1 h
- If glucose >20 mmol/L, then 0.9% NaCl at maintenance
- If glucose <20 mmol/L, then D5W + 0.9% NaCl at maintenance
- Add KCl once voiding

Hyperglycemia
- Do not omit insulin
- Use SC insulin unless acidotic (see Figure 15.2)
- If BG >11 mmol/L and ketonuria, give usual insulin plus RAI q4h (10–20% of total daily dose)

Hypoglycemia
- Do not omit insulin
- Decrease next insulin by 10–20%
- If not tolerating oral fluids, follow IV as per hypoglycemia guidelines (Figure 15.3)
- Otherwise encourage carbohydrate-containing fluids

Discharge
- Tolerating oral fluids
- No other reason for hospitalization
- Replace usual meal plan with carbohydrate-containing fluids

Observation and monitoring
- Input and output
- Blood glucose q2–4h (keep within 4–10 mmol/L)
- Urine for ketones q4h

Endocrinology

15

Figure 15.2 Diagnosis and Management of Diabetic Ketoacidosis

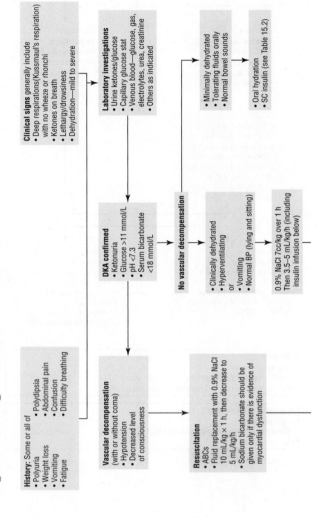

History: Some or all of
- Polyuria
- Weight loss
- Vomiting
- Fatigue
- Polydipsia
- Abdominal pain
- Confusion
- Difficulty breathing

Clinical signs generally include
- Deep respirations(Kussmaul's respiration) with no wheeze or rhonchi
- Ketones on breath
- Lethargy/drowsiness
- Dehydration—mild to severe

Laboratory investigations
- Urine ketones/glucose
- Capillary glucose stat
- Venous blood—glucose, gas, electrolytes, urea, creatinine
- Others as indicated

DKA confirmed
- Ketonuria
- Glucose >11 mmol/L
- pH <7.3
- Serum bicarbonate <18 mmol/L

No vascular decompensation
- Clinically dehydrated
- Hyperventilating
  or
- Vomiting
- Normal BP (lying and sitting)

0.9% NaCl 7cc/kg over 1 h
Then 3.5–5 mL/kg/h (including insulin infusion below)

- Minimally dehydrated
- Tolerating fluids orally
- Normal bowel sounds

- Oral hydration
- SC insulin (see Table 15.2)

Vascular decompensation (with or without coma)
- Hypotension
- Decreased level of consciousness

Resuscitation
- ABCs
- Fluid replacement with 0.9% NaCl 10 mL/kg × 1 h, then decrease to 5 mL/kg/h
- Sodium bicarbonate should be given only if there is evidence of myocardial dysfunction

Management
- If history of voiding and K^+ <5.5 mmol/L, add 40 mEq/L KCL to IV fluid
- Aim to keep K^+ between 4 and 5 mEq/L
- Continuous insulin infusion 0.1 units/kg/h = 1 mL/kg/h (of solution of 25 units regular insulin in 250 mL NS)
- Do not give bolus of insulin

Neurologic deterioration
- Headache, irritability, decreased level of consciousness, decreased HR
- First, rapidly exclude hypoglycemia by capillary BG measurement
- Then, treat for cerebral edema

Acidosis not improving (in 3–4 h)
- Check insulin delivery system
- Consider sepsis
- Contact tertiary pediatric diabetes center

Acidosis improving
- Blood glucose <15 mmol/L or glucose falls >5 mmol/L/h
- Change IV to D5W + 0.9% NaCl
- Decrease insulin to 0.05 units/kg/h
- Glucose <10 mmol/L, change IV to D10W + 0.9% NaCl

Improvement
- Clinically well
- Tolerating oral fluids
- pH >7.3
- HCO_3^- >18 mmol/L

- Start SC insulin
- Stop IV insulin 30 min after SC dose of Humalog or 1 h after SC dose of regular insulin
- Determine cause of DKA
- Contact regional pediatric diabetes education center

- 20% mannitol 5 mL/kg over 20 min
- If Na^+ has declined significantly, consider administration of 2–4 mL/kg of 3% 0.9% NaCl over 10–20 min, then 0.9% NaCl at maintenance IV rate
- Decrease insulin to 0.04–0.05 units/kg/h = 0.4–0.5 mL/kg/h of standard solution as above
- Contact tertiary pediatric diabetes center
- Admit to ICU

Observation and monitoring
- Hourly blood glucose (capillary)
- Aim for a decrease in blood glucose of 5 mmol/L/h
- Hourly documentation of fluid input/output
- Minimum hourly documentation of neurologic function
- Electrolytes, venous gas 2–4h after start of IV; then q2–4h
- Follow effective osmolality (2x measured Na^+ measured blood glucose)
- Avoid decrease of >2–3 mmol/L/h in effective osmolality by increasing IV Na^+ concentration

Hypoglycemia in Diabetes Mellitus

Clinical Features
- Mild: sweating, weakness, tachycardia, tremors, feelings of nervousness and/or hunger
- Severe: lethargy, irritability, confusion, behavior that is out of character, seizure, coma

Management of Minor Hypoglycemia
- Treat BG <4 mmol/L or 4–6 mmol/L accompanied by symptoms of hypoglycemia
- Treat with 10–15 g CHO (e.g., 125 mL juice or regular soft drink, 2–3 dextrose tablets, 250 mL milk, or 2 tsp sugar)
- Wait 10–15 min, recheck BG
- May re-treat with 10–15 g CHO

Glucagon Administration
- Indication: altered level of consciousness or seizure
- Families should have emergency glucagon kit at home
- Reconstitute glucagon crystals with fluid provided in kit
- SC injection: <6 yr, half vial (0.5 mg) or >6 yr, whole vial (1.0 mg)
- Avoid giving oral sugar until child is awake and alert
- Vomiting may occur after severe hypoglycemia, regardless of whether glucagon was given
- Go to emergency department if child has not completely recovered after an episode of severe hypoglycemia (Figure 15.3)

Management During Surgery
- Minor procedures (<1 h and expected to be tolerating oral fluids shortly after procedure)
  - Admit on day of surgery for IV insertion and preoperative monitoring
  - IV fluid should contain D5W or D10W + 0.9% NaCl
  - On day of surgery:
    - IAI: give ⅔ A.M. dose of IAI only (i.e., no RAI)
    - LAI: give 80% of LAI dose only (i.e., no RAI)
    - Pump: continue usual basal infusion rate only (i.e., no insulin boluses)
    - BG preoperatively and immediately postoperatively; monitor as necessary
    - RAI given postoperatively as necessary to maintain BG 5–15 mmol/L
    - Usual dose of insulin resumed when child able to take normal diet
- Major procedure (>1 h and/or not expected to tolerate oral fluids immediately after procedure)
  - May need to admit patient 1 d prior to procedure if poor glycemic control or patient not previously known; discuss plan with anesthesiologist
  - No SC insulin on day of procedure
  - NPO perioperatively

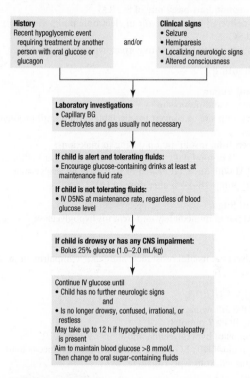

Figure 15.3 Emergency Room Management of Hypoglycemia

History
Recent hypoglycemic event requiring treatment by another person with oral glucose or glucagon

and/or

Clinical signs
• Seizure
• Hemiparesis
• Localizing neurologic signs
• Altered consciousness

Laboratory investigations
• Capillary BG
• Electrolytes and gas usually not necessary

If child is alert and tolerating fluids:
• Encourage glucose-containing drinks at least at maintenance fluid rate

If child is not tolerating fluids:
• IV D5NS at maintenance rate, regardless of blood glucose level

If child is drowsy or has any CNS impairment:
• Bolus 25% glucose (1.0–2.0 mL/kg)

Continue IV glucose until
• Child has no further neurologic signs
            and
• Is no longer drowsy, confused, irrational, or restless
May take up to 12 h if hypoglycemic encephalopathy is present
Aim to maintain blood glucose >8 mmol/L
Then change to oral sugar-containing fluids

Discharge only when child is
• Fully alert
• Tolerating oral fluids
• Free of neurologic signs

Observation and monitoring
• Try to determine cause of hypoglycemia
• Decrease all insulin doses by 20% for next 24 h
• Arrange for follow-up
• Renew prescription of glucagon if used

• IV with D5W or D10W + 0.9% NaCl
• Insulin infusion: 0.02 units regular insulin/kg/h
• Adjust insulin infusion to maintain BG at 8–15 mmol/L
• Monitor BG hourly intraoperatively, q4h postoperatively
• When tolerating fluids PO:
  1. Start SC insulin (⅔–¾ usual dose and increase as indicated; administer extra RAI as required)
  2. Discontinue insulin infusion 30 min after giving SC insulin

Insulin Pump
- Delivers continuous basal rate of SC RAI
- Insulin delivered from reservoir in electronic pump via tubing inserted SC
- Boluses given with CHO or to correct hyperglycemia

Troubleshooting

High Blood Sugar
- Check pump and pump site
- Change pump site or convert to injectable insulin until problem corrected
- To convert from insulin pump dosing to injections:
  - Give ⅔–¾ of total daily basal insulin dose as IAI at bedtime, then give RAI with any CHO eaten or to correct hyperglycemia
  - Restart pump 18–24 h after dose of IAI

Low Blood Sugar
- Suspend pump immediately and treat for hypoglycemia

TYPE 2
- Hyperglycemia, insulin resistance, and relative impairment in insulin secretion

Diagnostic Criteria
- One of the following:
  - Fasting BG $\geq$7 mmol/L
  - Symptoms of hyperglycemia and BG >11.1 mmol/L
  - Abnormal OGTT, BG >11.1 mmol/L 2 h after glucose load
- Distinguished from type 1 diabetes by
  - Obesity
  - Signs/symptoms of insulin resistance (e.g., acanthosis nigricans, hypertension, dyslipidemia, polycystic ovary syndrome)
  - Positive family history

Risk Factors
- Ethnicity: Aboriginal, Hispanic, Asian, South Asian, African descent
- Intrauterine factors: gestational diabetes, low birth weight

Clinical Presentation
- DKA (25%)
- Polyuria/polydipsia ± ketonuria

Management
- Nonpharmacologic goal: increase insulin sensitivity and secretion through weight reduction, increase in physical activity

- Pharmacologic medications:
  - To replace deficient insulin
  - To decrease hepatic glucose production and reduce insulin resistance (e.g., biguanides)
- Ideal approach is multidisciplinary, including physicians, nurses, dietitians, exercise physiologists, and mental health professionals

HHS or Nonketotic Hyperglycemia

Definition
- BG can be very high (>56 mmol/L), plasma osmolality as high as 380 mOsm/kg, and neurologic abnormalities may be present

Clinical Features
- Acidosis or ketonuria not usually present
- Neurologic signs (e.g., change in level of consciousness, focal deficits, seizures secondary to high osmolality)

Management
- Medical emergency, admit to hospital
- Initial treatment similar to DKA (no evidence-based treatment guidelines currently available)
- Rehydration with IV 0.9% NaCl to achieve hemodynamic stability
- Sodium bicarbonate not recommended: may induce hypokalemia and ventricular arrhythmias
- Monitor BG hourly
- Aim to reduce BG by ≤5 mmol/h; may be achieved by IV rehydration alone
- Need for insulin infusion best determined after initial IV fluid resuscitation
- ICU admission may be necessary because of high risk of hyperthermia, rhabdomyolysis, renal failure, worsening mental status, ventricular arrhythmias, and death in patients with HHS

HYPOGLYCEMIA

- See Chapter 25 and Figure 25.5

DIFFERENTIAL DIAGNOSIS
- See Table 15.3
- In <1 yr old, hyperinsulinemic hypoglycemia is most common cause of persistent hypoglycemia
- In >1 yr old, ketotic hypoglycemia is the most common cause

Table 15.3	Etiology of Hypoglycemia	
Endocrine Causes		**Nonendocrine Causes**
Ketotic hypoglycemia		Sepsis/shock
Primary hyperinsulinism		Inborn error of metabolism
Panhypopituitarism		Poisoning
GH deficiency		Birth asphyxia
Adrenal insufficiency		Prematurity
Addison disease		Liver disease
Maternal DM (in neonates)		

DIAGNOSIS

- Critical blood sample for BG, blood gas, electrolytes, FFAs, β-hydroxybutyrate, insulin, GH, cortisol, TSH, free T_4, acylcarnitine, quantitative amino acids, NH_4, lactate, urine organic acids
- Key investigation: urine for ketones; absence of ketonuria raises suspicion of hyperinsulinism or defects in fatty acid or ketone oxidation

TREATMENT

- Treat with glucose 0.5 g/kg (1 mL/kg of D50W or 2 mL/kg of D25W) IV bolus, then continuous infusion of sufficient glucose to maintain BG level in normal range
- More detailed investigation may require admission for monitored fasting challenge

THYROID DISORDERS

HYPOTHYROIDISM

Congenital Hypothyroidism

Etiology
- Thyroid dysgenesis—most common; accounts for 85%
- Dyshormonogenesis
- Hypopituitarism
- Hypothalamic deficiency
- Iatrogenic (inadvertent administration of radioiodine during pregnancy)

Clinical Manifestations
- Rarely seen because of neonatal screening
- Asymptomatic at birth because of transplacental passage of maternal T_4
- Prolonged neonatal jaundice
- Feeding difficulties, poor appetite
- Apneic episodes

Investigations
- TSH, free T$_4$
- Thyroid scan

Diagnosis
- TSH >40 mU/L on neonatal screening (days 2–3 of life)
- Note: TSH surge after birth can lead to false-positive results (TSH 20–40 mU/L); values need to be repeated if this occurs

Treatment
- Levothyroxine 10–14 mcg/kg body weight to the closest available dose: 25, 37.5, 44, or 50 mcg
- Dose adjustment: if TSH >5 mU/L, increase levothyroxine dose by 6–12.5 mcg increments

Prognosis
- Normal cognitive function if treated before 10 d of age

Follow-Up
- Monitor free T$_4$, TSH, and growth at
  - 2 wk after initiation of therapy; at 2, 3, 6, 9, 12 mo; q6mo until 3 yr; yearly after 3 yr
  - Annually by primary care MD for >6 yr of age with uncomplicated hypothyroidism

Acquired Hypothyroidism

Etiology
- Most commonly caused by lymphocytic thyroiditis (Hashimoto thyroiditis)
- Autoimmune thyroid disease with 2:1 female preponderance
- Trisomy 21, Turner, Klinefelter syndromes, other autoimmune diseases (e.g., celiac and DM1) at higher risk

Initial Investigations
- TSH, free T$_4$
- Bone age

Clinical Manifestations
- See Box 15.1

Treatment
- If asymptomatic or euthyroid, monitor
- If symptomatic or abnormal TSH/free T$_4$, treat with levothyroxine according to age (Table 15.4)

HYPERTHYROIDISM
- Graves disease most common; more rarely, thyroiditis (thyroid inflammation) and hashitoxicosis (silent or painless thyroiditis)
- Peak in adolescence; female-to-male ratio: 6:1

Box 15.1 Clinical Manifestations of Hypothyroidism

- Fatigue, lethargy, somnolence
- Cold intolerance; cool, dry extremities
- Linear growth failure; short stature
- Delayed or precocious puberty
- Constipation
- Dry skin, hair
- Diffuse goiter
- Bradycardia
- Muscle hypertrophy and weakness
- Delayed relaxation phase of deep tendon reflexes
- Myxedema

Table 15.4 Levothyroxine Dose Recommendations

Age	Dose (mcg/kg/d)
0–3 mo	10–15
3–6 mo	8–10
6–12 mo	6–8
1–3 yr	4–6
3–10 yr	3–4
10–15 yr	2–4
>15 yr	2–3

Adapted from Alario A. *Practical Guide to the Care of the Pediatric Patient.* St. Louis, Mo: Mosby; 1997.

Graves Disease

Etiology
- Autoimmune disorder (caused by TSIs causing hyperthyroidism); may also cause exophthalmos, myopathy, and dermopathy (rare in children)

Clinical Manifestations
- See Box 15.2

Investigations
- TSH, T_3 and T_4: elevated free T_4 and T_3 in presence of low TSH (if TSH normal, suggests abnormality of thyroid hormone binding)
- TSIs
- Thyroid ^{123}I scan indicated if nodule palpated

Box 15.2 Clinical Manifestations of Hyperthyroidism

- Palpitations
- Tremor
- Fatigue, weakness
- Sweating, heat intolerance
- Weight loss
- Increased appetite
- Exophthalmos
- Diarrhea

Management

Medical

- Propylthiouracil: 5–10 mg/kg/d divided q8h—inhibits conversion from T_4 to T_3 and inhibits thyroid hormone synthesis; or methimazole: 0.5–1.0 mg/kg/d q12h—inhibits thyroid hormone synthesis
- Side effects of both drugs include lupuslike syndrome, granulocytopenia, jaundice, rashes
- Remission rate with medical management up to 30% after 2 yr
- Propranolol: 0.5–2.0 mg/kg/d divided q6–8h—to block sympathetic hyperactivity, if severe

Ablation

- Radioiodine therapy with ^{131}I
- Remission may take weeks to months; therefore, interval antithyroid drug therapy is required
- Consequence is hypothyroidism

Surgery

- Immediate remission
- Subsequent hypothyroidism
- Risks: hypoparathyroidism, recurrent laryngeal nerve palsy, keloid formation

CALCIUM DISORDERS

HYPOCALCEMIA

Normal Calcium Range

- See Box 15.3

History

- Neck surgery/trauma; family history; diet; decreased sunlight exposure; GI, hepatobiliary, or pancreatic disease; renal disease

Box 15.3 Normal Total Calcium Range

Premature Infant
- 0–3 d: 1.8–2.5 mmol/L
- 3 d–2 mo: 2.0–2.75 mmol/L

Term Infant
- 0–2 mo: 2.0–2.75 mmol/L

Child
- 2.25–2.62 mmol/L

Adult
- 2.12–2.62 mmol/L

Corrected Calcium
- Plasma calcium concentration falls by 0.2 mmol/L for every 10 g/L fall in the plasma albumin concentration
- Measure ionized calcium if serum protein or pH abnormal

Signs/Symptoms

- Muscle cramps, carpopedal spasm (Trousseau sign), facial twitch (Chvostek sign), paresthesias, tetany, seizures, laryngeal stridor, ECG abnormalities (e.g., shortened QT, bradycardia, widened T waves)

Investigations

- PO_4^-, Mg^{2+}, ALP, PTH
- 25-(OH)-vitamin D
- 1,25-$(OH)_2$-vitamin D
- ± renal and liver function tests, serum pH, total protein/albumin

Differential Diagnosis

- See Boxes 15.4 and 15.5

Box 15.4 Differential Diagnosis of Neonatal Hypocalcemia

Early (within first 72 h of life)
- Maternal illness: diabetes mellitus, hyperparathyroidism
- Neonatal illness: prematurity, low birth weight, birth asphyxia

Late (after 72 h of life)
- Hypoparathyroidism (22q deletion syndrome, autosomal dominant and X-linked recessive)
- Pseudohypoparathyroidism
- Ingestion of high-phosphate milk
- Hypomagnesemia
- Vitamin D deficiency
- Renal insufficiency

Adapted from Sperling M. *Pediatric Endocrinology*. 2nd ed. Philadelphia, Pa: WB Saunders; 2002.

Hypoparathyroidism
- Impaired synthesis/secretion (genetic, autoimmune, postsurgical)
- Defect in the calcium-sensing receptor (autosomal dominant)
- End-organ resistance to PTH (pseudohypoparathyroidism type 1 and 2)

Hypovitaminosis D
Hypomagnesemia
Miscellaneous (pancreatitis, hyperphosphatemia)

Adapted from Jeha G, Kirkland J. Etiology of hypocalcemia in infants and children. *UpToDate*. 2007. Available at: http://www.uptodate.com/online/content/topic.do?topicKey=pediendo/6894&selectedTitle=1~150&source=search_result

Laboratory Findings
- See Table 15.5

Management
- Most mild hypocalcemia can be managed without IV Ca^{2+} infusion
- If IV Ca^{2+} infusion is required, administer as diluted solution (e.g., 10% Ca^{2+} gluconate diluted to 2% solution)
- Ca^{2+} gluconate is preferred over Ca^{2+} chloride to treat symptomatic hypocalcemia because of ↓ incidence of thrombophlebitis and tissue necrosis
- 10 mL of 10% Ca^{2+} gluconate contains 90 mg of elemental Ca^{2+} (2.25 mmol); add 10 mL of 10% Ca^{2+} gluconate to 40 mL of saline to obtain 2% solution; this dilution contains Ca^{2+} 0.04 mmol/mL
- For serious hypocalcemia (convulsions and arrhythmias), give Ca^{2+} 0.1 mmol/kg/h
- For less severe cases (muscle cramps, paresthesias), give Ca^{2+} 0.05 mmol/kg/h
- Never give IV bolus Ca^{2+} to correct hypocalcemia
- Adjust infusion rate q4h based on plasma Ca^{2+} levels; aim for >2 mmol/L; reduce infusion rate slowly, once desired level reached

Table 15.5 Laboratory Findings in Hypocalcemia

Diagnosis	Ca^{2+}	PO_4^-	25-(OH)-D_3	1,25-(OH)$_2$-D_3	PTH	Alkaline Phosphate
Vitamin D deficiency	↓	N or ↓	↓	N or ↑	↑	↑↑↑
Hypoparathyroidism	↓	↑	N	↓	↓	N or ↑
Pseudohypoparathyroidism	↓	↑	N	↓	↑	↑

Adapted from Alario A. *Practical Guide to the Care of the Pediatric Patient*. St. Louis, Mo: Mosby; 1997.

- All patients receiving IV Ca^{2+} should have cardiac monitoring
- Monitor IV site: high risk of extravasation burns and venous thrombosis
- Do not administer Ca^{2+} and $NaHCO_3$ in same IV tubing
- Ceftriaxone and Ca^{2+} should never be infused at the same time, even in different IV lines because fatal reactions with Ca^{2+}–ceftriaxone precipitates in lungs and kidneys of neonates have been reported
- Never give Ca^{2+} IM or SC
- Maintain oral intake of 100 mg elemental Ca^{2+}/kg/d; use supplement if needed (e.g., Ca^{2+} lactate/gluconate/carbonate)
- Start vitamin D metabolites: 1,25-$(OH)_2$-vitamin D_3 (calcitriol) or 1α-(OH)-vitamin D_3 if more than 3–4 d of IV Ca^{2+} are anticipated

HYPERCALCEMIA

Definition
- $Ca^{2+} > 2.75$ mmol/L

Signs/Symptoms
- Nonspecific weakness, anorexia, polyuria, polydipsia, mental status changes

Differential Diagnosis
- See Table 15.6

Table 15.6	Differential Diagnosis of Hypercalcemia	
Increased Intestinal Ca^{2+} Absorption	**Increased Resorption of Bone**	**Other**
Increased Ca^{2+} intake	Hyperparathyroidism	Thiazide diuretics
Hypervitaminosis D	Hyperthyroidism	Lithium
Granulomatous disease (subcutaneous fat necrosis in newborn, sarcoidosis)	Hypervitaminosis A	Pheochromocytoma
		Adrenal insufficiency
		Acute renal failure
		Rhabdomyolysis
		Familial hypocalciuric hypercalcemia
		Immobilization
		Total parenteral nutrition

Management
- Low-Ca^{2+}, high-fluid diet
- For emergency treatment, give IV fluids to increase ECF volume (0.9% NaCl at 2.5 × maintenance), followed by furosemide
- If unresponsive in 12–24 h, consider bisphosphonate ± calcitonin (2 doses max)
- Steroids may be useful in special circumstances of increased 1,25-$(OH)_2$-vitamin D production (e.g., sarcoidosis and lymphoma)

PUBERTY

NORMAL PUBERTAL DEVELOPMENT

- See Box 15.6
- See Box 15.7

Box 15.6   Normal Pubertal Development

Girls: Onset at 10.5 yr (range: 8–13 yr)
1. Thelarche
2. Pubarche
3. Peak growth velocity
4. Menarche (approximately 2 yr post-thelarche)

Boys: Onset at 11.5 yr (range: 9–14 yr)
1. Increased testicular volume
2. Pubarche
3. Elongation of penis
4. Peak growth velocity

Box 15.7   Tanner Staging

Boys: Genital Development

Stage 1: Preadolescent: testes, scrotum, and penis same size and proportion as early childhood

Stage 2: Enlargement of scrotum and testes; skin of scrotum reddens, changes in texture; little or no enlargement of penis

Stage 3: Enlargement of penis, mainly in length; further growth of testes and scrotum

Stage 4: Increased size of penis with growth in breadth and development of glans; testes and scrotum larger; scrotal skin darkened

Stage 5: Genitalia adult size and shape

Girls: Breast Development

Stage 1: Preadolescent: elevation of papilla only

Stage 2: Breast bud stage: elevation of breast and papilla as small mound; enlargement of areola diameter

Stage 3: Further enlargement and elevation of breast and areola, with no separation of their contours

Stage 4: Projection of areola and papilla to form a secondary mound above level of breast

Stage 5: Mature stage: projection of papilla only, due to recession of the areola to general contour of breast

Both Sexes: Pubic Hair

Stage 1: Preadolescent: no pubic hair

Stage 2: Sparse growth of long, slightly pigmented downy hair, straight or slightly curled, chiefly at base of penis or along labia

Stage 3: Considerably darker, coarser and more curled; hair spreads sparsely over junction of the pubes

Stage 4: Hair now adult type, but area covered still considerably smaller than in adult; no spreading to medial surface of thighs

Stage 5: Adult quantity and type; spreading to medial surface of thighs but not up linea alba or elsewhere above the base of the inverse triangle (spread up linea alba occurs late and is rated stage 6)

PRECOCIOUS PUBERTY

Definition
- Onset of puberty before age 8 yr in girls (may be age 6–7 yr for black or African descent) and 9 yr in boys

Differential Diagnosis
- See Table 15.7

Investigations
- Bone age
- LH, FSH, estradiol, testosterone, 17-hydroxyprogesterone
- Thyroid function studies
- LHRH stimulation test
- Pelvic and abdominal US
- Neuroimaging, if indicated by history and physical examination

Management
- Treat underlying cause
- To arrest pubertal development, GnRH analogue (e.g., Lupron) downregulates receptor response

DELAYED PUBERTY

Definition
- Lack of breast development in girls by age 13 yr or lack of testicular enlargement in boys by age 14 yr

Differential Diagnosis
- Constitutional delay
- Delayed but spontaneous pubertal development (functional hypogonadotropic hypogonadism)
- Permanent hypogonadotropic hypogonadism
- Permanent hypergonadotropic hypogonadism (primary gonadal failure)

Table 15.7	Differential Diagnosis of Precocious Puberty	
Benign Variants	**Central (Gonadotropin Dependent)**	**Peripheral (Gonadotropin Independent)**
· Premature thelarche · Premature adrenarche	· Idiopathic · CNS lesion (trauma, tumor, malformation) · Hypothalamic hamartoma · CNS irradiation · CNS infection	· Exogenous steroid ingestion · Adrenal cause (tumor, CAH) · Ovarian cause (cyst, tumor) · Testicular cause (tumor, testotoxicosis) · hCG-producing tumor (germinoma, teratoma) · Hypothyroidism · McCune-Albright syndrome

Adapted from Root AW. Precocious puberty. *Pediatr Rev.* 2000; 21:10–19.

Investigations

- Bone age
- Pelvic or testicular US if an ovarian or testicular mass is detected
- Pelvic US in girls to determine presence or absence of a uterus
- LH, FSH, estradiol (females), testosterone (males), prolactin, DHEAS
- TSH, free T_4
- Karyotype
- Brain MRI if associated neurologic symptoms/signs suggest a central process or if laboratory results suggest hypothalamic or pituitary disease

Management

- Treat underlying cause
- Watchful waiting for constitutional delay
- Gonadal steroid replacement: testosterone (boys >14 yr) or estrogen (girls >13 yr)

DISORDERS OF SEXUAL DEVELOPMENT

- Note: Infants with suspected DSD should be examined by a pediatrician or pediatric endocrinologist on an emergency basis; delay assignment of gender and naming until appropriate investigations reviewed

CLINICAL EVALUATION

- Family and prenatal history, complete physical examination (rule out other malformations)
- Clinical features suggestive of DSD:
  - Apparent female genitalia with clitoral enlargement, posterior labial fusion, or an inguinal/labial mass
  - Apparent male genitalia with bilateral undescended testes, micropenis (anthropometric measurements vary by ethnicity and gestational age), or isolated perineal hypospadias or mild hypospadias with undescended testis

INITIAL INVESTIGATIONS

- Karyotype and fluorescent in situ hybridization (FISH) for X and Y markers
- Abdominal/pelvic US
- 17-Hydroxyprogesterone, testosterone, gonadotropins, antimüllerian hormone, serum electrolytes

CLASSIFICATION OF DSD

- See Table 15.8

46 XX DSD

- Most commonly seen
- Up to 70% of cases of DSD

Table 15.8	Classification of DSD	
Sex Chromosome DSD	**46 XY DSD**	**46 XX DSD**
45 X (Turner syndrome) 47 XXY (Klinefelter syndrome) 45 X/46 XY (mixed gonadal dysgenesis, ovotesticular DSD) 46 XX/46 XY (chimeric, ovotesticular DSD)	Disorders of gonadal (testicular) development Disorders in androgen synthesis or action	Disorders of gonadal (ovarian) development Androgen excess (e.g., CAH)

Adapted from Lee PA, Houk CP, Faisal Ahmed S, Hughes IA, et al. Consensus statement on the management of intersex disorders. *Pediatrics*, 2006; 118: e488–e500.

Etiology
- CAH
- Maternal ingestion of androgens
- Maternal virilizing tumors

CAH
- Most common cause of DSD
- Autosomal recessive defects of enzymes of cortisol synthesis, including 21-hydroxylase deficiency, 11β-hydroxylase deficiency, 3β-hydroxysteroid dehydrogenase deficiency
- 21-Hydroxylase deficiency is most common defect and causes:
  - Increased ACTH secretion and subsequent hyperpigmentation
  - Adrenal hyperplasia, hypersecretion of adrenal androgens → masculinized external genitalia (degree of masculinization variable)
  - Impaired cortisol secretion; in complete severe form, no cortisol or aldosterone produced; consequent hyponatremia, hyperkalemia, dehydration, acidosis, and vascular collapse
- See pp. 276–277 for guidelines for management of intercurrent illness
- In milder form, mineralocorticoid activity is present; thus, no salt and water loss
- In both, increase in 17-hydroxyprogesterone, androstenedione, and testosterone
- Late-onset milder form exists

Management
- Delay gender assignment until expert evaluation in newborns
- Immediate referral to tertiary care center with multidisciplinary team: pediatrician, urologist, geneticist, endocrinologist, psychologist, social worker, and psychiatrist
- Open communication with patients and families
- Ensure patient and family concerns are addressed with sensitivity and that confidentiality is maintained
- Glucocorticoid ± mineralocorticoid replacement

46 XY DSD

Pathophysiology

- Insufficient testosterone production (enzyme defect in adrenal steroid synthesis; autosomal recessive, or rarely caused by Leydig cell dysgenesis or agenesis); all have bilateral testes found in varying locations
- Inability to convert testosterone (deficiency in 5α-reductase; autosomal recessive)
  - At puberty, normal adult testosterone levels may be reached with virilization
- Failure of target tissue to respond to DHT (androgen insensitivity)
  - X-linked
  - Complete form usually presents with primary amenorrhea

SEX CHROMOSOME DSD

- Includes karyotype 45 X (Turner syndrome), 45 X/46 XY (mixed gonadal dysgenesis, ovotesticular DSD), 46 XX/46 XY (chimeric, ovotesticular DSD)
- Have mix of streak gonad, ovarian, or testicular tissue
- May manifest signs of Turner syndrome (short stature, webbed neck, inverted nipples, shieldlike chest, coarctation of the aorta, VSD, hypoplastic nails)

Investigations

- Complete physical examination (rule out other malformations)
  - Presence of palpable gonads suggests undervirilized male
- Karyotype
- Electrolytes and BG levels should be evaluated, after day 3
- 17-hydroxyprogesterone levels, after day 3 (if clinically indicated)
- US to determine:
  - Presence of internal organs (e.g., uterus)
  - Presence of female internal genitalia suggests female with CAH
  - Anomalies of urinary tract
  - Anomalies of adrenal glands (hyperplasia in CAH)
- Plasma ratios of testosterone precursors to testosterone (DHEA, androstenedione), testosterone to DHT on day 2 of life aids in determining testicular function
- Exogenous stimulation with hCG
  - In normal testes, will produce plasma levels of testosterone and its precursors within normal adult range

Management

- Psychosocial sensitivity and support
- Early referral to tertiary care center with multidisciplinary team: pediatrician, urologist, geneticist, endocrinologist, psychologist, social worker, and psychiatrist

Medical Management
- Testosterone may be used in undervirilized male
- Glucocorticoids and mineralocorticoids in forms of CAH
- Sex steroid replacement therapy at puberty

Surgical Management
- External genitalia reconstruction later

Genetic Counseling
- Prenatal diagnosis and treatment of CAH (antenatal administration of dexamethasone controversial)

Basis of Gender Assignment
- Appearance of external genitalia
- Feasibility of genital reconstruction
- Future sexual functioning
- Risk of malignancy
- Fertility
- Parental wishes

ADRENAL DISORDERS

ADRENAL INSUFFICIENCY

Etiology
- See Box 15.8

Box 15.8	Adrenal Insufficiency

Primary Adrenal Insufficiency
Congenital causes:
- Congenital adrenal hyperplasia
- Congenital adrenal hypoplasia
- Adrenal unresponsiveness to ACTH

Acquired causes:
- Autoimmune
- Infection (fungal, bacterial, viral, AIDS)
- Adrenoleukodystrophy
- Amyloidosis
- Metastasis
- Hemorrhage

Secondary Adrenal Insufficiency
- Panhypopituitarism
- Result of prolonged glucocorticoid therapy

Adapted from Alario A. *Practical Guide to the Care of the Pediatric Patient.* St. Louis, Mo: Mosby; 1997.

Clinical Manifestations

- Skin and mucous membrane hyperpigmentation
- Hypotension
- Nausea, vomiting, abdominal pain
- Anorexia, weight loss
- Slowing of linear growth
- Muscular weakness, fatigue
- Adrenal crisis (acute onset or exacerbation of insufficiency with electrolyte abnormalities, metabolic acidosis, and shock)

Investigations

- Electrolytes, urea, creatinine
- Morning (8 A.M.) cortisol
- ACTH stimulation test
  - Measure serum cortisol at time 0
  - Administer cosyntropin (Cortrosyn) 0.035 mg/kg (max 0.25 mg) IV
  - Measure serum cortisol in 60 min
  - Normal response is a doubling of baseline cortisol in 60 min with peak >500 nmol/L

Management

Immediate

- 0.9% NaCl 20 mL/kg bolus for resuscitation
- Hydrocortisone 100 mg/m^2 IV bolus, then 100 mg/m^2/d divided q4–6 h
- Treat underlying illness

Long-Term

- Hydrocortisone 6–9 mg/m^2/d in three divided doses
- For CAH, may require higher dose (10–15 mg/m^2/d) to suppress ACTH
- For infants, use 9α-fludrocortisone acetate (Fluorinef) 0.05 to 0.1 mg/d (up to 0.2 mg)

Intercurrent Illnesses

- Triple usual hydrocortisone dose; no changes to mineralocorticoid dose
- If patient vomiting, requires parenteral hydrocortisone
- IM hydrocortisone in emergency situation
- For surgery, 100 mg/m^2/d divided q6h, beginning on call to operating room and continuing for 48 h thereafter

CUSHING SYNDROME

- Cushing syndrome is the result of abnormally high serum levels of glucocorticoids

Etiology

- Iatrogenic most common cause by far (prolonged administration of glucocorticoids)
- Functioning adrenocorticoid tumor (most commonly found in infants)
- Disturbances of hypothalamic–pituitary axis
  - Congenital in infants with midline defects
  - Acquired (e.g., cranio/spinal radiation, as a complication of neurosurgery)
  - Cushing disease (pituitary ACTH-secreting tumors): extremely rare in children

Clinical Manifestations

- Hyperglycemia
- Hypertension
- Weight gain
- Linear growth retardation
- Osteoporosis
- Suppression of endogenous glucocorticoid production
- Note: These patients require increased doses of steroid with illness/stress

Investigations

- 24-h urine cortisol
- Dexamethasone suppression test
  - Administer 20 mcg/kg to a maximum dose of 1 mg dexamethasone the preceding night and measure early-morning cortisol level

SHORT STATURE

- Definition: < 3rd percentile for height
- May be normal variant vs. pathologic (Table 15.9)
- For normal growth parameters, see p. 394
- Investigate if height < 3rd percentile, abnormal growth rate, or height significantly less than genetic potential

EVALUATION

- History of prenatal insult
- History of disproportionate growth
- Growth velocity based on growth curve
- Assessment of bone age

INITIAL INVESTIGATIONS

- CBC and ESR
- Thyroid function tests: TSH, free T_4
- Urea, creatinine
- Karyotype in girls or any child with dysmorphic features

Table 15.9	Differential Diagnosis of Short Stature		
Prenatal onset	· IUGR: placental disease, teratogens (e.g., ethanol, medications), congenital infection · Chromosomal disorder (e.g., Turner, Down syndromes) · Syndrome (e.g., Russell-Silver)		
Postnatal onset	Disproportionate growth*	· Skeletal dysplasia (e.g., achondroplasia) · Rickets	
	Proportionate growth	Normal growth velocity	· Constitutional growth delay (bone age < chronologic age) · Familial short stature (bone age = chronologic age) · Idiopathic short stature (height below 2 SD of the mean for age, and no endocrine, metabolic, or other diagnosis made)
		Abnormal growth velocity	· Chronic disease (e.g., GI, renal, cardiac) · Malnutrition · Endocrinopathies: hypothyroidism, GH deficiency, excess glucocorticoid · Psychosocial · Drugs (e.g., glucocorticoids)

*To measure proportion, measure (1) lower body segment: distance from top of pubic symphysis to the floor and (2) upper body segment: subtract lower body segment from total standing height. Normal upper:lower proportion ranges from 1.7 in neonate to slightly below 1.0 in the adult.

- Urinalysis
- Radiologic investigations: bone age, head imaging if CNS disorder suspected

GH DEFICIENCY

Diagnosis

- History of short stature with abnormal growth velocity and absence of chronic disease
- Delayed bone age but otherwise normal initial investigation
- Failure to secrete GH on two pharmacologic stimulation tests

Indications for GH Treatment

- GH deficiency
- Turner syndrome
- Renal failure
- Other: Prader-Willi, idiopathic short stature (relative indication)

Complications of GH Treatment

- Benign intracranial hypertension (pseudotumor cerebri)
- Slipped capital femoral epiphyses
- Increase in the growth and pigmentation of nevi
- Glucose intolerance and DM2

- Consider possible hormonal disturbances in children who have underlying conditions or who have had interventions that may disturb the HPA:
  - Hypothyroidism, GH deficiency, diabetes insipidus, cortisol deficiency
  - Midline defects, postcraniospinal radiation, neurosurgery for CNS tumors

INITIAL INVESTIGATIONS

- TSH, free T_4, cortisol, prolactin, GH, urine SG, Na^+, and ACTH stimulation test

DISORDERS OF ANTIDIURETIC HORMONE SECRETION

DIABETES INSIPIDUS

- See Box 15.9

Box 15.9	Etiology of Diabetes Insipidus
Central	**Nephrogenic**
• Genetic	• Genetic
• Trauma	• Drug induced
• Neurosurgical intervention	• Neoplasm
• Congenital anatomic defect	• Renal failure
• Neoplasm	• Fanconi syndrome
• Infiltrative disease	• Obstructive uropathy
• Infection	• Sarcoidosis
	• Sickle cell disease/trait

Clinical Characteristics

- ↑ Urine output
- Enuresis/nocturia
- Excessive thirst
- Dehydration if no access to water
- Large amounts of dilute urine (urine SG <1.010)
- Hypernatremia
- ↑ Serum osmolality
- Inappropriately ↓ urine osmolality

Diagnosis

- Confirmed with water deprivation test (Table 15.10)
- Consultation with endocrinologist recommended

Endocrinology

15

Table 15.10 — Diagnosing Diabetes Insipidus Using the Water Deprivation Test

	Basal State				After Water Deprivation	After ADH
	Daily Urine Volume	Serum Na⁺ (mEq/L)	Serum Osmolality (mOsm/kg H_2O)	Urine SG	Urine Osmolality (mOsm/kg H_2O)	Change in Urine Osmolality
Normal	0.5-1.0	135-145	280	>1.010	>800	<5%
Central DI	4-10	>145	>300	<1.010	<200	>50%
Nephrogenic DI	4-10	>145	>300	<1.005	<200	<50%
Psychogenic polydipsia	2-20	140	<280	<1.020	600	<5%

Adapted from Saborio P, Tipton GA, Chan JCM. Diabetes insipidus. *Pediatr Rev.* 2000;21:122–129.

Management

Central
- DDAVP can be given by intranasal, SC, or oral routes

Nephrogenic
- Low-solute diet; thiazide diuretics

SIADH

Etiology
- Intracranial causes
  - Infection
  - Trauma
  - Neoplasm
  - Other: status epilepticus, hydrocephalus
- Malignancy
- Pulmonary disease
- Psychiatric disease (e.g., psychogenic polydipsia)
- Drugs
  - Barbiturates
  - Carbamazepine
  - Vincristine, cyclophosphamide
  - Salicylates, indomethacin, other NSAIDs
- Pain/stress

Clinical Characteristics
- May be asymptomatic
- Oliguria
- Volume expansion
- Symptoms associated with Na^+ depletion (see p. 290)

Diagnosis
- Hyponatremia
- Urine osmolality usually > plasma osmolality
- Urinary Na^+ >20 mmol/L
- Urinary osmolality and Na^+ higher than expected for serum levels

Management

Fluid Restriction
- Restrict to insensible losses (400 mL/m^2) + 50–100% urine output
- 3% NaCl with symptomatic hyponatremia (e.g., seizures)
- Drugs such as demeclocycline very rarely used in pediatrics

FURTHER READING

Daneman D, Frank M, Perlman K. *When a Child Has Diabetes*. Toronto, Ontario, Canada: Key Porter Books; 2002.

Foley TP. Hypothyroidism. *Pediatr Rev.* 2004;25:94–100.

Hughes IA, Houk C, Ahmed SF, et al. Consensus statement on management of intersex disorders. *Arch Dis Child.* 2006;91:554–562.

Kaufman FR. Type 1 diabetes mellitus. *Pediatr Rev.* 2003;24:291–300.

Nesmith D. Type 2 diabetes mellitus in children and adolescents. *Pediatr Rev.* 2001;22:147–152.

Root AW. Precocious puberty. *Pediatr Rev.* 2000;21:10–19.

Sperling MA. *Pediatric Endocrinology.* 2nd ed. Philadelphia, Pa: WB Saunders; 2002.

USEFUL WEB SITES

American Diabetes Association. Available at: **www.diabetes.org**

Canadian Diabetes Association. Available at: **www.diabetes.ca**

International Society for Pediatric and Adolescent Diabetes. Available at: **www.ispad.org**

Chapter 16 Fluids, Electrolytes, and Acid–Base

Mathieu Lemaire

Seetha Radhakrishnan

Christoph Licht

Chapter 16 Fluids, Electrolytes, and Acid–Base

COMMON ABBREVIATIONS

ATN	acute tubular necrosis
BSA	body surface area
DI	diabetes insipidus
DKA	diabetic ketoacidosis
ECF	extracellular fluid
ECF_{Osm}	ECF osmolality
F&E	fluid and electrolytes
FE	fractional excretion
GFR	glomerular filtration rate
HCO_3^-	bicarbonate ion
ICF	intracellular fluid
ICF_{Osm}	ICF osmolality
IV	intravenous
NG	nasogastric
ORT	oral rehydration therapy
P_{CO_2}	partial pressure of carbon dioxide
PO_4^-	phosphate
P_{Na^+}	plasma sodium
P_{Osm}	plasma osmolality
PTH	parathyroid hormone
RDI	recommended daily intake
RTA	renal tubular acidosis
SAG	serum anion gap
SIADH	syndrome of inappropriate antidiuretic hormone
TBW	total body water
TRP	tubular reabsorption of phosphate
TTKG	transtubular potassium gradient
U_{Cl^-}	urinary chloride
U_{K^+}	urinary potassium
U_{Na^+}	urinary sodium
UAG	urinary anion gap
UNC	urinary net charge
U_{Osm}	urinary osmolality
VF	ventricular fibrillation
VT	ventricular tachycardia

GENERAL APPROACH TO ABNORMALITIES
OF FLUID AND ELECTROLYTES

- Emergencies (e.g., seizures) managed in parallel to the following steps:
  - Cardiac monitoring (many F&E disorders associated with arrhythmias)
  - Determine patient's fluid status: hypovolemic, euvolemic, hypervolemic
  - If hypovolemic, consider administering 0.9% NaCl bolus
  - Repeat test with abnormal result and add relevant blood and urine tests (see following sections)
  - Thoroughly review F&E history for all previous inputs and outputs:
    1. Inputs = enteral + parenteral fluids
    2. Outputs = urine losses + insensible losses + other losses

INSENSIBLE LOSSES

- Include sweat, evaporation, and breathing
- 300 mL/m^2 × BSA (ventilated); 400 mL/m^2 × BSA (not ventilated)
- 500–600 mL/m^2 × BSA for neonates (↑ with overhead heaters)

$$BSA = \sqrt{\frac{weight \times height}{3600}}$$

weight (kg); height (m)

OTHER LOSSES

- Diarrhea, NG aspiration, surgical drains

TREATMENT

- Identify type of physiologic fluid lost (Table 16.1)
- Choose IV fluid that approximates expected losses (Table 16.2)

Table 16.1	Approximate Electrolyte Composition* of Body Fluids				
Fluid	[H$^+$]	[Na$^+$]	[K$^+$]	[Cl$^-$]	[HCO$_3^-$]
Gastric	80	40 (20–80)	20 (5–20)	150 (100–150)	0
Diarrhea	0	40 (10–90)	40 (10–80)	40 (10–110)	40
Sweat	0	10	5	15	0

*In mmol/L; ranges appear in parentheses.

Table 16.2	Commonly Used Intravenous Fluid Solutions					
Fluid	[Na⁺]	[K⁺]	[Cl⁻]	Lactate	Dextrose	Tonicity vs. Plasma
D5W	0	0	0	0	5 g/100 mL	Hypotonic
D10W	0	0	0	0	10 g/100 mL	Hypotonic
0.9% NaCl	154	0	154	0	0	Isotonic
0.45% NaCl	77	0	77	0	0	Half-isotonic
0.2% NaCl	33	0	33	0	0	Hypotonic
⅔–⅓	45	0	45	0	3.33 g/100 mL	Hypotonic
Ringer's	130	4	128	28	0	Isotonic

Note: All concentrations in mmol/L; any dextrose solution may be mixed with any of the NaCl solutions; KCl may be added at 10, 20, or 40 mmol/L.

MAINTENANCE REQUIREMENTS

- Based on estimated daily F&E requirements (Table 16.3)
- H_2O requirements ↑ in fever, ↓ in ventilator or incubator use (see Insensible Losses section)

Table 16.3	Recommended Daily Intake of Na⁺, K⁺, and H₂O		
Parameter	Weight Range	RDI	Example: for a 47-kg Child
Na⁺	Any weight	2–3 mmol/kg/d	94–141 mmol/d
K⁺	Any weight	1–3 mmol/kg/d	47–141 mmol/d
H₂O	1 to 10 kg	100 mL/kg	1000 mL
	11 to 20 kg	50 mL/kg	500 mL
	Additional kg >20 kg	20 mL/kg	540 mL
	The values above are additive		Total = 2040 mL/d

GENERAL PRINCIPLES OF IV MAINTENANCE FLUIDS

- Na^+ requirements calculated this way may result in use of hypotonic solutions; all hospitalized children requiring IV fluids are at risk of SIADH (SIADH → iatrogenic ↓Na^+)
- See Table 16.4 for guidelines on IV maintenance fluids
- Include oral fluids (mostly hypotonic) in fluid balance
- Choose IVF [Na⁺] based on current P_{Na^+} levels (Table 16.5)
- Both volume and [Na⁺] of IVF contribute to dysnatremias: reassess maintenance fluid if this occurs

Table 16.4	Guidelines for Fluid and Electrolyte Administration in Pediatric Patients
Indications	· Maintenance fluid therapy · Bolus fluid therapy · Fluid therapy to replace abnormal losses
Contraindications	These guidelines do not apply to children with: · Cardiac, renal, and hepatic failure (chronic hyponatremia) · Current severe electrolyte abnormalities
Initial assessment	· Baseline serum electrolytes (Na^+, K^+, glucose, creatinine, urea) · Weight, BP
Starting IV fluid therapy	· Hypotonic solutions (see Table 16.2) should *not* be used as maintenance fluid, unless ordered in CCU, NICU, or by nephrologist · Isotonic fluids should be used while waiting for baseline laboratory results · Infants and young children have limited glycogen stores: use IV fluid solutions with dextrose to prevent hypoglycemia and ketosis
Monitoring	Patients receiving >50% maintenance fluid by IV route should have at least daily: · Measurements of serum electrolytes and glucose · Accurate record of input and output · Weight measurement

© The Hospital for Sick Children, 2007. Adapted from *The Hospital for Sick Children Hospital-Wide Patient Care Clinical Practice Guideline – F&E Administration in Children.*

Table 16.5	Intravenous Fluid Maintenance Recommendations Based on Current Plasma Na^+ Level
Specific Indications	**Recommended IV Fluid**
Na^+ <138 mmol/L	Isotonic IV solutions
Na^+ = 138–144 mmol/L	Isotonic or half-isotonic IV solutions
Na^+ = 145–154 mmol/L	Half-isotonic IV solution
Na^+ >154 mmol/L	See p. 292 (consider Nephrology consultation for advice)
Perioperative period	Isotonic IV solutions

© The Hospital for Sick Children, 2007. Adapted from *The Hospital for Sick Children Hospital-Wide Patient Care Clinical Practice Guideline—F&E Administration in Children.*

ORAL REHYDRATION THERAPY

GENERAL CONCEPTS

- See Table 16.6
- ORT as effective as IV therapy for mild to moderate dehydration; first choice in these patients
- Children with mild diarrhea and no dehydration should be fed a regular diet
- Glucose enhances Na^+ and H_2O transport across intestinal mucosa, which remains intact in viral or enteropathogenic bacterial diarrhea

Table 16.6	Composition of Glucose–Electrolyte Solutions and "Clear Liquids"				
Solution	Carbohydrate (mmol/L)	Na$^+$ (mmol/L)	K$^+$ (mmol/L)	Base (mmol/L)	Osmolality (mOsm/L)
Pedialyte	140	45	20	30	250
WHO/UNICEF	111	90	20	30	310
Cola	700	2	0	13	750
Apple juice	690	3	32	0	730
Chicken broth	0	250	8	0	500
Sports beverage	255	20	3	3	330
Ginger ale	500	3	1	4	540

EARLY REFEEDING

- Commence 6–12 h into therapy; breastfeeding should continue despite diarrhea
- Extra ORT solution may be given (5–10 mL/kg) after each stool if diarrhea persists
- Appropriate foods: complex carbohydrates, lean meat, yogurt, fruits, vegetables
- *Do not use* BRAT diet (**b**anana, **r**ice, **a**pplesauce, **t**ea); *avoid* foods high in simple sugars

PROBLEMS

Vomiting

- Administer small volume of ORT solution frequently (5 mL every 1–2 min)
- As dehydration and electrolyte imbalances correct, vomiting will decrease
- If vomiting continues, IV hydration is indicated
- Antiemetic use controversial; not currently recommended in home setting

Refusal to Take ORT Solution

- Give solution in small amounts to get used to salty taste
- NG tube may be used to administer fluids
- Add 30 mL of juice to 120 mL of ORT to improve compliance

SALT AND WATER

IMPORTANT CONCEPTS

Osmolality

- Osmolality proportional to number of dissociated particles (solute) in H_2O (units: mOsm/kg H_2O)
- Main constituents: Na^+, accompanying anions, urea, and glucose
- P_{Na^+} is by far the most important plasma osmole under normal circumstances
- P_{Osm} either measured in the laboratory or calculated:

$$P_{Osm} = 2 \times P_{Na^+} + \text{urea} + \text{glucose (all in mmol/L)}$$

Water

- As percentage of body weight, TBW varies inversely with age: in utero (85%); term infants (70%), toddlers/children (65%), adolescents/adults (60%)
- TBW contained in two main compartments: ICF (⅔ of TBW) and ECF (⅓ of TBW)
- ECF further subdivided into interstitial fluid (80%) and plasma volume (20%)

Sodium

- Na^+ *content* is 60 mmol/kg
- Normal $[Na^+]$ are very different for ECF (135–145 mmol/L) and ICF (10–20 mmol/L)

Dynamics of Fluid Shifts Between Compartments

- At equilibrium, $ECF_{Osm} = ICF_{Osm}$
- Change in P_{Osm} in either compartment causes rapid H_2O shifts until $ECF_{Osm} = ICF_{Osm}$
- Generally, acute changes (minutes) in P_{Osm} occur only in the ECF; ICF_{Osm} changes occur slowly (hours to days) and are never the primary problem
- Changes in P_{Na^+} always result in proportional alterations in ICF_{volume}:
  - Hypernatremia → ICF_{volume} contraction (water shifts from ICF to ECF)
  - Hyponatremia → ICF_{volume} expansion (water shifts from ECF to ICF)

HYPONATREMIA

- Most common electrolyte abnormality in hospitalized patients
- Caused by too much Na^+ loss, too much water retention, or combination
- May be acute (<48 h) or chronic (>48 h)

Clinical Manifestations

- Most patients with mild hyponatremia are asymptomatic
- Symptoms imply cerebral edema: headache, lethargy, ataxia, psychosis, abdominal discomfort, diminished level of consciousness; requires emergent management (rapid $\downarrow$ECF$_{Osm}$ has caused H_2O to shift to the ICF)
- Severe symptoms: seizure or coma (P$_{Na^+}$ usually <120 mmol/L)
- Hyponatremia may exaggerate signs of hypovolemia because fluid shifts from ECF to ICF; circulatory compromise occurs earlier than expected

Approach to Diagnosis

- See Figure 16.1 for diagnostic algorithm
- Physical examination: hydration status (weight, BP, mucous membranes, general appearance, capillary refill)
- Laboratory: plasma and urine Na$^+$, K$^+$, creatinine, urea, and osmolality (or specific gravity)
- Useful information: all inputs and outputs

General Management

- Based on etiology, severity of symptoms, and timing (acute or chronic)

General Principles

- Hypovolemic hyponatremia: give Na$^+$
- Other hyponatremias: restrict water
- Do not exceed increase in P$_{Na^+}$ of 12 mmol/L/d (see Dangers to Anticipate from Therapy section)

Acute Symptomatic Hyponatremia

- Immediate goal: prevent cerebral edema by acutely increasing P$_{Na^+}$ by ~6–8 mmol/L, to >130 mmol/L, or until resolution of symptoms

Acute Phase

- Give hypertonic saline (3% NaCl) at 2–3 mL/kg over 30–60 min (stop other IV fluids)
- Once immediate goal reached, stop or slow 3% NaCl infusion

Intermediate Phase

- Intermediate goal: $\uparrow$P$_{Na^+}$ by a maximum of 0.5 mmol/L/h (12 mmol/L/d)
- H_2O restriction ± 0.9% NaCl infusion as maintenance IV fluid
- Other treatment options:
  - Mannitol (1 g/kg) if 3% NaCl not available (to prevent brain swelling)
  - Coadministration of furosemide (to promote diuresis)
- Note: Similar approach used for treatment of acute or chronic hyponatremia

Figure 16.1 Diagnostic Algorithm for Hyponatremia

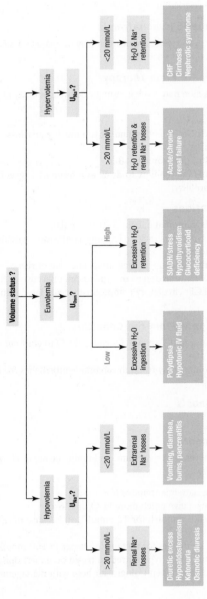

Adapted from Pomeranz AJ, Busey SL, Sabnis S, et al. *Pediatric Decision-Making Strategies to Accompany Nelson Textbook of Pediatrics* (16th ed.). Philadelphia: WB Saunders, 2002 (p. 337).

Fluids, Electrolytes, and Acid–Base

16

Acute Asymptomatic Hyponatremia

- Management: H_2O restriction

Chronic Asymptomatic Hyponatremia

- Management: H_2O restriction (extreme thirst may decrease compliance)
- Other treatment options: furosemide

Dangers to Anticipate From Therapy

- Too rapid P_{Na^+} correction may result in osmotic demyelination syndrome

HYPERNATREMIA

- Caused by too much Na^+ retention and/or too much water loss (renal or extrarenal)
- May be acute (<48 h) or chronic (>48 h)
- Usually >1 problem (i.e., inability to drink as a result of $\downarrow$ level of consciousness or mobility)

Clinical Manifestations

- Most patients are asymptomatic if Na^+ <160 mmol/L
- At >160 mmol/L, symptoms include lethargy, confusion, twitching, seizures, stupor, and coma
- Severity of symptoms depends on magnitude and rate of rise
- Hypernatremia may minimize signs of hypovolemia because of fluid shifts from ICF to ECF; circulatory compromise occurs later than expected

Dangers to Anticipate From the Condition

- Cerebral desiccation: rapid $\uparrow$ in ECF_{Osm} causes H_2O to shift *out* of the ICF
- Rapid $\downarrow$ in brain volume may result in cerebral hemorrhages from blood vessel tearing

Approach to Diagnosis

- See Figure 16.2

General Management

- Based on etiology, severity of symptoms, and timing (acute or chronic)

General Principles

- Hypervolemic hypernatremia: remove Na^+
- Other hypernatremias: give much more H_2O than Na^+
- Do not $\downarrow$ P_{Na^+} by >0.5 mmol/h (or 12 mmol/L/d) because of risk of cerebral edema
- No evidence-based guidelines for therapy for severe (>160 mmol/L) or extreme (>175 mmol/L) hypernatremia; based on expert opinion only (consider consulting a nephrologist for help with management)

Figure 16.2 Diagnostic Algorithm for Hypernatremia

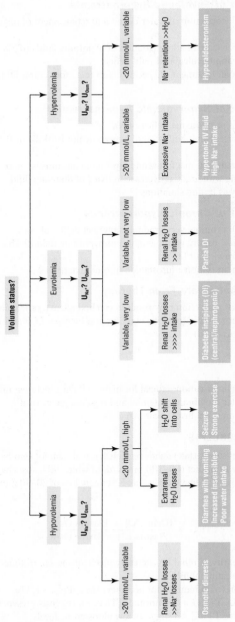

Adapted from Pomeranz AJ, Busey SL, Sabnis S, et al. *Pediatric Decision-Making Strategies to Accompany Nelson Textbook of Pediatrics* (16th ed.). Philadelphia: WB Saunders, 2002 (p. 331).

Fluids, Electrolytes, and Acid-Base

16

Management of Euvolemic Hypernatremia
- Primary goal: correction of water deficit and replacement of ongoing losses
- Fluid of choice: careful administration of hypotonic fluids (0.2% NaCl) according to calculated fluid deficit
- Secondary goal: treatment of specific defect (e.g., for central DI use DDAVP)

Management of Hypervolemic Hypernatremia
- Primary goal: promote net deficit of Na^+
- Fluids of choice: careful infusion of hypotonic fluids (0.2% or 0.45% NaCl)
- Other treatment options: furosemide (promote natriuresis), peritoneal dialysis with gradual decrease in $[Na^+]$ of dialysate fluid, or hemodialysis in dire situations

Management of Chronic Hypernatremia
- Primary goal: promote very gradual (slow) net deficit of Na^+
- Fluid of choice: careful administration of hypotonic fluid (0.45% NaCl, with or without D5W)
- Other treatment options: furosemide (promote natriuresis)

Dangers to Anticipate From Therapy
- Too rapid P_{Na^+} correction may result in cerebral edema, especially in chronic hypernatremia (osmotic equilibration between ECF and ICF has already occurred)

POTASSIUM
- Major intracellular cation; crucial for many cellular functions: maintaining cellular membrane potential and regulating electrical excitability (muscles, heart, neurons)

IMPORTANT CONCEPTS
- K^+ balance (at steady state) tightly regulated, usually aim for zero balance
- Input mainly from diet (60–100 mmol/d, of which 90% absorbed)
- Output mainly via kidneys: obligatory K^+ urinary loss of 20–30 mmol/d

TTKG

$$TTKG = \frac{[Urine\ K^+] \times Plasma\ Osm}{[Plasma\ K^+] \times Urine\ Osm}$$

- Assesses integrity of renal K^+ excretory mechanisms, controlling for renal concentrating ability
- Interpretation (requirements for accuracy: $U_{Osm}/P_{Osm} > 1$, $U_{Na^+} > 25$ mmol/L): TTKG = 6 is normal; TTKG > 6 suggests presence of aldosterone; TTKG < 5 suggests low aldosterone levels

HYPOKALEMIA

- Observed with either K^+ loss (urine or GI) or ↑ shifts of K^+ to the intracellular compartment

Clinical Manifestations

- Clinical: weakness, cramping, myalgia, restless legs syndrome, rhabdomyolysis, respiratory failure
- ECG: ↓ST segments, ↓T waves, U waves, ↑QT intervals, VF, other arrhythmias

Approach to Diagnosis

- See Figure 16.3
- Characteristic ECG changes mandate rapid treatment
- Laboratory: plasma Na^+, K^+, Mg^{2+}, creatinine, urea, osmolality, pH, HCO_3^-; urinary Na^+, K^+, pH
- In hypokalemia, TTKG is expected to be < 6 if renal loss is not the cause

Management

- Cardiac monitoring
- Symptomatic or K^+ < 2.9 mmol/L: strongly consider parenteral treatment, including adding K^+ to IV fluid; chronic and/or stable: may consider enteral treatment
- Symptomatic and K^+ > 3.0 mmol/L: enteral or slow IV K^+ supplementation
- Treat underlying cause
- If hypokalemia persists despite supplementation, measure urine electrolyte levels (to determine extent of K^+ loss) and plasma Mg^{2+} (see Magnesium section on p. 301)

Dangers to Anticipate From Therapy

- Hyperkalemia
- Caution: concomitant acidosis corrected with bicarbonate will worsen hypokalemia secondary to transcellular shifts

HYPERKALEMIA

- Occurs mainly in three situations:
  - ↓ Urinary K^+ excretion (e.g., renal failure)
  - ↑ GI absorption of K^+ or ↑ intake
  - Cellular lysis resulting in spilling of ICF K^+ into the ECF

Clinical Manifestations

- ECG: tall and peaked T waves, decreased amplitude of P waves, QRS widening, VT, VF

Figure 16.3 Diagnostic Algorithm for Hypokalemia

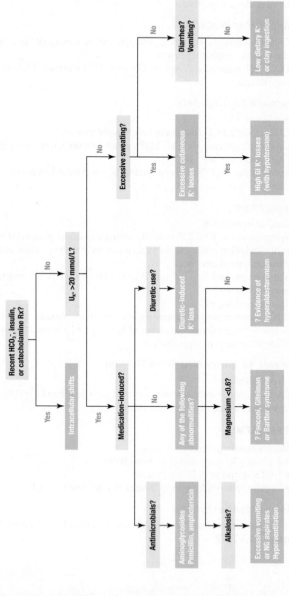

© The Hospital for Sick Children, 2009. New artwork created by The Hospital for Sick Children for *The Hospital for Sick Children Handbook of Pediatrics*, 11th edition.

Approach to Diagnosis

- See Figure 16.4
- Characteristic ECG changes mandate rapid treatment
- Laboratory: same as hypokalemia (see previous section); may add CPK and CBC/differential
- TTKG is expected to be >6; values <5 consistent with ↓ aldosterone activity (↓ plasma aldosterone levels or lack of renal response to aldosterone)

Figure 16.4 Diagnostic Algorithm for Hyperkalemia

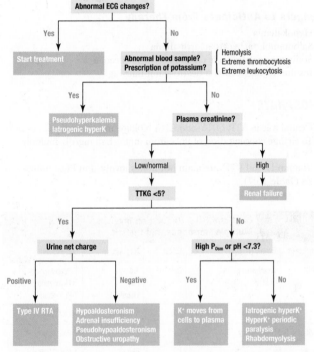

© The Hospital for Sick Children, 2009. New artwork created by The Hospital for Sick Children for *The Hospital for Sick Children Handbook of Pediatrics*, 11th edition.

Management

- Cardiac monitoring
- Stop any K^+ infusion or supplementation
- Cardiac stabilizer: calcium gluconate 10% solution (0.5 mL/kg over 10 min)
- Immediate shifts into cells: salbutamol (2.5–5 mg inhaled × 3 doses), $NaHCO_3$ (1–2 mmol/kg IV over 30 min), dextrose with insulin (bolus: 0.5–1 g/kg glucose and insulin 0.1–0.2 units/kg; continuous infusion: D10W 5 mL/kg/h and insulin 0.1 unit/kg/h)
- Promotion of K^+ excretion: diuretics or K^+-binding resin, such as sodium polystyrene sulfonate (Kayexalate)
- Definitive therapy: dialysis

Dangers to Anticipate From Therapy

- Hypokalemia
- Salbutamol: tachycardia, arrhythmia
- Sodium bicarbonate: acute ionized hypocalcemia
- Insulin: hypoglycemia if dextrose not infusing

PHOSPHATE

- Central role in ATP, DNA, and RNA biology; major constituent of bone
- To change concentration of PO_4^- from mmol/L to mg/dL, multiply by 3.1
- Vitamin D and PTH are main hormones involved in PO_4^- homeostasis (Table 16.7)

Table 16.7	Ca^{2+} and PO_4^- Regulation Involves Multiple Hormones and Organs			
Hormones	**Origin (Trigger)**	**Effect**	**Target(s)**	**End Result**
↑PTH	Parathyroid gland ($\downarrow Ca^{2+}$, $\uparrow PO_4^-$)	Ca^{2+}	Kidney Bone Vitamin D	↑ Reabsorption ↑ Mobilization ↑ Production
		PO_4^-	Kidney	↑ Excretion
↑ Vitamin D	Liver/kidney ($\uparrow$PTH, $\downarrow PO_4^-$ ↑ calcitonin)	Ca^{2+}	GI tract	↑ Reabsorption
		PO_4^-	GI tract Kidney	↑ Absorption ↑ Reabsorption
Calcitonin	C cells (thyroid gland)	Ca^{2+}	GI tract Kidney Bone	↓ Reabsorption ↓ Reabsorption ↓ Osteoclasts
		PO_4^-	Kidney	↑ Reabsorption

HYPOPHOSPHATEMIA

- Most commonly seen in patients with diabetes or anorexia (refeeding syndrome)

Etiology

- $\uparrow$ Urinary PO_4^- loss
- $\downarrow$ GI absorption of PO_4^- (70% of dietary PO_4^- is absorbed)
- PO_4^- shifts from extracellular to intracellular compartment

Clinical Manifestations

- Most patients with mild hypophosphatemia are asymptomatic
- Chronic severe hypophosphatemia ($PO_4^- < 0.35$ mmol/L): muscle weakness and myalgia

Dangers to Anticipate From the Condition

- $\uparrow$ Risk of gram-negative sepsis (especially if immunosuppressed)
- Respiratory and/or cardiac failure

Approach to Diagnosis

- See Figure 16.5
- Laboratory: plasma Na^+, K^+, Cl^-, creatinine, urea, PO_4^-, Ca^{2+}, pH, HCO_3^-, PTH, vitamin D; urinary PO_4^-, Ca^{2+}, creatinine

Management

- Based on etiology and severity of symptoms
- If tolerated, oral supplementation is preferable; most hospitalized patients require IV PO_4^-
- Stop PO_4^- binders

HYPERPHOSPHATEMIA

- Most commonly seen in patients with renal failure or cellular lysis

Etiology

- $\downarrow$ Urinary PO_4^- loss
- $\uparrow$ GI absorption of PO_4^-
- PO_4^- shifts from intracellular to extracellular compartment

Clinical Manifestations

- No obvious symptoms: check plasma PO_4^- if evidence of renal failure
- Observed when GFR is < 25 mL/min (normal 120 mL/min)
- Often associated with hypocalcemia
- Chronic $\uparrow PO_4^-$ is associated with $CaHPO_4$ precipitation (metastatic calcifications)

Figure 16.5 Diagnostic Algorithm for Hypophosphatemia

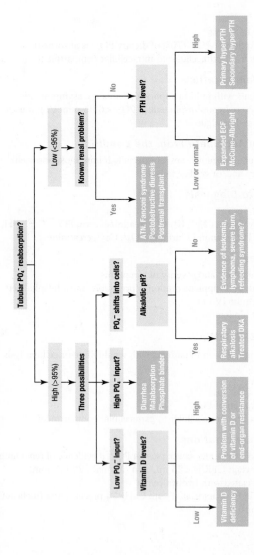

$TRP = 1 - FE - PO_4^-$, where: $FE - PO_4^- = \dfrac{U_{PO_4^-} \times P_{Creat}}{U_{Creat} \times P_{PO_4^-}}$

© The Hospital for Sick Children, 2009. New artwork created by The Hospital for Sick Children for *The Hospital for Sick Children Handbook of Pediatrics*, 11th edition.

Dangers to Anticipate From the Condition
- Increased risk of severe hypocalcemia (acute) or metastatic calcifications (chronic)

Approach to Diagnosis
- See Figure 16.6
- Laboratory: same as for hypophosphatemia; add CBC/differential/smear, CPK, urine dipstick (for hemoglobinuria/myoglobinuria)

Management
- Treat underlying cause
- ↓GI absorption by ↓ dietary PO_4^- intake or by ↓ absorption with PO_4^- binders (calcium carbonate, aluminum-based salts, sevelamer hydrochloride)
- ↑ Urinary PO_4^- excretion with ECF volume expansion
- Use dialysis if severe ↑PO_4^-, especially in context of end-stage renal failure
- With cellular lysis, counteract PO_4^- shifts out of cells by using insulin and glucose

Dangers to Anticipate From Therapy
- Vascular calcifications from long-term administration of calcium carbonate
- If severe hypocalcemia (symptomatic or not) presents with concomitant hyperphosphatemia, disregard risks of calcification because emergency treatment may be life saving

MAGNESIUM

- Central role in oxidative phosphorylation, muscle, and modulation of Ca^{2+} and K^+ channels
- No regulating hormone
- To change concentration of Mg^{2+} from mmol/L to mg/dL, multiply by 2.4

IMPORTANT CONCEPTS
- Input mainly from diet (20–40 mmol/d, of which 30% is absorbed)
- Output mainly via kidneys (outputs usually match inputs)
- Important for both Ca^{2+} and K^+ homeostasis

HYPOMAGNESEMIA

Etiology
- ↑ Urinary Mg^{2+} loss
- ↓GI absorption of Mg^{2+} or ↓ intake

Figure 16.6 Diagnostic Algorithm for Hyperphosphatemia

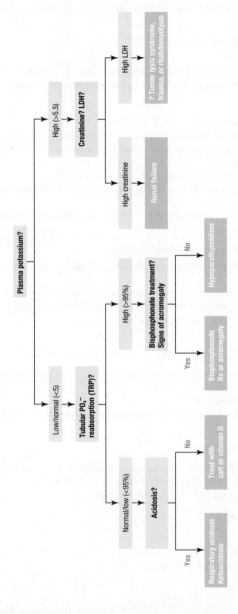

$$TRP = 1 - FE\text{-}PO_4^-; \text{ where: } FE - PO_4^- = \frac{U_{PO_4^-} \times P_{creat}}{U_{creat} \times P_{PO_4^-}}$$

© The Hospital for Sick Children, 2009. New artwork created by The Hospital for Sick Children for *The Hospital for Sick Children Handbook of Pediatrics*, 11th edition.

Clinical Manifestations

- Usually asymptomatic
- ECG: prolonged QT, torsades de pointes
- Often associated with hypokalemia and/or hypocalcemia (with their associated symptoms)

Dangers to Anticipate From the Condition

- Cardiac arrhythmias, increased risk of hypokalemia and/or hypocalcemia

Approach to Diagnosis

- See Figure 16.7
- Laboratory: plasma Mg^{2+}, K^+, Ca^{2+}, creatinine, urea; urinary Mg^{2+} (usually timed collection), Ca^{2+} (spot or timed), creatinine

Management

- Symptomatic: parenteral treatment: 0.2 mL/kg of 50% $MgSO_4$ over 30 min
- Asymptomatic: enteral Mg^{2+} supplements
- Chronic hypomagnesemia implies decrease in both intracellular and extracellular Mg^{2+} pools: long-term supplementation necessary

Dangers to Anticipate From Therapy

- If abnormal renal function exists, hypermagnesemia may occur (excretion of excess Mg^{2+} impaired)

HYPERMAGNESEMIA

- Most commonly observed in renal failure

Etiology

- ↓ Urinary Mg^{2+} loss
- ↑ GI absorption of Mg^{2+} or ↑ intake

Clinical Manifestations

- Mild hypermagnesemia: asymptomatic, cutaneous flushing, mild hypotension
- Severe hypermagnesemia (> 2.5 mmol/L): muscle weakness, hyporeflexia, ↓BP, ECG abnormalities (bradycardia, prolonged QT, increased QRS duration), nausea, vomiting, paralytic ileus, hypocalcemia
- Extreme hypermagnesemia (> 15 mmol/L) associated with complete heart block and respiratory muscle paralysis

Approach to Diagnosis

- See Figure 16.8
- Similar investigations as for hypomagnesemia
- Expected FE-Mg^{2+} is $> 5\%$; lower implies suboptimal renal Mg^{2+} excretion

Figure 16.7 Diagnostic Algorithm for Hypomagnesemia

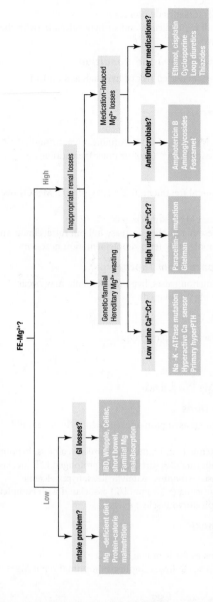

Fractional excretion of Mg^{2+} (FE–Mg^{2+}): low <5%; high >5%

© The Hospital for Sick Children, 2009. New artwork created by The Hospital for Sick Children for *The Hospital for Sick Children Handbook of Pediatrics*, 11th edition.

Figure 16.8 Diagnostic Algorithm for Hypermagnesemia

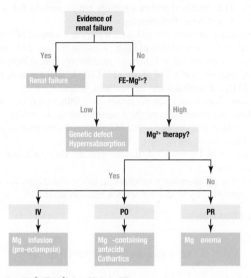

Fractional excretion of Mg^{2+} (FE–Mg^{2+}): low <5%; high >5%
© The Hospital for Sick Children, 2009. New artwork created by The Hospital for Sick Children for *The Hospital for Sick Children Handbook of Pediatrics*, 11th edition.

Management

- Stop Mg^{2+} infusion or supplementation
- IV Ca^{2+} infusion may counteract the effects of hypermagnesemia
- For rapid correction, dialysis may also be considered

ACID–BASE

GENERAL CONCEPTS

- pH determined by plasma CO_2 tension and HCO_3^- concentration:
  - CO_2: regulated by pulmonary system ("respiratory" component)
  - HCO_3: regulated by the renal system ("metabolic" component)
- Bicarbonate–carbon dioxide buffer system: $H^+ + HCO_3^- \leftrightarrow H_2CO_3 \leftrightarrow CO_2 + H_2O$
- pH calculated using the Henderson–Hasselbach equation:

$$pH = 6.1 + \log \left[\frac{[HCO_3^-]}{0.03 \times PaCO_2} \right]$$

BASIC PHYSIOLOGY

- Plasma pH maintained within a narrow range (around 7.4)
- Two main acid–base disturbances:
  1. Acidosis: ↓ extracellular pH (i.e., a gain or excess of H^+ ions)
  2. Alkalosis: ↑ extracellular pH (i.e., a loss or deficit of H^+ ions)
- pH changes prevented by buffering systems: control of P_{CO_2} via ventilation changes, control of plasma HCO_3^- via changes in renal excretion of H^+, extracellular and intracellular buffers
- Acid–base disturbances further subdivided; fifth type is mixed acid–base disturbance (more than one process is occurring)
- Compensatory responses distinct from primary disturbance; help re-establish acid–base homeostasis
  - Further the pH is from 7.4, the stronger the drive to return to homeostasis
  - Secondary compensatory mechanism rarely overshoots 7.4 (e.g., compensation for acidosis does not result in alkalosis)

USEFUL EQUATIONS

SAG

$$SAG = \{[Na^+]\} - \{[Cl^-] + [HCO_3^-]\}$$

- Useful in determining etiology of metabolic acidosis (normal, 12 ± 2 mmol/L)
- Corresponds to quantity of unmeasured anions/cations in plasma
- Note: serum albumin is an unmeasured anion: ↓ 2.5 mmol/L SAG for every ↓ 1g/dL albumin

UNC/UAG

$$UNC = \{[U_{Na^+}] + [U_{K^+}]\} - \{[U_{Cl^-}]\}$$

- Useful in clarifying whether the renal response to acidosis is appropriate (normal ≥0)
- Measures quantity of unmeasured anions and cations in the urine

Serum Osmolal Gap

- Serum osmolal gap = measured osmolality – calculated osmolality
- Calculated osmolality = $2 \times Na^+$ + glucose + urea
- Helps to determine whether additional unmeasured osmotically active molecules are present
- Normal <10 mOsm/Kg H_2O

Bicarbonate Deficit

$$HCO_3^- \text{ deficit} = (nHCO_3^- - cHCO_3^-) \times 0.6 \times TBW$$
$$(n = normal; c = current)$$

- Calculates the amount of HCO_3^- necessary to return to homeostasis

16

Base Excess

- Amount of acid required to return the blood pH to 7.4
- Calculated and reported; normal value, –2 to 2 mmol/L

APPROACH TO BLOOD GAS INTERPRETATION

- See Figure 16.9

METABOLIC ACIDOSIS

- Concomitant finding of low blood pH (<7.4) and low plasma HCO_3^-
- Compensatory hyperventilation should occur (resulting in $\downarrow P_{CO_2}$)
- Caused by a process that generates either a gain of H^+ or a loss of HCO_3^- from plasma

Clinical Manifestations

- Acute acidemia: tachypnea
- Chronic acidemia: dyspnea, anorexia, nausea, weight loss, poor weight gain, muscle weakness

Approach to Diagnosis

- See Figure 16.10

Management

- Specific to underlying cause of acidosis
- Usually acute metabolic acidosis is treated with HCO_3^- only if plasma pH <7.0, plasma $[HCO_3^-] <12$, or to replace significant ongoing renal HCO_3^- losses (does not apply to DKA, see Chapter 3)
- Use previous equation to calculate the HCO_3^- deficit
- Rate of correction depends on target HCO_3^- and clinical scenario: typically start with 1–2 mmol/kg followed by half of calculated HCO_3^- deficit over the next 24 h

Dangers to Anticipate From Therapy

- Hypokalemia and ionized hypocalcemia

Renal Tubular Acidosis

- See Table 16.8
- Hyperchloremic metabolic acidosis secondary to impaired urinary acidification
- Suspect in child with failure to thrive and/or normal anion gap metabolic acidosis

Figure 16.9 **Algorithm to Distinguish the Primary Acid-Base Disturbances**

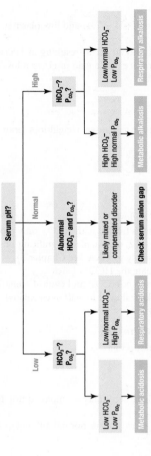

Adapted from Halperin ML, Goldstein MB. *Fluid, Electrolyte, and Acid-Base Physiology: A Problem-Based Approach.* 3rd ed. Philadelphia, Pa: WB Saunders; 1999.

Figure 16.10 Diagnostic Algorithm for Acidosis

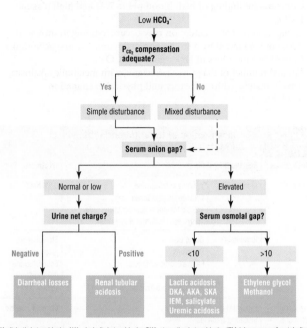

DKA, diabetic ketoacidosis; AKA, alcoholic ketoacidosis; SKA, starvation ketoacidosis; IEM, inborn error of metabolism.
© The Hospital for Sick Children, 2009. New artwork created by The Hospital for Sick Children for *The Hospital for Sick Children Handbook of Pediatrics*, 11th edition.

Table 16.8	Types of Renal Tubular Acidosis		
RTA Type	Problem	Diagnostics	Treatment
Type 1	Deficiency in H⁺ secretion by the distal tubule resulting in ↓NH₄⁺ urinary excretion and ↑HCO₃⁻ urinary losses	Urine pH > 5.8 Positive UNC Low serum K⁺ U-B P_{CO_2} < 15	Alkali therapy with Na⁺ or K⁺ salts
Type 2	Proximal HCO₃⁻ reabsorption defect causing bicarbonaturia	Urine pH < 5.6 Negative UNC Low serum K⁺ U-B P_{CO_2} > 25	K⁺ supplementation
Type 4	↓ Production or response to aldosterone	Urine pH < 5.5 Negative UNC High serum K⁺ U-B P_{CO_2} < 15	Treat hyperkalemia K⁺ restriction Fludrocortisone

U-B P_{CO_2} = urine P_{CO_2} – blood P_{CO_2}.

METABOLIC ALKALOSIS

- Concomitant finding of high blood pH (>7.4) and high plasma HCO_3^-
- Compensatory hypoventilation may occur (resulting in increased PCO_2) but is limited by a strong competing interest (oxygenation)
- Caused by either loss of H^+ or gain of HCO_3^-
- Limited number of diagnoses associated with metabolic alkalosis; usually diagnosed from history and physical examination
- See Table 16.9

Table 16.9	Classification of the Differential Diagnosis for Metabolic Alkalosis		
Mechanisms	**Specific Diagnoses**		**Treatment**
Loss of H^+	GI losses	Vomiting or NG suction	0.9% NaCl
		Chloride-losing diarrhea	
		Antacid therapy in patients taking sodium polystyrene sulfonate (Kayexalate)	
	Renal losses	Diuretics	Stop diuretics
		Penicillins	Stop antibiotics
		Mineralocorticoid excess	Spironolactone
		Hypercalcemia	0.9% NaCl
		Postchronic hypercapnia*	Time
Transcellular shift of H^+	Hypokalemia		Correct K^+ deficit
	Refeeding syndrome		
HCO_3^- excess	NaHCO$_3$ administration		Stop NaHCO$_3$
	Massive blood transfusion (citrate)†		Time
	Milk–alkali syndrome		
Contraction alkalosis	Diuretics		Stop diuretics
	Sweat losses in cystic fibrosis		0.9% NaCl
	Gastric losses in patients with achlorhydria		

*Postchronic hypercapnia occurs in chronic respiratory acidosis with metabolic alkalosis compensation.
†Citrate is metabolized to HCO_3^-.
Adapted from Rose BD, Post TW. *Clinical Physiology of Acid-Base and Electrolyte Disorders*. 5th ed. New York: McGraw-Hill; 2001.

Management

- Correct any volume, K^+, and/or Cl^- deficit(s) and treat underlying etiology

RESPIRATORY ACIDOSIS

- Defined by $\downarrow$pH and $\uparrow$PCO$_2$
- Caused by $\downarrow$ in alveolar ventilation
- Chronic respiratory acidosis leads to $\uparrow$ renal reabsorption of HCO_3^-

Clinical Manifestations

- CNS: drowsiness, somnolence (due to hypercarbia), restlessness, irritability, confusion, headache, fatigue, sweating
- Respiratory: compensatory tachypnea (if able), irregular breathing, cyanosis
- Cardiac: tachycardia

Complications

- Long-term complications depend on underlying cause of respiratory acidosis
- Respiratory failure, acute or chronic

Approach to Diagnosis

- See Table 16.10

Table 16.10	Systematic Approach to Differential Diagnosis of Respiratory Acidosis	
Major Problem	**Anatomic Correlate**	**Differential Diagnoses**
Breathing problem	Central control of breathing	Anesthetics, sedatives, opioids, brain injury, congenital central hypoventilation syndrome
	Respiratory muscles	Spinal cord injury, Guillain-Barré syndrome, myasthenia gravis, botulism, tetanus, poliomyelitis, spinal cord tumors, organophosphate poisoning
	Chest wall weakness	Muscular dystrophy, spinal muscular atrophy
	Chest wall restriction	Kyphoscoliosis, extreme obesity, contracted chest burn scars
Lung failure	Lung restriction	Pulmonary fibrosis, sarcoidosis, pneumothorax, massive pleural effusion
	Parenchyma	Pneumonia, pulmonary edema
	Airway	Severe acute asthma, chronic obstructive pulmonary disease

Adapted from Rose BD, Post TW. *Clinical Physiology of Acid-base and Electrolyte Disorders*, 5th ed. New York: McGraw-Hill; 2001.

Management

- Support ventilation (see pp. 5–9)
- Ultimate goal: identify and treat the underlying cause

RESPIRATORY ALKALOSIS

- Defined by plasma $\uparrow$pH and $\downarrow$PCO_2
- Caused by $\uparrow$ in minute ventilation and "blowing off" of CO_2

Clinical Manifestations and Dangers to Anticipate

- Depends on underlying etiology
- Risk of respiratory muscle fatigue with prolonged increased work of breathing

Approach to Diagnosis

- CNS activation (anxiety with tachypnea, encephalitis, meningitis, tumor)
- Drugs (salicylates, certain hormones)
- Fever, bacteremia
- Pulmonary diseases (acute asthma exacerbation, pulmonary embolism)
- Overventilation with mechanical ventilator

Management

- Treat the underlying cause

FURTHER READING

Dubose T, Hamm L. *Acid–Base and Electrolyte Disorders—A Companion to Brenner & Rector's The Kidney.* Philadelphia, Pa: WB Saunders; 2002.

Halperin ML, Goldstein MB. *Fluid, Electrolyte, and Acid-Base Physiology: A Problem-Based Approach.* 3rd ed. Philadelphia, Pa: WB Saunders; 1999.

Reilly RF, Perazella MA. *Instant Access—Acid-Base, Fluids and Electrolytes.* New York, NY: Lange McGraw-Hill; 2007.

Rose BD. *Clinical Physiology of Acid-Base and Electrolyte Disorders.* 5th ed. New York, NY: McGraw-Hill; 2000

Whittier FC, Rutecki GW. *Fluids and Electrolytes: The Guide for Everyday Practice—The Little Yellow Book.* Columbus, Ohio: Anadem Publishing; 2000.

USEFUL WEB SITES

Schrier R, ed. Atlas of Diseases of the Kidney. Vol 1. Available at: http://kidneyatlas.org/segments.htm

Nephrology calculator. Available at: www.tinkershop.net/nephro.htm

Up to date. Available at: www.uptodate.com

Hypertension dialysis and clinical nephrology. Available at: www.hdcn.com/ch/acid/

Chapter 17 Gastroenterology and Hepatology

Catharine M. Walsh
Ewurabena A. Simpson
Mary Zachos

COMMON ABBREVIATIONS

5-ASA	5-aminosalicylate
AA	amino acids
α-1-AGP	alpha-1 acid glycoprotein
ALP	alkaline phosphatase
ANCA	antinuclear cytoplasmic antibody
ASCA	antisaccharomyces cerevisiae antibody
α1-AT	alpha-1 antitrypsin
AXR	abdominal X-ray
CBC	complete blood cell count
CD	Crohn disease
C. difficile	Clostridium difficile
CF	cystic fibrosis
CMPI	cow's milk protein intolerance
CMV	cytomegalovirus
CRP	C-reactive protein
C&S	culture and sensitivity
EM	electron microscopy
EMA	antiendomysial antibody
ESR	erythrocyte sedimentation rate
FAP	functional abdominal pain
FTT	failure to thrive
GER	gastroesophageal reflux
GERD	gastroesophageal reflux disease
GGT	gamma-glutamyl transpeptidase
G tube	gastrostomy tube
HCC	hepatocellular carcinoma
HSP	Henoch-Schönlein purpura
HUS	hemolytic uremic syndrome
IBD	inflammatory bowel disease
Ig	immunoglobulin
INR	international normalized ratio
LFT	liver function test
LGI	lower gastrointestinal
MCT	medium chain triglycerides
NEC	necrotizing enterocolitis
NG	nasogastric
O&P	ova and parasites (stool culture)
PEG	polyethylene glycol
Pi	protease inhibitor
PPI	proton pump inhibitor
PTT	partial thromboplastin time

PUD	peptic ulcer disease
SBFT	small bowel follow-through
SBP	spontaneous bacterial peritonitis
SLE	systemic lupus erythematosus
TPN	total parenteral nutrition
TORCH	congenital infections including *t*oxoplasmosis, *o*ther agents, *r*ubella, *c*ytomegalovirus, *h*erpes
TSH	thyroid-stimulating hormone
UC	ulcerative colitis
UGI	upper gastrointestinal

GASTROINTESTINAL EMERGENCIES

ACUTE GI BLEEDING

- UGI bleeding caused by bleeding proximal to ligament of Treitz; LGI bleeding distal
- Hematemesis: emesis of blood
- Melena: black, tarry, foul-smelling stool caused by degradation of blood in LGI tract
- Hemtatochezia: bloody stools; seen with LGI bleeding or with vigorous UGI bleeding
- See Table 17.1 for differential diagnosis
- See Figure 17.1 for approach to GI bleeding

Table 17.1	Differential Diagnosis of Gastrointestinal Bleeding		
Age	**Infant**	**Child**	**Adolescent**
Common causes	· Infectious enterocolitis (bacterial > viral) · Allergic gastroenteritis (CMPI most common) · Intussusception · Swallowed maternal blood · Anal fissure · Lymphoid hyperplasia	· Infectious enterocolitis (bacterial > viral) · Anal fissure · Colonic polyps · Intussusception · PUD/gastritis · Epistaxis · Mallory-Weiss syndrome	· Infectious enterocolitis (bacterial > viral) · IBD · PUD/gastritis · Mallory-Weiss syndrome · Colonic polyps
Less common causes	· Volvulus · NEC · Meckel diverticulum · Stomach ulcer · Coagulopathy (hemorrhagic disease of the newborn)	· Esophageal varices · Esophagitis · Meckel diverticulum · Lymphoid hyperplasia · HSP · Foreign body · Vascular malformation · Hemangioma · Trauma/abuse · HUS · IBD · Coagulopathy	· Hemorrhoids · Esophageal varices · Esophagitis · Telangiectasia-angiodysplasia · Graft-versus-host disease

From Berhman RE, Kliegman RM, Jenson HB. *Nelson's Textbook of Pediatrics.* 17th ed. Philadelphia, Pa: Elsevier Science; 2004.

Figure 17.1 Approach to Gastrointestinal Bleeding

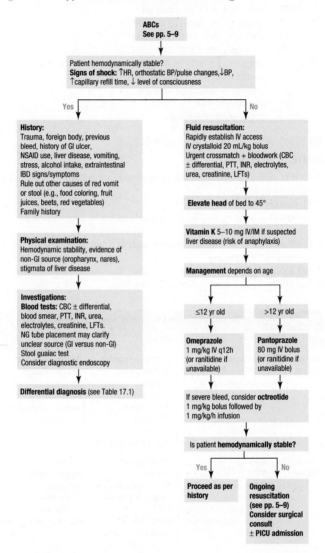

ABCs
See pp. 5–9

Patient hemodynamically stable?
Signs of shock: ↑HR, orthostatic BP/pulse changes, ↓BP, ↑capillary refill time, ↓ level of consciousness

Yes

History:
Trauma, foreign body, previous bleed, history of GI ulcer, NSAID use, liver disease, vomiting, stress, alcohol intake, extraintestinal IBD signs/symptoms
Rule out other causes of red vomit or stool (e.g., food coloring, fruit juices, beets, red vegetables)
Family history

Physical examination:
Hemodynamic stability, evidence of non-GI source (oropharynx, nares), stigmata of liver disease

Investigations:
Blood tests: CBC ± differential, blood smear, PTT, INR, urea, electrolytes, creatinine, LFTs.
NG tube placement may clarify unclear source (GI versus non-GI)
Stool guaiac test
Consider diagnostic endoscopy

Differential diagnosis (see Table 17.1)

No

Fluid resuscitation:
Rapidly establish IV access
IV crystalloid 20 mL/kg bolus
Urgent crossmatch + bloodwork (CBC ± differential, PTT, INR, electrolytes, urea, creatinine, LFTs)

Elevate head of bed to 45°

Vitamin K 5–10 mg IV/IM if suspected liver disease (risk of anaphylaxis)

Management depends on age

≤12 yr old

Omeprazole
1 mg/kg IV q12h
(or ranitidine if unavailable)

>12 yr old

Pantoprazole
80 mg IV bolus
(or ranitidine if unavailable)

If severe bleed, consider **octreotide** 1 mg/kg bolus followed by 1 mg/kg/h infusion

Is patient **hemodynamically stable?**

Yes

Proceed as per history

No

Ongoing resuscitation (see pp. 5–9)
Consider surgical consult
± PICU admission

ACUTE ABDOMINAL PAIN

- See Figure 17.2

Figure 17.2 Approach to Acute Abdominal Pain

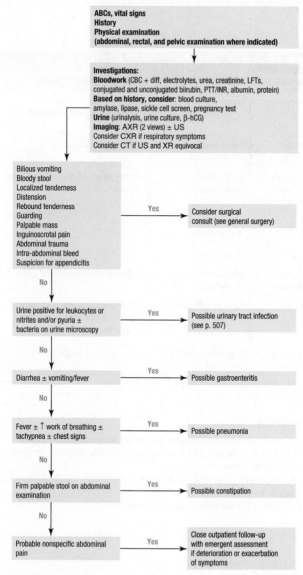

ABCs, vital signs
History
Physical examination
(abdominal, rectal, and pelvic examination where indicated)

Investigations:
Bloodwork (CBC + diff, electrolytes, urea, creatinine, LFTs, conjugated and unconjugated bilirubin, PTT/INR, albumin, protein)
Based on history, consider: blood culture, amylase, lipase, sickle cell screen, pregnancy test
Urine (urinalysis, urine culture, β-hCG)
Imaging: AXR (2 views) ± US
Consider CXR if respiratory symptoms
Consider CT if US and XR equivocal

Bilious vomiting
Bloody stool
Localized tenderness
Distension
Rebound tenderness
Guarding
Palpable mass
Inguinoscrotal pain
Abdominal trauma
Intra-abdominal bleed
Suspicion for appendicitis

Yes → Consider surgical consult (see general surgery)

No ↓

Urine positive for leukocytes or nitrites and/or pyuria ± bacteria on urine microscopy

Yes → Possible urinary tract infection (see p. 507)

No ↓

Diarrhea ± vomiting/fever

Yes → Possible gastroenteritis

No ↓

Fever ± ↑ work of breathing ± tachypnea ± chest signs

Yes → Possible pneumonia

No ↓

Firm palpable stool on abdominal examination

Yes → Possible constipation

No ↓

Probable nonspecific abdominal pain

Yes → Close outpatient follow-up with emergent assessment if deterioration or exacerbation of symptoms

Gastroenterology and Hepatology

17

Adapted from *Policy Directive: Children and Infants with Acute Abdominal Pain—Acute Management.* North Sydney, Australia: New South Wales Government, Dept of Health; 2004.

- See Table 17.2

Table 17.2	Common Investigations on Stool	
Investigation	**Indications**	**Preparation/Results/Comments**
Culture	Suspected infection	· C&S, O&P, virology, *C. difficile* · *C. difficile* not indicated <1 yr (about 50% colonized)
Serology	Rule out infection in setting of terminal ileitis	*Yersinia* and amebic titers
Fat (3-d collection with record of dietary fat intake)	Suspected fat malabsorption	· Newborn period: nonabsorbed fat is 10–15% · Adult: normal is <7%
WBC	Suspected infection or inflammation	
Eosinophils	Suspected CMPI	
Stool-reducing substances	Suspected carbohydrate malabsorption	Detects most dietary sugars except sucrose
Stool pH	Suspected carbohydrate malabsorption	pH <6 if carbohydrate intolerant (caused by organic acids from bacterial breakdown of nonabsorbed sugar)
α-1-AT	Suspected protein-losing enteropathy	Need serum α-1-AT at same time

From Berhman RE, Kliegman RM, Jenson HB. *Nelson's Textbook of Pediatrics.* 17th ed. Philadelphia, Pa: Elsevier Science; 2004.

DYSPHAGIA

- Difficulty swallowing secondary to either abnormal esophageal motility (both liquids and solids affected) or mechanical obstruction (relieved by vomiting)
- Odynophagia: pain with swallowing; indicates esophageal mucosal disease
- See Table 17.3 for differential diagnosis

Table 17.3	Differential Diagnosis of Dysphagia	
Mechanism	**Etiology**	**Description**
Mechanical	Achalasia	Functional obstruction of esophagogastric junction
	External compression	
	Esophageal stricture	Often past history of GERD or caustic ingestion
	Lower esophageal (Schatzki) ring	Intermittent dysphagia; can be acute with large food bolus
	Foreign body	
Motor dysfunction	Infectious esophagitis (*Candida*, HSV)	Severe odynophagia; often unable to swallow saliva
	GERD	See section in text
	Caustic ingestion	May lead to erosive esophagitis and stricture formation
	Eosinophilic esophagitis	Often associated with atopic history
	Collagen vascular disease	Classically associated with scleroderma
Other	Globus hystericus	Difficulty swallowing between meals; usually with emotional stress

VOMITING

- See Figure 17.3 for differential diagnosis
- History (presence of other GI and systemic symptoms, quality, timing, presence of bile/blood in vomitus) key for determining etiology
- Investigations guided by history and physical and may include:
  - Blood tests: CBC, differential, ESR, electrolytes, blood gas, urea, creatinine, glucose, LFTs, amylase, further metabolic workup depending on history
  - Urine: dip, microscopy, culture
  - Stool: virology (EM), occult blood, eosinophils
  - Radiology: AXR (2 views), UGI radiography ± SBFT, gastric emptying time, head CT
  - pH probe, upper endoscopy

CHRONIC ABDOMINAL PAIN

- See Figure 17.4 for approach to chronic abdominal pain
- See Box 17.1 for red flags when evaluating abdominal pain

17

Figure 17.3 **Differential Diagnosis of Vomiting**

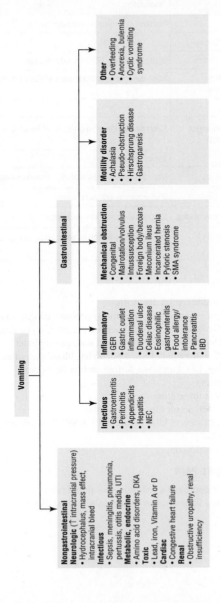

Vomiting

Nongastrointestinal

Neurologic (↑ intracranial pressure)
• Hydrocephalus, mass effect, intracranial bleed

Infectious
• Sepsis, meningitis, pneumonia, pertussis, otitis media, UTI

Metabolic, endocrine
• Amino acid disorders, DKA

Toxic
• Lead, iron, Vitamin A or D

Cardiac
• Congestive heart failure

Renal
• Obstructive uropathy, renal insufficiency

Gastrointestinal

Infectious
• Gastroenteritis
• Peritonitis
• Appendicitis
• Hepatitis
• NEC

Inflammatory
• GER
• Gastric outlet inflammation
• Duodenal ulcer
• Celiac disease
• Eosinophilic gastroenteritis
• Food allergy/intolerance
• Pancreatitis
• IBD

Mechanical obstruction
• Congenital
• Malrotation/volvulus
• Intussusception
• Foreign body/bezoars
• Meconium ileus
• Incarcerated hernia
• Pyloric stenosis
• SMA syndrome

Motility disorder
• Achalasia
• Pseudo-obstruction
• Hirschsprung disease
• Gastroparesis

Other
• Overfeeding
• Anorexia, bulemia
• Cyclic vomiting syndrome

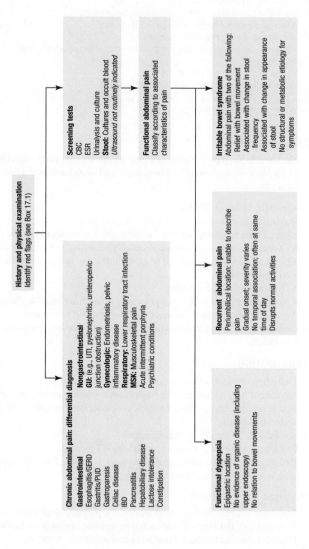

Figure 17.4 Approach to Chronic Abdominal Pain

History and physical examination
Identify red flags (see Box 17.1)

Chronic abdominal pain: differential diagnosis

Gastrointestinal
Esophagitis/GERD
Gastritis/PUD
Gastroparesis
Celiac disease
IBD
Pancreatitis
Hepatobiliary disease
Lactose intolerance
Constipation

Nongastrointestinal
GU: (e.g. UTI, pyelonephritis, ureteropelvic
junction obstruction)
Gynecologic: Endometriosis, pelvic
inflammatory disease
Respiratory: Lower respiratory tract infection
MSK: Musculoskeletal pain
Acute intermittent porphyria
Psychiatric conditions

Screening tests
CBC
ESR
Urinalysis and culture
Stool: Cultures and occult blood
Ultrasound not routinely indicated

Functional abdominal pain
Classify according to associated
characteristics of pain

Functional dyspepsia
Epigastric location
No evidence of organic disease (including
upper endoscopy)
No relation to bowel movements

Recurrent abdominal pain
Periumbilical location: unable to describe
pain
Gradual onset; severity varies
No temporal association; often at same
time of day
Disrupts normal activities

Irritable bowel syndrome
Abdominal pain with two of the following:
Relief with bowel movement
Associated with change in stool
frequency
Associated with change in appearance
of stool
No structural or metabolic etiology for
symptoms

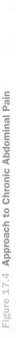

Gastroenterology and Hepatology

17

- Well-localized pain away from umbilicus
- Pain awakening patient from sleep
- Radiation of pain to back, shoulder, scapula, lower extremities
- Altered bowel pattern (diarrhea, constipation) or vomiting
- Involuntary weight loss or growth deceleration
- GI bleeding, constitutional symptoms (e.g., fever, arthralgias, rash) or unexplained physical findings
- Consistent sleepiness after pain attacks
- Positive family history of peptic ulcer, IBD, celiac disease

Adapted from Walker WA, Durie PR, Hamilton JR, Walker Smith JA, Watkins JB. *Pediatric Gastrointestinal Disease.* 3rd ed. Hamilton, Ontario, Canada: BC Decker Inc; 2000:132.

FAP Syndromes

- No identifiable pathologic cause; may be due to abnormal reactivity of enteric nervous system to physiologic and stressful stimuli (visceral hyperalgesia)

Diagnostic Criteria (ROME III)

- Symptom onset at least 6 mo before diagnosis
- Meets all the following criteria for the 3 mo leading up to diagnosis:
  - Constant, nearly constant, or frequently recurring abdominal pain
  - No clear physiologic pattern (e.g., with menses, eating, defecation)
  - No malingering
  - Decreased daily functioning
  - Symptoms do not meet criteria for any other functional GI disorder
- Avoid overinvestigation; focus on explanation and reassurance
- Goal is return to normal function rather than complete symptom resolution

CONSTIPATION

- Definition: difficult and infrequent passage of hard stool
- Significant normal variation in bowel movement frequency; diagnosis best based on changes from baseline and associated symptoms (e.g., abdominal pain)
- See Table 17.4 for differential diagnosis
- Organic disease more common in infants <3 mo old
- Red flags on history: abdominal distension, vomiting, fever, anorexia, weight loss, poor weight gain, blood in stool

Physical Examination

- Red flags: abdominal distension/tenderness, palpable fecal mass, sacral dimpling/tuft, flat buttocks, abnormal neurologic examination findings
- Digital rectal examination (anal tone and sensation, rectal size, rectal stool)
- Tight empty rectum in presence of abdominal fecal mass and/or explosive stool on withdrawal of finger suggests Hirschsprung disease

Table 17.4	Differential Diagnosis of Constipation	
Neonate (<1 mo)	**Infant**	**Child/Adolescent**
Hypothyroidism	CMPI	Functional
Meconium ileus/plug (must rule out CF)	Hirschsprung disease	Developmental (cognitive, ADHD)
	Botulism	Situational (phobia, abuse)
Intestinal atresia or stricture/stenosis	Drugs (e.g., opiates, phenobarbital, anticholinergics)	Depression
Hirschsprung disease		Constitutional (colonic inertia, genetic predisposition)
CMPI	Spinal cord pathology	
Anal stenosis	Visceral myopathies/ neuropathies	Drugs (e.g., opiates, phenobarbital, anticholinergics, antidepressants, sympathomimetics)
Imperforate anus		
Spinal cord pathology (e.g., spinal muscle atrophy, tethered cord)		
Visceral myopathies/neuropathies		

Investigations

- Consider further investigation if <3 mo, no response to conventional treatment, or concerning red flags
- Exclude UTI, which can complicate chronic constipation

Management

- See Table 17.5

DIARRHEA

- See Figure 17.5 for differential diagnosis

Table 17.5	Management of Constipation
Intervention	**Description**
Education	Scheduled toilet attempts, proper position, positive reinforcement
Dietary	Increase fiber (whole grains, fruits, vegetables) and fluids; reduce complex carbohydrates (rice, pasta, white bread)
Medical therapy (two phases):	· Initial options include mineral oil, lactulose, PEG-3350 stimulant laxatives
1. Initial disimpaction: oral or rectal approach	· Use suppositories intermittently (e.g., glycerin in infants, bisacodyl in older children)
	· Severe cases: enemas (saline, 10–20 mL/kg) or GI lavage (NG electrolyte and polyethylene glycol solution [PegLyte], 10–12 mL/kg)
2. Maintenance therapy	· Mineral oil 15 mL/15 kg, increase by 5 mL every 3 d until oil leaking from anus
	· Continue 4–6 mo before weaning
	· Avoid in <1 yr or neurologically impaired (risk of aspiration)
	· Lactulose (may cause transient cramping due to undigested sugars), PEG-3350
	· Long-term stimulant laxative use not recommended; however, may be necessary intermittently to avoid recurrence of impaction (rescue therapy)

Figure 17.5 Differential Diagnosis of Acute and Chronic Diarrhea

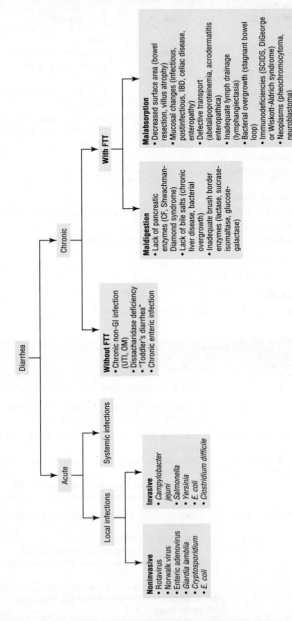

Noninvasive
- Rotavirus
- Norwalk virus
- Enteric adenovirus
- Giardia lamblia
- Cryptosporidium
- E. coli

Invasive
- Campylobacter jejuni
- Salmonella
- Yersinia
- E. coli
- Clostridium difficile

Without FTT
- Chronic non-GI infection (UTI, OM)
- Dissacharidase deficiency
- "Toddler's diarrhea"
- Chronic enteric infection

Maldigestion
- Lack of pancreatic enzymes (CF, Shwachman-Diamond syndrome)
- Lack of bile salts (chronic liver disease, bacterial overgrowth)
- Inadequate brush border enzymes (lactase, sucrase-isomaltase, glucose-galactase)

Malabsorption
- Decreased surface area (bowel resection, villus atrophy)
- Mucosal changes (infectious, postinfectious, IBD, celiac disease, enteropathy)
- Defective transport (abetalipoproteinemia, acrodermatitis enteropathica)
- Inadequate lymph drainage (lymphangiectasia)
- Bacterial overgrowth (stagnant bowel loop)
- Immunodeficiencies (SCIDS, DiGeorge or Wiskott-Aldrich syndrome)
- Neoplasms (pheochromocytoma, neuroblastoma)
- Other (laxatives, heavy metal poisoning)

Acute Diarrhea

- Intestinal infections most common cause

Investigations

- History and physical examination; assess degree of dehydration
- Stool: examination for consistency, fecal leukocytes (microscopy), virology (EM and cultures); bacterial cultures, O&P, and *C. difficile* toxin, depending on clinical situation
- Blood tests (if severe diarrhea): consider CBC, differential, blood film, electrolytes, blood gas, urea, creatinine, blood culture, *Yersinia* and ameba titers
- Urine: microscopy, culture

Management

- Prevention and treatment of dehydration most important: replacement of fluid deficit + maintenance + ongoing losses; see pp. 285–288 for both oral rehydration therapy and IV management
- Transient lactose intolerance possible, secondary to villus damage; avoidance of lactose-containing formulas and foods may be required for 48–72 h
- Antidiarrheal medications not indicated; potentially harmful
- Antibiotic therapy for specific organisms, if indicated (see Chapter 24)

Chronic Diarrhea

- Definition: diarrhea lasting > 14 d

Investigations

- Serial height, weight, growth percentiles
- Stool examination
- Specific investigations as per differential (see Figure 17.5)

Management

- Nonspecific diarrhea of infancy (toddler's diarrhea): no specific therapy; avoid elimination diets, but restrict high sorbitol–containing fruit juices; stools usually form by 3 yr and/or when toilet trained
- Pathologic chronic diarrhea may require electrolyte, water, and nutrient replacement
- Specific therapy as required

MALABSORPTION

- May be caused directly by impaired nutritional uptake from intestine or indirectly as a result of incomplete enzymatic digestion of macronutrients
- May be accompanied by FTT, chronic diarrhea/steatorrhea, abdominal pain, edema, and ascites
- Suspect in FTT even in absence of chronic diarrhea, especially if adequate intake
- Differential diagnosis: can be classified according to the phase of digestion and absorption (luminal, mucosal, postabsorptive) (Table 17.6)

Table 17.6	Differential Diagnosis for Nutrient Malabsorption	
Phase	**Mechanism**	**Etiology**
Luminal phase	Impaired nutrient hydrolysis; leads to impaired fat and protein absorption	· Pancreatic insufficiency (chronic pancreatitis, CF, Shwachman-Diamond syndrome, pancreatic resection) · Decreased luminal transit time (intestinal resection, short-bowel syndrome) · Decreased enzyme activation (rare: trypsinogen and/or enterokinase deficiencies)
	Impaired micelle formation; leads to impaired fat absorption	· Decreased bile acid production (parenchymal liver disease, fatty liver disease, liver cirrhosis) · Decreased bile acid secretion (TPN cholestatic liver disease, biliary atresia, primary biliary cirrhosis, primary sclerosing cholangitis) · Impaired enterohepatic bile circulation (intestinal resection) · Increased bile acid deconjugation (bacterial overgrowth)
	Decreased luminal substrate availability	Bacterial overgrowth
Mucosal phase	Impaired brush border enzyme activity	Disaccharidase deficiency (primary or postinfectious), IgA deficiency
	Impaired nutrient absorption	· Congenital (e.g., galactosemia, fructosemia, immunodeficiency syndromes, abetalipoproteinemia, cystinuria) · Acquired (e.g., short-bowel syndrome, celiac disease, IBD, AIDS enteropathy, lymphoma)
Postabsorptive phase	Lymphatic obstruction	· Congenital (intestinal lymphangiectasia) · Acquired (lymphoma, TB, Whipple disease)

Investigations

- Assess caloric intake and requirements (calorimetry)
- Stool: consistency, pH, reducing substances, and color (pink color may indicate phenolphthalein, present in some laxatives); microscopy for fecal leukocytes, fat globules, and RBCs (also test for occult blood); O&P (min. 3 samples), C&S, *C. difficile* toxin, 3-d fecal fat collection, α1-AT clearance, electrolytes
- Urinalysis, urine C&S

- Blood tests: CBC, differential, ESR, blood film, electrolytes, total protein, albumin, Igs, fat-soluble vitamins (A and E most commonly measured), INR (vitamin K), Ca^{2+}, PO_4^-, Mg^{2+}, Zn, iron, ferritin, folate
- If indicated: celiac testing, LFTs, cholesterol, triglycerides, trypsinogen, thyroid function tests, urine VMA and HVA, HIV testing, and lead levels
- Specialized tests: upper endoscopy with small-bowel biopsy, exocrine pancreatic testing

GASTROESOPHAGEAL REFLUX

- History and physical examination sufficient for diagnosis in majority of cases
- May be benign, manifesting as effortless nonbilious emesis after some or every feeding ("happy spitter"); requires no investigation
- If complicated by FTT, dysphagia, or respiratory symptoms (e.g., chronic cough), then known as GERD

INVESTIGATIONS

- UGI series and abdominal US to rule out anatomic causes (pyloric stenosis, malrotation, annular pancreas, hiatal hernia, esophageal stricture); not sensitive or specific for GER
- 24-h pH probe when presence of GER not obvious clinically or to assess efficacy of therapy
- Medical trial of therapy often diagnostic
- Upper endoscopy and esophageal biopsies in refractory or complicated cases

MANAGEMENT

- Smaller volume and more frequent feeding, positioning, dietary changes (thickening of feeds, trial of hypoallergenic formula)
- Empiric medical therapy (acid suppressant)
  - See Table 17.7
  - PPI superior to H_2 receptor antagonist; choice based on formulation available for different age groups, feeding tube use, and cost
  - Prokinetic medications (e.g., cisapride) may be considered but, due to concerns about the potential for serious cardiac arrhythmias, appropriate patient selection and monitoring as well as proper use (correct dosage and avoidance of coadministration of contraindicated medications) are important.

Table 17.7	Commonly Used Pediatric Acid Suppressant Medications
Drug (Class)	**Formulation and Dose**
Ranitidine (H₂ receptor antagonist)	· Available in capsules and liquid suspension · Maintenance for infants and older children: 2–6 mg/kg/d PO qd · Maximum 300 mg/d
Omeprazole (PPI)*	· Available in 10-, 20- and 40-mg delayed-release capsules · Initial dosage: 0.7–1.4 mg/kg/d PO qd and titrate to therapeutic effect · Can be mixed with feeds for administration through G tube but may cause clogging

Lansoprazole (PPI)	· Available in 15- and 30-mg capsules, disintegrating tablets, and liquid suspension
	· Dosage:
	  · <10 kg: 7.5 mg PO qd
	  · 10–30 kg: 15 mg PO qd
	  · ≥30 kg: 30 mg PO qd
	· Maximum: 1.6 mg/kg/d or 30 mg/d, whichever is less
	· Suspension can be administered through G tube, but may cause clogging

Pantoprazole (PPI)*	· Available in IV formulation only · Dosage: 1–1.5 mg/kg IV qd · Maximum: 40 mg/dose

Note: Other available PPIs include esomeprazole and rabeprazole.
*Available in IV form when rapid gastric acid inhibition is desired (e.g., NPO, UGI bleeding).

INFLAMMATORY BOWEL DISEASE

- See Table 17.8 and Figure 17.6 for clinical manifestations
- Differential diagnosis includes infectious, inflammatory (HUS, HSP, eosinophilic gastroenteritis), and other causes (e.g., allergic colitis)
- History: positive family history in a first-degree relative is a major risk factor for the development of IBD

INVESTIGATIONS

- To rule out other causes and differentiate between CD and UC, the following may be required:
  - Blood tests: CBC, differential, culture, ESR, CRP, albumin, total protein, *Yersinia* and ameba titers, CMV serology
  - Stool cultures: bacterial, *C. difficile* toxin, O&P
  - TB skin test (depending on risk factors)
  - Specific serologic tests (low sensitivity): α1-AGP, ANCA, ASCA
  - Radiology: UGI series and SBFT, US (to identify abscess), MRI (to assess perianal or fistulizing disease)
  - Upper and lower endoscopies with biopsies

| Table 17.8 | Crohn Disease Versus Ulcerative Colitis | |

Investigations	CD	UC
Clinical History, physical examination	· Mean age 13 yr · Often present with GI symptoms: abdominal pain, weight loss, vomiting, diarrhea (may be bloody if colonic involvement) · May also present with growth failure, pubertal delay, anemia, weight loss, fever of unknown origin · Extraintestinal manifestations common (see Figure 17.6) · Perianal lesions common (skin tags, fissures, abscesses, fistulae)	· Mean age 11 yr · Classically presents with bloody diarrhea ± abdominal pain with defecation · Extraintestinal manifestations
Laboratory Serologic markers (ASCA, ANCA) limited use in differentiation of IBD Note: Laboratory findings can be normal or minimally abnormal in perianal disease	· ↑ESR, CRP, platelets · ↓ serum protein, albumin · Iron deficiency anemia	· ↑ESR, CRP, platelets · Serum protein, albumin results normal unless severe · Iron deficiency anemia
Radiology UGI with SBFT	Mucosal inflammation of any part of small bowel, most commonly terminal ileum	Normal
Endoscopy Note: CD may resemble UC with continuous colonic involvement	· Affects any part of GI tract · Classically, segmental GI disease with skip lesions; relative rectal sparing	· No small-bowel disease · Begins in rectum and extends continuously proximally for variable distance (25% pancolitis)
Histopathology	· Focal transmural inflammation · Fissures, fistulae · Noncaseating granulomas	· Diffuse mucosal inflammation
Complications	· Abscess, fistula, stricture leading to bowel obstruction · Toxic megacolon with severe colonic involvement · Increased colon cancer risk	· Toxic megacolon · Severe abdominal pain, tenderness, vomiting, fever · Monitor with serial AXR · Increased colon cancer risk
Management (See Table 17.9 for medical treatment)	· Goals: reduce symptoms, achieve mucosal healing, optimize nutrition, bone health, and growth · Surgery reserved for complications (e.g., obstruction, abscesses); *not* curative	· Avoid opioid-derived analgesia in fulminant colitis · Colectomy indicated for fulminant and medically refractory disease or complications associated with colitis ("curative")

Adapted from Zachos M, Critch J, Jackson R. Gastroenterology and hepatology. In: Laxer RM, ed. *The Hospital for Sick Children Atlas of Pediatrics*. Philadelphia, Pa: Current Medicine LLC; 2005:401.

TREATMENT

- Choice of therapy is individualized based on disease location, severity, and comorbidities (e.g., growth delay, medication allergies) (see Table 17.8)
- See Figure 17.7
- See Table 17.9

Figure 17.6 **Extraintestinal Manifestations of Inflammatory Bowel Disease**

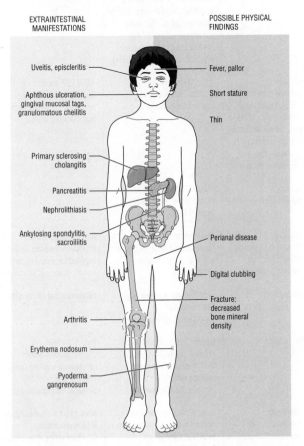

EXTRAINTESTINAL MANIFESTATIONS

- Uveitis, episcleritis
- Aphthous ulceration, gingival mucosal tags, granulomatous cheilitis
- Primary sclerosing cholangitis
- Pancreatitis
- Nephrolithiasis
- Ankylosing spondylitis, sacroiliitis
- Arthritis
- Erythema nodosum
- Pyoderma gangrenosum

POSSIBLE PHYSICAL FINDINGS

- Fever, pallor
- Short stature
- Thin
- Perianal disease
- Digital clubbing
- Fracture: decreased bone mineral density

CELIAC DISEASE

- Gluten sensitivity syndrome secondary to immune-mediated enteropathy in genetically susceptible patients

Figure 17.7 Treatment Pyramid for Inflammatory Bowel Disease

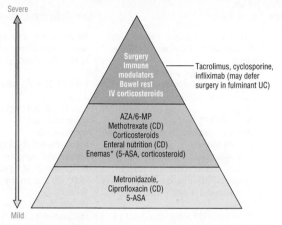

Severe

Surgery
Immune
modulators
Bowel rest
IV corticosteroids

Tacrolimus, cyclosporine, infliximab (may defer surgery in fulminant UC)

AZA/6-MP
Methotrexate (CD)
Corticosteroids
Enteral nutrition (CD)
Enemas* (5-ASA, corticosteroid)

Metronidazole,
Ciprofloxacin (CD)
5-ASA

Mild

*For distal disease or adjuncts in extensive disease.
5-ASA, 5-aminosalicyclic acid; AZA, azathioprine; CD, Crohn disease; IV, intravenous; 6-MP, 6-mercaptopurine; UC, ulcerative colitis.
Adapted from Walker WA, Durie P, Hamilton JR, et al. eds. Pediatric Gastrointestinal Disease: Pathophysiology, Diagnosis and Management. 3rd ed. Hamilton, Ontario, Canada: BC Decker; 2000.

CLINICAL MANIFESTATIONS

- GI: diarrhea, FTT, vomiting, abdominal distension, abdominal pain, constipation
- Non-GI: dermatitis herpetiformis, osteopenia, osteoporosis, delayed puberty, iron deficiency anemia unresponsive to treatment, dental enamel hypoplasia

DIAGNOSIS

- History and physical examination, serologic testing, small intestinal biopsy (gold standard)

Serologic Testing

- False-negative serologic testing in patients with selective IgA deficiency (check IgA levels simultaneously)
- Antitissue transglutaminase (TTG) IgA: sensitivity 90–98%, specificity 94–97%
- EMA: sensitivity 89–98%, specificity 97–100%
- Antigliadin antibody no longer recommended because of poor sensitivity and specificity

Table 17.9 — Medical Management Options for Inflammatory Bowel Disease

Disease	Active Disease	Maintenance of Remission
CD	· Nutritional therapy: exclusive elemental/polymeric formula feedings × 4–6 wk, usually by NG tube Steroids · Prednisone 1 mg/kg/d to max 40–60 mg daily · Controlled ileal release budesonide (9 mg/d) for ileal and right colonic disease ASA · Oral 5-ASA (50–100 mg/kg/d to max 4 g daily) · Mesalamine (Pentasa or Salofalk) for small-bowel or colonic disease · Mesalamine (Asacol) for distal small-bowel or colonic disease · Sulfasalazine[†] (50–75 mg/kg/d to max 3–4 g daily) · 5-ASA enemas[‡] (1–4 qnightly or bid) Antibiotics · Metronidazole[‡] (10–20 mg/kg/d to max 1 g daily) · Ciprofloxacin[‡] (20 mg/kg/d) Immunosuppression · Methotrexate (10–25 mg SC once weekly) with 1 mg/d supplemental folic acid For severe luminal, fistulizing, and/or perianal CD · Infliximab (5 mg/kg IV at time 0, 2 wk, 6 wk for induction of remission of active disease) · Adalimumab (80–160 mg SC for induction of remission)	· Nutritional therapy: 5 nights/wk of supplemental nutrition (in addition to regular daily intake) ASA · Oral 5-ASA (50 mg/kg/d to max 3 g daily) · 5-ASA enemas[*] (1–4 g nightly or every other night) Immunosuppression · 6-Mercaptopurine[†] (1–1.5 mg/kg/d) · Azathioprine[†] (2 mg/kg/d) · Methotrexate[†] (10–25 mg SC once weekly) with 1 mg/d supplemental folic acid · Infliximab (5 mg/kg IV q8wk after 3-dose induction) · Adalimumab (40–80 mg SC q2wk)
UC	5-ASA · Oral 5-ASA (50–100 mg/kg/d to max 4 g daily) · Sulfasalazine (50–75 mg/kg/d to max 3–4 g daily) · 5-ASA enemas (1–4 g nightly or twice daily) Steroids · Prednisone 1 mg/kg/d to max 40–60 mg daily · Hydrocortisone/budesonide enemas For fulminant or severe colitis: · Infliximab (5 mg/kg IV at time 0, 2 wk, 6 wk for induction of remission of active disease) · Tacrolimus/cyclosporine	5-ASA · Oral 5-ASA/sulfasalazine (50 mg/kg/d to max 3 g daily) Immunosuppression · Azathioprine[†] (2 mg/kg/d) · Infliximab (5 mg/kg IV q8wk after 3-dose induction)

[*]Randomized placebo-controlled trial not supportive of benefit in maintenance of remission.
[†]Delayed onset of action.
[‡]No controlled clinical trials.
Adapted from Zachos M, Critch J, Jackson R. Gastroenterology and hepatology. In: Laxer RM, ed. *The Hospital for Sick Children Atlas of Pediatrics*. Philadelphia, Pa: Current Medicine LLC; 2005:402.

Intestinal Biopsy
- Blunting/atrophy of small intestinal villi; crypt elongation, intraepithelial lymphocytes
- To confirm diagnosis when TTG or EMA elevated
- Patient must be on gluten-containing diet at time of biopsy for optimal diagnostic accuracy.

TREATMENT
- Lifelong gluten-free diet, if biopsy positive
- Reverses biopsy changes; normalizes serologic markers

PROTEIN-LOSING ENTEROPATHY
- Hypoproteinemia secondary to GI protein leakage; implies intestinal mucosal integrity loss

CLINICAL MANIFESTATIONS
- Diarrhea, FTT, abdominal distension, ascites, abdominal pain
- Edema, hypoproteinemia, but no proteinuria (i.e., exclude renal causes)

INVESTIGATIONS
- Blood tests: CBC, differential, blood film, ESR, albumin, Igs, iron, ferritin, serum α1-AT
- Urinalysis
- Fecal α1-AT clearance: endogenous protein not normally excreted in stool; therefore, detection in stool abnormal
- Specific testing, as needed

ETIOLOGY
- Common causes: cow's milk or soy protein intolerance, celiac disease, IBD
- Less common causes: Hirschsprung disease, Ménétrier disease, HSP, lymphangiectasia, CHF, restrictive pericarditis, eosinophilic gastroenteritis

CMPI
- Most common cause of protein-losing enteropathy in infancy
- Precipitated by cow's milk protein (also soy and/or goat's milk protein)
- Do not confuse with lactose intolerance (result of mucosal lactase deficiency)

Clinical Features
- Classically presents at 10–18 mo: edema, hypoalbuminemia, iron deficiency anemia
- Younger infants (2–4 mo) most often present with proctocolitis
- Broad spectrum: irritability, vomiting, diarrhea, GER, hives, facial swelling, food-associated wheezing, eczema, anaphylaxis

Investigations
- CBC ± differential, PTT/INR, albumin, urea, creatinine
- Stool for culture, microscopy for eosinophils
- Blood tests: IgE and RAST usually normal; may have peripheral eosinophilia
- Skin prick testing unreliable, but atopy patch testing may be useful

Management
- Quick response to removal of antigenic proteins; 50% also react to soy protein
- Hypoallergenic diets: extensively hydrolyzed or AA-based formula
- Elimination of cow's milk from maternal diet helpful in breastfed infants
- Prognosis: most tolerate cow's milk by 2 yr; rarely persist >3 yr

PANCREATITIS

- Present with abdominal pain that may radiate to back or shoulder, vomiting
- See Box 17.2 for etiology

INVESTIGATIONS
- Serum amylase often but not always elevated (↑ amylase also found in pancreatic pseudocyst, parotitis, biliary tract disease, duodenal ulcer, peritonitis, renal failure, burns, stress)
- Lipase, trypsinogen, LFTs, conjugated and unconjugated bilirubin, Ca^{2+}, glucose, venous gas, CBC, differential, blood C&S
- US useful in detecting obstruction (e.g., stones), but CT provides better imaging of pancreas

MANAGEMENT
- NPO, analgesia, NG suction, IV fluids, control of metabolic complications (i.e., glucose, Ca^{2+}); closely monitor reintroduction of clear fluids to solids

EVALUATION OF LIVER DISEASE

LABORATORY EVALUATION OF THE LIVER
- See Table 17.10 for details
- Serum markers suggestive of hepatocellular necrosis: AST, ALT (transaminases)
- Serum markers suggestive of cholestasis: bilirubin (total, conjugated/direct), GGT, ALP
- Tests of liver synthetic function:
  - ↓: albumin, clotting factors (I, II, V, VII, IX, X), cholesterol, glucose
  - ↑: INR, PTT, ammonia

Box 17.2 Etiology of Acute Pancreatitis

Trauma

Infection
- Virus (e.g., mumps, coxsackievirus B, EBV, hepatitis A, influenza A)
- Bacteria
- Parasites (e.g., malaria)

Drugs
- Furosemide
- Steroids
- Azathioprine

Obstruction
- Gallstones
- Choledochal cyst
- Pancreas divisum
- Sclerosing cholangitis

Systemic Diseases
- CF (pancreatic sufficient)
- IBD
- Vasculitis (HSP, SLE)
- Hyperparathyroidism, hypercalcemia
- Hyperlipoproteinemia I, IV

Idiopathic

NORMAL (AVERAGE) LIVER SIZE

- Upper border of liver should be between the fourth and sixth inter-costal space at the midclavicular line
- See Table 17.11 for age-related variables

EVALUATION OF INFANT WITH CONJUGATED (DIRECT) HYPERBILIRUBINEMIA

- Measure total, conjugated/direct, and unconjugated/indirect bilirubin to rule out conjugated hyperbilirubinemia in all jaundiced infants at 2–4 wk of age or earlier, or if they have pale stools or dark urine
- Conjugated/direct bilirubin considered abnormal if
  - >18 mmol/L (1 mg/dL) if the total bilirubin is <85 mmol/L (5 mg/dL)
  - >20% total bilirubin if total bilirubin is >85 mmol/L (5 mg/dL)
- Hepatologic emergency! Timely, accurate diagnosis important for prognosis
- See Figure 17.8 and Table 17.12
- Treatment depends on specific etiology

Table 17.10 Laboratory Evaluation of the Liver

Lab	Source	Increased	Comments
ALT (SGPT) AST (SGOT)	Predominantly liver but also Heart Skeletal muscle Kidney Pancreas Lung Brain Leukocytes Erythrocytes	Hepatocellular inflammation Muscle disease Rhabdomyolysis Hemolysis Anorexia nervosa Celiac disease (mild)	· ALT more sensitive than AST for detecting liver damage · Concurrent increase in CPK, LDH, or aldolase suggests primary muscle source · AST > ALT in hemolysis, muscle disorders
ALP	Liver Bone Intestine Kidney Placenta Leukocytes	Cholestasis Infiltrative liver disease Bone growth or disease Trauma Pregnancy	· Must differentiate from bone source (i.e., history/ examination suggestive of bone disease, no elevation in GGT) · Subnormal levels in Wilson disease
GGT	Liver Kidney Pancreas Seminal vesicles Spleen Heart Brain	Cholestasis Newborn period Drug induced (e.g., phenytoin, phenobarbital, erythromycin, nitrofurantoin, alcohol)	· Most *sensitive* indicator of biliary tract disease · Not present in bone
INR (PT)		Liver disease Vitamin K deficiency Factor II, V, VII, X, or fibrinogen deficiency Dysfibrinogenemia	Factor VII earliest to be depleted in liver disease; therefore, PT (INR) prolonged before PTT

Table 17.11 Normal Liver Size

Age	Maximum Normal Projection of Liver Edge Below Costal Margin at Midclavicular Line
0–6 mo	3.5 cm
6 mo–4 yr	3.0 cm
>4 yr	2.0 cm

From Wolf AD, Lavine JE. Hepatomegaly in neonates and children. *Pediatr Rev.* 2000;21:303–310.

Figure 17.8 **An Approach to Conjugated Hyperbilirubinemia**

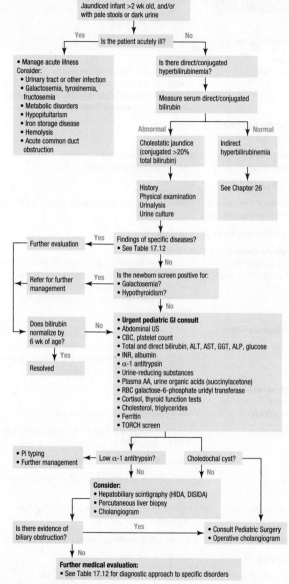

Adapted from Moyer V, Freese DK, Whitington PF, et al. Guideline for the evaluation of cholestatic jaundice in infants: Recommendations of the North American Society of Pediatric Gastroenterology, Hepatology and Nutrition. *J Pediatr Gastroenterol Nutr.* 2004;38:115–128.

Table 17.12 Differential Diagnosis of Cholestasis in Infants Younger Than 2 Months

Disease	Major Diagnostic Strategy
Obstructive Cholestasis	
Structural	
Biliary atresia	Diagnose and treat <60 d for optimal outcome! Hepatobiliary scan—premedicate with phenobarbital 5 mg/kg/d × 5 d (positive = delayed/absent excretion), liver biopsy (biliary obstruction on histologic examination)
Choledochal cyst or other congenital bile duct anomaly	US, cholangiogram
Caroli disease and congenital hepatic fibrosis	US, cholangiogram, liver biopsy Renal US (associated abnormalities)
Gallstones or biliary sludge	US
Inspissated bile (secondary to severe or prolonged hemolysis)	Coombs test (+ve), other evidence for hemolysis, dilated bile ducts
Neonatal sclerosing cholangitis	Cholangiogram
Duct paucity syndrome	
Alagille syndrome (paucity of intrahepatic bile ducts)	Echocardiogram (peripheral pulmonic stenosis), eye examination (posterior embryotoxin), CXR (butterfly vertebrae), liver biopsy (paucity of small ducts), typical facial appearance (broad forehead, pointed chin, elongated nose with bulbous tip), genetic testing
Hepatocellular Cholestasis	
Idiopathic neonatal hepatitis	Rule out other causes, liver biopsy (multinucleated giant cells, variable inflammation with infiltration of lymphocytes, neutrophils, and eosinophils; little/no bile duct proliferation)
Genetic and metabolic disorders	
α1-AT deficiency	$\downarrow \alpha$1-AT level, Pi typing (ZZ, Znul, nul deficient)
Galactosemia	Non–glucose-reducing substances (+ve), $\downarrow$ galactose 1-phosphate uridyl transferase in RBCs Associated with *Escherichia coli* sepsis
Tyrosinemia	$\uparrow$ Serum tyrosine and methionine, $\uparrow$ alpha fetoprotein, urine succinylacetone (+ve)
Hereditary fructosemia	Hepatic fructose-1-phosphate aldolase B ($\downarrow$/absent), liver biopsy: EM
Neonatal hemochromatosis	$\uparrow$ Ferritin, $\downarrow$ total iron binding capacity, liver biopsy: iron stain
Cystic fibrosis	Sweat chloride test (+ve)
Inborn errors of bile acid synthesis	Urinary/serum bile acid intermediates by *FAB–MS

(continued)

Table 17.12 | **Differential Diagnosis of Cholestasis in Infants Younger Than 2 Months (continued)**

Disease	Major Diagnostic Strategy
Progressive familial intrahepatic cholestasis	Liver biopsy, GGT ($\downarrow$/normal in types 1 and 2, $\uparrow$ in type 3), genetic testing
Endocrine	
Hypothyroidism	$\uparrow$TSH, $\downarrow$ free T$_4$
Panhypopituitarism	$\downarrow$ cortisol, $\downarrow$TSH, $\downarrow$T$_4$
Toxic/secondary	
Parenteral nutrition–associated cholestasis	See p. 419
Drugs (e.g., acetaminophen, anticonvulsants)	Urine and serum toxicology screen, in vitro lymphocyte testing for specific drugs
Infectious	
Toxoplasmosis	IgM antibodies, chorioretinitis (eyes), head CT (intracranial calcification), viral isolation (CSF, liver)
Rubella	IgM antibodies, viral isolation (CSF, liver, urine, pharyngeal secretions), cataracts
CMV	Urine for viral culture, IgM antibodies, chorioretinitis, head CT (intracranial calcification)
HSV	EM/viral culture of vesicle scrapings
HIV	HIV DNA PCR, Igs, CD4 count
Syphilis	VDRL, STS, FTA-ABS*, long-bone films (osteochondritis, periostitis)
Urinary tract infection	Urine cultures
Sepsis	Blood cultures

*FAB–MS, fast-atom bombardment–mass spectroscopy; FTA-ABS, fluorescent treponemal antibody, absorbed.

ACUTE LIVER FAILURE

- See Figures 17.9, 17.10, and 17.11

DEFINITION

- Children: biochemical evidence of acute liver injury and hepatic-based coagulopathy not responsive to vitamin K (PT ≥15 s or INR ≥1.5 with clinical hepatic encephalopathy or PT ≥20 s or INR ≥2.0, regardless of clinical hepatic encephalopathy) and no clinical evidence of chronic liver disease
- Neonates (perinatal): severe hepatic dysfunction with coagulopathy, metabolic instability, and signs of liver damage in the first 60 d of life

Figure 17.9   Acute Liver Failure: Signs, Symptoms, and Laboratory Assessment

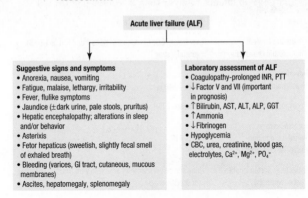

Acute liver failure (ALF)

Suggestive signs and symptoms
- Anorexia, nausea, vomiting
- Fatigue, malaise, lethargy, irritability
- Fever, flulike symptoms
- Jaundice (± dark urine, pale stools, pruritus)
- Hepatic encephalopathy; alterations in sleep and/or behavior
- Asterixis
- Fetor hepaticus (sweetish, slightly fecal smell of exhaled breath)
- Bleeding (varices, GI tract, cutaneous, mucous membranes)
- Ascites, hepatomegaly, splenomegaly

Laboratory assessment of ALF
- Coagulopathy-prolonged INR, PTT
- ↓ Factor V and VII (important in prognosis)
- ↑ Bilirubin, AST, ALT, ALP, GGT
- ↑ Ammonia
- ↓ Fibrinogen
- Hypoglycemia
- CBC, urea, creatinine, blood gas, electrolytes, Ca^{2+}, Mg^{2+}, PO_4^-

Figure 17.10   Acute Liver Failure: Investigations

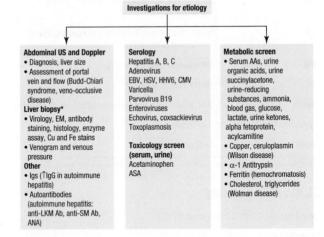

Investigations for etiology

Abdominal US and Doppler
- Diagnosis, liver size
- Assessment of portal vein and flow (Budd-Chiari syndrome, veno-occlusive disease)

Liver biopsy*
- Virology, EM, antibody staining, histology, enzyme assay, Cu and Fe stains
- Venogram and venous pressure

Other
- Igs (↑IgG in autoimmune hepatitis)
- Autoantibodies (autoimmune hepatitis: anti-LKM Ab, anti-SM Ab, ANA)

Serology
Hepatitis A, B, C
Adenovirus
EBV, HSV, HHV6, CMV
Varicella
Parvovirus B19
Enteroviruses
Echovirus, coxsackievirus
Toxoplasmosis

Toxicology screen (serum, urine)
Acetaminophen
ASA

Metabolic screen
- Serum AAs, urine organic acids, urine succinylacetone, urine-reducing substances, ammonia, blood gas, glucose, lactate, urine ketones, alpha fetoprotein, acylcarnitine
- Copper, ceruloplasmin (Wilson disease)
- α-1 Antitrypsin
- Ferritin (hemochromatosis)
- Cholesterol, triglycerides (Wolman disease)

*Consider transjugular biopsy if percutaneous biopsy contraindicated because of coagulopathy.

Figure 17.11 Acute Liver Failure: Complications and Supportive Care

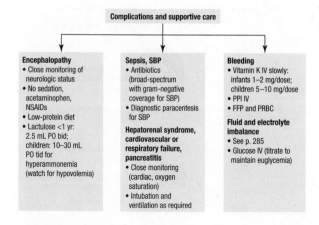

Complications and supportive care

Encephalopathy
- Close monitoring of neurologic status
- No sedation, acetaminophen, NSAIDs
- Low-protein diet
- Lactulose <1 yr: 2.5 mL PO bid; children: 10–30 mL PO tid for hyperammonemia (watch for hypovolemia)

Sepsis, SBP
- Antibiotics (broad-spectrum with gram-negative coverage for SBP)
- Diagnostic paracentesis for SBP

Hepatorenal syndrome, cardiovascular or respiratory failure, pancreatitis
- Close monitoring (cardiac, oxygen saturation)
- Intubation and ventilation as required

Bleeding
- Vitamin K IV slowly: infants 1–2 mg/dose; children 5–10 mg/dose
- PPI IV
- FFP and PRBC

Fluid and electrolyte imbalance
- See p. 285
- Glucose IV (titrate to maintain euglycemia)

CHRONIC LIVER FAILURE

- See Figure 17.12

GOALS OF THERAPY

- Slow or reverse progression of liver disease
- Prevent additional liver insults
  - Immunizations: scheduled vaccines, hepatitis A and B vaccines
  - Avoid hepatotoxic medications (e.g., acetaminophen, NSAIDS, methotrexate, valproic acid)
- Prevent and treat complications (Table 17.13)
- Early assessment with transplant team for listing

Figure 17.12 Stigmata of Chronic Liver Failure

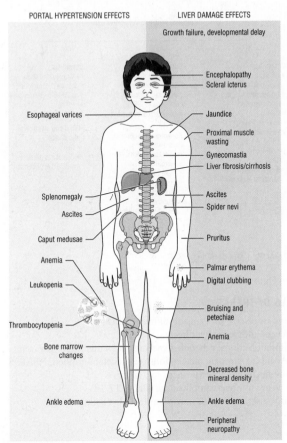

PORTAL HYPERTENSION EFFECTS | LIVER DAMAGE EFFECTS

Growth failure, developmental delay

Encephalopathy
Scleral icterus

Esophageal varices

Jaundice

Proximal muscle wasting

Gynecomastia
Liver fibrosis/cirrhosis

Splenomegaly

Ascites
Spider nevi

Ascites

Caput medusae

Pruritus

Anemia

Palmar erythema
Digital clubbing

Leukopenia

Bruising and petechiae

Thrombocytopenia

Anemia

Bone marrow changes

Decreased bone mineral density

Ankle edema

Ankle edema

Peripheral neuropathy

Adapted from Zachos M, Critch J, Jackson R. *Hospital for Sick Children Atlas of Pediatrics*. Philadelphia, Pa: Current Medicine LLC; 2005:390–413.

Table 17.13	Complications and Management of Chronic/End-Stage Liver Disease
Problem	**Approach**
Malnutrition and growth failure*	· Adequate calories (MCT and branch chain AA supplementation)
Fat-soluble vitamin deficiency	· Vitamin A, D, E, K supplementation
Cholestasis (jaundice, pruritus, xanthomas, xanthelasma)	· Choleretic agents (ursodiol, cholestyramine) · Antihistamines, rifampin

(continued)

Table 17.13 Complications and Management of Chronic/End-Stage Liver Disease (continued)

Problem	Approach
Bleeding · Thrombocytopenia (hypersplenism) · Coagulopathy (prolonged INR ± PTT) · Vitamin K deficiency · Esophageal varices (portal hypertension)	· Avoid antiplatelet drugs (ASA, NSAIDs) · Vitamin K · FFP and activated factor VIIa for active bleeding · PPIs/octreotide (UGI bleeding) · Endoscopic sclerotherapy/banding, portosystemic shunting for varices
Ascites (± edema/pleural effusions)[†]	· Sodium restriction · Diuretics: spironolactone (Aldactazide), furosemide · Water restriction (insensible losses + output) if dilutional hyponatremia prominent · Albumin (0.5–1 g/kg/d) + furosemide in cases of azotemia and intravascular volume depletion · Paracentesis for respiratory distress
Increased susceptibility to infections	· Prevention (vaccination) · Appropriate antibiotic treatment
SBP · Presentation: subtle (± fever, abdominal pain, ↓ bowel sounds, altered mental status) · Diagnosis: ascitic fluid PMN count ≥ 250/mm^3 ± positive culture	· Early recognition and treatment (third-generation cephalosporin)
Renal insufficiency	· Prerenal failure: volume expansion · ATN: ± dialysis · Hepatorenal syndrome: treatment is expectant (no predictably effective therapy); must rule out treatable causes (diagnosis of exclusion)
Impaired drug clearance · Hepatic and renal failure, portal–systemic shunting, hypoalbuminemia	· Reduce dosage, monitor toxicity, choose alternative agents
Hepatic encephalopathy · Precipitating factors · GI hemorrhage · Hypokalemia (especially with alkalosis) · Sepsis, SBP · High-protein diet · Constipation · Sedative-hypnotic medications (diazepam safest: 25–50% normal dose) · Azotemia · Pancreatitis · Surgery (especially portosystemic shunts)	· Identify, remove/correct, and avoid precipitants · Tight fluid and electrolyte control · Dietary: protein restriction (0.5–1 g/kg/d) · Lactulose (PO/PR): ↓ ammonia resorption · Antibiotics (neomycin, metronidazole): ↓ available bacterial urease

*May require supplemental NG feedings or TPN to prevent catabolic state, rickets, ataxia syndrome, coagulopathy, xerophthalmia.
†Fluid is transudative; ↑ serum-ascitic albumin gradient (≥ 11 g/L).

ACUTE CHOLANGITIS

- Clinical syndrome characterized by fever, jaundice, and right upper quadrant abdominal pain as a result of stasis or obstruction and infection in the biliary tract
- Associations: biliary atresia, biliary calculi, benign stricture, sclerosing cholangitis, post liver transplant
- Diagnosis: ↑WBC count, cholestatic pattern of LFTs, blood C&S, US
- Treatment: broad-spectrum antibiotics to cover gram-negative bacteria and enterococci ± anaerobes (e.g., ampicillin, gentamicin, and metronidazole); biliary drainage in select cases (e.g., cholangitis secondary to biliary calculi)

TPN-ASSOCIATED LIVER DISEASE

- Associated factors: young age, prematurity, low birth weight, duration of TPN, sepsis, absence of enteral intake, excessive AA intake, multiple operative procedures, bacterial sepsis, GI mucosal disease
- Onset: 10–180 d (earlier in premature infants)
- Laboratory tests: conjugated/direct hyperbilirubinemia, ± ↑AST, ALT, GGT, ALP
- ± Liver biopsy: steatosis, steatohepatitis, cholestasis, progression to fibrosis and cirrhosis
- Clinical impact: increased rates of sepsis, cirrhosis, and death

Treatment

- Promote enteral feeding, minimize TPN
  - ± Ursodeoxycholic acid
  - ± Fat emulsion containing primarily omega-3 (vs. omega-6) fatty acids (experimental), ± n-acetylcysteine (experimental)

VIRAL HEPATITIS

- See Table 17.14 for a comparison of hepatotropic viruses
- See Figure 17.13 for the serologic course of hepatitis B

Table 17.14	Comparison of Major Hepatotropic Viruses		
	Hepatitis A	**Hepatitis B**	**Hepatitis C**
Type of virus	Picornavirus (RNA)	Hepadnavirus (DNA)	Flavivirus (RNA)
Transmission	Fecal-oral	Parenteral, sexual, vertical	Parenteral, sexual, vertical
Incubation	15–50 d	60–180 d	14–180 d
Risk factors	· Personal contact · Outbreak · International travel · Male homosexual activity · Injection drug use	· More likely to transmit infection if HBeAg +ve (higher HBV DNA load) · Personal contact · Multiple sexual partners · Male homosexual activity · Injection drug use · From endemic area · Frequent blood product exposure	· Personal contact · Injection drug use · Frequent blood product exposure
Diagnostic tests	· Anti-HAV IgM (recent infection) · Total anti-HAV	See Figure 17.13 for diagnostic tests	· Anti-HCV IgG (80% +ve within 15 wk of exposure) · HCV RNA (NAA test, +ve within 1–2 wk of exposure)
Presentation	· Acute self-limited illness · Fulminant hepatic failure (<1%)	· Asymptomatic infection to fulminant hepatitis	· Asymptomatic to clinical hepatitis · Fulminant hepatic failure (rare)
Signs and symptoms of acute infection	· Fever, malaise, jaundice, anorexia, nausea, abdominal discomfort	· Nonspecific: fatigue, jaundice, arthralgias, arthritis, rashes · Young children: usually asymptomatic	· Nonspecific · Onset usually mild and insidious, often asymptomatic, <20% jaundiced
Chronic infection	No	Yes	Yes
Definition of chronic infection		· HBsAg +ve for 6 mo or HBsAg in person who tests –ve for anti-Hep B core antibody (anti-HBc)	Persistence of +ve HCV RNA
Characteristics of infection by age	· Children <6 yr: 30% symptomatic (2–3 wk), few jaundiced · Older children/adults: most symptomatic (lasting 1 wk to 6 mo), >70% jaundiced	Higher rates of chronic infection in younger individuals; neonates: >90%; 1–5 yr: 25–50%; older children and adults: 2–6%	Chronic infection in 50–60% children, 60–70% adults (usually asymptomatic)

(continued)

Table 17.14	Comparison of Major Hepatotropic Viruses (continued)		
	Hepatitis A	**Hepatitis B**	**Hepatitis C**
Monitoring		· AST/ALT q6–12 mo · HBeAg and anti-HBe q6–12 mo · Alpha fetoprotein yearly (at risk for HCC) · Liver US periodically	· AST/ALT q6–12 mo · Liver US periodically · Alpha fetoprotein yearly (at risk for HCC) · Quantitative HCV RNA assay
Vaccine available	Yes*	Yes*	No
Treatment	· Supportive	· Counseling · Surveillance for disease progression and complications · Lamivudine and interferon in select cases (may consider if persistent ALT >2× normal or advanced histologic features)	· Counseling · Surveillance for disease progression and complications · Adult trials: interferon-alfa or peginterferon-alfa ± ribavirin (may consider if severe disease, advanced histologic features)
Prevention	· Pre/postexposure immunization	· Pre/postexposure immunization · Blood donor screening · Risk behavior modification	· Blood donor screening · Risk behavior modification
Prophylaxis available	Yes*	Yes*	No
Long-term complications and prognosis		· Cirrhosis · HCC (increased if HBeAg +ve) · 1–2% adults and <1% children clear HBsAg and develop anti-HBs annually	· Cirrhosis · HCC

*See Chapter 24 for details on immunization and immunoprophylaxis.

anti-HAV, hepatitis A virus antibody; *anti-HBe*, hepatitis B e antibody; *anti-HBs*, hepatitis B surface antibody; *anti-HCV*, hepatitis C virus antibody; *HBeAg*, hepatitis B e antigen; *HBsAg*, hepatitis B surface antigen; *HBV*, hepatitis B virus; *HCV*, hepatitis C virus; *NAA*, nucleic acid amplification; *RNA*, ribonucleic acid.

Figure 17.13 Interpretation of Serologic Course of Viral Hepatitis B

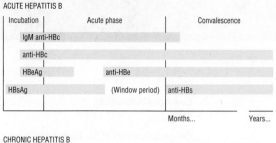

ACUTE HEPATITIS B

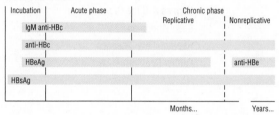

CHRONIC HEPATITIS B

Adapted from Willems B, Vincelette J. *Les hépatites virales*. In: Turgeon F, Steben M, eds. *Les maladies transmissible sexuellement*. PUM; 1994:188. Available at: http://www.phac-aspc.gc.ca/publicat/std-mts98hls/std98hse.html. Reprinted with the permission of the Minister of Public Works and Government Services Canada.

FURTHER READING

Moyer V, Freese DK, Whitington PF, et al. Guideline for the evaluation of cholestatic jaundice in infants: Recommendations of the North American Society of Pediatric Gastroenterology, Hepatology and Nutrition. *J Pediatr Gastroenterol Nutr.* 2004;38:115–128.

Pickering LK, Baker CJ, Long SS, McMillan JA, eds. *Red Book: 2006 Report of the Committee on Infectious Diseases*. 27th ed. Elk Grove Village, Ill: American Academy of Pediatrics; 2006.

Suchy FJ, Sokol RJ, Ballistreri WF: *Liver Disease in Children*. 3rd ed. New York, NY: Cambridge University Press; 2007.

Walker WA, Kleinman RE, Sherman PM, Shneider BL, Sanderson IR. *Pediatric Gastrointestinal Disease*. 4th ed. Hamilton, Ontario, Canada: BC Decker Inc; 2004.

USEFUL WEB SITES

North American Society for Pediatric Gastroenterology, Hepatology, and Nutrition (clinical guidelines/position statements). Available at: **www.naspghan.org**
Pediatric hepatology. Available at: **www.pedihepa.net**

Chapter 18 General Surgery

Glenda N. Bendiak

Georges Azzie

Chapter 18 General Surgery

COMMON ABBREVIATIONS

AXR	abdominal X-ray
NG	nasogastric
RLQ	right lower quadrant
RUQ	right upper quadrant
SMA	superior mesenteric artery
SMV	superior mesenteric vein
UGI	upper gastrointestinal (series)
VACTERL	*v*ertebral defects, *a*nal atresia, *c*ardiac anomalies, *t*racheoesophageal fistula with *e*sophageal atresia, *r*enal anomalies, *l*imb anomalies

OBSTRUCTION

NEONATAL

Intestinal Atresia
- See Table 18.1

Esophageal Atresia and Tracheoesophageal Fistula
- See Figure 18.1
- 55% have associated anomalies
- VACTERL association

Presentation
- History of maternal polyhydramnios
- Excessive oral secretions
- Choking/cyanosis with feeding
- Unable to pass catheter into stomach (except H type)
- Recurrent aspiration pneumonia (H type)

Investigations
- CXR: upper esophageal pouch dilated with air (for two most common types)
- Contrast studies are unnecessary; diagnosis based on inability to pass NG tube

	Duodenal Atresia	**Jejunoileal Atresia**	**Colonic Stenosis**
Table 18.1	**Duodenal, Jejunoileal, and Colonic Atresias**		
Incidence	· 1/5000–10,000 live births	· 1/1500 live births	1/15,000–20,000 live births
Associations	· Maternal polyhydramnios and trisomy 21 · 50% also have cardiac, renal, or other GI anomalies	· Maternal polyhydramnios and cystic fibrosis	
Presentation	· Bilious vomiting (85%) shortly after birth; often precedes feeding · May have upper abdominal distension (if not decompressed) · Failure to pass meconium in first 24 h of life	· Bilious vomiting (85%) · Abdominal distension with increasingly distal obstruction · Jaundice (30%) · Failure to pass meconium in first 24 h of life	· Bilious vomiting · Abdominal distension · Failure to pass meconium in first 24 h of life
Investigations	· AXR shows marked distension of stomach and proximal duodenum (double bubble sign) with no air distally · UGI can be done to verify diagnosis and exclude volvulus or malrotation	· AXR shows air–fluid levels and increasing distension with more distal obstruction · If suspected on plain AXR (distal bowel obstruction), contrast enema required to rule out associated colonic atresia ("micro-colon" on contrast enema lends more weight to diagnosis of small bowel atresia)	· AXR shows dilated intestine and air–fluid levels · Contrast enema shows a blind distal end of a microcolon
Management	· Decompression of upper GI tract with NG tube (may use suction at physician's discretion) · Maintenance IV fluids · Consider IV antibiotics based on grade of obstruction and physician's discretion · Rule out associated anomalies	· Decompression of upper GI tract with NG tube · Maintenance IV fluids · Consider IV antibiotics · Rule out cystic fibrosis (10% incidence)	· Decompression of upper GI tract with NG tube · Maintenance IV fluids · Consider IV antibiotics
Further comments	· Most common site of atresia/stenosis distal to entry of common bile duct	· Atresia most common (95%), stenosis (5%)	

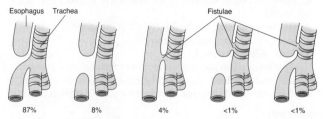

Esophagus Trachea   Fistulae

87%   8%   4%   <1%   <1%

Adapted from Behrman RE, Kliegman RM, Jenson HB, eds. *Nelson Textbook of Pediatrics.* 16th ed. Philadelphia, Pa: WB Saunders; 2000.

Management
- NPO
- Replogle tube set to low suction (instill 2 mL air q2h to keep tube patent)
- Maintenance IV fluids
- Consider IV antibiotics if aspiration pneumonia is present
- Delay primary repair until VACTERL screen completed, unless significant respiratory compromise (may then require emergent ligation of fistula)
- Complications: reflux, esophageal stricture, anastomotic disruption, tracheomalacia

Hirschsprung Disease
- Male:female (4:1)
- Absence of ganglion cells beginning at anorectal junction and extending proximally for variable distance (may be as far as duodenum)
- Rectosigmoid (75%), colonic extension (15–20%), total colon (5%)
- Associated with trisomy 21, Waardenburg syndrome, cardiovascular anomalies
- Rare in very premature infants

Presentation
- 94% fail to pass meconium in first 24 h
- Abdominal distension
- Vomiting
- Hirschsprung enterocolitis (triad of explosive diarrhea, abdominal distension, and fever with lethargy or shock)
- Late presentation with refractory constipation
- Rectal examination: may have explosive release of stool and gas

General Surgery

18

Investigations
- AXR findings same as in distal bowel obstruction (many loops of uniformly dilated bowel with air–fluid levels on upright X-ray); not specific
- Anorectal manometry can be used to aid in diagnosis
- Contrast enema can suggest diagnosis:
  1. Small-caliber rectum
  2. Dilation of colon proximal to narrowed (aganglionic) segment (diameter of colon > diameter of rectum) with transition zone
- Gold standard: rectal biopsy showing absence of ganglion cells

Management
- Usually responds to anal stimulation or rectal irrigations (not enemas) initially
- Most common surgical treatment is one-stage pull-through procedure
- If enterocolitis present: IV fluid resuscitation, antibiotics, rectal irrigations to decompress; may require urgent diverting ostomy if no response

Meconium Ileus
- Majority (>95%) associated with cystic fibrosis

Presentation
- Abdominal distension
- Bilious emesis
- Failure to pass stools

Investigations
- AXR: dilated loops of small bowel without air–fluid levels, ground-glass appearance within intestinal lumen proximal to obstruction
- Contrast enema: small pellets of meconium outlined by contrast material in terminal ileum

Management
- Water-soluble enemas to relieve obstruction; repeated until clear
- Surgery, if enemas unsuccessful
- "Complicated" meconium ileus (perforation with meconium peritonitis, intestinal atresia) requires surgical exploration

Anorectal Malformation/Imperforate Anus
- Spectrum of severity
- VACTERL association in 15% of cases; also associated with duodenal atresia, trisomy 21, and spinal cord anomalies
- Look for meconium excreted from urethra, vagina, or at perineum (due to presence of fistula)
- Three-stage treatment: colostomy in first days of life, posterior sagittal anorectoplasty at 3 mo, and colostomy closure at 6 mo; some patients may be amenable to single-stage procedure

Malrotation With Volvulus
- See the Acute Abdomen section (p. 359)

EARLY INFANCY

Hypertrophic Pyloric Stenosis
- Males > females (4:1), firstborn, familial tendency

Presentation
- 1–12 wk of age
- Nonbilious projectile vomiting followed by desire to feed
- Failure to gain weight or weight loss, dehydration
- Hypochloremic hypokalemic metabolic alkalosis with paradoxic aciduria
- Upper abdominal peristaltic waves (late finding)
- Gastritis (late finding)

Physical Examination
- To enhance palpation of epigastric "olive" (i.e., the hypertrophied pylorus):
  1. PO sugar water, NG tube
  2. Elevate legs to relax abdominal muscles
  3. Deep palpation using first three fingers of right hand directed cephalad

Investigations
- Suggestive features on US: thickness >4 mm, length >16 mm (sensitivity, 91–100%; specificity, 100%); different parameters in premature infants
- UGI if US not available

Management
- NPO
- NG tube (optional)
- Fluid resuscitation preoperatively with 20 mL/kg 0.9%NaCl bolus, then 1.5 × maintenance fluids (may require 48–72 h to correct electrolyte abnormalities and fluid deficit)
- Pyloromyotomy

Malrotation With Volvulus
- See the Acute Abdomen section (p. 359)

CHILDHOOD

Intussusception
- Telescoping or invagination of proximal portion of intestine into more distal portion
- Male:female (3:2)
- Most common from 3 mo to 3 yr of life

18

- Lead point: usually increased GI lymphatic tissue from viral infection; pathologic lead points: Meckel diverticulum, appendix, polyps, duplications, submucosal hemorrhage (e.g., Henoch-Schönlein purpura), tumors
- Within typical age range, further investigations to look for pathologic lead point generally unnecessary

Presentation
- Cyclic abdominal pain q5–30min
- Child screams, flexes at waist, draws legs up to abdomen, appears pale
- Calm or somnolent appearance between episodes
- Vomiting can occur; may be bilious
- "Red currant jelly" stools occur later due to intestinal mucosal congestion, ischemia, or mucosal sloughing
- RUQ or RLQ mass may be palpable

Investigations
- US: 97% sensitivity, 95% specificity when intussuscepted

Treatment
- Ileoileal or jejunoileal intussusceptions usually not significant; generally no treatment necessary (usually incidental US finding)
- Ileocolic (most common) and colocolic (very rare) intussusceptions should be treated
- Air enema reduction in radiology suite; combined with delayed repeat enema in stable patients, >95% success rate
- Barium enema can be used but is associated with more complications if intestine perforates and has lower success rate
- Immediate surgery without attempt at radiologic reduction for patients who are unstable, have peritonitis, or have obvious perforation
- Recurrence risk: 5–10% after nonoperative reduction, 1–4% after surgical reduction

Bowel Obstruction
- Congenital causes of obstruction as already described
- Additional causes: constricting bands, intra-abdominal hernias, duplications
- 5% lifetime risk of adhesive small-bowel obstruction for postsurgical patients
- Most common in first 2 yr after abdominal surgery

Presentation
- Level (small vs. large bowel)
  1. Small-bowel obstruction: large-volume frequent bilious emesis, epigastric pain relieved by vomiting, minimal distension if proximal, more distended if distal

2. Large-bowel obstruction: abdominal distension, emesis that is progressively feculent, diffuse abdominal pain
- Note: fundoplication patients are unable to vomit
- Obstipation (complete obstruction) vs. loose stools (incomplete obstruction)
- Complicated (peritonitis) vs. uncomplicated
- Peritonitis (surgical emergency) should be suspected if patient develops fever, tachycardia, hypotension, hematemesis, bleeding from rectum, or clinical signs (pain, guarding, peritoneal signs)
- Mechanical vs. functional: distinguished on basis of history, physical examination, and special investigations

Investigations
- AXR (at least two views: flat and upright views or flat and left lateral decubitus): dilated loops of bowel, air–fluid levels, paucity of gas in colon

Management
- NPO
- NG tube
- IV fluids
- CBC, electrolytes
- AXR
- Consider antibiotics
- Surgical consultation
- Indications for operation: peritonitis, free air on AXR, radiologic evidence of nonevolving gas pattern

CONGENITAL DEFECTS OF THE ABDOMINAL COMPARTMENT

CONGENITAL DIAPHRAGMATIC HERNIA

Bochdalek Hernia
- Herniation through posterolateral foramen of Bochdalek
- Left-sided defects most common (70–85%); occasionally bilateral (<5%)
- Associated anomalies (15–25%): CNS lesions, esophageal atresia, omphalocele, cardiac lesions, trisomy 21, lethal syndromes

Presentation
- Most common: antenatal diagnosis on routine US
- Severe respiratory distress in first hours of life
- Absent breath sounds on affected side with chest wall prominence; shifted heart sounds
- Scaphoid abdomen

Investigations
- CXR/AXR: loops of air-filled intestine within thoracic cavity, absence of intestine in abdominal cavity, shifted mediastinum, NG tube in chest (if stomach above diaphragm)

Management
- Major management issues: pulmonary hypoplasia and pulmonary hypertension (neither managed surgically)
- NG tube to low suction
- Spontaneous ventilation with permissive hypercapnia
- Endotracheal intubation, if necessary
- Avoid bag and mask ventilation: will fill intestine in thorax with air
- Depending on difficulty with oxygenation, may require high frequency oscillation ventilation, pulmonary vasodilators (e.g., nitric oxide), extracorporeal membrane oxygenation
- Operative repair when stable

Morgagni Hernia
- Accounts for <2% of all congenital diaphragmatic hernias
- Herniation of bowel through anterior foramen of Morgagni
- Usually incidental CXR finding; rarely presents in older infants or children with symptoms of intestinal obstruction
- Once identified, repaired to avoid small risk of incarceration

GASTROSCHISIS AND OMPHALOCELE
- See Table 18.2

Table 18.2	Characteristics of Gastroschisis and Omphalocele	
Factor	Gastroschisis	Omphalocele
Definition	Abdominal contents free on anterior abdominal wall; defect almost always to right of umbilical cord	Abdominal contents herniated onto anterior abdominal wall but are encased in sac (unless ruptured)
Umbilical cord	Separate, to left of defect (usually)	Included in defect
Size of defect	Small (2-3 cm)	Variable (2-15 cm)
Contents	Bowel; occasionally bladder; ovaries, testes	Bowel; frequently liver
Membrane	Never	Always (may rupture)
Rotational anomaly	Yes	Yes
Intestinal function	Prolonged ileus	Usually normal
Associated defects	Intestinal atresia (10-15%)	Cardiac (20-25%), chromosomal (5-15%)

Adapted from Levine BA, Copeland EM III, Howard RJ, Sugerman HJ, Warshaw AL. *Current Practice of Pediatric Surgery.* New York, NY: Churchill Livingstone; 1994.

Management
- For gastroschisis, immediately position in right lateral decubitus position
- Insert nasogastric/orogastric tube to low continuous suction
- Cover viscera with sterile saline-soaked gauze and cellophane wrap
- Fluid resuscitation with 20 mL/kg 0.9%NaCl, then maintain crystalloid infusion at 6 mL/kg/h until urine output ≥ 1 mL/kg/h
- Prophylactic antibiotics
- Avoid hypothermia (use overhead warmer)
- Search for associated defects, especially in omphalocele

HERNIAS AND THE GROIN

DIASTASIS RECTI ABDOMINIS
- Lateral displacement of rectus muscles above umbilicus
- No fascial defect present, no risk of incarceration
- No need for surgical intervention

UMBILICAL HERNIA
- Due to incomplete closure of umbilical ring after cord separation
- Almost never incarcerate; majority close by 3 yr of age
- Unlikely to close spontaneously after 5 yr of age; these require surgical repair

HYDROCELE
- Continuum of patent processus vaginalis → hydrocele → inguinal hernia
- Processus vaginalis fails to undergo spontaneous obliteration in approximately 10% of children
- Hydrocele: fluid remains in patent portion of processus vaginalis

Presentation
- Soft, nontender fluid-filled sac along tract of processus vaginalis
- Sac may transilluminate
- If patent connection at internal ring, fluid in hydrocele may communicate with peritoneal cavity, leading to fluctuation in size of hydrocele

Management
- Noncommunicating hydroceles and small communicating hydroceles often involute in first 12 mo of life
- Larger communicating hydroceles, or those that persist beyond 12 mo of life, require surgical intervention

INGUINAL HERNIA

- Incidence 1–5% of males, 30% in extreme preterm infants; male > female (6:1)
- Right-sided (60%), left-sided (25%), bilateral (15%)
- Factors associated with increased incidence: hydrops, chylous ascites, meconium peritonitis, abdominal wall defects, bladder exstrophy, hypospadias, ventriculoperitoneal shunts, connective tissue disorder

Presentation

- Bulging in groin or scrotal sac, increased with crying or straining

Incarceration

- Incarceration (hernia sac is not reducible, but contents are viable) occurs in 30% of inguinal hernias in the first year of life and in 12% of all children with inguinal hernias
- Note: *true incarceration is a medical emergency*

Signs of Incarceration

- Irritability
- Signs of intestinal obstruction (abdominal distension, vomiting, obstipation)
- Firm, tender mass in inguinal region or scrotum

Strangulation

- Strangulation (compromise of bowel blood supply) can occur within 2 h

Signs of Strangulation

- Erythematous, hard, fixed, and painful mass
- Fever
- Dehydration may be present

Investigations

- AXR may reveal bowel loop in inguinal region
- US can be helpful in diagnosis of incarcerated hernia
- Transilluminant mass does not rule out incarcerated hernia

Treatment

- Attempt reduction, refer to surgeon for elective repair if reducible
- While awaiting surgery, counsel parents regarding need for medical attention should symptoms of incarceration/strangulation develop
- Unsuccessful reduction requires urgent surgical correction (medical emergency)

CRYPTORCHIDISM

- Testicle not present in normal intrascrotal position
- Incidence 1–4% of boys, 20–30% of premature boys
- Higher incidence in infants with the following: neural tube defects, bladder exstrophy, prune-belly syndrome, hypospadias, abdominal wall defects

- Unilateral (90% of cases); usually right side (70%)
- Undescended testes can lead to infertility, torsion, or malignancy
- To determine location of testicle (in decreasing order of sensitivity and specificity): laparoscopy, MRI, US
- Note: most testes can be palpated by experienced examiner under ideal conditions; repeated examinations may be required
- Refer to surgeon before 2 yr of age to improve fertility; orchidopexy for easier monitoring for malignancy (does not decrease risk of malignancy)

ACUTE ABDOMEN

NEONATAL NECROTIZING ENTEROCOLITIS
- See p. 592

MALROTATION/VOLVULUS WITH BOWEL ISCHEMIA
- Spectrum of illness from malrotation to malrotation with volvulus (latter causes gut ischemia and infarction and is a *true medical emergency*)
- 30% of patients with symptomatic malrotation present in first week of life, >50% in first month, but may present at any age

Presentation
- Must be ruled out in previously healthy infant/child who presents with bilious vomiting, sudden onset of abdominal pain
- Symptoms more vague in older children:
  1. Chronic intermittent vomiting
  2. Crampy abdominal pain
  3. Failure to thrive
  4. Constipation
  5. Bloody diarrhea
  6. Hematemesis with persistent vomiting
- Abdominal distension not usually present until very late
- 50% have normal physical examination
- Signs of progression from ischemia to infarction and necrosis: fever, peritonitis, abdominal distension, dehydration, vascular instability, metabolic acidosis, septic appearance

Investigations
- Many have normal AXR
- UGI is gold standard in stable patient:
  1. Malrotation: ligament of Treitz is not left of midline and not at or higher than level of pylorus
  2. Malrotation with volvulus: duodenum does not cross midline, stays to right of spine, and demonstrates duodenal obstruction with no filling of jejunum or a "corkscrew" filling pattern down right side of spine
- Contrast enema may confirm position of cecum (not in the RLQ in malrotation)
- Can use US to check relationship of SMA to SMV (mesenteric inversion)

Management

- Fluid resuscitation
- NPO
- NG tube
- Broad-spectrum IV antibiotics
- Immediate radiologic assessment (if stable)
- Laparotomy

APPENDICITIS

- Peak incidence 10–12 yr of age
- Perforation may occur 36–48 h after onset of symptoms

Classic Presentation

- Periumbilical dull constant pain, followed by anorexia and vomiting
- Pain moves to the RLQ (but 15% have atypically located appendix) as inflammation progresses
- May be accompanied by constipation or small amounts of watery diarrhea, low-grade fever (max 38°C/100.4°F), which increases after perforation
- Generalized peritonitis may occur with perforation
- RLQ tenderness with localized peritonitis is most valuable finding on examination

Investigations

- Check urinalysis to rule out urinary tract infection, and in adolescent females, β-hCG to rule out pregnancy
- CBC may be helpful (elevated WBC or left shift)
- AXR may show calcified fecalith in 15% of patients
- US, CT scan, or overnight observation helpful after surgical consultation if diagnosis unclear
- Do not give antibiotics until diagnosis made

Management

- IV fluids
- IV antibiotics before appendectomy:
  1. Cefoxitin if not perforated
  2. Ampicillin, gentamicin, and metronidazole if perforated

Perforated Appendicitis
(when immediate surgery is not indicated)

- Treat empirically at least until afebrile with ampicillin, gentamicin, and metronidazole
- End therapy if clinical improvement without fever, nausea, vomiting, or pain and with consultation with general surgeon
- If no clinical improvement: obtain additional imaging, consider drainage, and additional antibiotics
- Interval appendectomy after 6–8 wk

BILIARY ATRESIA

- Progressive obliterative cholangiopathy

Presentation

- Progressive jaundice; pale stools
- Biliary atresia must be ruled out in infant with conjugated hyper-bilirubinemia (see p. 335)
- Associated anomalies in 10–35% of cases, including situs inversus viscerum, dextrocardia, congenital heart defects, polysplenia, preduo-denal portal vein

Investigations

- US to rule out choledochal cyst
- Findings on US suggestive of biliary atresia: absence of ductal dilata-tion, cirrhotic liver, absent or small shrunken gallbladder, "triangular cord sign"
- Biliary scan (Tc^{99m}-DISIDA scan) and/or percutaneous cholangiogra-phy to delineate ductal anatomy/atresia after pretreatment with phe-nobarbital (5–6 mg/kg PO daily or divided bid for 5 d)
- Liver biopsy to differentiate from neonatal hepatitis or metabolic diseases

Management

- Hepatoportoenterostomy (Kasai procedure), ideally before 8 wk of age
- Liver transplantation if Kasai fails (rising bilirubin, continued pale stools)

GALL BLADDER DISEASE

- Cholelithiasis can occur at any age
- Associated with hemolytic disorders, polycythemia, prematurity, par-enteral nutrition, cystic fibrosis, sickle cell disease, distal bowel resec-tion, sepsis, obesity

Presentation

- Nonspecific RUQ pain and nausea with meals
- Fatty-food intolerance is rare
- Suspect choledocholithiasis in a healthy jaundiced child
- Acute cholecystitis: localized RUQ pain, nausea, vomiting, fever

General Surgery

18

Investigations
- US most useful diagnostic test for cholelithiasis

Management
- Nonoperative therapy for asymptomatic gallstones
- Cholecystectomy for stones causing symptoms or complications (acute cholecystitis, cholangitis, pancreatitis)
- Surgery recommended for children with sickle cell disease and cholelithiasis

FURTHER READING

O'Neill JA, Grosfeld JL, Fonkalsrud EW, Coran AG, Caldamone AA. *Principles of Pediatric Surgery*. 2nd ed. St. Louis, Mo: Mosby-Year Book; 2003.

Rowe MI, O'Neill JA, Grosfeld JL, Fonkalsrud EW, Coran AG. *Essentials of Pediatric Surgery*. St. Louis, Mo: Mosby-Year Book; 1995.

General Surgery

18

Chapter 19 Genetics

Daniela S. Ardelean

Sharan Goobie

Roberto Mendoza-Londono

Chapter 19 Genetics

COMMON ABBREVIATIONS

AD	autosomal dominant
AR	autosomal recessive
AVSD	atrioventricular septal defect
CAH	congenital adrenal hyperplasia
CGH	comparative genomic hybridization
CHARGE	*c*oloboma, *h*eart disease, *a*tresia choanae, *r*etarded growth and development, *g*enital hypoplasia, and *e*ar anomalies and/or deafness
7-DHC	7-dehydrocholesterol
FISH	fluorescent in situ hybridization
FTT	failure to thrive
HC	head circumference
Hib	*Haemophilus influenzae* type B
IBD	inflammatory bowel disease
JIA	juvenile idiopathic arthritis
MPS	mucopolysaccharides
OGTT	oral glucose tolerance test
PCKD	polycystic kidney disease
TAPVD	total anomalous pulmonary venous drainage
TEF	tracheoesophageal fistula
TOF	tetralogy of Fallot
TORCH	*t*oxoplasmosis, *o*ther agents, *r*ubella, *c*ytomegalovirus, and *h*erpes simplex
UPJ	ureteropelvic junction
VCUG	voiding cystourethrogram
XR	X-ray

COMMON TERMS

Association: nonrandom group of developmental anomalies seen more frequently than expected by chance; not caused by a sequence or syndrome (e.g., VACTERL)

FISH: technique to identify presence of specific chromosome or chromosomal regions through hybridization (attachment) of fluorescent-labeled DNA probes to denatured chromosomal DNA; used to detect known microdeletion/microduplication syndromes or chromosomal aneuploidy

Karyotype: cytogenetic technique on skin, blood, or other tissues to determine number and structure of chromosomes within cells

Microarray analysis: technique used to detect DNA copy number abnormalities (microdeletions and microduplications) not visible on regular karyotype; also known as array CGH

Mosaicism: presence of two or more genotypically different cell populations in same individual (e.g., mosaic Down syndrome)

Sequence: series of developmental abnormalities caused by a single primary defect (e.g., Potter sequence)

Syndrome: recognizable pattern of developmental anomalies with single etiology (e.g., Down syndrome)

DYSMORPHOLOGY TERMS

- See Box 19.1

PHYSICAL EXAMINATION OF CHILDREN WITH DYSMORPHISM

- Full history including three-generation family tree (consanguinity, similarly affected relatives, miscarriages, newborn deaths)
- Suggestive findings for genetic syndromes: one major anomaly (e.g., bilateral cleft lip and palate) or ≥ three minor anomalies (e.g., ear tags/pits)
- Measure growth variables (HC, length, weight); plot on appropriate growth chart (e.g., achondroplasia, Down, Turner, Williams growth charts)

Box 19.1	Common Dysmorphology Terms

Head and Neck
- Brachycephaly: disproportionate anteroposterior shortening of head
- Hypertelorism: increased distance between orbits (pupils)
- Low-set ears: superior attachment of pinna below a hypothetical line connecting the inner and outer canthi and extending to the occipital prominence
- Nuchal: pertaining to back of neck
- Palpebral fissure orientation:
  - Upslanting: lateral corner of eyelid above medial corner
  - Downslanting: lateral corner below medial corner

Extremities
- Arachnodactyly: abnormally thin, long fingers and toes
- Clinodactyly: lateral or medial curvature of a digit
- Camptodactyly: flexure contracture of a digit
- Polydactyly: supernumerary digit
  - Postaxial: lateral to fifth finger/toe
  - Preaxial: lateral to the thumb
- Syndactyly: webbing/fusion of part/whole of two or more consecutive digits

- Skull: symmetry, shape, fontanelle (size), sutures (patency), scalp
- Hair: implantation (anterior and posterior hairline), texture, pattern
- Eyes: intercanthal distance, orientation, coloboma, eyelashes, palpebral fissures
- Mouth: cleft, shape of palate, lips (pits), tongue (size, texture), teeth (eruption time, quality, number)
- Philtrum: shape, length
- Nose: shape of nasal root, bridge, and tip; shape and position of nostrils
- Ears: size, shape, placement, pits/tags
- Neck: length, shape, webbing, pits/fistulas
- Thorax: shape, size, position of nipples, pectus deformities
- Spine: curvature, vertebral anomalies, sacral dimple
- Limbs: proportions, reductions/amputations, missing parts
- Hands and feet: creases, nails, digits (shape, number)
- Genitalia: hypoplasia, cryptorchidism, ambiguous genitalia, hypospadias
- Anus: patency, localization
- Viscera: size, shape, localization, extra masses

MODES OF INHERITANCE

- See Table 19.1

COMMON SEQUENCES

- See Table 19.2

COMMON ASSOCIATIONS

- See Table 19.3

COMMON SYNDROMES

- See Tables 19.4 through 19.7

Table 19.1   Characteristics of Different Modes of Genetic Inheritance

Inheritance	Affected Gender	Risk of Having an Affected Child With Each Pregnancy	Characteristics	Examples
Mendelian				
AD	M = F	· 50% (1:2) for affected individual · Unaffected parents have low risk of recurrence · 1–2% if gonadal mosaicism	· Phenotype occurs in every generation · M to M transmission possible	Myotonic dystrophy, neurofibromatosis, tuberous sclerosis
AR	M = F	· 25% (1:4) for carrier parents of affected child	· Disease occurs only in homozygous · Parents obligate carriers	Cystic fibrosis, CAH, sickle cell disease
X-linked	M > F	· Affected M passes mutated gene to all daughters · Affected F: 50% of M and F offspring inherit mutated copy of chromosome X · Carrier's risk of disease depends on underlying condition and pattern of X inactivation	· Generally severe or lethal in M · Heterozygous F carriers range from unaffected to less severe, based on X inactivation pattern · No M to M transmission	Incontinentia pigments, Rett syndrome, Duchenne muscular dystrophy, fragile X syndrome, hemophilia A
Nonmendelian				
Multifactorial	Unequal M:F	· Nonmendelian pattern of inheritance	· Multiple genetic, environmental factors · Risk of recurrence related to disease incidence	Cleft lip/palate, neural tube defect, club feet, diabetes mellitus type 1
Mitochondrial	M = F	· All (100%) maternal offspring are affected	· Maternal inheritance of mitochondrial DNA · Phenotypic variability (threshold effect) · Males do not pass disease to offspring · Characteristically affects high-energy tissues such as muscles, nerves, optic tract	MELAS (**m**itochondrial myopathy, **e**ncephalopathy, **l**actic **a**cidosis, **s**trokelike episodes), Leigh syndrome, MERRF (**m**yoclonic **e**pilepsy with **r**agged **r**ed **f**ibers)
Chromosomal	M = F	· Dependent on chromosomal abnormality and degree of fertility	· Offspring of balanced translocation carriers at risk of unbalanced translocations · Chromosomal abnormalities tend to be sporadic	Down syndrome

Genetics

19

Table 19.2 Common Sequences

Type	Inheritance	Clinical Manifestations	Initially	Later	Characteristics
Pierre Robin	· ⅔ isolated , ⅓ syndromic (e.g., Stickler)	· Cleft palate · Glossoptosis · Micrognathia	· Upper airway obstruction · Feeding difficulties	· Favorable prognosis	Primary anomaly: mandibular retrognathia
Potter (oligohydramnios sequence)	· Etiology often unknown · 20% due to bilateral renal agenesis/dysgenesis · M > F, 2–3:1	· Potter facies: flattened nose, retrognathia, wide-set eyes, large low-set ears · Bilateral pulmonary hypoplasia · Limb positioning defects · Growth deficiency	· Respiratory failure secondary to pulmonary hypoplasia · Acute renal failure	· Chronic lung disease · Chronic renal failure	Due to renal anomalies, obstructive uropathy, or prolonged leakage of amniotic fluid → oligohydramnios → deformation by constraint

Table 19.3

Table 19.3	Common Associations		
Type	**Inheritance**	**Clinical Manifestations**	**Investigations**
VACTERL Diagnostic: ≥3 anomalies	· Sporadic · Recurrence risk: 2–3%	**V** = vertebral defects **A** = anal atresia/stenosis **C** = cardiac anomalies (80%) (most common: VSD, ASD, TOF) **T** = tracheoesophageal fistula **E** = esophageal atresia **R** = renal anomalies (80%) (most common: PCKD, horseshoe kidney) **L** = limb defects (radial anomalies) Development usually normal	· Echocardiogram, renal US · Consider XR of the spine and upper extremities

Genetics

19

Table 19.4 Common Chromosomal Abnormalities

Type	Inheritance	Clinical Features	Later	Investigations	Attention
Trisomy 21 (Down syndrome)	· 95%: three copies of chromosome 21 · 5%: unbalanced translocation between chromosome 21 and another chromosome (often 14) · 1–2%: mosaicism · Recurrence risk: 1% or maternal age-adjusted risk, whichever is higher, Much higher risk if translocation in carrier parents	· Distinct facial features (epicanthal folds, upslanting palpebral fissures) · Patent posterior fontanelle · Brachycephaly · Brushfield spots, myopia · Furrowed, protruding tongue · Single palmar crease · Clinodactyly fifth finger · Sandal gap · Hypotonia · Hip dysplasia · Cardiac defects (50% [e.g., VSD, AVSD, ASD, PDA]) · GI anomalies (12% [e.g., TEF, duodenal atresia/stenosis, pyloric stenosis, Hirschsprung]) · Hypothyroidism (20–40%) · Transient leukemoid reactions, polycythemia (18%)	· Developmental delay · Asymptomatic atlantoaxial subluxation (12%) · Obstructive sleep apnea · Conductive hearing loss (otitis media) · Acute lymphoblastic leukemia (1–2%) · Obesity · Hip abnormalities (8%): dislocation, slipped capital femoral epiphysis, avascular necrosis *Adults:* · Early Alzheimer · Infertility (primary gonadal deficiency) · Cataracts	· FISH for chromosome 21 (for rapid diagnosis) · Karyotype in patient and parents · Echocardiogram, ophthalmologic, hearing assessment · Thyroid function (yearly), CBC, differential · ± Cervical XR Note: Follow health supervision guidelines	· Use Down growth charts · Careful neurologic examination: any change in bowel/bladder function, loss of ambulatory skills, neck posturing; neck pain: rule out spinal cord compression · Early intervention and special education

(continued)

Table 19.4 Common Chromosomal Abnormalities *(continued)*

Type	Inheritance	Clinical Features	Later	Investigations	Attention
Trisomy 13 (Patau)	· Majority have three copies of chromosome 13 · Rarely mosaicism; partial trisomy 13 · Risk of recurrence: 0.5% (increases with maternal age)	· Dysmorphic features (low-set ears, microcephaly, depressed nasal bridge) · Cutis aplasia · Micro/anophthalmia (60–70%) · Holoprosencephaly (60–70%) · Hearing defects · Cleft lip/palate (60–70%) · Low birth weight (40%) · Heart defects (80% [e.g., ASD, VSD]) · Polydactyly (60–70%) · Clenched fist · Omphalocele · Renal malformations (PCKD, horseshoe kidney)	· Growth retardation · Severe/profound mental retardation · Seizures	· Karyotype · Echocardiogram · Head US	· Median survival 7–10 d · Very poor outcome in surviving infants
Trisomy 18 (Edwards)	· Majority have three copies of chromosome 18 (risk increases with maternal age) · Rarely mosaicism, partial trisomy 18 · 80% are female	· Dysmorphic features (narrow bifrontal diameter, small mouth, micrognathia) · Prominent occiput · Short sternum · Overriding fingers · Rocker-bottom feet · Heart anomalies (90%: usually VSD ± polyvalvular dysplasia) · Renal (PCKD, horseshoe kidney) · Cryptorchidism · Hypertonia · Apneic episodes · Feeding issues	· Growth retardation · Severe to profound developmental delay	· Karyotype · Echocardiogram · Renal US	· Median survival 4 d · Very poor outcome in surviving infants · Increased risk of Wilms tumors and hepatoblastomas in survivors

(continued)

Genetics

19

371

Table 19.4 Common Chromosomal Abnormalities (continued)

Type	Inheritance	Clinical Features	Later	Investigations	Attention
Monosomy X (Turner)	· 50%: 45 X (haploinsufficiency) · 25%: mosaicism · 25%: structural abnormalities of second chromosome X · Most often: sporadic · Recurrence risk: very low	· Low posterior hairline · Short, webbed neck · Cystic hygroma · Puffiness of hands and feet (congenital lymphedema) · Broad chest, widely spaced nipples · Left-sided heart defects (15–50% [e.g., bicuspid aortic valve, coarctation of aorta, mitral valve prolapse]) · Renal abnormalities (%): horseshoe kidney · Developmental dysplasia of the hip	· Short stature · Strabismus, glaucoma · Hypertension (40%) · Aortic root dilatation (3–8%) · Primary ovarian failure · No pubertal growth spurt · Minimal breast development · Ovarian dysgenesis (90%) · Infertility · Hypothyroidism · Glucose intolerance · Hyperlipidemia · Normal intelligence	· Karyotype (5–10% will have Y chromosome material in all/some cells) · FISH for chromosomes X and Y · Echocardiogram · Renal US · Hearing assessment · Thyroid function · ± Glucose tolerance test	· Turner growth charts · Growth hormone therapy at early age · Later: estrogen therapy · Increase risk for autoimmune diseases (IBD, thyroiditis, JIA, celiac disease) · Increase risk for gonadoblastoma or dysgerminoma (7–10%)

Table 19.5 Mendelian Inheritance

Types	Inheritance	Clinical Features	Later	Investigations	Attention
Achondroplasia	· AD · 75–90%: sporadic · Recurrence risk: if sporadic, <1%	· Short to normal length at birth · Proximal shortening (rhizomelic) · Brachydactyly with trident hands · Short vertebral pedicles · Square-shaped pelvis · Mild hypotonia	· Short stature · Macrocephaly · Recurrent otitis media · Delayed gross motor milestones · Bowing of lower legs *Rare (2–5%):* · Hydrocephalus · Cervicomedullary junction compression in first year (due to narrow foramen magnum): <3% · Upper airway obstruction *Adults:* · Kyphosis · Lumbosacral spinal stenosis · Normal intelligence and life expectancy	· XR of bones · Targeted mutation testing in *FGFR3* (atypical cases) · CT/MRI (assess foramen magnum size) in first year of life · Polysomnography in first year of life; repeat if apneas	· Measure HC · Achondroplasia-specific growth chart · If large fontanelle or rapid ↑ in HC or symptoms of raised intracranial pressure: head imaging

(continued)

Table 19.5 Mendelian Inheritance *(continued)*

Types	Inheritance	Clinical Features	Later	Investigations	Attention
CHARGE	· AD · Most cases sporadic · Recurrence rate: 1%	**C** = coloboma, bilateral (80%) **H** = heart defects (50–85% [e.g. conotruncal defects, ASD, VSD, coarctation]) **A** = atresia choanae (58%) **R** = retarded growth and/or development delay (70–80%) **G** = genital hypoplasia: micropenis, cryptorchidism (75% in males) **E** = ear anomalies and/or deafness (88%); abnormal semicircular canals · CNS anomalies (55–85%) · I (hypo/anosmia), VII (facial palsy), VIII (hypoplasia of auditory nerve), IX/X (swallowing difficulties and aspiration) · Holoprosencephaly · TEF: 15–20% · Cleft lip/palate: 15–20%	· Short stature · Delayed/absent puberty (hypogonadotropic hypogonadism) · ± Learning disabilities · Scoliosis (60%)	· Molecular analysis: mutation within *CHD7* gene (⅔ cases) · CT temporal bones (semicircular canal malformation) · Echocardiogram · Renal US	· Clinical diagnosis (3C triad = *coloboma, abnormal semicircular canals, atresia choanae*, highly predictive) *Neonate:* · Feeding issues (risk of aspiration) *Surveillance:* · Eye examinations, audiologic evaluations · Hormonal replacement, if delayed puberty

(continued)

Table 19.5 Mendelian Inheritance (continued)

Types	Inheritance	Clinical Features	Later	Investigations	Attention
Fragile X	· X-linked · M: 1:1250–2500 · F: 1:1600–5000	*Infancy/childhood:* · Poor eye contact · Developmental delay · Seizures (20%) · Mental retardation (milder in affected females) · ADHD, autism · Strabismus, myopia	*Puberty:* · Relative macrocephaly · Prominent forehead and jaw, large protuberant ears · Macro-orchidism · Joint hypermobility *Adults:* · Mitral valve prolapse (50%), aortic dilatation	· DNA molecular analysis for trinucleotide repeat size of the *FMR1* gene (99% rate of detection)	· Developmental pediatrician · Mothers obligate carriers; at risk of premature ovarian failure
Marfan	· AD · 25–35% sporadic	· Joint laxity, contractures · Neonatal presentation rare, but diagnosis can be made if positive family history	*Systemic involvement as per Ghent criteria:* · Lens dislocation, myopia · Heart: aortic root dilatation and dissection, mitral valve prolapse · Spontaneous pneumothorax (4–11%), apical blebs · Joint hypermobility/dislocations, scoliosis, pectus carinatum/excavatum · Recurrent hernias, striae · Lumbosacral dural ectasis (95% by MRI)	· DNA molecular analysis for *FBN1* gene (less frequently *TGFβR1* or *TGFβR2* genes) · Periodic echocardiograms · Slit-lamp examination · Monitor BP · If symptoms, pelvic XR (detects protrusion of acetabulae)	· Clinical diagnosis (Ghent criteria less reliable in childhood) · Avoid isometric exercise, contact sports, and scuba diving · Consider β-blockade as prophylaxis for aortic dilatation in children and adults

(continued)

Table 19.5 Mendelian Inheritance (continued)

Types	Inheritance	Clinical Features	Later	Investigations	Attention
Noonan	· AD	· Wool-like hair (curly) · Low-set, posteriorly rotated ears · Downslanting palpebral fissures, ptosis · Neck webbing · Heart defect (50–80% [e.g., pulmonary valve stenosis]); hypertrophic cardiomyopathy, 20%) · Hypotonia · Bilateral cryptorchidism (60%) · Mild renal abnormalities (11%: dilatation of renal pelvis, cysts)	*Infancy:* · FTT *Later:* · Short stature · Developmental delay · Strabismus, refractive errors · Bleeding diathesis (50%): thrombocytopenia, platelet dysfunction	· Molecular genetic test (mutation in *PTPN11* gene: 50%; *SOS1* gene: 10%; *RAF1* gene: 10%; *KRAS* gene: 5%) · Echocardiogram, ophthalmologic examination, renal US · CBC, coagulation screen	· Clinical diagnosis · May have malignant hyperthermia · Tumor risk slightly increased
Smith–Lemli–Opitz	· AR · ↓ Levels of 7-DHC reductase	· Microcephaly · Holoprosencephaly (5%) · Cleft palate (37–52%) · Ptosis, congenital cataracts, demyelination of optic nerve · Postaxial polydactyly (50%) · 2,3 syndactyly of toes (95%) · Heart defects (36–38%: AVSD, TAPVD) · Pyloric stenosis, Hirschsprung · Renal anomalies (UJP obstruction, renal cystic dysplasia, renal agenesis) · Hypospadias and/or cryptorchidism (90–100%)	· Growth and mental retardation	· ↑ 7-DHC in blood · ↑ Ratio of 7-DHC: cholesterol · ± ↓ Cholesterol (90% cases) · Mutation + sequence analysis of *DHCR7* gene for prenatal diagnosis and carrier detection · Echocardiogram, renal US	· Clinical + biochemical diagnosis

Table 19.6 Microdeletion/Duplications

Type	Inheritance	Neonate	Later	Investigations	Attention
DiGeorge	· 94%: sporadic deletion 22q11 · Rare: deletion 10p14 · If familial, behaves like AD	· Cleft palate/velopharyngeal insufficiency · Heart disease (75%: VSD, aortic arch anomalies, TOF) · Immunodeficiency (thymus hypoplasia) · Hypocalcemia (parathyroid dysfunction) · Renal tract anomalies (36%)	· Short stature · Feeding difficulties · Hypernasal speech · Learning difficulties (68%)	· Karyotype · MLPA* to exclude microdeletions of the 22q11 region (replaces FISH) · FISH (22q11 deletion) · Echocardiogram, renal US, audiogram · Monitor Ca²⁺, CBC, platelets · Lymphocyte subset testing (exclude impaired T-cell maturation and function), serum immunoglobulins, tetanus, diphtheria, Hib antibody titers	· No live vaccines until immune function checked · If transfusion necessary, CMV negative and irradiated if < 6 mo of age or if CD4 count <500 · Infant development program
Williams	· >90%: sporadic deletion 7q11 · If familial, behaves like AD	· Wide mouth, full lips · Hoarse voice · Heart anomalies (80%): supravalvular aortic stenosis (75%), peripheral pulmonary artery stenosis (50–75%), supravalvular pulmonary stenosis (25%) · Idiopathic hypercalcemia · Renal artery stenosis and hypertension, urethral stenosis, small solitary and/or pelvic kidney · Hypotonia · Feeding issues	· FTT · Mild cognitive impairment · Hypercalciuria (30%), nephrocalcinosis · Hypothyroidism (10%) · Refractive errors, strabismus · Recurrent otitis media · Partial anodontia · Lordosis, scoliosis, kyphosis · Inguinal hernias, rectal prolapse · Chronic constipation, diverticulosis, cholelithiasis *Adults:* · Abnormal OGTT · Anxiety (80%) · Cataracts	· FISH (contiguous deletion on 7q11 [99% patients]) · Echocardiogram, renal US · Eye examination, hearing test · Urinalysis, Ca²⁺/creatinine ratio, renal function · Monitor serum Ca²⁺, thyroid function	· Williams growth chart · Increased incidence of celiac disease (9%) · Do not give vitamin D

*MLPA, multiplex ligation-dependent probe amplification; molecular diagnostic technique used to better characterize microdeletion size and position.

Genetics

19

Table 19.7 Imprinting Defects

Type	Inheritance	Neonate	Later	Investigations	Attention
Angelman	· Majority sporadic · Loss of maternally imprinted genetic contribution at 15q11.2–q13 (AS/PWS) region · Rare: maternal inheritance of mutation in *UBE3A* gene	· Normal HC and weight at birth · Weak suck · Feeding problems	· Severe developmental delay (starting at 6–12 mo) · Early-onset seizures · Strabismus (42%), refractive errors, nystagmus · Decreased sleep · Ataxia/tremulousness · Autistic features	· DNA methylation analysis of chromosome 15 (greatest detection rate) · FISH for 15q11.2–q13 deletion (75%) · *UBE3A* mutation (25%) · EEG (if needed)	· Microcephaly by 1 yr (50%)
Beckwith–Wiedemann	· 85% sporadic · 10% AD pedigrees · Few chromosomal abnormalities involve 11p15	· Macrosomia · Macroglossia · Visceromegaly · Omphalocele · Hemihypertrophy *Neonatal:* · Hypoglycemia (30–50%) · Polycythemia · Hypercalciuria	· Embryonal tumors (6.5%) *Rare:* · Cardiomyopathy	· Karyotype (11p15 dup) · DNA methylation of 11p15 region · Uniparental disomy studies of 11p15 · Surveillance for · Wilms tumor: renal US every 3 mo to 8 yr · Hepatoblastoma: serum alpha fetoprotein every 3 mo to 4 yr	*Rare:* · Rabdomyosarcomas · Gonadoblastomas · Adrenal carcinomas

(continued)

Table 19.7 Imprinting Defects *(continued)*

Type	Inheritance	Neonate	Later	Investigations	Attention
Prader-Willi	· Majority sporadic · 75–80%: deletion of paternal chromosome 15q11–15q13 · 15%: uniparental disomy of chromosome 15q11 · <5%: imprinting defect · Recurrence risk: ≤1%	· Severe central hypotonia (improves with age) · Poor suck · Delicate facial features (narrow bifrontal diameter, almond-shaped eyes, triangular mouth) · Small hands and feet · Genital hypoplasia, cryptorchidism (80–90%)	*Infancy:* · FTT *Toddler:* · Food foraging *Childhood:* · Rapid weight gain between 1–6 yr · Strabismus · Global developmental delay *Later:* · Short stature · Scoliosis · Ritualistic behavior (80%) · Delayed, incomplete puberty *Adult:* · Morbid obesity · Hypogonadism · Infertility	· DNA methylation analysis (detects defect in >99% cases) · Karyotype · FISH for 15q11.2–q13 deletion · Eye examination	· Early growth hormone therapy beneficial for body composition, even if growth normal · Adolescents need testosterone replacement therapy · Prone to diabetes

Genetics

19

EAR ABNORMALITIES

- Full physical examination to determine whether ear abnormality is isolated: preauricular ear pits, ear tags, cupped ears, microtia, iris or lid colobomas, malar hypoplasia, epibulbar dermoid, skin tags along line between ear and angle of mouth, branchial cleft sinuses or cysts, heart murmur, imperforate anus, rectovaginal fistula, polydactyly, asymmetry of thenar muscle group, triphalangeal or abnormal thumbs
- See Figure 19.1

MICROCEPHALY

- Confirm microcephaly: HC <2 SD below mean
- Pregnancy history: HC, IUGR
- Exclude secondary causes: TORCH infections, maternal PKU, exposure to alcohol or drugs, birth trauma or hypoxia, craniosynostosis
- Family history: parental microcephaly, developmental delay, seizures, consanguinity
- Neurodevelopmental status: developmental delay, seizures, vision, ataxia

Physical Examination

- Growth variables: prenatal or postnatal onset
- Skull shape: craniosynostosis
- Dysmorphic features
- Cardiac: murmur

Investigations

- Head US/brain MRI
- Ophthalmologic examination
- Routine karyotype
- Metabolic testing: urine organic acids, serum amino acids, very long chain fatty acids
- Virology: TORCH infections
- Bank DNA

Approach to Microcephaly

- See Figure 19.2

Figure 19.1 Approach to Structural Ear Abnormalities

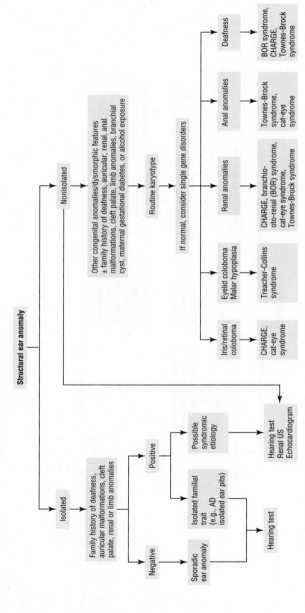

© The Hospital for Sick Children, 2009. New artwork created by The Hospital for Sick Children for *The Hospital for Sick Children Handbook of Pediatrics*, 11th edition.

Figure 19.2 **Approach to Microcephaly**

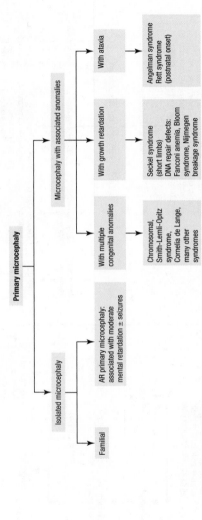

Primary microcephaly

Isolated microcephaly
- Familial
- AR primary microcephaly: associated with moderate mental retardation ± seizures

Microcephaly with associated anomalies
- With multiple congenital anomalies
  - Chromosomal, Smith-Lemli-Opitz syndrome, Cornelia de Lange, many other syndromes
- With growth retardation
  - Seckel syndrome (short limbs) DNA repair defects: Fanconi anemia, Bloom syndrome, Nijmegen breakage syndrome
- With ataxia
  - Angelman syndrome Rett syndrome (postnatal onset)

© The Hospital for Sick Children, 2009. New artwork created by The Hospital for Sick Children for *The Hospital for Sick Children Handbook of Pediatrics*, 11th edition.

MACROCEPHALY

- Confirm macrocephaly: HC >2 SD above mean
- Prenatal history: HC (fetal US, birth)
- Family history: macrocephaly, malignancy (breast, basal cell), thyroid disorders, consanguinity
- Parental HCs
- Neurodevelopmental status: developmental delay, seizures, regression

Physical Examination

- Growth variables: isolated/relative macrocephaly vs. macrosomia (all growth variables large)
- Abnormal skull shape: craniosynostosis
- Dysmorphic/coarse facial features
- Limb asymmetry
- Skin: café au lait spots, hypopigmented lesions, lipomas, hemangiomas, papillomata around nose

Investigations

- Head US/MRI, if neurologic impairment
- Routine karyotype
- Metabolic testing: urine organic acids, urine MPS, urine oligosaccharides
- Bank DNA: fragile X testing in boys with developmental delay ± autism

Approach to Macrocephaly

- See Figure 19.3

CLEFT LIP AND PALATE

- See Figure 19.4

Figure 19.3 Approach to Macrocephaly

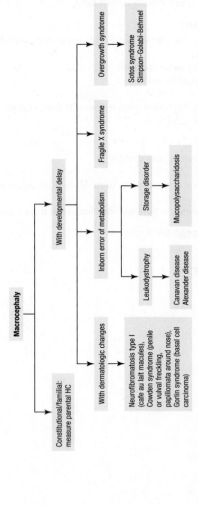

Macrocephaly

- Constitutional/familial: measure parental HC
- With dermatologic changes
  - Neurofibromatosis type I (cafe au lait macules), Cowden syndrome (penile or vulval freckling, papillomata around nose), Gorlin syndrome (basal cell carcinoma)
- With developmental delay
  - Inborn error of metabolism
    - Leukodystrophy
      - Canavan disease
      - Alexander disease
    - Storage disorder
      - Mucopolysaccharidosis
  - Fragile X syndrome
  - Overgrowth syndrome
    - Sotos syndrome
    - Simpson-Golabi-Behmel

© The Hospital for Sick Children, 2009. New artwork created by The Hospital for Sick Children for *The Hospital for Sick Children Handbook of Pediatrics*, 11th edition.

Figure 19.4 Approach to Cleft Lip and/or Palate

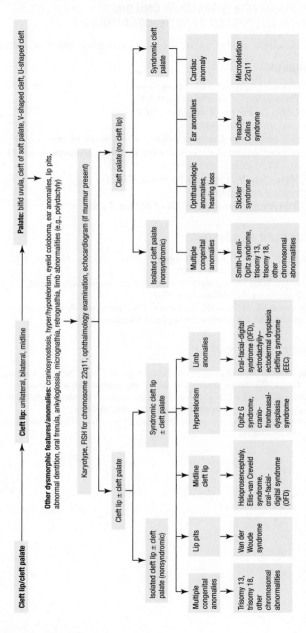

© The Hospital for Sick Children, 2009. New artwork created by The Hospital for Sick Children for The Hospital for Sick Children Handbook of Pediatrics, 11th edition.

Genetics

19

PERIMORTEM WORKUP IN CHILDREN WITH SUSPECTED GENETIC CONDITIONS

- Indication: sudden, unexplained death in children with dysmorphisms

WORKUP

- Blood: two spots on filter paper
- Plasma: 5 mL (heparinized sample)
- Urine: 30 mL (to be frozen at –20°C)
- CSF: 1 mL (to be frozen)
- Skin biopsy (for fibroblast culture): 4-mm punch biopsy; place in cell culture medium or sterile saline (keep at room temperature if < 24 h or +4°C if longer; do not freeze)
- Muscle and liver biopsies (frozen at –70°C)
- Clinical photographs
- Babygram (skeletal XR) ± XR of the hands and feet

FURTHER READING

Firth HV, Hurst JA. *Oxford Desk Reference: Clinical Genetics*. New York, NY: Oxford University Press; 2005.

Jones KL. *Smith's Recognizable Patterns of Human Malformation*. 5th ed. Philadelphia, Pa: WB Saunders; 1997.

Nussbaum RL, McInnes RR, Huntington FW. *Thompson & Thompson Genetics in Medicine*. 6th ed. Philadelphia, Pa: WB Saunders; 2004.

USEFUL WEB SITES

Health supervision of children with achondroplasia, Down, fragile X, Marfan, Turner, Williams syndrome. Available at: http://aappolicy.aappublications.org

National Center for Biotechnology Information, Online Mendelian Inheritance in Man. Available at: www.ncbi.nlm.nih.gov/sites/entrez?db=OMIM

Genetest/Geneclinics. Funded by the National Institutes of Health. Available at: www.genetests.org

Genetics

19

Chapter 20 Growth and Nutrition

Deena Savlov

Alène A. Toulany

Stacey Bernstein

Chapter 20 Growth and Nutrition

COMMON ABBREVIATIONS

AST	aspartate aminotransferase
BMI	body mass index
CBC	complete blood count
CVL	central venous line
EBM	expressed breast milk
FTT	failure to thrive
GER(D)	gastroesophageal reflux (disease)
GIR	glucose infusion rate
IBW	ideal body weight
MCT	medium-chain triglycerides
PN	parenteral nutrition
TFI	total fluid intake
TNA	total nutrient admixture

NUTRITIONAL REQUIREMENTS

- Most rapid growth and highest nutritional requirement occur during first year of life
- Estimated energy requirements and dietary reference intakes (DRIs): see Tables 20.1 through 20.4

ASSESSMENT OF GROWTH

- Minimum parameters of growth assessment: weight, height, head circumference (Table 20.5)
- Single measurements can be compared with normal population values by plotting on appropriate growth chart (Figures 20.1 to 20.8, pp. 396–403)
- Serial measurements also provide information on growth velocity and can show changes in growth pattern over time
- For premature infants (<37 wk), use corrected gestational age until 2 yr to monitor growth parameters
- Growth charts have been developed for a number of conditions for which growth patterns are altered (e.g., trisomy 21, Prader-Willi syndrome, Turner syndrome, and achondroplasia) (see relevant growth charts at http://aappolicy.aappublications.org/)

Table 20.1		Summary of Estimated Energy Requirement (EER) for Infants and Children			
		Estimated Energy Requirement (EER)* (kcal/kg/d)			
Age	**Sex**	**Physical Activity Level (PAL)†**			
Infants (mo)					
0–2	M	107			
	F	104–102			
3–6	M	95–82			
	F	95–82			
7–9	M	79–80			
	F	80			
10–20	M	79–82			
	F	82			
21–35	M	82–83			
	F	83			
		Sedentary	**Low Active**	**Active**	**Very Active**
Children (yr)					
3–4	M	81–75	93–86	104–97	117–109
	F	78–72	89–83	100–94	118–111
5–6	M	69–64	80–74	90–84	103–97
	F	66–62	77–72	87–82	104–97
7–8	M	60–57	70–66	80–75	92–87
	F	57–53	67–62	75–71	90–85
9–10	M	54–50	63–59	71–67	83–78
	F	49–45	57–53	65–60	78–72
11–12	M	47–44	55–52	64–60	74–70
	F	41–39	49–46	56–53	67–64
13–14	M	42–41	50–48	57–56	67–64
	F	37–35	44–41	50–47	60–57
15–16	M	40–38	47–45	54–52	62–60
	F	33–32	40–38	45–44	55–54
17–18	M	37–36	43–42	50–49	58–57
	F	31–30	37–36	43–42	52–51

(continued)

Table 20.1 — Summary of Estimated Energy Requirement (EER) for Infants and Children (continued)

EER (kcal/day)	
Infants	
0–3 mo	EER = (89 × weight [kg] – 100) + 175
4–6 mo	EER = (89 × weight [kg] – 100) + 56
7–12 mo	EER = (89 × weight [kg] – 100) + 22
13–36 mo	EER = (89 × weight [kg] – 100) + 20
Children	
Boys	
3–8 yr	EER = (88.5–61.9 × age[y]) + PA x (26.7 × weight [kg] + 903 × height [m]) + 20
9–18 yr	EER = (88.5–61.9 × age[y]) + PA x (26.7 × weight [kg] + 903 × height [m]) + 25
Girls	
3–8 yr	EER = (135.3–30.8 × age[y]) + PA × (10.0 × weight [kg] + 934 × height [m]) + 20
9–18 yr	EER = (135.3–30.8 × age[y]) + PA × (10.0 × weight [kg] + 934 × height [m]) + 25

Physical Activity (PA) Coefficients Used in EER Equations				
	Sedentary	**Low Active**	**Active**	**Very Active**
Boys 3–18 yr	1.00	1.13	1.26	1.42
Girls 3–18 yr	1.00	1.16	1.31	1.56

*EER (kcal/kg) calculated based on equations divided by reference weights.
†PAL for infants not determined.
Reference weights for Infants 0–35 mo and reference weights and heights for children 3–18 yr used for calculations. Adapted from Kuczmarski RJ, Ogden CL, Grummer-Strawn LM. Flegal KM, et al. CDC growth charts: United States. *Adv Data.* 2000; 314, 1–28; and Food and Nutrition Board, Institute of Medicine-National Academy of Sciences. *Dietary Reference Intakes for Energy, Carbohydrate, Fiber, Fat, Fatty Acids, Cholesterol, Protein, and Amino Acids (Macronutirents).* 2005. Available at http://www.nap.edu.

Table 20.2 Summary of Dietary Reference Intakes (DRIs): Macronutrients for Infants and Children

Age	Sex	Protein (g/kg/d)	Carbohydrate (Digestible) (g/d)	Total Fat (g/d)	Linoleic Acid (g/d)	Linolenic Acid (g/d)	Total Fiber (g/d)	Total Water (g/d)
Infants								
0–6 mo	Both	1.52*	60*	31*	4.4*	0.5*	ND	0.7*
7–12 mo	Both	1.2	90*	30*	4.6*	0.5*	ND	0.8*
Children								
1–3 yr	Both	1.05	130	ND	7*	0.7*	19*	1.3*
4–8 yr	Both	0.95	130	ND	10*	0.9*	25*	1.7*
9–13 yr	M	0.95	130	ND	12*	1.2*	31*	2.4*
	F	0.95	130	ND	10*	1.0*	26*	2.1*
14–18 yr	M	0.85	130	ND	16*	1.6*	38*	3.3*
	F	0.85	130	ND	11*	1.1*	26*	2.3*

Recommended daily allowances (RDAs) in bold type and adequate intakes (AIs) in ordinary type followed by an asterisk (*). ND, not determinable.
Adapted from Food and Nutrition Board, Institute of Medicine-National Academy of Sciences. *Dietary Reference Intakes for Energy, Carbohydrate, Fiber, Fat, Fatty Acids, Cholesterol, Protein, and Amino Acids (Macronutrients)*. 2005. Available at http://www.nap.edu.

Table 20.3 Summary of Dietary Reference Intakes (DRIs) for Infants and Children: Vitamins

Age	Sex	Vit A (mcg/d)	Vit C (mg/d)	Vit D (mcg/d)	Vit E (mg/d)	Vit K (mcg/d)	Thiamin (mcg/d)	Riboflavin (mcg/d)	Niacin (mg/d)	Vit B₆ (mcg/d)	Folate (mcg/d)	Vit B₁₂ (mcg/d)	Pantothenic (mg/d)	Biotin (mcg/d)	Choline (mg/d)
Infants															
0-6 mo	Both	400*	40*	5*	4*	2.0*	0.2*	0.3*	2*	0.1*	65*	0.4*	1.7*	5*	125*
7-12 mo	Both	500*	50*	5*	5*	2.5*	0.3*	0.4*	4*	0.3*	80*	0.5*	1.8*	6*	150*
Children															
1-3 yr	Both	300	15	5*	6	30*	0.5	0.5	6	0.5	150	0.9	2*	8*	200*
4-8 yr	Both	400	25	5*	7	55*	0.6	0.6	8	0.6	200	1.2	3*	12*	250*
9-13 yr	M	600	45	5*	11	60*	0.9	0.9	12	1.0	300	1.8	4*	20*	375*
	F	600	45	5*	11	60*	0.9	0.9	12	1.0	300	1.8	4*	20*	375*
14-18 yr	M	900	75	5*	15	75*	1.2	1.3	16	1.3	400	2.4	5*	25*	550*
	F	700	65	5*	15	75*	1.0	1.0	14	1.2	400	2.4	5*	25*	400*

Recommended daily allowances (RDAs) in bold type and adequate intakes (AIs) in ordinary type followed by an asterisk (*). ND not determinable.
Adapted from Food and Nutrition Board, Institute of Medicine-National Academy of Sciences: Dietary Reference Intakes for Water, Potassium, Sodium, Chloride, and Sulfate, 2004; Dietary Reference Intakes for Vitamin A, Vitamin K, Arsenic, Boron, Chromium, Copper, Iodine, Iron, Manganese, Molybdenum, Nickel, Silicon, Vanadium, and Zinc, 2000; Dietary Reference Intakes for Vitamin C, Vitamin E, Selenium, and Carotenoids, 2000; Dietary Reference Intakes for Thiamin, Riboflavin, Niacin, Vitamin B6, Folate, Vitamin B12, Pantothenic Acid, Biotin, and Choline, 1998; and Dietary and Reference Intakes for Calcium, Magnesium, Vitamin D, and Fluoride, 1997. Available at: http://www.nap.edu.

Table 20.4		Summary of Dietary Reference Intakes (DRIs) for Infants and Children: Minerals														
Age	Sex	Ca²⁺ (mg/d)	Chromium (mcg/d)	Cu (mcg/d)	Fl (mg/d)	I (mcg/d)	Fe (mg/d)	Mg²⁺ (mg/d)	Manganese (mg/d)	Molybdenum (mcg/d)	PO₄⁻ (mg/d)	Selenium (mcg/d)	Zinc (mg/d)	P (g/d)	Na (g/d)	Cl (g/d)
Infants																
0–6 mo	Both	210*	0.2*	200*	0.01*	110*	0.27*	30*	0.003*	2*	100*	15*	2*	0.4*	0.12*	0.18*
7–12 mo	Both	270*	5.5*	220*	0.5*	130*	11	75*	0.6*	3*	275*	20*	3	0.7*	0.37*	0.57*
Children																
1–3 yr	Both	500*	11*	340	0.7*	90	7	80	1.2*	17	460	20	3	3.0*	1.0*	1.5*
4–8 yr	Both	800*	15*	440	1.0*	90	10	130	1.5*	22	500	30	5	3.8*	1.2*	1.9*
9–13 yr	M	1300*	25*	700	2*	120	8	240	1.9*	34	1250	40	8	4.5*	1.5*	2.3*
9–13 yr	F	1300*	21*	700	3*	120	8	240	1.6*	34	1250	40	8	4.7*	1.5*	2.3*
14–18 yr	M	1300*	35*	890	2*	150	11	410	2.2*	43	1250	55	11	4.5*	1.5*	2.3*
14–18 yr	F	1300*	24*	890	3*	150	15	360	1.6*	43	1250	55	9	7*	1.5*	2.3*

Recommended daily allowances (RDAs) in bold type and adequate intakes (AIs) in ordinary type followed by an asterisk (*). ND, not determinable.

Food and Nutrition Board, Institute of Medicine-National Academy of Sciences: *Dietary Reference Intakes for Water, Potassium, Sodium, Chloride, and Sulfate,* 2004; *Dietary Reference Intakes for Vitamin A, Vitamin K, Arsenic, Boron, Chromium, Copper, Iodine, Iron, Manganese, Molybdenum, Nickel, Silicon, Vanadium, and Zinc,* 2000; *Dietary Reference Intakes for Vitamin C, Vitamin E, Selenium, and Carotenoids,* 2000; *Dietary Reference Intakes for Thiamin, Riboflavin, Niacin, Vitamin B6, Folate, Vitamin B12, Pantothenic Acid, Biotin, and Choline,* 1998; and *Dietary and Reference Intakes for Calcium, Magnesium, Vitamin D, and Fluoride,* 1997. Available at: http://www.nap.edu.

Table 20.5	Average Growth Parameters and Rate of Growth	
	Birth	**Rate of Growth**
Weight	3–4 kg	2 × birth wt by 4–5 m 3 × birth wt by 1 yr 4 × birth wt by 2 yr
Height	50 cm	25 cm in first yr 12 cm in second yr 2 × birth ht by age 4 yr, then 5–8 cm/yr until puberty
Head circumference	35 cm	2 cm/m until 3 m 1 cm/m from 3–6 m 0.5 cm/m from 6–12 m

WEIGHT

- Infant weights done with clothes and diaper removed; on same scale, if possible
- Term neonates may lose up to 10% of birth weight in first week of life; should regain weight by 10 d of age, then approximately 180 g/wk until 4–5 mo
- To estimate weight for children >1 yr (kg): (age in yr × 2) + 8

LENGTH/HEIGHT

- Measure supine length until age 2 yr, then standing height
- To estimate child's adult height from parental heights:
  - Boy's height: ([father's height in cm + mother's height in cm]/2) + 6.5 cm
  - Girl's height: ([father's height in cm + mother's height in cm]/2) − 6.5 cm

HEAD CIRCUMFERENCE

- Should be measured up to 3 yr
- Measure over the most prominent part of the back of the head (occiput) and just above the eyebrows (supraorbital ridge) to try and obtain the largest anterior/posterior diameter

WEIGHT FOR HEIGHT

- Given normal variance in height, important to consider weight in relation to height
- Several measures of weight for height are used; examples include %IBW and BMI
- To calculate %IBW:
  - Step 1: plot child's height to determine height percentile
  - Step 2: find the same percentile and record weight (IBW)
  - Step 3: (child's actual body weight/IBW) × 100
  - Note: if child's height plots <3rd percentile or >97th percentile, IBW can only be estimated
- BMI: weight in kg/height^2 in m^2
- See Table 20.6 and Figures 20.7 and 20.8

Table 20.6	BMI Weight Status Categories
BMI	**Weight Status**
<15	Starvation
15–18.5	Underweight
18.5–25	Normal
25–30	Overweight
30–40	Obese
>40	Morbidly obese

Adapted from Centers for Disease Control and Prevention (2007). Available at: http://www.cdc.gov/nccdphp/dnpa/bmi/index.htm

Figure 20.1 Boys, Birth–36 Months: Length-for-Age and Weight-for-Age Percentiles

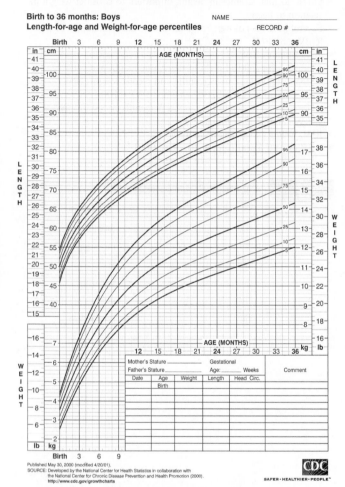

From Kuczmarski RJ, Ogden CL, Guo SS, et al. *2000 CDC Growth Charts for the United States: Methods and Development.* National Center for Health Statistics. Vital Health Statistics. Series II, Number 246. May 2002. Accessed at: http://www.cdc.gov/growthcharts

Figure 20.2 Girls, Birth–36 Months: Length-for-Age and Weight-for-Age Percentiles

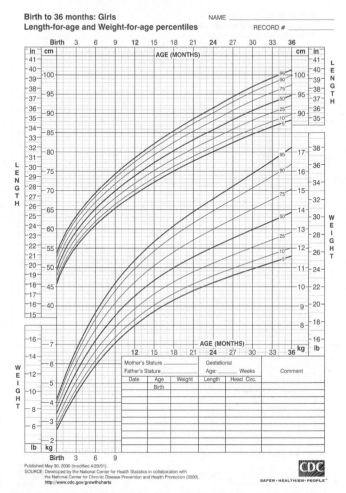

From Kuczmarski RJ, Ogden CL, Guo SS, et al. *2000 CDC Growth Charts for the United States: Methods and Development.* National Center for Health Statistics. Vital Health Statistics. Series II, Number 246. May 2002. Accessed at: http://www.cdc.gov/growthcharts

Figure 20.3 Boys, Birth–36 Months: Head Circumference-for-Age and Weight-for-Length Percentiles

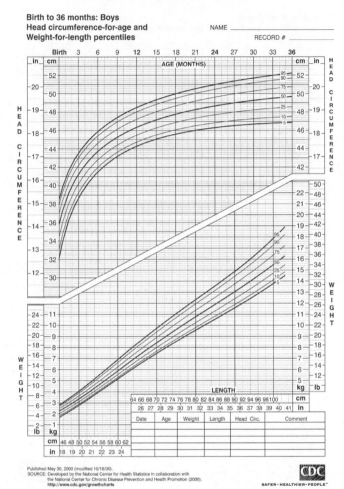

Birth to 36 months: Boys
Head circumference-for-age and
Weight-for-length percentiles

NAME _____

RECORD # _____

Published May 30, 2000 (modified 10/16/00).
SOURCE: Developed by the National Center for Health Statistics in collaboration with
the National Center for Chronic Disease Prevention and Health Promotion (2000).
http://www.cdc.gov/growthcharts

From Kuczmarski RJ, Ogden CL, Guo SS, et al. 2000 CDC Growth Charts for the United States: Methods and Development. National Center for Health Statistics. Vital Health Statistics. Series II, Number 246. May 2002. Accessed at: http://www.cdc.gov/growthcharts

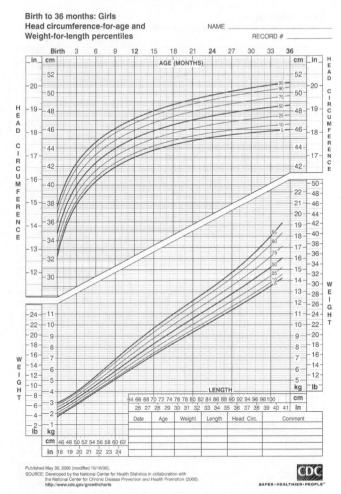

Birth to 36 months: Girls
Head circumference-for-age and
Weight-for-length percentiles

Published May 30, 2000 (modified 10/16/00).
SOURCE: Developed by the National Center for Health Statistics in collaboration with
the National Center for Chronic Disease Prevention and Health Promotion (2000).
http://www.cdc.gov/growthcharts

From Kuczmarski RJ, Ogden CL, Guo SS, et al. 2000 CDC Growth Charts for the United States: Methods and
Development. National Center for Health Statistics. Vital Health Statistics. Series II, Number 246. May 2002.
Accessed at: http://www.cdc.gov/growthcharts

Growth and Nutrition

20

Figure 20.5 Boys, 2–20 Years: Stature-for-Age and Weight-for-Age Percentiles

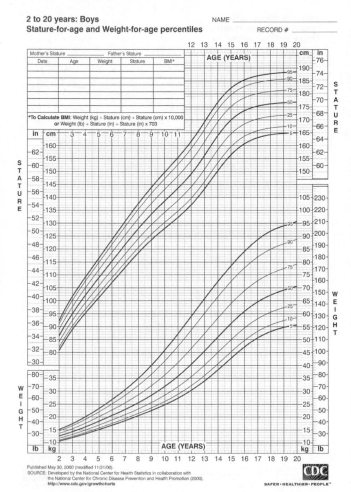

From Kuczmarski RJ, Ogden CL, Guo SS, et al. *2000 CDC Growth Charts for the United States: Methods and Development.* National Center for Health Statistics. Vital Health Statistics. Series II, Number 246. May 2002. Accessed at: http://www.cdc.gov/growthcharts

Figure 20.6 Girls, 2–20 Years: Stature-for-Age and Weight-for-Age Percentiles

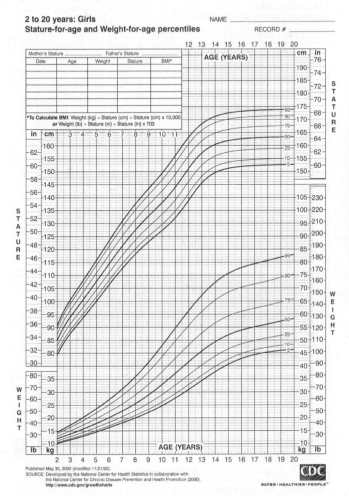

2 to 20 years: Girls
Stature-for-age and Weight-for-age percentiles

NAME _____
RECORD # _____

Published May 30, 2000 (modified 11/21/00).
SOURCE: Developed by the National Center for Health Statistics in collaboration with
the National Center for Chronic Disease Prevention and Health Promotion (2000).
http://www.cdc.gov/growthcharts

From Kuczmarski RJ, Ogden CL, Guo SS, et al. *2000 CDC Growth Charts for the United States: Methods and Development.* National Center for Health Statistics. Vital Health Statistics. Series II, Number 246. May 2002.
Accessed at: http://www.cdc.gov/growthcharts

Growth and Nutrition

20

Figure 20.7 Boys, 2–20 Years: Body Mass Index-for-Age Percentiles

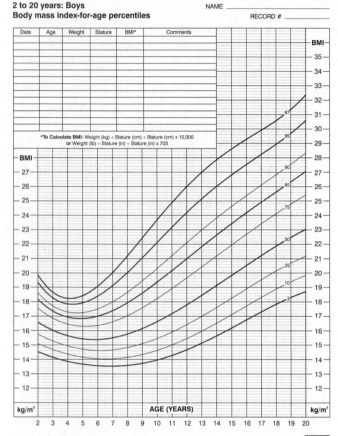

2 to 20 years: Boys
Body mass index-for-age percentiles

NAME _____

RECORD # _____

*To Calculate BMI: Weight (kg) ÷ Stature (cm) ÷ Stature (cm) x 10,000
or Weight (lb) ÷ Stature (in) ÷ Stature (in) x 703

Published May 30, 2000 (modified 10/16/00).
SOURCE: Developed by the National Center for Health Statistics in collaboration with
the National Center for Chronic Disease Prevention and Health Promotion (2000).
http://www.cdc.gov/growthcharts

From Kuczmarski RJ, Ogden CL, Guo SS, et al. *2000 CDC Growth Charts for the United States: Methods and Development.* National Center for Health Statistics. Vital Health Statistics. Series II, Number 246. May 2002. Accessed at: http://www.cdc.gov/growthcharts

Figure 20.8 Girls, 2–20 Years: Body Mass Index-for-Age Percentiles

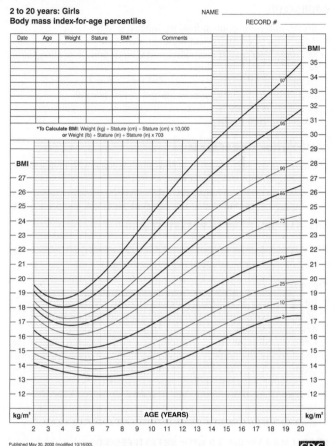

2 to 20 years: Girls
Body mass index-for-age percentiles

NAME _____

RECORD # _____

*To Calculate BMI: Weight (kg) ÷ Stature (cm) ÷ Stature (cm) x 10,000
or Weight (lb) ÷ Stature (in) ÷ Stature (in) x 703

Published May 30, 2000 (modified 10/16/00).
SOURCE: Developed by the National Center for Health Statistics in collaboration with
the National Center for Chronic Disease Prevention and Health Promotion (2000).
http://www.cdc.gov/growthcharts

Form Kuczmarski RJ, Ogden CL, Guo SS, et al. *2000 CDC Growth Charts for the United States: Methods and
Development.* National Center for Health Statistics. Vital Health Statistics. Series II, Number 246. May 2002.
Accessed at: http://www.cdc.gov/growthcharts

Growth and Nutrition

20

COUNSELING

- Breast milk is the optimal food for infants
- Advantages: maternal–infant bonding, sterile, convenient, economical, protection against respiratory and GI infections, low allergenicity, and low renal solute load
- Exclusive breastfeeding recommended for the first 6 mo of life
- Breastfeeding may continue for up to 2 yr and beyond
- Both breasts should be offered at each feeding, for a minimum of 10 min on each breast

COMPOSITION OF BREAST MILK

- Colostrum for first 24–48 h: yellow, small volume with high protein, immunoglobulin and low-fat content
- Breast milk energy: 67 kcal/100 mL
- Composed of carbohydrate (40% calories), fat (55%), and protein (5%)

CONTRAINDICATIONS TO BREASTFEEDING

Baby

- Inborn errors of metabolism (e.g., galactosemia)

Mother

- Infections such as HIV/AIDS, herpes in breast region, or active, untreated tuberculosis (may not be absolute contraindications in developing world)
- Certain medications (e.g., chemotherapy, metronidazole, tetracycline, cyclosporine, doxorubicin, ergotamine, lithium); refer to Motherrisk (http://www.motherrisk.org) for complete list
- Radioactive materials for diagnosis or treatment
- Alcohol/drug abuse
- Note: maternal CMV, hepatitis, and antibiotic-treated mastitis are *not* contraindications; most medications safe to take while breastfeeding

PROBLEMS ASSOCIATED WITH BREASTFEEDING

- See Table 20.7

ENTERAL NUTRITION

FEEDING SELECTION (<1 YR OLD)

- If breast milk unavailable, contraindicated, or mother chooses not to breastfeed, best alternative is commercially available infant formula (Table 20.8)

Table 20.7	Onset, Characteristics, and Management of Common Problems Associated With Breast Feeding		
	Onset	**Characteristics**	**Management**
Baby			
Breastfeeding jaundice	Usually in the first week of life	Exaggeration of physiologic jaundice due to poor intake and dehydration. Baby usually >10% below birth weight	Encourage frequent breast-feeding; lactation consultant; may need lactation aid and phototherapy
Breast milk jaundice	Usually after the first week of life	Caused by an enzyme (glucuronidase) in breast milk which inhibits the conjugation of bilirubin in the liver. Bilirubin usually normalizes over 3–10 wk; may persist longer	Early onset jaundice is NOT breast milk jaundice and must be investigated and treated appropriately. Ensure no conjugated hyperbiliru-binemia (see p. xx). No need to stop breastfeeding
Oral candidiasis/ thrush		Appears as white plaques on buccal mucosa, palate, tongue, or the oropharynx	Treat baby with antifungal (nystatin, gentian violet). Treat mother's nipples topically
Mother			
Sore/cracked nipples	Anytime	May lead to bloody stool in the baby. Normal nipple sensitivity typically subsides within 1 min of suckling	Ensure proper positioning and good latch. Apply breast milk to nipples after each feed and allow to air dry. Avoid soap. May apply creams (e.g., lanolin)
Breast engorgement	Occurs most often in the first week	Due to accumulated milk. May be exaggerated by poor feeding	Encourage more frequent feeding; may require pumping
Mastitis	Anytime	Infection of the breast, usually due to *S. aureus*. Typically presents as a hard, red, tender, swollen area of one breast associated with fever	Continue breastfeeding, ensure adequate emptying of affected side. Treat mother with antibiotics, compresses. Monitor for abscess which may require drainage

Table 20.8 Nutrition Content per Liter of Infant Feed*

	Milk		Cow's Milk–Based Formulas					Soy-Based Formulas		Premature		Common Therapeutic Formulas				
		Human	Enfamil A+	Similac Advance	Goodstart	Enfalac LF	Enfamil A+ for Babies Who Spit Up	Isomil	ProSobee	Similac Advance Special Care (20)	Similac Advance Neosure	Nutramigen	Alimentum	Pregestimil	Portagen	Neocate (Elemental)
Indication(s)	Optimal		Term, Preterm >2000 g & Breast Milk Not Available		Risk Cow's Milk Protein Allergy	Lactose Intolerance	Mild to Moderate GERD	Lactose Intolerance, Risk of Cow's Milk Protein Allergy, Galactosemia		Preterm <2000 g	Transitional for ELBW Infants at Term	Cow's Milk Protein Allergy	Protein ± Fat Malabsorption		Fat Malabsorption	Malabsorption
Calories	680	680	680	680	670	680	680	680	680	680	750	680	680	680	670	670
Protein (g)	10	10	14.5	14	15	14	17	17	17	18	20	19	19	19	24	21
Whey:casein	70:30	70:30	60:40	48:52	100:0	18:82	18:82	–	–	60:40	50:50	0:100	0:100	0:100	0:100	–
Fat (g)	39	39	36	37	34	35	34	37	36	37	41	34	38	38	32	30
CHO (g)	72	72	74	73	75	73	74	70	72	72	77	75	69	69	77	78
Na+ (mmol)	7.8	7.8	8	7	7.8	8.7	11.7	13	10.4	15.2	10.8	11	13	12	15	11
K+ (mmol)	13.5	13.5	18.7	18	18.5	19	18.7	18.7	21	21.2	27.4	19	21	19	22	27

(continued)

Table 20.8   Nutrition Content per Liter of Infant Feed* (continued)

	Milk	Cow's Milk–Based Formulas					Soy-Based Formulas		Premature		Common Therapeutic Formulas				
	Human	Enfamil A+	Similac Advance	Goodstart	Enfalac-LF	Enfamil A+ for Babies Who Spit Up	Isomil	ProSobee	Similac Advance Special Care (20)	Similac Advance Neosure	Nutramigen	Alimentum	Pregestimil	Portagen	Neocate (Elemental)
Indication(s)	Optimal	Term, Preterm >2000 g & Breast Milk Not Available		Risk Cow's Milk Protein Allergy	Lactose Intolerance	Mild to Moderate GERD	Lactose Intolerance, Risk of Cow's Milk Protein Allergy, Galactosemia		Preterm <2000 g	Transitional for ELBW Infants at Term	Cow's Milk Protein Allergy	Protein ± Fat Malabsorption		Fat Malabsorption	Malabsorption
Ca²⁺ (mmol)	7	13.2	13.2	10.7	13.7	13.2	17.5	17.8	25.2	19.8	15.7	17.8	15.7	15.8	20.8
Fe (mg)	0.4	12	12	10	12	12	12	12	2.5	14	12	12	12	13	10
Vit D (mcg)	5	10.2	10	10	10	10	10	10.2	25.5	13.3	7.5	7.5	8	5	8.7
Osmolality (mOsm/kg/H₂O)	290	300	300	265	200	230	240	200	240	250	294	370	330	230	375

*Note: Not all electrolytes and vitamins are listed above.

© The Hospital for Sick Children. Adapted from Hospital for Sick Children. *Formulary of Infant and Enteral Formulas.* Toronto, Ontario, Canada: Hospital for Sick Children; 2006.

FEEDING FREQUENCY AND VOLUME

- See Table 20.9

Table 20.9	Feeding Frequency and Volume	
Age	Feeds/Day	Approximate Quantity/Feed
Birth-1 wk	6-10	2-3 oz (60-90 mL)
1 wk-1 mo	6-8	3-4 oz (90-120 mL)
1-3 mo	5-6	4-6 oz (120-180 mL)
3-7 mo	4-5	6-7 oz (180-210 mL)
7-12 mo	3-4	7-8 oz (210-240 mL)

Adapted from Kalnins D, Saab J. *Better Baby Food: Your Essential Guide to Nutrition, Feeding and Cooking for All Babies and Toddlers.* Toronto, Ontario, Canada: Robert Rose Inc.; 2001: 23.

FEEDING SELECTION (>1 YR OLD)

- For children >1 yr of age, determine appropriate feeding selection for children requiring nutritional supplementation (Table 20.10)

INCREASING ENERGY/NUTRIENT DENSITY OF FEED

- Indications for increasing caloric content of feeds: fluid restriction, increased energy requirements, feeding difficulties, weight loss/poor weight gain
- Nutrients such as fat (corn oil, Microlipid, MCT oil), carbohydrates (Caloreen, Polycose), and/or protein (ProMod) may be used
- Concentrating infant feedings increases energy density and provides additional nutrients; however, it also increases osmolality and renal solute load
- Precaution: infant feeds should only be concentrated to a *max* of 4 g protein/kg unless warranted by medical condition because of risk of renal impairment from high solute load
- Energy density of breast milk and standard full-strength infant formulas = 2800 kJ/L = 67 kcal/100 mL = 20 kcal/fl oz
- Most standard pediatric enteral formulas for children >1 yr of age come ready to feed and contain 4200 kJ/L = 100 kcal/100 mL = 30 kcal/fl oz
- Breast milk caloric and nutrient content may be increased with commercially available human milk fortifier
- Follow recommended stepwise progression of energy density in enteral feeding (Table 20.11)

Table 20.10 Nutrient Content per Liter of Enteral Formulas*

	Tube Feeds				Oral Supplements			Malabsorption				Renal	
	Nutren Junior	Nutren Junior Fiber With Prebio	Isosource HN	Isosource HN With Fiber	Resource	Resource Plus	Resource Fruit Beverage	Peptamen/ Peptamen Jr	Tolerex	Vital HN	Vivonex Pediatric	Suplena	Novasource Renal
Indication(s)	Can Use Orally	3.6 g/L Prefiber 2 g/L Prebio (Probiotic), Can Use Orally	High Protein	12 g/L Soy Fiber, High Protein	Can Use as Tube Feed	Energy Dense; Can Tube Feed	Use as Clear Fluid	Impaired GI Function, Oral/Tube Feed	Impaired GI Function, Tube Feed			Restricted Protein	High Protein Needs
Ages	Children 1-2 yr		Children 2-12 yr		Children >12 yr			"Jr" = Children 1-9 yr			Children 1-9 yr	Children >4 yr	
Calories	1000	1000	1200	1200	1060	1520	770	1000/1000	1000	1000	800	2000	2000
Protein (g)	30	30	53	53	38	55	37	40/30	21	42	24	30	74
Fat (g)	50	50	42	42	25	46	2	39/38	1.5	11	24	96	100
CHO (g)	110	110	151	157	170	220	150	128/136	230	186	130	250	200
Na$^+$ (mmol)	20	20	49	49	40	57	13	24/20	20	25	17	30	39
K$^+$ (mmol)	34	34	46	46	38	50	1.1	38/34	30	36	31	28	21
Ca^{2+} (mmol)	25	25	25	25	37	32	14	20/25	14	17	24	35	32.5

(continued)

Growth and Nutrition

Table 20.10 Nutrient Content per Liter of Enteral Formulas* (continued)

	Tube Feeds				Oral Supplements			Malabsorption				Renal	
	Nutren Junior	Nutren Junior Fiber With Prebio	Isosource HN	Isosource HN With Fiber	Resource	Resource Plus	Resource Fruit Beverage	Peptamen/ Peptamen Jr	Tolerex	Vital HN	Vivonex Pediatric	Suplena	Novasource Renal
Indication(s)	Can Use Orally	3.6 g/L Prefiber 2 g/L Prebio (Probiotic), Can Use Orally	High Protein	12 g/L Soy Fiber, High Protein	Can Use as Tube Feed	Energy Dense; Can Tube Feed	Use as Clear Fluid	Impaired GI Function, Oral/Tube Feed	Impaired GI Function, Tube Feed			Restricted Protein	High Protein Needs
Ages	Children 1-2 yr		Children 2-12 yr		Children >12 yr			"yr" = Children 1-9 yr			Children 1-9 yr	Children >4 yr	
Fe (mg)	14	14	12	12	19	19	9.5	18/14	10	12	10	19	18
Vit D (mcg)	7.5	7.5	6.75	6.75	8.5	10.5	5.3	6.75/7.5	5.5	7	8	2	2
Osmolality (mOsm/kg/H2O)	350	350	435	435	600	870	700	270/360	550	460	360	600	700
Free water (mL)	850	850	813	813	840	766	881	850/850	864	867	893	719	709

*Note: Not all electrolytes and vitamins are listed above.
© The Hospital for Sick Children. Adapted from Hospital for Sick Children. Formulary of Infant and Enteral Formulas. Toronto, Ontario, Canada: Hospital for Sick Children; 2006.

Table 20.11	Stepwise Progression for Energy Density of Enteral Feedings	
Kilojoules/Liter	**Kilocalories/Milliliter**	**Kilocalories/Fluid Ounce**
2800	0.67	20
3300	0.8	24
3800	0.9	27
4200	1.0	30
4600	1.1	33
5000	1.2	36

© The Hospital for Sick Children. From Hospital for Sick Children. *Guidelines for the Administration of Enteral and Parenteral Nutrition in Pediatrics.* Toronto, Ontario, Canada: Hospital for Sick Children; 2007.

THICKENING FEEDS

- Indications to thicken feeds: known or suspected aspiration risk (failed feeding study, history of aspiration/suspected aspiration pneumonia, choking/gagging with feeds, severe neurologic impairment)
- If aspiration from above suspected, feeding assessment by occupational therapist recommended
- GER symptoms may improve with thickened feeds
- 1 tbsp of infant cereal/30–120 mL of infant formula is recommended for GER management
  - Note: EBM does not thicken with infant cereal

VITAMIN AND MINERAL SUPPLEMENTATION

Vitamin D

- Preterm infants (until 1 yr): 200-400 IU/d intake from all sources
- Full-term infants: 400 IU/d, with an increase to 800 IU/d between October and April in northern communities
- Commercially available formulas fortified with vitamin D; supplementation not required
- Minimum recommended dietary vitamin D intake for children >1 yr = 400 IU/d

Iron Deficiency

- Iron stores normally adequate for first 4–6 mo of life
- Breastfed infants require alternate iron source by 6 mo, usually provided by iron-fortified infant cereals
- Formula-fed infants should use iron-fortified formulas; no evidence of increased GI symptoms
- Preterm infants: start iron supplements by 8 wk of age
- Recommended daily iron intake: 7 mg/d for term infants 5–12 mo, 6 mg/d for toddlers 1–3 yr, 8 mg/d for children 4–12 yr
- Risk factors for iron-deficiency anemia in infants: premature birth, early feeding of cow's milk, poor dietary consumption of iron-containing first foods
- Risk factors for iron deficiency anemia in older children: consumption of large amounts (>16–20 oz/d) of milk with minimal solid food intake, prolonged breastfeeding, vegan or vegetarian diets
- Cow's milk should not be introduced until 9–12 mo of age

Fluoride Supplementation

- Supplementation required for infants 6 mo–2 yr if water fluoride concentration <0.3 ppm

NURSING BOTTLE CARIES

- Common causes: use of bottle with sugar-containing beverage (milk/juice) during sleep, pacifiers dipped in sugar/syrup/honey, bottle-feeding >12 mo of age
- Prevention: avoid bottles during sleep time (unless water only), discourage long-term use of baby bottles beyond approximately 12 mo

TRANSITION TO SOLIDS

- See Table 20.12
- 6-mo-olds usually physiologically and developmentally ready for new foods and textures
- Do not give skimmed/partly skimmed milk to children <2 yr; some guidelines suggest role for lowfat milk at 1 yr in children at very high risk of obesity
- Avoid egg whites and added sugar or salt until 1 yr
- Avoid peanut products until 18–24 mo
- Single new foods should not be introduced more frequently than every 3 d—slower if family history of allergy; combination foods added after known whether the single foods are tolerated
- Progression to safe finger and table foods takes place at ~9–12 mo when developmentally ready to feed self
- By 12 mo, should be eating foods from all four food groups and be on schedule of three meals and two to three snacks a day

Table 20.12 Transition to Solid Foods

Food	0–6 mo	6–7 mo	7–9 mo	9–12 mo
Iron-fortified infant cereal and other grains	–	May start to introduce infant cereals: rice, barley, or oatmeal; feed with a spoon; start with 1–2 teaspoons, progress to 2–4 tablespoons twice daily	Continue with infant cereal, 2–4 tablespoons twice daily; introduce other grain products such as baby biscuits, unsalted crackers, pasta	Continue with infant cereal. Introduce other plain cereals, bread, rice, and pasta, 8–10 tablespoons a day
Vegetables and fruits	–	–	Offer pureed cooked vegetables. Progress to soft mashed cooked vegetables, 4–6 tablespoons a day. Offer pureed cooked fruits, very ripe mashed fruit (banana), 6–7 tablespoons a day	Offer mashed or diced cooked soft vegetables, 6–10 tablespoons a day. Offer soft fresh fruits, peeled, seeded, and diced or canned fruit, 7–10 tablespoons a day
Meat and alternatives	–	–	After vegetables and fruit, offer pureed cooked meat, fish, chicken, tofu, mashed beans, egg yolk, 1–3 tablespoons a day	Offer ground or chopped meat, fish, chicken, tofu, beans, egg yolk, 3–4 tablespoons a day
Milk and dairy products	–	–	Offer plain yogurt (3.25% MF or higher), cottage cheese, or grated hard cheese, 1–2 tablespoons a day.	Introduce whole (homogenized) cow's milk. Progress from bottle to cup. Continue with plain yogurt, cottage or other cheese, 2–4 tablespoons a day

Adapted from Kalnins D, Saab J. Better Baby Food: Your Essential Guide to Nutrition, Feeding and Cooking for All Babies and Toddlers. Toronto, Ontario, Canada: Robert Rose Inc; 2001: 36; and from Feeding Your Baby [pamphlet]; and from Dairy Farmers of Ontario. 1999.

Growth and Nutrition

20

OTHER FLUIDS

- Tap water, well water meeting safety standards, and commercially bottled water (not mineral or carbonated) are generally suitable for infants to reconstitute powdered formula
- Bring all water for feeding infants <4 mo to boil for at least 2 min
- Limit use of fruit juice to avoid interfering with intake of milk and nutrient-containing foods
- Herbal teas and other beverages are of no known benefit to an infant and may be harmful

FOOD SAFETY

- To prevent infant botulism, honey should not be fed to infants <1 yr of age
- To prevent salmonella poisoning, eggs should be cooked well; products made with raw eggs should not be fed to infants <1 yr of age
- Hard, small, round, smooth, and sticky solid foods present potential choking and aspiration risk in children <4 yr of age; unsafe foods include hot dogs, grapes, peanuts, raisins, and raw vegetables and fruits not cut in small pieces
- Infants and children should not be left unattended at mealtime and should eat while in an upright position, not while walking, running, or lying down

VEGETARIAN DIET

- Well-planned vegetarian diet with adequate nutrients and energy can meet growth and nutrition needs at any age
- Commercial soy-based formula is recommended until 2 yr of age for vegan infants who are not breastfed; after 2 yr of age, fortified or enriched soy-based milk should be used
- Monitor intake of total calories, protein, iron, vitamin B_{12}, zinc, calcium, and vitamin D

PARENTERAL NUTRITION

- Indications: unable to ingest and/or absorb enterally delivered nutrition for significant period of time ($\geq$2–3 d in infants, $\geq$4–5 d in older children), chylothorax not managed by MCT formulas (20% and 30% lipids may be used because they do not enter the lymphatic system)
- Newborns who are not expected to feed enterally until $\geq$2–3 d of life should be started on electrolyte-free PN within the first hours of life
- PN may provide full nutrition or partial supplementation
- PN is routinely administered as TNA; amino acids, glucose, and lipids delivered in single bag

- In areas where specialized electrolyte and mineral additions may affect stability of solution (e.g., bone marrow transplantation unit, NICU), PN is delivered as separate amino acid/glucose and lipid solutions (Table 20.13)
- Solutions containing ≤12.5% glucose *and* with an osmolality <1050 mOsm/L can be delivered through peripheral venous access

Table 20.13	Composition of Parenteral Nutrition Solutions				
Variable	P-5/-7.5	P-10*	PI-10*	I-10*/I-20*†	C-30†
Calories (kcal/mL)	0.23/0.31	0.42	0.42	0.46/0.80	1.22
Amino acids (g/L)	15	20	20	30	50
Dextrose (g/L)	50/75	100	100	100/200	300
Sodium (mmol/L)	20	20	30	30	30
Potassium (mmol/L)	20	20	30	30	30
Chloride (mmol/L)	21.1	17.2	31.3	32.1	30.0
Calcium (mmol/L)	9	12	12	9	9
Phosphate (mmol/L)	9	12	12	9	9
Magnesium (mmol/L)	3	4	4	4	4
Zinc (µmol/L)	46	46	46	46	46
Copper (µmol/L)	6.3	6.3	6.3	6.3	6.3
Manganese (µmol/L)	1.8	1.8	1.8	5	5
Iodide (µmol/L)	0.47	0.47	0.47	0.47	0.47
Chromium (µmol/L)	0.076	0.076	0.076	0.076	0.076
Selenium (µmol/L)	0.25	0.25	0.25	0.25	0.25
Iron (µmol/L)	Nil	Nil	Nil	18	18
Acetate (mmol/L)	1.4	Nil	5.4	6.1	81.5
Osmolarity (mOsm/L)	485/611	769	824	874/1378	2101
pH (approximate)	5.97/5.91	5.85	5.91	5.62/5.50	5.85

*Available as TNA, containing 20% fat emulsion. Note: 1.2-µL in-line filter must be used during administration.
†Must be administered via CVL only.
© The Hospital for Sick Children. From Hospital for Sick Children. *Guidelines for the Administration of Enteral and Parenteral Nutrition in Pediatrics.* Toronto, Ontario, Canada: Hospital for Sick Children; 2007.

Growth and Nutrition

20

NUTRITIONAL REQUIREMENTS

- PN should be initiated in stepwise fashion to minimize complications associated with overdelivery
- Energy requirements vary but approximately 10–15% less than with enteral feedings (minimal energy requirement of digestion)
- Sufficient calories from nonprotein sources (fats and carbohydrates) ensure amino acids are used for anabolism and not as source of energy
- PN lipids are isotonic; 20% lipid emulsion should be used for all patients except those who are severely fluid restricted, in whom 30% lipid emulsion may be necessary to meet needs (Table 20.14)
- Note: do *not* give IV lipids to patients with allergy to egg or soy

Table 20.14	Composition of Lipid Emulsions	
	20% Lipids	**30% Lipids**
Calories (kcal/mL)	2	3
Fat (g/mL)	0.2	0.3

© The Hospital for Sick Children. From Hospital for Sick Children. *Guidelines for the Administration of Enteral and Parenteral Nutrition in Pediatrics.* Toronto, Ontario, Canada: Hospital for Sick Children; 2007.

APPROACH TO ORDERING PN

1. Based on patient's weight and desired TFI, determine max total fluid rate per hour (TFI [mL/kg/d] × weight [kg] ÷ 24 h)
2. Summate hourly rate of other fluids (if applicable) and subtract from hourly max rate to determine rate available for PN
3. If ordering lipids separate from amino acid/glucose solution, start with 1 g/kg lipids; in general, fat emulsion 20% if fluid liberalized, fat emulsion 30% if fluid restricted; example for a 10-kg baby: fat emulsion 20% contains 200 g lipids per 1000 mL: (1 g/kg × 10 kg) × 1000 mL/200 g ÷ 24 h/d = desired rate (mL/h)
4. If using a premixed amino acid/glucose solution, select an appropriate PN for age (P, preterm; I, infant; C, child)
5. Determine recommended protein intake for age (see Table 20.1); similar calculation as for lipids; preterm standard solutions contain 20 g amino acids per 1000 mL (30 g amino acids per 1000 mL for infant and child solutions); example for a 10-kg baby: (1 g/kg × 10 kg) × 1000 mL/30 g ÷ 24 h/d = desired rate (mL/h)
6. See Table 20.15 for recommendations on initiation and advancement of PN

	Amino Acid (g/kg/d)	Fat (g/kg/d)	Carbohydrate (mg/kg/min)
Table 20.15 Guidelines for Initiating and Advancing Parenteral Nutrition			
Stage			
Preterm infants:			
Initial	1	0.5–1*	5–8
Daily advancement	0.5–1	0.5–1	1–2
Maximum	2.7–3.5	3–4	11–12
Term infants/children:			
Initial	1–1.5	1	7–9
Daily advancement	1	1	1–3
Maximum	2.5–3	4	11–12
Older children and adolescents:			
Initial	1.5–2	1	3–5
Daily advancement	–	1	1–3
Maximum	1.5–2	2–4	5–8

*Small preterm infants <1 kg should be started at smaller dose.
© The Hospital for Sick Children. From Hospital for Sick Children. *Guidelines for the Administration of Enteral and Parenteral Nutrition in Pediatrics*, Toronto, Ontario, Canada: Hospital for Sick Children; 2007.

CONSIDERATIONS IN MANAGEMENT

Weaning From PN

- Rate of PN solution should be tapered at a 1:1 ratio as enteral intake increases
- When rate of solution approximates 25% of original order, PN may be discontinued and replaced by appropriate solution (D5W or D10W) to account for the remaining fluid
- Lipids may be stopped completely without tapering the rate

Cycling PN

- Cycling may decrease risk of cholestasis, allow administration of incompatible medications, increase patient freedom for ambulation, help wean off PN
- Note: sudden cessation of PN solution with high glucose concentration (>15%) may result in rebound hypoglycemia; tapering should take place over 1–2 h, with half the full PN rate given over the first ½–1 h and one quarter of full rate over the second ½–1 h
- Calculations for infused nutrients should be made over total amount of time infusion is running, not over 24 h (e.g., calculate over 20 h if patient is off for 4 h)

Monitoring PN
- See Table 20.16
- Daily weights and fluid balance
- PN blood tests (as recommended in Table 20.16) may not be necessary if done in previous 24 h, if enteral feedings exceed 50% of total fluid intake, or in long-term PN patients (weekly monitoring may be sufficient)

COMPLICATIONS OF PN

Short-Term

Hyperglycemia
- Most commonly seen in infants <1000 g or receiving steroid therapy or excess glucose intake in the infusion, or with physiologic stressors (postoperative or trauma patients)
- Determine glucose intake based on the GIR (mg/kg/min):

$$\frac{\text{Volume per 24 h of amino acid/dextrose solution (L)} \times \text{dextrose (g)/solution (L)} \times 1000 \text{ mg/g}}{\# \text{ hours of infusion} \times 60 \text{ min/h} \times \text{patient's weight (kg)}}$$

- Treatment options: decrease PN glucose (and substitute with fat calories); decrease the rate of PN; use a solution with less dextrose to make up TFI
- Rarely, insulin treatment required if unable to deliver sufficient nutrition or glucocorticosteroids necessary

Hypoglycemia
- At risk: glucose infusion is abruptly decreased, small-for-gestational-age infants, low rate of PN delivery
- Management: ensure gradual weaning from PN to avoid rebound hypoglycemia, ensure minimum GIR is provided, may slowly increase rate or concentration of glucose from 6 mg/kg/min to 11–12 mg/kg/min over 4–5 d, as indicated

Hyperlipidemia
- Lipid clearance may be decreased in premature infants and some malnourished, septic, and/or acutely ill patients; excess fat may interfere with host defenses
- Sepsis is not an absolute contraindication for IV lipid use; however, careful monitoring is imperative for determining clearance
- If intralipid level 1.0–1.5 g/L: cut lipid dose in half and repeat level
- If intralipid level >1.5 g/L: hold lipid dose for 24 h and repeat level
- For hematology/oncology patients: hold dose if intralipid level >1.0 g/L due to potential lipid effect on platelet function; restart at lower dose when intralipid level <1.0 g/L

Table 20.16	Monitoring Schedule for Stable Patients on Parenteral Nutrition		
Parameter	**At Start of Therapy**	**Monday**	**Thursday**
Glucose	Yes	Yes	Yes
Electrolytes	Yes	Yes	Yes
Intralipid level	No	Yes	Yes
Complete blood count	No	Yes	No
Urea, PO_4^-, Ca^{2+}, conjugated bilirubin, albumin, Mg^{2+}	Yes	Yes	No
Aspartate aminotransferase (AST), alkaline phosphatase, creatinine, blood gas	Yes	If indicated	If indicated

© The Hospital for Sick Children. From Hospital for Sick Children. *Guidelines for the Administration of Enteral and Parenteral Nutrition in Pediatrics,* Toronto, Ontario, Canada: Hospital for Sick Children; 2007.

Electrolyte and/or Mineral Imbalances

* May be necessary to alter electrolyte and/or mineral content of standard PN solutions to meet increased or decreased needs of specific nutrients
* May require CVL access for administration of higher concentrations of certain electrolytes

Long-Term

PN Cholestasis

* Patients most at risk: lack of enteral nutrition, previously or currently receiving long-term PN, previous GI surgery, history of prematurity and/or recurrent sepsis
* Can be reversed on introduction to enteral nutrition and weaning, cycling, discontinuing PN; consider discontinuing manganese, as can be hepatotoxic

FAILURE TO THRIVE

* FTT: weight <3rd percentile, or decrease in growth velocity resulting in weight and/or height crossing ≥2 percentiles, or weight <80% predicted weight for height
* Nonorganic/primary FTT: no other chronic disease or illness present
* Organic/secondary FTT: occurs in presence of, or associated with, chronic disease
* May be mixed causes: medical illness + psychosocial factors

FTT DIFFERENTIAL DIAGNOSIS

* See Figure 20.9

Figure 20.9 Differential Diagnosis of Failure to Thrive

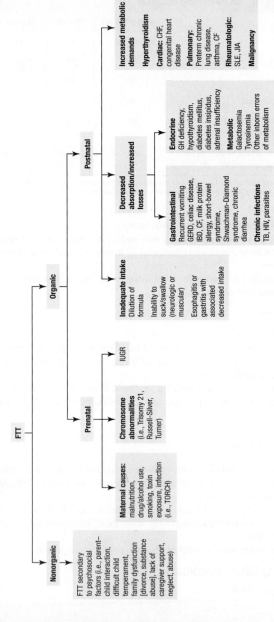

TORCH, toxoplasmosis, other agents, rubella, cytomegalovirus, and herpes simplex virus; *IUGR*, intrauterine growth restriction; *GERD*, gastroesophageal reflux disease; *IBD*, inflammatory bowel disease; *CF*, cystic fibrosis; *TB*, tuberculosis; *HIV*, human immunodeficiency virus; *GH*, growth hormone; *CHF*, congestive heart failure; *SLE*, systemic lupus erythematosus; *JIA*, juvenile idiopathic arthritis.

APPROACH TO FTT

History

- Detailed diet history: duration/quantity of feeds, dilution of formula, juice intake
- Emesis, diarrhea, urinary frequency, fevers, prior growth velocity
- Past medical history, developmental milestones, detailed social history (i.e., caregivers, psychosocial stressors, parental mental illness/substance abuse, social services involvement), parental heights/weights, thorough review of systems
- Birth history: small for gestational age, intrauterine growth restriction, prematurity, intrauterine infections, maternal substance abuse

Physical Examination

- Plot height, weight, head circumference (compare to prior measurements)
- Full physical examination with special attention to hydration status, dysmorphic features, wasting, signs of chronic disease, signs of abuse/poor hygiene
- Observe parent–child interaction and child's temperament

Investigations

- Feeding observation, diet journal, 3-d food records
- Assessment by occupational therapist/social worker, as indicated; consider hospitalization to assess weight gain/observe feeding
- CBC, electrolytes, urinalysis, urea, creatinine, liver enzymes and function, albumin
- Other tests, as indicated by history and physical examination, may include sweat chloride, tissue transglutaminase, thyroid function tests, immunoglobulins, 72-h fecal fat collection, α1-AT clearance, fat-soluble vitamin levels, carotene, stool for reducing substances, stool for ova and parasites, Mantoux test, HIV testing, pH probe for GERD, gastric emptying studies, and indirect calorimetry, if suspect elevated metabolic rate

Treatment

- Variable, depending on etiology
- Increase energy density of feedings (see Table 20.11)
- Energy-boosting techniques: add butter, margarine, whipping cream to foods to increase energy density of everyday foods; use high-energy drinks
- Involvement of psychologist/social worker, if issues with parent–child interactions
- Behavioral therapy related to feeding, if available
- Assess for tube feeding if attempts at increasing energy intake orally are unsuccessful

FURTHER READING

Committee on Nutrition, American Academy of Pediatrics. *Pediatric Nutrition Handbook*. 4th ed. Elk Grove Village, Ill: American Academy of Pediatrics; 1998.

Kalnins D, Saab J. *The Hospital for Sick Children. Better Baby Food*. Toronto, Ontario, Canada: Robert Rose; 2001.

Tsang RC, Zlotkin SH, Nichols BL, et al. *Nutrition During Infancy, Principles and Practice*. 2nd ed. Cincinnati, Ohio: Digital Educational Publishing; 1997.

USEFUL WEB SITES

Nutrition for healthy term infants—statement of the Joint Working Group: Canadian Paediatric Society, Dieticians of Canada, and Health Canada (2005). Available at: www.hc-sc.gc.ca/fn-an/pubs/infant-nourrisson/nut_infant_nourrisson_term_e.html#table

American Dietetic Association. Available at: www.eatright.org

American Society for Parenteral and Enteral Nutrition. Available at: www.nutritioncare.org

Growth and Nutrition

20

Chapter 21 Gynecology

Dalia Alabdulrazzaq

Lisa M. Allen

Chapter 21 Gynecology

COMMON ABBREVIATIONS

AFP	alpha fetoprotein
β-hCG	β-human chorionic gonadotropin
BV	bacterial vaginosis
DHEAS	dehydroepiandrosterone
DUB	dysfunctional uterine bleeding
EBV	Epstein-Barr virus
EUA	examination under anesthesia
FSH	follicle-stimulating hormone
GU	genitourinary
IUD	intrauterine device
LDH	lactate dehydrogenase
LH	luteinizing hormone
NAAT	nucleic acid amplification testing
NSAIDs	nonsteroidal anti-inflammatory drugs
OCP	oral contraceptive pill
PCOS	polycystic ovary syndrome
PID	pelvic inflammatory disease
STI	sexually transmitted infection
TP-PA	*Treponema pallidum* particle agglutination
TSH	thyroid-stimulating hormone
VDRL	Venereal Disease Research Laboratory

ANATOMY OF THE EXTERNAL GENITALIA

- See Figure 21.1

GENITAL EXAMINATION OF PEDIATRIC AND ADOLESCENT FEMALES

GENITAL EXAMINATION OF THE PREPUBERTAL CHILD

- Put child at ease with caregiver visible and appropriate draping and lighting
- Two common techniques:
  1. Frog-leg position: supine with feet together and knees apart either on examination table or caregiver's lap; inspect external genitalia; apply gentle separation and traction on the labia minora in a lateral and slightly posterior direction to allow visualization of the lower third of vagina and hymenal ring

Figure 21.1 **The Vulva and Perineum**

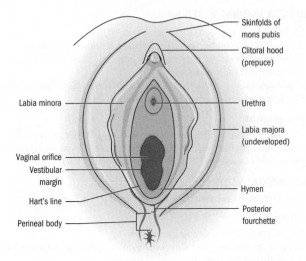

Skinfolds of mons pubis

Clitoral hood (prepuce)

Labia minora

Urethra

Labia majora (undeveloped)

Vaginal orifice

Vestibular margin

Hart's line

Hymen

Posterior fourchette

Perineal body

Gynecology

2. Knee–chest position: allows inspection of the upper vagina and possibly cervix

- Depending on necessity of examination and anxiety of patient, may require topical anesthetics, midazolam, ice pack, cool compresses, or an EUA
- *Never* force an examination
- Speculums not used in prepubertal children; if better visibility required, cystoscope or vaginoscope may be used (under anesthesia or conscious sedation)

GENITAL EXAMINATION OF THE ADOLESCENT

- Discuss each part of examination with patient; offer chaperone
- Inspect external genitalia, noting Tanner stage (see Chapter 15)
- Modify pelvic examination according to sexual activity; in virginal patients: vaginal swabs, hymenal inspection, and rectoabdominal palpation may be appropriate, depending on complaint; in sexually active patients: speculums and bimanual vaginal–abdominal examinations to palpate adnexa and uterus

21

VAGINAL BLEEDING

NEONATAL VAGINAL BLEEDING
- Usually occurs between day of life 5 and 10
- Most often physiologic: maternal estrogen withdrawal leads to endometrial shedding; may see other estrogen effects (breast buds, pale engorged vaginal mucosa)
- Other rare causes: hematuria, gynecologic disease (infection, tumor), bleeding diathesis, urethral prolapse, sexual abuse

Management
- Observe; workup indicated only if suspicious of other causes: CBC, coagulation profile, vaginal swab, urine culture, referral to gynecologist to rule out lesions of upper and lower genital tract

PREPUBERTAL VAGINAL BLEEDING
- For differential diagnosis and clues on history, see Box 21.1

Examination
- Follow previous examination principles
- General examination including vital signs and dermatologic examination (petechiae, bruising, signs of trauma)
- Gynecologic examination (following previous principles) including Tanner staging and appropriate use of rectal and rectoabdominal examinations; external perineal examination usually sufficient
- Irrigation with warm saline to wash away collected vaginal blood may help visualization

Box 21.1	Differential Diagnosis of Prepubertal Vaginal Bleeding

- Trauma
  - Straddle injury
  - Penetrating injury (accidental vs. intentional/abuse)
- Vulvovaginitis—history of vaginal discharge
  - Nonspecific vulvitis—history of poor hygiene
  - Vaginitis secondary to infection (group A β-hemolytic streptococcus, *H. influenzae*, less commonly STIs)
- Foreign body
- Urethral mucosal prolapse—history of excessive Valsalva
- Lichen sclerosis
- Endocrine conditions
  - Precocious puberty—history of accelerated growth and pubertal development
  - Precocious menarche
- Exogenous hormone preparations
- Condyloma acuminatum
- Blood dyscrasia—history of bleeding from other sites
- Hemangioma
- Ovarian tumors (benign or malignant)
- Uterine/vaginal pathology (rare; benign or malignant)

Trauma

- Distinguish between straddle injury (force of body falling on an object) and penetrating injury
- High level of suspicion for nonaccidental injury required (see Chapter 10); ensure mechanism of injury on history matches examination; ask parents to bring in object involved in accident to help determine pattern of injuries
- Straddle injuries may result in ecchymoses of vulva and periclitoral folds, vulvar hematomas, lacerations of labia minora and periurethra; hymenal tear implies penetrating injury (accidental or abuse)
- Apply perineal pressure with ice pack for 15–20 min, then irrigate; penetrating injury usually requires EUA to document full extent; may extend through vaginal fornices into broad ligament; in extreme cases, may cause an acute abdomen
- Assess ability to void after trauma; deep lacerations or large hematomas may require Foley catheter
- Management depends on extent of injury, associated injuries, amount of bleeding, ability to void, predicted anatomic healing
- Superficial abrasion: treat with ice and compression
- Small laceration: may require suturing with sedation, 1–2% lidocaine, 4-0 Vicryl
- Deep lacerations, inability to visualize extent of hymenal laceration, and uncooperative child: refer to gynecologist for assessment
- Hematomas: conservative management with ice and compression, unless rapidly expanding

Precocious Puberty

- See Chapter 15

Urethral Prolapse

- History of increased intra-abdominal pressure or Valsalva (constipation, acute/chronic cough)
- Diagnosis on external genital examination: friable annular mass with urethra at center, separate from hymen and vagina
- Management: reassurance, estrogen creams, sitz baths; surgical excision required if large or persistent after medical treatment
- Treat initiating precipitant

Lichen Sclerosis

- Hourglass pattern around labia and perineum, often surrounding clitoris, vagina, and anus
- White and atrophic, parchmentlike, with possible excoriations, subepithelial hemorrhages; chronic ulceration, eventual loss of normal external architecture may occur
- No biopsy required if diagnostic appearance
- Symptoms include pruritus, pain, dysuria, dyschezia, constipation, encopresis

- Treatment: medium- to high-potency topical steroid ointment daily; may be tapered depending on response; often maintenance doses of low- to midpotency topical steroids required; avoid vulvar irritants such as perfumed lotions
- Secondary infection may require treatment with oral antibiotics

Foreign Body
- Persistent or recurrent vaginal discharge; often bloody
- Most common foreign body is toilet paper
- Rectal examination: may palpate foreign body in vagina
- Treatment: flushing of vagina with catheter or feeding tube; EUA may be required to remove any nonvisualized foreign bodies

POSTMENARCHAL VAGINAL BLEEDING
- See Box 21.2 for differential diagnosis
- Menorrhagia requiring admission most often secondary to DUB or coagulation disorders

Box 21.2	Differential Diagnosis of Abnormal Vaginal Bleeding in the Postmenarchal Adolescent

DUB
- Immaturity of hypothalamic–pituitary axis (within 2 yr of menarche onset)
- Anovulatory bleeding

PCOS

Pregnancy Complications
- Threatened, incomplete, or complete abortion
- Ectopic pregnancy

Blood Dyscrasia (e.g., ITP, von Willebrand disease)

Infections
- STIs
- PID
- Endometritis, cervicitis, vaginitis

Endocrine Disorders
- Hyperprolactinemia
- Hypo/hyperthyroidism
- Late-onset congenital adrenal hyperplasia
- Others

Chronic Illness

Medications
- Hormonal contraceptives
- Anticoagulants
- Androgens
- Spironolactone

Structural Lesion

Trauma (accidental vs. abuse)

Neoplasms (ovarian, vaginal, cervical)

- DUB: prolonged heavy irregular bleeding from endometrium in absence of structural or systemic disease
- Full history required: sexual history, medical conditions, pubertal development including menarche and menstrual history, medications, bleeding history
- Always consider pregnancy

Investigations
- Full physical examination
- CBC, coagulation profile, β-hCG, type and screen, TSH; consider prolactin, DHEAS, testosterone, FSH, LH, depending on clinical history
- Cervical swabs for *Chlamydia* and *Neisseria gonorrhoeae*, if sexually active
- Pelvic US if concern over structural abnormality or ovarian pathology

Management
- Based on etiology with goal of stopping acute bleeding and preventing recurrence and long-term sequelae
- See Box 21.3 for management of DUB

VULVOVAGINITIS
- See Table 21.1

Box 21.3 | **Management of Dysfunctional Uterine Bleeding**

Mild (no anemia: Hb >120)
- Reassurance, menstrual calendar, iron supplementation
- NSAIDs if dysmenorrhea (30–50% effective)
- OCP if require contraception or prefer cycle regulation

Moderate (anemia: Hb 80–120)
- Combined hormonal contraceptive agent (usually 30–35 mcg ethinyl estradiol dose of an OCP or transdermal contraceptive patch), prescribed either cyclically (28-d cycle) or continuous (extended regimen to avoid frequent withdrawal bleeding)
  OR
  Progestin (medroxyprogesterone acetate 5–10 mg or micronized progestin 100 mcg) daily for 10–14 d of the month: either day 1–14 of the month or day 14–27 of the month
- Iron supplementation

Severe (significant anemia: Hb <80 or unstable, ongoing bleeding)
- IV conjugated estrogen (Premarin) 25 mg IV q4–6h, max 4 doses in 24 h (followed by combined OCP to maintain endometrial stability)
  OR
  Ovral (50 mcg ethinyl estradiol) two tablets PO bid × 3 d, taper to one tablet PO bid, then taper to one tablet PO od to end of pack; immediately begin second pack of low-dose OCP either cyclically or continuously
- Need concomitant antiemetic therapy
- Transfuse, if clinically indicated
- Other options include DDAVP, antifibrinolytics (tranexamic acid), and surgical therapy (dilatation and curettage—extremely rare)

Table 21.1   Clinical and Laboratory Features of Common Causes of Vulvovaginitis

Clinical/Laboratory Features	Physiologic	Candida	Trichomonas	BV
Appearance of discharge	White, gray, or clear	White, with curdlike quality	Yellow, green, or gray	Gray or white
Vulvar/vaginal inflammation	None	Present	Occasional	Rare
pH of discharge	<4.5	<4.5	>4.5	>4.5
Microscopy	Epithelial cells, few WBCs, lactobacilli	WBCs; KOH: pseudohyphae and budding yeast in some patients	WBCs; saline prep: motile trichomonads in some patients	Few WBCs; saline prep: "clue cells" (vaginal epithelial cells)
Risk factors	Secretion of estrogen	Menstruation, antibiotics, diabetes, heat, moisture, OCPs, topical steroids, immunodeficiency	Other STIs	Sexual activity, douching, previous BV
Other clinical signs and symptoms	None	Itching, dysuria, dyspareunia	Vulvar itching, burning, dysuria, pelvic discomfort	Fishy odor
Whiff test (strong fishy odor on addition of 10% KOH to vaginal sample)	Negative	Negative	Sometimes positive	Positive
Management	Reassurance	Miconazole nitrate or clotrimazole intravaginally × 3–7 nights; terconazole for resistant strains Diflucan 150 mg PO × 1 dose for adolescent	Metronidazole 500 mg PO bid × 7 d	Metronidazole 500 mg PO bid × 7 d OR metronidazole gel 0.75%, applicator (5 g) once a day intravaginally for 5 d

Adapted from Zitelli BJ, Davis HW. Atlas of Pediatric Physical Diagnosis. 3rd ed. London, England: Mosby Wolfe; 1997.

PREPUBERTAL VULVOVAGINITIS

- See Box 21.4
- 85% of cases before puberty nonspecific
- Present with symptoms of nonbloody discharge, pruritus, frequency/dysuria, and erythema

---

Box 21.4 | **Differential Diagnosis of Prepubertal Vulvovaginitis**

Noninfectious
- Nonspecific vulvovaginitis (poor hygiene)
- Foreign body
- Contact dermatitis (chemical irritant)
- Trauma or abuse
- Dermatologic conditions

Infectious
- Group A β-hemolytic streptococcus, *H. influenzae* most common
- Pinworms
- STIs
- *Candida* uncommon before perimenarchal hormonal changes unless immunocompromised/hospitalized
- *E. coli* considered a nonpathogen

Investigations

- Perineal examination should include consideration of vaginal cultures (use moistened urethral swab or calgiswab)
- Note: gonoccocal and chlamydial testing in prepubertal girls should be done by vaginal culture and not NAAT
- Also include saline preparation for *Trichomonas*, if profuse purulent discharge or sexual assault
- Gynecology referral for vaginoscopy if bloody discharge, suspicion of foreign body after attempt of gentle saline irrigation, recurrence or persistence of symptoms

Treatment

- Hygiene education (cotton underwear, no underwear to bed, appropriate voiding posture, wiping front to back)
- Sitz baths three times a day
- Avoid perfumed soaps/products (e.g., bubble baths or other irritants)
- Remove foreign bodies
- Treat specific organisms, if indicated
- For severe inflammation, consider topical estrogen or steroid cream

POSTPUBERTAL VULVOVAGINITIS

- See Box 21.5 for differential diagnosis and Table 21.1 for a comparison of the most common causes

Physiologic Leukorrhea
- Normal vaginal discharge (midcycle)
- May be more profuse post thelarche before onset of menses
- ↑ Estrogen states (e.g., pregnancy, OCPs)

Noninfectious
- Contact dermatitis
- Poor hygiene
- Retained tampon
- Dermatologic disorders (e.g., psoriasis)

Infectious
- BV
- *Candida*
- *Trichomonas*
- STIs
- Condylomata acuminata: external genital warts
- Parasites: scabies, pediculosis pubis

Investigations
- Perineal and gynecologic examination including bimanual examination to rule out PID, if sexually active
- Vaginal swabs prepared as per Table 21.1
- If sexually active, should perform NAAT on cervical swabs for *N. gonorrhoeae* and *Chlamydia* (unless sexual assault, in which culture should be used)

Treatment
- No treatment for physiologic leukorrhea; reassurance only
- Hygiene education
- Treat specific infectious causes
- Condylomata: referral to gynecologist

GENITAL ULCERATION
- See Box 21.6
- Full history focusing on multiple or single lesions; presence or absence of pain; recurrence (herpes, Behçet); associated symptoms, for example, fever, malaise (EBV, herpes), GI symptoms (Crohn); sexual activity; medications
- Full physical examination
- Investigations: culture (viral, bacterial, fungal), dark-field examination, CBC, ESR, C-reactive protein, ANA, complement, VDRL, EBV serology, others as indicated
- Consider biopsy of large ulcer or if unclear diagnosis

Box 21.6   Differential Diagnosis of Genital Ulceration

Infectious
- Venereal

  Painful
  - Herpes (herpes simplex virus)
  - Chancroid (*Haemophilus ducreyi*)

  Painless
  - Syphilis (*T. pallidum*)
  - Granuloma inguinale (*Calymmatobacterium granulomatis*)
  - Lymphogranuloma venereum (*C. trachomatis* serotypes L1–3)
- Nonvenereal
  - Viral: varicella, EBV
  - Fungal: actinomycosis
  - Bacterial: *Pseudomonas aeruginosa*, diphtheria, typhoid
  - Other: amebiasis, brucellosis

Noninfectious
- Apthous ulcer
- Lichen planus
- Trauma
- Foreign body
- Behçet disease
- Pyoderma gangrenosum
- Adverse drug reaction
- Crohn disease

SEXUALLY TRANSMITTED INFECTIONS

- See Table 21.2
- Always include in differential of abdominal pain and urethral or vaginal discharge in adolescence
- Chlamydia and gonorrhea often occur together (20–30%); therefore, empiric treatment for chlamydia if positive diagnosis of gonorrhea
- Suspect child abuse in all prepubescent and nonsexually active post-pubescent children with STIs
- Need to report to public health department for contact tracing
- Partners should be treated simultaneously
- Presence of one STI should raise suspicion for others

PID

- Ascending GU infection, resulting in uterine, adnexal, or cervical motion tenderness
- May also cause fever or abnormal vaginal discharge
- Acquired sexually, postabortal, or postinstrumentation
- Polymicrobial infection including STIs (*C. trachomatis*, *N. gonorrhoeae*), endogenous organisms (*Mycoplasma genitalium*, *Mycoplasma hominis*, *Ureaplasma urealyticum*), anaerobic organisms (*Bacteroides* sp, *Peptostreptococcus* sp), facultative bacteria (*Escherichia coli*, *Gardnerella*, *Haemophilus influenzae*, *Streptococcus* sp)

Table 21.2	Treatment of Common Sexually Transmitted Infections	
Disease	Treatment	Alternatives*
Chlamydia, 1 mo–9 yr	Azithromycin 12–15 mg/kg PO single dose (max dose 1 g/d)	Erythromycin 40 mg/kg/d PO in divided doses (max 500 mg qid for 7 d or 240 mg qid for 14 d) OR Sulfamethoxazole 75 mg/kg/d PO in divided doses for 10 d (max 1 g bid)
Chlamydia, 9–18 yr	Doxycycline 5 mg/kg/d PO in divided doses for 7 d (max 100 mg bid) OR Azithromycin 12–15 mg/kg (max 1 g/d; single dose if poor compliance)	Erythromycin 40 mg/kg/d PO in divided doses (max 500 mg qid for 7 d or 240 mg qid for 14 d) OR Sulfamethoxazole 75 mg/kg/d PO in divided doses for 10 d (max 1 g bid)
Gonorrhea, <9 yr	Cefixime 8 mg/kg PO in a single dose (max 400 mg) OR Ceftriaxone 125 mg IM in a single dose	Spectinomycin 40 mg/kg IM (max 2 g) in a single dose
Gonorrhea, nonpregnant/ not breastfeeding	Cefixime 400 mg PO in a single dose OR Ciprofloxacin 500 mg PO in a single dose (unless quinolone resistant) OR Ofloxacin 400 mg PO in a single dose OR Ceftriaxone 125 mg IM in a single dose	Azithromycin 2 g PO in a single dose OR Spectinomycin 2 g IM in a single dose
Primary, secondary, early latent syphilis (<1 yr duration) –nonpregnant	Benzathine penicillin G 2.4 million units IM as single dose	Doxycycline 100 mg PO bid for 14 d OR Ceftriaxone 1 g IV or IM daily for 10 d

*Use alternates only if use of quinolones not recommended and cephalosporin allergy OR immediate/anaphylactic penicillin allergy.

- Consequences: chronic PID, chronic pain, infertility, ectopic pregnancy, tubo-ovarian abscess, perihepatitis
- Low index of suspicion required; treat often and early, as needed; remember to evaluate and treat all sexual contacts
- Hospitalize if concerns about compliance, diagnosis, immunodeficiency, pregnancy, unable to tolerate oral medications, no response to outpatient regimen
- If patient treated in ambulatory setting, *must* be followed up for improvement in 48–72 h

SPECIFIC CAUSES

C. trachomatis

- Most commonly reported STI
- May cause urethritis, vaginitis, cervicitis, endometritis, salpingitis, perihepatitis, epididymitis, lymphogranuloma venereum, and various non-GU infections
- Often asymptomatic; may either coexist with gonorrhea or present after gonorrhea treated
- Diagnosis: vaginal swabs for culture (children, sexual abuse); NAAT (PCR) or direct fluorescent antibody test (adolescents) unless sexual abuse suspected, then culture

N. gonorrhoeae

- May be asymptomatic or cause urethritis, endocervicitis, salpingitis, perihepatitis, bartholinitis, PID, or epididymitis
- Can cause non-GU infections, particularly disseminated gonococcal infection (arthritis, dermatitis, endocarditis, and meningitis), conjunctivitis, and neonatal disease
- Gram stain and culture
- Cultures should be obtained from endocervical, vaginal, rectal, urethral, and pharyngeal locations, depending on gender and type of sexual activity
- Cultures obtained <48 h after exposure can be negative
- Urine PCR if culture swab not available
- All patients should return 3–7 d after therapy for clinical evaluation and follow-up cultures

Treponema pallidum

- Primary syphilis: painless ulcer on cervix (chancre) with regional lymphadenopathy
- Secondary syphilis: any rash, fever, malaise, lymphadenopathy, mucous lesions, condyloma lata, alopecia, meningitis, headaches, uveitis, retinitis
- Latent syphilis: asymptomatic; may last 10–30 yr
- Tertiary syphilis presents with cardiovascular or neurologic manifestations
- Diagnosed by dark-field examination; spirochetes in material from primary chancre or skin and mucocutaneous lesions
- Serologic tests: initial screening by nontreponemal tests (e.g., VDRL); if positive, treponemal assays (e.g., TP-PA) or enzyme immunoassays should be done
- Use of only one type of test insufficient for diagnosis because of false-positive results of nontreponemal tests (e.g., in lupus)
- Serology may be negative early
- Follow-up: report to public health department for contact tracing; repeat VDRL at 3, 6, and 12 mo to follow response to treatment

- May be acute, chronic, or cyclic
- See Box 21.7 for differential diagnosis
- History: last menstrual period, menstrual history, contraceptive use, sexual history, history of the pelvic/abdominal pain itself
- Physical examination must include musculoskeletal and abdominal examinations; gynecologic examination, if appropriate
- Rectoabdominal or bimanual examination may document cervical/adnexal tenderness or presence of adnexal masses

INVESTIGATIONS

- CBC with differential, urinalysis, urine culture, cervical/vaginal cultures for gonococcus and *Chlamydia*, if sexually active, β-hCG
- Pelvic US, if inadequate examination or mass/uterine anomaly suspected
- Adolescents may not disclose sexual activity if parent present or if abused; therefore, β-hCG necessary
- If etiology of pain unclear and pain persistent, diagnostic laparoscopy warranted

ADNEXAL TORSION

- Infants and children may have torsion of normal adnexa; in post-menarchal patients, ovarian torsion is usually associated with adnexal mass (neoplasm or functional cysts)
- May be complete or intermittent
- History: "waves" of acute pain ± nausea; usually afebrile, normal to mildly elevated WBC
- Doppler US may demonstrate mass, increased diameter of ovarian vessel proximal to occlusion or absence of flow, but torsion *not* ruled out with normal Doppler
- Ultimately, *clinical* diagnosis
- Management: laparoscopic detorsion ± ovarian cystectomy; no current evidence to support oophoropexy of contralateral ovary

Box 21.7	Differential Diagnosis of Pelvic Pain

Gynecologic
- PID/tubo-ovarian abscess
- Ovarian cysts (ruptured, hemorrhagic)
- Adnexal torsion
- Primary dysmenorrhea
- Endometriosis
- Pregnancy complications: ectopic pregnancy, spontaneous abortion
- Müllerian anomalies with obstruction
- Mittelschmerz

Nongynecologic
- See pp. 316–319 for further details on nongynecologic causes of abdominal pain

Gynecology

21

MITTELSCHMERZ

- Ovulatory pain theoretically due to irritation of pelvic peritoneum from follicular fluid release at rupture
- Midcycle, generally recurrent, crampy pain that localizes to one lower quadrant
- Duration typically 6–8 h; rarely may last 2–3 d
- Exclude other causes of pain
- Management: reassurance, NSAIDs

ENDOMETRIOSIS

- Presence of endometrial glands and stroma outside of uterus
- Symptoms: dysmenorrhea, chronic pelvic pain, dyspareunia (pain with sexual activity)
- Usually at a mild stage in adolescents; true "endometriomas" rare at this age
- Etiologic factor in ⅔ of adolescents with chronic pain unresponsive to initial management (NSAIDs and cyclic OCPs)
- Requires laparoscopy with biopsy and histologic confirmation for diagnosis

OVARIAN MASSES

- May be functional cysts (20–50%) or neoplastic masses (either benign or malignant)
- Ovarian follicles up to 2 cm (adolescents) and 5 mm (children) considered physiologically normal

FETAL/NEONATAL OVARIAN CYSTS

- Present either as abdominal mass or detected on routine US
- Most likely secondary to maternal and fetal gonadotropin stimulation
- Differential mainly includes nongynecologic entities that should be ruled out
- Spontaneous regression for simple and complex ovarian cysts common; therefore, management often involves observation
- Risks to fetus: intracystic hemorrhage, rupture, torsion, abdominal dystocia for large masses
- Regression usually by 4 mo postdelivery; if not, consider tumor (rare) or previous torsion with hemorrhage or necrosis
- Potential role for postnatal aspiration of simple ovarian cysts >5 cm to reduce risk of torsion
- Surgical intervention should be considered for size >5 cm, enlargement, or nonresolution

PREPUBERTAL

- Present either as asymptomatic abdominal mass, chronic abdominal pain, sense of abdominal fullness, or acute abdominal pain (torsion/hemorrhage/rupture)
- Majority are functional (if cystic)
- May be hormonally active and cause pseudoprecocious puberty (vaginal bleeding, breast development)
- Other differentials include ovarian neoplasms, paraovarian/paratubal cysts, mesothelial cysts, true precocious puberty

Management

- Observation acceptable for purely cystic masses; repeat US in 4–6 wk: 90% will resolve
- Persistence or concerning US features mandate workup for malignancy: tumor markers (β-hCG, AFP, LDH), CT scan, surgical removal, and pathologic examination
- Surgery may be required for torsion causing acute pain or continued hemorrhaging

POSTMENARCHAL

- If simple on US (unilocular, thin-walled with no echoes) and <10 cm, conservative therapy warranted (follow-up US in 6–8 wk)
- OCP will not help resolution of ovarian cyst but may prevent new cyst formation
- Corpus luteal cyst/hemorrhagic cyst: observation, analgesia, follow-up US for resolution up to 3 mo
- If complex on US, differential includes functional cysts (hemorrhagic, corpus luteal), benign neoplasms, malignant neoplasms
- Usually require surgical management if functional cyst excluded, although majority will be benign
- Generally conservative surgical approach possible (i.e., laparoscopy vs. laparotomy, cystectomy vs. oophorectomy)
- Tumor markers helpful in differentiating malignant tumor: β-hCG, AFP, LDH, CA-125

AMENORRHEA

- See Box 21.8
- Defined as either primary (absence of menses by age 16 yr) or secondary (absence of menses for >6 mo after documented menarche or for >3 consecutive cycles)
- Full history crucial with emphasis on menarche, other signs of puberty, growth, medications, sexual activity, chronic or systemic illness, eating disorders, visual field defects, galactorrhea, and headache
- Full physical examination emphasizing Tanner staging and neurologic examination; consider pelvic examination

Box 21.8 Differential Diagnosis of Amenorrhea

Anatomic
- Pregnancy
- Imperforate hymen
- Transverse septum
- Agenesis of vagina, cervix, uterus (müllerian agenesis)
- Androgen insensitivity syndrome
- Uterine synechiae

Ovarian
- Gonadal dysgenesis—mixed, pure
- Premature ovarian failure
  - Turner syndrome
  - Autoimmune
- Fragile X

Endocrine
- Thyroid disease
- Cushing disease
- Hypothalamic (e.g., Kallmann syndrome)
- Anorexia, stress, illness, obesity, drugs, exercise
- Gonadotropin deficiency (e.g., Prader-Willi syndrome)
- Hypopituitarism
  - CNS tumor
  - Infiltration/infarction
- Hyperandrogenism
  - PCOS
  - CAH
- Ovarian/adrenal tumor

Medications
- Chemotherapy
- OCPs

INVESTIGATIONS

- Laboratory tests: CBC, β-hCG, LH, FSH, estradiol, testosterone, prolactin, T_4, TSH, karyotype (if elevated gonadotropins), 17-OHP (if clinical/biochemical hyperandrogenism), DHEAS
- Progesterone challenge to assess estrogen status; responsive withdrawal bleeding implies adequate endogenous estrogen and functional outflow tract
- Combined estrogen and progesterone challenge: no bleeding implies obstructed outflow tract
- High levels of endogenous gonadotropins seen in premature ovarian failure; low levels seen in hypopituitarism
- US for pelvic anatomy and MRI of head may be indicated
- Management depends on specific etiology

PCOS

- Inappropriate signals to hypothalamic–pituitary axis secondary to insulin resistance, androgen excess, and abnormal gonadotropin dynamics
- Most common cause of persistent irregular menses, usually occurring between ages 15 and 35
- Suggestive clinical features include hyperandrogenism (hirsutism, acne, virilization), menstrual dysfunction, obesity, and acanthosis nigricans
- Diagnosis based on Rotterdam criteria; two of the following three: irregular menses, clinical or biochemical hyperandrogenism, and polycystic ovaries on US in absence of any other etiology
- Biochemical findings: ↑DHEAS, ↑ testosterone, ↑LH, ↓ or normal FSH
- Treatment directed at symptom relief and prevention of long-term sequelae
- Behavior modification (reduce weight, diet, exercise) may decrease androgen secretion
- Prevent endometrial hyperplasia: cyclic medroxyprogesterone acetate (Provera) q35–60d, OCP, contraceptive patch or ring
- Prevent hirsutism: OCP, spironolactone
- If pregnancy desired: clomiphene citrate, Pergonal
- Metformin may help reduce hyperinsulinemia, hyperandrogenism, and cardiovascular risk, but not considered first-line therapy in adolescents

21 CONTRACEPTION

METHODS

- See Table 21.3 for list of methods of contraception that should be discussed when counseling an adolescent about contraception
- Counseling should include a complete history and physical examination and pelvic examination, if sexually active
- Maintain high suspicion of pregnancy; contraception often sought after pregnancy scare
- Investigations may include Pap smear, pregnancy test, urinalysis; screening for gonorrhea, chlamydia, HIV, syphilis should be offered
- Counseling is an opportunity for sexual education and anticipatory guidance

MISSED PILLS ADVICE

- One pill missed: take pill once remembered (may mean taking two pills in 1 d)
- Two pills missed in a row: take two pills once remembered and two pills the next day (use backup birth control method [e.g., condom])
- Three or more pills missed in a row: start new pack with backup birth control method

Table 21.3

Table 21.3　Methods of Contraception

Method	Failure Rate (%)*	Benefits	Risks/Contraindications
Combined Hormonal			
Oral Transdermal (EVRA) Vaginal ring	2.5–6.0 0.7–1.3 0.7–1.8	· Mechanism of action: ovulation suppression, atrophic endometrium, thickening in cervical mucus · Intercourse independent · Rapid reversibility · Daily, weekly, or monthly dosing options · Decrease risk of dysmenorrhea, iron deficiency anemia, ovarian and uterine cancers, ovarian cysts, acne, ectopic pregnancy, benign breast disorders	Side effects/risks: · Thromboembolism · Cerebrovascular accidents · Hypertension · Worsening of migraines · Nausea · Breast tenderness · Breakthrough bleeding · Depression · No STI protection · Drug interactions Absolute contraindications: · Thromboembolic disorders · Cerebrovascular accident · Coronary artery disease · Breast/gynecologic estrogen-dependent malignancy · Pregnancy · Undiagnosed genital bleeding · Active liver disease Relative contraindications: · Hypertension · Diabetes mellitus · Sickle cell disease · Impaired liver function within last year · Acute-phase mononucleosis · Cardiac or renal disease · Depression · Epilepsy (pill may not be as effective) · Lipid disorders · Migraine · Smoking
Progestin Only			
Depo-Provera (IM q3m) Progestin pill	0.3 3.0–10.0	· Intercourse independent · Can be used while breastfeeding · No estrogen · Decrease risk of ovarian/ uterine cancer · Pill has rapid reversibility	· Menstrual irregularity · Weight gain · Osteopenia · Mood changes · Breast tenderness · Headaches · No STI protection · Depo-Provera has delayed return to fertility

(continued)

Table 21.3		Methods of Contraception *(continued)*	
Method	**Failure Rate (%)***	**Benefits**	**Risks/Contraindications**
IUD			
Copper T380A (nonhormonal)	0.7	· Decrease ectopic pregnancy	· Practitioner placement/removal required
Levonorgestrel IUS (Mirena)	0.1	· Intercourse independent · Rapidly reversible · Discrete · Less user dependent	· No STI protection · Most appropriate for women at low risk for STI (parous and monogamous) · May increase chance of PID or colonization (nonhormonal IUD) · Increase menstrual bleeding and cramping (nonhormonal IUD) · Expulsion, perforation, or embedment
Barrier			
Condom	12.0	· Low cost · Nonprescription · Single use ONLY · Male involvement · STI protection	· Decreased sensation · Repeated use with each act of coitus · Requires male cooperation
Diaphragm with contraceptive cream or jelly	16.0–18.0	· Most effective female barrier method · Reduces risk of STI · May be placed in anticipation · Single insertion for multiple acts of intercourse	· Professional fitting and prescription only · Requires motivation, preparation, and access · Messy · Increase risk of UTI · Small risk for toxic shock syndrome
Female condom	21.0–26.0	· May be inserted up to 8 h before intercourse	· Complex and difficult to place · Low efficacy · No STI protection · Expensive · Use with each action of coitus · Associated noise
Other			
Withdrawal Spermicide	19.0 40.0		
No method	85.0		

*Failure rate (%): chance of pregnancy within 1 yr of use.
Note: The following methods generally not recommended for adolescents: progestin-only pills, female condom, withdrawal, spermicides, natural family planning.

EMERGENCY CONTRACEPTION

- Contains 0.75 mg levonorgestrel (sold in Canada as "Plan B")
- Pregnancy rate 0.4% if taken within 24 h of intercourse, 1.2% within 25–48 h, and 2.7% within 49–72 h; can be taken up to 120 h after intercourse, but effectiveness decreases further
- Taking two pills at one time (levonorgestrel 1.5 mg) as effective as the old regimen of one pill and then another 12 h later
- Contraindications: known pregnancy, undiagnosed abnormal vaginal bleeding
- Alternatives include two high-dose norgestrel–ethinyl estradiol tablets at presentation and 12 h later
- Side effects: nausea, vomiting (should prescribe antiemetics), abdominal pain, fatigue, headache, dizziness, breast tenderness
- Most teens will get their period within 21 d of treatment

CONTRACEPTION IN CHRONIC DISEASE

- See Table 21.4
- In each case, must balance the risks of contraception with the risks of pregnancy

Table 21.4	Methods of Contraception in Complex Medical Conditions*	
Condition	**Special Considerations**	**Possibilities**
Lupus	· Avoid OCPs and other estrogen-containing birth control if history of vascular disease, thrombosis, CNS disease, nephritis, antiphospholipid antibodies (lupus anticoagulant; anticardiolipin) · OCPs can interact with corticosteroids: ↑ steroid side effects · Depo-Provera may potentiate bone loss from concurrent use with steroids	· OCPs, patch, ring, if lupus well-controlled and no special considerations · Progesterone only (minipill, Depo-Provera) · Barrier methods · Hormonal IUD (Mirena) · Nonhormonal IUD may be less effective while taking steroids, ↑ infection risk
Transplant recipients	· Liver transplant is a relative contraindication to OCPs as estrogen is cholestatic and has been associated with hepatocellular adenoma and thrombosis of hepatic and portal veins · OCPs may increase corticosteroid and immunosuppressant levels and increase toxic effects · Avoid nonhormonal IUD due to risk of infection from immunosuppression · OCPs safe after kidney or heart transplant as long as no other contraindications (hypertension, thrombosis); ideally delay until 1 yr post-transplant, but more important to prevent unplanned pregnancy	· OCPs, patch, ring in absence of special considerations · Progesterone only (minipill, Depo-Provera) · Hormonal IUD (Mirena) · Barrier methods

(continued)

Table 21.4	Methods of Contraception in Complex Medical Conditions* *(continued)*	
Condition	**Special Considerations**	**Possibilities**
Bleeding disorders and sickle cell anemia	· Nonhormonal IUD not recommended due to increased risk of bleeding and infection	· OCPs, patch, ring · Progesterone only (minipill, Depo-Provera) · Hormonal IUD (Mirena) · Barrier methods
Inflammatory bowel disease	· OCPs may not be absorbed adequately and may cause irritation of GI tract · OCPs may increase levels of corticosteroids and cyclosporine, leading to increased side effects	· Combined patch, ring · Progesterone only (minipill, Depo-Provera) · Hormonal IUD (Mirena) · Barrier methods
Cystic fibrosis	· Theoretical risk that OCPs may thicken respiratory secretions; however, it does not seem to worsen symptoms · Malabsorption and certain antibiotics may decrease effectiveness of OCPs	· OCPs, patch, ring · Progesterone only (minipill, Depo-Provera) · Hormonal IUD (Mirena) · Barrier methods
Congenital heart disease	· OCPs contraindicated if risk of thromboembolic event (cyanotic heart disease, atrial/ventricular dilatation, pulmonary hypertension, prosthesis, shunting) · Nonhormonal IUD not recommended due to risk of endocarditis	· Progesterone only (minipill, Depo-Provera) · Hormonal IUD (Mirena) · Barrier methods

*Table courtesy of Drs. Miriam Kaufman and Ellie Vyver (see Chapter 7).

USEFUL WEB SITES

Contraception Online. Available at: www.contraceptiononline.org/

Public Health Agency of Canada. Canadian guidelines on sexually transmitted infections. 2006 ed. Available at: www.phac-aspc.gc.ca/std-mts/sti_2006/sti_intro2006_e.html

Emergency contraception. Available at: www.cps.ca/english/statements/AM/ah03-01.htm

Chapter 22 Hematology

Vicky R. Breakey

Alisha Kassam

Nisha Thampi

Melanie-Ann Kirby

Chapter 22 Hematology

COMMON ABBREVIATIONS

ACS	acute chest syndrome
APCR	activated protein-C resistance
BMA	bone marrow aspirate
BMT	bone marrow transplant
CMV	cytomegalovirus
CVL	central venous line
DAT	direct antiglobulin test
DIC	disseminated intravascular coagulation
DVT	deep vein thrombosis
EBV	Epstein-Barr virus
FEP	free erythrocyte protoporphyrin
FFP	fresh frozen plasma
FVIII:C	factor VIII coagulant
HIT	heparin-induced thrombocytopenia
HUS	hemolytic uremic syndrome
ICH	intracranial hemorrhage
INR	international normalized ratio
ITP	idiopathic thrombocytopenic purpura
IVIG	intravenous immunoglobulin
LMWH	low molecular weight heparin
MCV	mean corpuscular volume
MDS	myelodysplastic syndrome
MTHFR	methylene tetrahydrofolate reductase
NAITP	neonatal alloimmune thrombocytopenic purpura
NATP	neonatal autoimmune thrombocytopenic purpura
PE	pulmonary embolism
PLT	platelets
PNH	paroxysmal nocturnal hemoglobinuria
PTT	partial thromboplastin time
SLE	systemic lupus erythematosus
TIBC	total iron-binding capacity
TCT	thrombin time
TTP	thrombotic thrombocytopenic purpura
UFH	unfractionated heparin
VOC	vaso-occlusive crisis
V/Q	ventilation/perfusion
VWD	von Willebrand disease
VWF	von Willebrand factor

ANEMIA

- See Figure 22.1 for diagnostic approach
- See Table 22.1 for laboratory features of various types of anemia

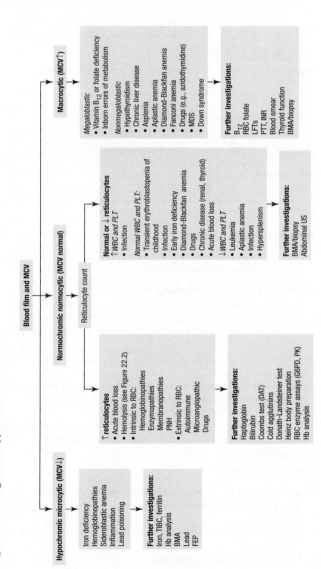

Figure 22.1 Diagnostic Approach to Anemia

Blood film and MCV

Hypochromic microcytic (MCV↓)

- Iron deficiency
- Hemoglobinopathies
- Sideroblastic anemia
- Inflammation
- Lead poisoning

Further investigations:
- Iron, TIBC, ferritin
- Hb analysis
- BMA
- Lead
- FEP

Normochromic normocytic (MCV normal)

Reticulocyte count

↑reticulocytes
- Acute blood loss
- Hemolysis (see Figure 22.2)
  - Intrinsic to RBC:
    - Hemoglobinopathies
    - Enzymopathies
    - Membranopathies
    - PNH
  - Extrinsic to RBC:
    - Autoimmune
    - Microangiopathic
    - Drugs

Further investigations:
- Haptoglobin
- Bilirubin
- Coombs test (DAT)
- Cold agglutinins
- Donath-Landsteiner test
- Heinz body preparation
- RBC enzyme assays (G6PD, PK)
- Hb analysis

Normal or ↓ reticulocytes

↑WBC and PLT:
- Infection

Normal WBC and PLT:
- Transient erythroblastopenia of childhood
- Infection
- Early iron deficiency
- Diamond-Blackfan anemia
- Drugs
- Chronic disease (renal, thyroid)
- Acute blood loss

↓WBC and PLT:
- Leukemia
- Aplastic anemia
- Infection
- Hypersplenism

Further investigations:
- BMA/biopsy
- Abdominal US

Macrocytic (MCV↑)

Megaloblastic
- Vitamin B₁₂ or folate deficiency
- Inborn errors of metabolism

Nonmegaloblastic
- Hypothyroidism
- Chronic liver disease
- Asplenia
- Aplastic anemia
- Diamond-Blackfan anemia
- Fanconi anemia
- Drugs (e.g., azidothymidine)
- MDS
- Down syndrome

Further investigations:
- B₁₂
- RBC folate
- LFTs
- PTT, INR
- Thyroid function
- Blood smear
- BMA/biopsy

Hematology

22

447

Table 22.1		Laboratory Features of Various Types of Anemia*				
Test	Aplastic Anemia	Thalassemia Major	Thalassemia Minor	Iron Deficiency Anemia	Anemia of Chronic Disease
Hb	↓	↓	↓	↓	↓
MCV	↑	↓	↓	↓	N or ↓
MCH	N	↓	↓	↓	N
RDW	N or ↑	↑	N	↑	N
Iron	N	↑	N or ↑	↓	N or ↓
TIBC	N	↓	N	↑	↓
Ferritin	N	↑	N or ↑	↓	N or ↑
Transferrin	N	↓	N	↑	↓
Reticulocyte count	↓	↑	N	↓	N or ↓

*Additional variables may be helpful: ↑RBC count in thalassemia, ↑FEP in iron deficiency anemia and lead poisoning. N, normal; ↑, increased; ↓, decreased; Hb, hemoglobin; MCH, mean corpuscular hemoglobin; RDW, red cell distribution width.

IRON DEFICIENCY ANEMIA

- Most common pediatric anemia, especially in toddlers, secondary to excessive milk intake/poor oral iron

Treatment of Iron Deficiency Anemia

- Dietary counseling and education to ensure compliance essential
- Therapeutic trial of iron supplementation in toddlers with hypochromic, microcytic anemia without further investigation (if typical history)
- 6 mg elemental iron/kg/d PO divided tid on empty stomach ½ h before meals
- Expect reticulocyte response at 7–10 d; check Hb in 1 mo to ensure response and compliance; after Hb becomes normal, treat for 2–3 mo to replenish iron stores
- If failed response to therapy, investigate for chronic inflammatory diseases, chronic blood loss, thalassemias, sideroblastic anemias, or noncompliance

HEMOLYTIC ANEMIA

- History: jaundice, anemia, painful crisis, gallstones, transfusions, splenectomy, family history, medications
- Symptoms
  - Acute: fatigue, headache, dizziness, fainting, fever, abdominal or back pain
  - Chronic: gallbladder symptoms

- Signs: tachycardia, dyspnea, pallor, jaundice, splenomegaly, dark or red urine, growth retardation, thalassemic facies, leg ulcers
- See Figure 22.2 for approach to hemolytic anemia

HEMOGLOBINOPATHIES

Thalassemia

- Result of impaired synthesis of one or more globin chains
- Features of thalassemia syndromes (Table 22.2)

Sickle Cell Disease

- Diagnosis suggested by anemia with blood smear (sickle cells, target cells, polychromasia) and confirmed by Hb analysis (Table 22.3)
- See Table 22.4 for clinical manifestations

Management of Patients With Sickle Cell Disease

Perioperative Management
- See Figure 22.3
- Hematologist to see 2 wk before procedure
- Admit day before procedure for assessment and blood work: CBC, reticulocytes, extended crossmatch (request blood on hold for surgery and postoperatively)

Figure 22.2 Approach to Hemolytic Anemia

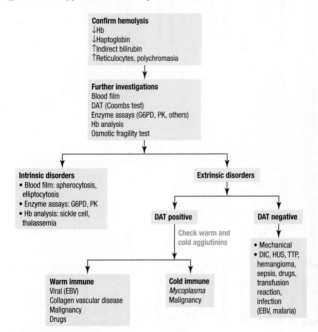

Table 22.2 Features of Thalassemia Syndromes

Genetic Abnormality	% Hb			Other	Clinical Syndrome	Therapy
	HbA	HbA₂	HbF			
Normal α₂β₂	90-98	2-3	2-3	–	None	
β-Thalassemias						
Thalassemia major β⁰/β⁰	0	2-5	95	–	Diagnosed in late infancy (↓ γ-chain synthesis): severe anemia, pallor, FTT, hepatosplenomegaly, poor growth	Regular transfusion Iron elimination therapy BMT Family counseling
Thalassemia intermedia β⁺/β⁺	20-40	–	60-80	–	Moderate-severe anemia beyond infancy; anisocytosis, poikilocytosis	No or irregular transfusion ± Iron chelation Family counseling
Thalassemia minor β/β⁰ or β/β⁺	90-95	5-7	2-10	↑RBC count	Asymptomatic mild anemia; hypochromic/microcytic smear; basophilic stippling	Family counseling
α-Thalassemias						
Homozygous α-thalassemia –/–	–	–	–	HbH (β₄) Hb Bart (γ₄) 80-90%	Hydrops fetalis, stillborn	Prenatal transfusion Regular transfusion Iron chelation BMT Family counseling

(continued)

Table 22.2   Features of Thalassemia Syndromes *(continued)*

Genetic Abnormality	% Hb			Other	Clinical Syndrome	Therapy
	HbA	HbA₂	HbF			
HbH disease $--/-\alpha$	60-90	2-5	2-5	HbH 30-40	Neonatal microcytic anemia (Hb 70-100), Heinz bodies	Transfusion in hemolytic/aplastic crisis ± splenectomy Folic acid Family counseling
α-Thalassemia trait $-\alpha/-\alpha,$ $\alpha\alpha/--$	90-98	2-3	2-3	—	Hypochromic/microcytic smear, no anemia	Family counseling
Silent carrier $-\alpha/\alpha\alpha$	90-98	2-3	2-3	—	Normal	Family counseling

Classified according to globin chain produced at reduced rate: α, β, δβ, and γδβ types; if no α or β chains are produced, thalassemias are described as α° or β°.

Table 22.3 Hemoglobin Analysis in Sickle Cell Disease

Hb Variant	Hb (g/L)	MCV	% Hb				
			HbA	HbS	HbA$_2$	HbF	Other
Hb-SA Sickle cell trait	Normal	N	55–60	30–40	2–3	–	–
Hb-SS Sickle cell anemia	60–80	N or ↑	0	85–95	2–3	5–15	–
HbS β^0-thalassemia	70–90	↓	0	70–80	3–5	10–20	–
HbS β$^+$-thalassemia	90–120	↓	10–20	60–75	3–5	10–20	–
Hb-SC disease	100–140	N	0	45–50	–	–	HbC 45–50

Adapted from Driscoll MC. Sickle cell disease. *Pediatr Rev.* 2007;28:259–268.

Table 22.4 Clinical Manifestations of Sickle Cell Disease

Clinical Manifestation	Description	Management
ACS	Infection and/or infarction, severe hypoxemia, infiltrates on CXR, dyspnea, rales	See Figure 22.3
Anemia	Chronic, onset 3–4 mo of age, hematocrit usually 18–26% May see further hemolysis with G6PD deficiency, malaria	
Aplastic crisis	Parvovirus infection, reticulocytopenia	Supportive care and transfusion
Cardiomyopathy	Heart failure (fibrosis, rare)	
Cerebral vascular accidents	Sickling and thrombosis in large and small vessels (stroke)	Monitoring: annual transcranial Doppler US; chronic transfusions if flow velocity >200 cm/s Acutely: head CT, transfusion (exchange) if stroke suspected
Chronic lung disease	Pulmonary fibrosis, restrictive lung disease, cor pulmonale	
Dactylitis	Swelling of dorsal aspects of hands and feet, presents at 6–12 mo (< age 5 yr)	Analgesia, hydration
Gall bladder disease	Bilirubin stones, cholecystitis	Elective cholecystectomy for recurrent cholecystitis and gallstones
Growth failure, delayed puberty		May respond to nutritional supplements

(continued)

Table 22.4 Clinical Manifestations of Sickle Cell Disease (continued)

Clinical Manifestation	Description	Management
Infections	Encapsulated bacteria (pneumococcus, meningococcus); osteomyelitis with *Salmonella*, *Staphylococcus aureus*; aplastic crises with parvovirus B19; *Escherichia coli* in infants	Prophylactic penicillin and immunizations Acute: see Figure 22.3
Leg ulceration	Unilateral or bilateral, medial and lateral malleolar area	
Ocular problems	Retinopathy, hyphema	Ophthalmic evaluation
Priapism	Eventual impotence if prolonged	Hydration, α-adrenergic agents (oral/intracavernosal); transfusion, oxygen, corpora cavernosa-to-spongiosa shunt
Psychological problems	Narcotic addiction or dependence unusual; chronic illness	
Renal problems	Hematuria, papillary necrosis, renal-concentrating defect, nephropathy, enuresis	
Splenic sequestration crisis	Seen in Hb-SS <3 yr old; Hb-SC or HbS-β at any age; massive splenomegaly, Hb decrease >20 g/L with reticulocytosis, breathlessness, shock	Volume expansion and transfusion; consider splenectomy after two or more events
VOC affecting bone	Consider other diagnoses: osteomyelitis, avascular necrosis	Analgesia (Table 22.5), hydration, watch for complications (e.g., ACS with abdominal/back VOC)

G6PD, glucose-6-phosphate dehydrogenase.

Acute Painful Crisis/VOC
- See Table 22.5 for pain management

ACS
- Defined as:
  - New infiltrate(s) on CXR and
  - One or more of the following new symptoms: fever, cough, dyspnea, sputum production, or hypoxia
- Past ACS increases risk of subsequent episodes and results in early mortality
- Multiple causes: pulmonary infarction secondary to sickling, hypoventilation secondary to rib/sternal bone infarction, fat embolism, infection, pulmonary edema (fluid overload), hypoventilation (narcotics) (see Figure 22.3 for special considerations in management)

Figure 22.3 Management of Ill Patients With Sickle Cell Disease

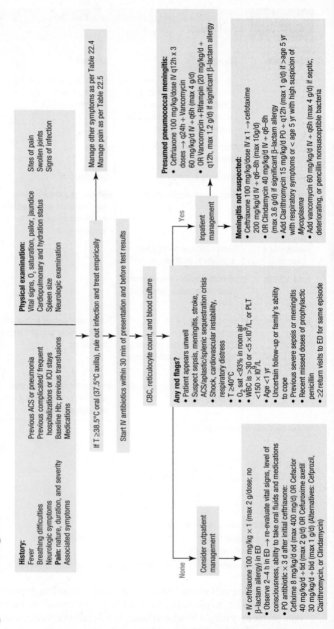

History:
Fever
Breathing difficulties
Neurologic symptoms
Pain: nature, duration, and severity
Associated symptoms

Previous ACS or pneumonia
Previous complicated/frequent
hospitalizations or ICU stays
Baseline Hb: previous transfusions
Medications

Physical examination:
Vital signs, O₂ saturation, pallor, jaundice
Cardiopulmonary and hydration status
Spleen size
Neurologic examination

Sites of pain
Swollen joints
Signs of infection

If T ≥38.5°C oral (37.5°C axilla), rule out infection and treat empirically

Manage other symptoms as per Table 22.4
Manage pain as per Table 22.5

Start IV antibiotics within 30 min of presentation and before test results

CBC, reticulocyte count, and blood culture

Any red flags?
• Patient appears unwell
• Suspect sepsis, meningitis, stroke,
  ACS/aplastic/splenic sequestration crisis
• Shock, cardiovascular instability,
  respiratory distress
• T ≥40°C
• O₂ sat <93% in room air
• WBC is >30 or <5 ×10⁹/L, or PLT
  <150 ×10⁹/L
• Age <1 yr
• Uncertain follow-up or family's ability
  to cope
• Previous severe sepsis or meningitis
• Recent missed doses of prophylactic
  penicillin
• ≥2 return visits to ED for same episode

None → Consider outpatient management

Yes → Inpatient management

Presumed pneumococcal meningitis:
• Ceftriaxone 100 mg/kg/dose IV q12h × 3
  doses → q24h + Vancomycin
  60 mg/kg/d IV + q6h (max 4 g/d)
• OR Vancomycin + Rifampin (20 mg/kg/d +
  q12h, max 1.2 g/d) if significant β-lactam allergy

Presumed pneumococcal meningitis:
• Ceftriaxone 100 mg/kg/dose IV × 1 →cefotaxime
  200 mg/kg/d IV + q6–8h (max 10g/d)

Meningitis not suspected:
• Ceftriaxone 100 mg/kg/dose IV × 1 →cefotaxime
  200 mg/kg/d IV + q6–8h (max 10g/d)
• OR Clindamycin 40 mg/kg/d IV + q6–8h
  (max 3.6 g/d) if significant β-lactam allergy
• Add Clarithromycin 15 mg/kg/d PO + q12h (max 1 g/d) if >age 5 yr
  with respiratory symptoms or < age 5 yr with high suspicion of
  Mycoplasma
• Add vancomycin 60 mg/kg/d IV + q6h (max 4 g/d) if septic,
  deteriorating, or penicillin nonsusceptible bacteria

• IV ceftriaxone 100 mg/kg × 1 (max 2 g/dose; no
  β-lactam allergy in ED
• Observe 2–4 h in ED → re-evaluate vital signs, level of
  consciousness, ability to take oral fluids and medications
• PO antibiotic × 3 d after initial ceftriaxone:
  Cefixime 8 mg/kg od (max 400 mg/d) OR Cefaclor
  40 mg/kg/d + tid (max 2 g/d) OR Cefuroxime axetil
  30 mg/kg/d + bid (max 1 g/d) (Alternatives: Cefprozil,
  Clarithromycin, or Clindamycin)

Special considerations in ACS:
- Avoid fluid overload: IV fluid maintenance
- Diuretics (furosemide 0.5–1 mg/kg IV, max 60 mg/dose as needed)
- Consider bronchodilators
- Enforce incentive spirometry
- Avoid oversedation with narcotics
- Follow O_2 sat, CBC, blood gas, CXR
- Simple transfusion early if moderately severe disease and Hb 15 g/L below baseline: pRBCs 10–15 mL/kg (avoid transfusing to Hb >100 g/L or > Hct 30%)
- Consider exchange transfusion if severe disease: extensive infiltrates, worsening ABGs, ↑need for O_2 (40% O_2) and ↓O_2 sat, not responding to simple transfusion

- Initial vital signs minimum q4h
- O_2 to keep saturation ≥94%
- IV fluids: consider 10 mL/kg 0.9% NaCl bolus → D5W–0.9% NaCl at 1.5× maintenance day 1 → maintenance (PO + IV) as improves
- Analgesia as per Table 22.5
- Incentive spirometry (>age 4 yr)
- Encourage ambulation
- CBC, reticulocyte count as clinically indicated
- If 48 h cultures negative, stop antibiotics unless focal infection or persistent fever

Other investigations as indicated:

Labs:
- ABG
- Electrolytes & renal function
- Crossmatch if pallor, respiratory or neurologic symptoms, or splenic enlargement (Phenotypically matched blood preferred)

Microbiology:
- Cultures: urine, throat, stool
- Nasopharyngeal swab
- Lumbar puncture (baseline & repeat if not improved after 48 h of therapy)
- *Mycoplasma* PCR from throat swab and serology

Imaging:
- CXR if cough, tachypnea, hypoxemia chest pain, fever >40°C
- Evaluation for osteomyelitis
- CT head for new focal neurologic symptoms

Other discharge criteria:
- Afebrile >24 h, with negative cultures at 48 h
- Pulmonary symptoms, if any, have resolved, off supplemental O_2

General discharge criteria:
- Tolerating fluids and medications by mouth
- Adequate pain control on oral medications
- Follow-up arranged with patient's primary care/sickle cell team member

Other discharge criteria:
- Follow-up of blood culture results arranged

Table 22.5	Pain Management in Vaso-Occlusive Crisis	
Pain Severity*	**Medication**	**Comments**
Mild to moderate	Acetaminophen and/or codeine or morphine ± ibuprofen PO	Encourage patients to drink If pain relief adequate in 30–60 min, discharge on oral analgesics
Moderate to severe	Morphine 0.1–0.15 mg/kg/dose IV bolus	Max 7.5 mg/dose Administer IV fluids Repeat once 60 min later if inadequate pain relief Acetaminophen + codeine if 2 h of pain relief after ≤2 doses of intermittent morphine Hospitalize if require >2 doses
Severe (hospitalized)	Morphine infusion 40 mcg/kg/h IV Morphine bolus 0.05 mg/kg IV q1–2h prn PCA pump, if appropriate Oral morphine (equivalent dose) if stable Docusate sodium 5 mg/kg/d od or ÷ tid Antihistamines prn pruritus	Titrate by 10–20 mcg/kg/h to max 100 mcg/kg/h for pain relief Decrease by 10 mcg/kg/h, as tolerated after pain controlled Administer IV fluids **Step-down**: acetaminophen + codeine/morphine PO ± ibuprofen

*See Chapter 5 for pain assessment scales.
PCA, patient-controlled analgesia

THROMBOCYTOPENIA

- See Figure 22.4 for approach to isolated thrombocytopenia

ITP

- Isolated immune-mediated thrombocytopenia
- Incidence peaks at 2–4 yr of age (usual range, 1–10 yr old)
- Sudden onset of minor bleeding (e.g., epistaxis), bruising, and purpura in otherwise well child; sometimes 1–4 wk after viral infection (e.g., URTI/chickenpox)
- No history of systemic symptoms (e.g., bone pain) or systemic findings such as hepatosplenomegaly or lymphadenopathy
- Broadly divided into acute (80–90%), relapsing, and chronic (lasting >6 mo, in 10–20%)

Investigations

- CBC and differential: normal apart from ↓PLT
- Blood smear: ↓PLT—various sizes, some larger due to increased production
- For atypical or chronic ITP: ANA, immunoglobulin levels, Coombs test (DAT), C3, C4, blood group and type
- BMA indicated if more than one cell line affected or significant symptoms or findings (e.g., lymphadenopathy, hepato/splenomegaly)
- BMA may be normal or show abundant megakaryocytes

Figure 22.4 Approach to Thrombocytopenia

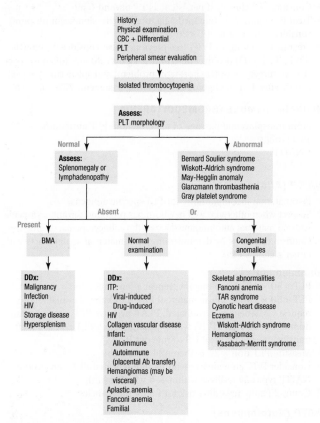

TAR, thrombocytopenia–absent radius; Ab, antibody.
Modified from Hastings CA, Lubin BH. Blood. In Rudolph AM, Kamel RK, (eds.). *Rudolph's Fundamentals of Pediatrics*, 2nd ed. Norwalk, Conn.: Appleton & Lange, 1998: 441–490. Reprinted with permission of The McGraw-Hill Companies, Inc.

Treatment Options

- Observation only (when PLT $> 20 \times 10^9$/L and no bleeding)
- IVIG 1 g/kg for 1–2 doses infused over 4–6 h each; repeat PLT count after 24 h before giving second dose if no response
- Steroids (various regimens available): prednisone 4 mg/kg/d (max 60 mg/dose or 200 mg/L/d) in 3–4 divided doses × 4 d (no taper)
- In case of life-threatening bleeding (e.g., intracranial), treat with IVIG, IV steroids, and PLT transfusion ± emergency splenectomy
- May give steroids (without BMA) provided that history, examination, and laboratory investigations are in keeping with typical ITP

Chronic ITP
- Consider ITP chronic if persistent ↓PLT beyond 6 mo
- Treat if symptomatic (menorrhagia, nosebleeds, significant purpura); consider treatment if PLT < 20×10^9/L
- Treatment: steroids or IVIG (see previous); also consider IV anti-Rho (D) Ig if Rho (D) positive: 50–75 mcg/kg over 30 min (often to cover elective surgery or other short-term problem) and splenectomy (usually only after 1 yr of ongoing ITP requiring treatment; 75% effective)

NEONATAL IMMUNE THROMBOCYTOPENIA
- From transplacental passage of maternal anti-PLT antibodies
- Two groups:
  - NAITP
  - NATP

NAITP (Alloimmune)
- Fetomaternal incompatibility for PLT-specific antigens
- Suspect when otherwise well newborn has profound thrombocytopenia with no maternal autoimmune disease, thrombocytopenia, or drug use
- Confirm diagnosis by demonstrating that maternal serum reacts with father's/child's PLT

Management
- PLT > 50×10^9/L: no therapy; repeat a few days later
- PLT < 50×10^9/L: infuse maternal PLT into baby, if available, or request CMV-negative, irradiated, PLA$_1$–negative PLT (may give random donor PLT and IVIG while waiting); check PLT count 1 h after transfusion; obtain head US to rule out ICH
- Measure PLT q6h × 24 h, then q2d once stable
- Consider IVIG in neonates who require repeated PLT transfusions
- NAITP typically resolves within 4–6 wk after birth
- Counsel family regarding risk for future pregnancies

NATP (Autoimmune)
- Maternal autoantibodies (IgG) cross placenta and cause passive ITP in fetus/neonate (transient)
- Clinically similar to NAITP but treatment different: maternal PLT destroyed if transfused
- History of maternal ITP, SLE, or autoimmune disease with low maternal PLT before delivery

Treatment Options
- Postnatal treatment like childhood ITP (i.e., IVIG)
- Steroids to mother 10–14 d before delivery may reduce need for cesarean section
- Can also give IVIG to mother antepartum or to child postpartum
- Note: mild asymptomatic maternal thrombocytopenia does not constitute ITP, and only 50% of children of mothers with ITP have thrombocytopenia

NEUTROPENIA

- See approaches to acute neutropenia (Figure 22.5) and chronic neutropenia (Figure 22.6)

Figure 22.5 Approach to Acute Neutropenia

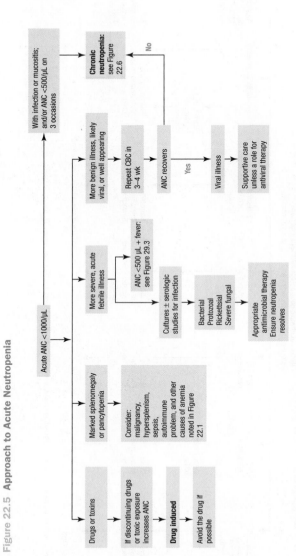

Adapted from Boxer LA. Neutropenia. In Sills RH, ed. *Protocol Algorithms on Pediatric Hematology and Oncology.* Albany, NY: Karger; 2003:42.

Figure 22.6 Approach to Chronic Neutropenia

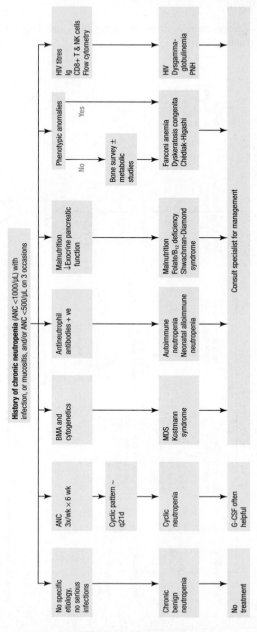

History of chronic neutropenia (ANC <1000/µL) with
infection, or mucositis, and/or ANC <500/µL on 3 occasions

| No specific etiology, no serious infections | ANC 3x/wk × 6 wk | BMA and cytogenetics | Antineutrophil antibodies + ve | Malnutrition ↓Exocrine pancreatic function | Phenotypic anomalies | HIV titres Ig CD8+ T & NK cells Flow cytometry |

Cyclic pattern ~ q21d

Yes / No

Bone survey ± metabolic studies

| Chronic benign neutropenia | Cyclic neutropenia | MDS Kostmann syndrome | Autoimmune neutropenia Neonatal alloimmune neutropenia | Malnutrition Folate/B₁₂ deficiency Shwachman–Diamond syndrome | Fanconi anemia Dyskeratosis congenita Chédiak-Higashi | HIV Dysgamma-globulinemia PNH |

| No treatment | G-CSF often helpful | | | | | |

Consult specialist for management

Adapted from Boxer LA, Neutropenia. In Sills RH, ed. *Protocol Algorithms on Pediatric Hematology and Oncology*. Albany, NY: Karger; 2003:42.

BLEEDING DISORDERS

- See Figure 22.7

- See Figure 22.7

Figure 22.7 **Simplified Pathway of Blood Coagulation**

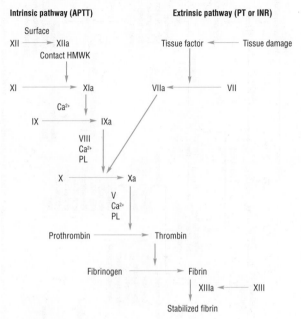

HMWK, high molecular weight kininogen; *PL*, phospholipid.

APPROACH TO PATIENTS WITH HEMOSTATIC DISORDERS

- Obtain history: bleeding postcircumcision, delayed bleeding from umbilical stump, hematomas after immunizations, previous transfusions, surgeries, trauma, or dental extractions, menstrual history
- Types/sites of bleeding (bruising, petechiae, epistaxis, menorrhagia; gingivae, muscles, joints, GI/GU), duration and amount; mucocutaneous bleeding suggests a primary hemostasis disorder; deep hematomas suggest a secondary hemostasis disorder
- Drug use (aspirin, NSAIDs)
- Family history (bleeding or bleeding tendency, excessive postpartum bleeding, menorrhagia)
- See Figure 22.8

SCREENING TESTS

- See Table 22.6 for screening tests for bleeding disorders

Figure 22.8 Laboratory Evaluation of the Child With a Bleeding Disorder

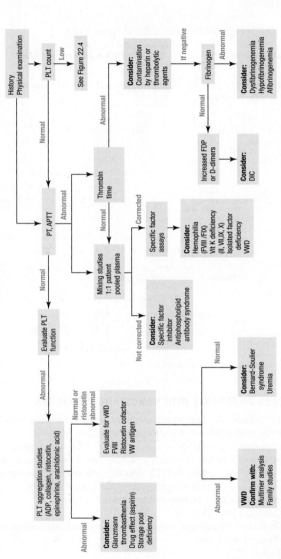

ADP adenosine triphosphate; *FDP* fibrin degradation products.
Adapted from Hastings CA, Lubin BH. Blood. In: Rudolph AM, Kamel RK, eds. *Rudolph's Fundamentals of Pediatrics.* 2nd ed. Norwalk, Conn: Appleton & Lange: 1998:441–490. Reprinted with permission of The McGraw-Hill Companies, Inc.

Table 22.6 — Screening Tests for Bleeding Disorders*

Laboratory Investigation	Measure/Process Assessed	Disorder
Blood smear	PLT number and morphology, RBC morphology, WBC inclusions	Large PLT: peripheral destruction or congenital PLT disorders Small PLT: Wiskott-Aldrich Fragmented, bizarre RBC morphology: microangiopathic process (e.g., HUS, TTP, hemangioma, DIC)
BT PFA preferable to BT if available	Primary hemostasis PLT function	PLT dysfunction, thrombocytopenia, VWD, aspirin (affects PFA for 7–10 d postingestion)
PT or INR	Extrinsic and common pathways	Defect in vitamin K–dependent factors; hemorrhagic disease of newborn, malabsorption, liver disease, DIC, oral anticoagulants, ingestion of rat poison
APTT, PTT	Intrinsic and common pathway	Hemophilia A or B, VWD, heparin, DIC, deficient FXI and FXII, lupus anticoagulant
TCT	Fibrinogen-to-fibrin conversion	↓ plasma fibrinogen (hypo/afibrinogenemia), dysfunctional fibrinogen (dysfibrinogenemia), heparin, DIC
Fibrinogen	Quantitative fibrinogen level	↓ plasma fibrinogen (hypo/afibrinogenemia), DIC
D-dimer	Thrombin generation and lysis of cross-linked fibrin	↑ in DIC, clots
Factor assays	Quantitative factor level	FII, FVII, FIX, FX, proteins C and S are vitamin K dependent All factors produced in liver except FVIII FXIII does not affect PTT or INR FVII has shortest half life FXII deficiency does not cause clinical bleeding
1:1 Mixing study (1:1 mix of patient's plasma and normal pooled plasma)	Cause of PTT prolongation	Repeat PTT prolonged: presence of factor inhibitor (heparin, lupus anticoagulant most common) Repeat PTT normalizes: factor deficiency

*Refer to Section III for laboratory reference values.
BT, bleeding time; PFA, PLT function assay.

PRIMARY AND SECONDARY HEMOSTASIS DISORDERS

- See Table 22.7

Table 22.7 Overview of Primary and Secondary Hemostasis Disorders

Types	Description	Investigations	Management
Primary Hemostasis Disorders			
Quantitative PLT abnormalities	See Figure 22.4		
Qualitative PLT abnormalities	Consider Bernard-Soulier syndrome, Glanzmann thrombasthenia, storage pool deficiency, uremia, drug effect		
VWD	Autosomal dominant; some cases very mild		
Type I: reduced VWF	↑ Bruising, bleeding	PTT, VWF antigen, ristocetin cofactor activity, FVIII:C	DDAVP 0.3 mg/kg IV in 0.9% NaCl at 0.5 mg/mL to max 20 mg over 20 min; may consider SC; intranasal not used for bleeding May use adjuvant tranexamic acid for minor surgery (e.g., dental): 7-10 mg/kg/dose IV preprocedure and q8h until able to take PO 25 mg/kg/dose qid × 5-7 d postprocedure
Type II (a, b): abnormal VWF	↑ Bruising, bleeding	As with type I + multimeric analysis	IIa: DDAVP mostly ineffective IIb: DDAVP *contraindicated* as abnormal forms aggregate PLT → thrombocytopenia Tranexamic acid per Type I
Type III: absent VWF	Hemarthroses, hematomas	As with type I; ↓FVIII:C	Humate-P (VWF-rich concentrate); if unavailable, use cryoprecipitate DDAVP ineffective Tranexamic acid per Type I

(continued)

Table 22.7 Overview of Primary and Secondary Hemostasis Disorders (*continued*)

Types	Description	Investigations	Management
Secondary Hemostasis Disorders			
FVIII deficiency (classic hemophilia/hemophilia A)	X-linked; 30% spontaneous	DNA analysis	Treat bleeding early; physiotherapy; consider prophylactic factor use Avoid IM injections, anti-PLT drugs Prophylactic dental care and preoperative planning Surveillance for hepatitis (recommend immunizations) and HIV
Mild (FVIII:C >5%)	Bleeding with trauma/surgery	↑PTT, ↓FVIII:C, normal VWF and ristocetin cofactor activity	Consider DDAVP as above (DDAVP responder: achieves FVIII:C ~30%); may repeat q24h; monitor for hyponatremia
Moderate (FVIII:C 2–5%)	Bleeding with minor trauma	↑PTT, ↓FVIII:C, normal VWF and ristocetin cofactor activity	Recombinant FVIII (1 unit/kg ↑ activity by 2%, half-life 8–12 h); take history of FVIII used (e.g. Kogenate FS by Bayer or Advate by Baxter)
Severe (FVIII:C <2%)	Spontaneous bleeding into joints, muscles, tissues	↑PTT, ↓FVIII:C, normal VWF and ristocetin cofactor activity	Consult hemophilia specialist if FVIII inhibitors present (10–20% patients)
FIX deficiency (Christmas disease or hemophilia B)	X-linked; FIX vitamin K dependent: lower at birth; early diagnosis harder	↑PTT, ↓FIX, normal FVIII:C, VWF and ristocetin cofactor activity	Preventive care as above FIX concentrates (1 unit/kg ↑ activity by 0.6–1%, half-life 18–24h)
DIC	Clinical problem mainly bleeding, although small-vessel thrombosis occurs	↑INR, PTT, TCT, D-dimers ↓ fibrinogen, PLT	Treat underlying disorder Supportive replacement: PLT, FFP, pRBC, cryoprecipitate or fibrinogen concentrate
Vitamin K deficiency	Affects FII, FVII, FIX, FX, proteins C and S	↑INR >PTT, ↓FII, FVII, FIX, FX	FFP if bleeding, Vitamin K₁ 1 mg SC or slow IV push (risk anaphylaxis) or 2–5 mg/d PO
FXIII deficiency	Delayed bleeding (umbilical cord, spontaneous ICH)	Normal INR, PTT	Monthly FXIII concentrate, or FFP if unavailable

Hematology

22

465

THROMBOSIS

DVT

- See Table 22.8

Table 22.8   **Risk Factors for Venous Thrombosis**

Inherited Thrombophilias	Acquired Disorders
FV Leiden mutation	Presence of CVL (most common cause in children)
Prothrombin gene mutation	Malignancy
Protein S deficiency, protein C deficiency	Immobilization
Homocystinuria	Surgery, especially orthopedic
Antithrombin deficiency	Inflammatory bowel disease
Heparin cofactor II deficiency	Decreased cardiac function
Dysfibrinogenemia/hypofibrinogenemia	Antiphospholipid antibody syndrome
	Myeloproliferative disorders
	Leukocytosis in acute leukemia
	Trauma
	Pregnancy
	Nephrotic syndrome
	Hemolytic anemia
	Estrogen

Adapted from Kenneth B, Gregory L. Overview of the causes of venous thrombosis. *UpToDate*. Available at: http://www.utdol.com/utd/content/topic.do?topicKey=coagulat/6864&selectedTitle=3~150&source=search_result. Accessed September 14, 2007.

Investigations for DVT

Imaging
- Suspect DVT in upper central venous system: venography (US only 20% sensitive)
- Suspect clot in jugular veins: US (venography relatively insensitive)
- Suspect DVT in lower proximal venous system: Doppler US may be sufficient; if normal, perform venography
- Suspect PE: CXR and V/Q scan; consider spiral CT

Thrombotic Workup
- CBC, INR, PTT, creatinine, prothrombotic workup
- Prothrombotic workup (baseline or after completion of anticoagulation therapy): antithrombin, protein C, protein S, APCR, FV Leiden, prothrombin gene defect, MTHFR gene variant, lupus anticoagulant antibodies, anticardiolipin antibodies, fasting lipoprotein (a), fasting homocysteine, plasminogen, reptilase time, TCT ± FVIII, FIX, and FXI

Management of DVT

Initial Therapy
- After ABCs: start anticoagulation before imaging if suspicion of thrombosis high or life/limb threatening
- UFH or LMWH for min of 5 d, 10–14 d if extensive DVT or PE

Duration of Therapy for DVT
- Ongoing therapy with either LMWH or warfarin
- Usual min duration: 3 mo for DVT after acquired insult, 6 mo for idiopathic DVT, indefinite for recurrent DVT

GUIDELINES FOR UFH THERAPY
- At concentrations ≥1000 units/mL or any concentrations in large enough volume, heparin is potentially toxic
- UFH may be administered IV or SC

IV UFH Dose
- Loading dose: 75 units/kg (usual max dose 5000 units) IV over 10 min; do not give a bolus in neonates or children with strokes or high risk of bleeding
- Initial maintenance dose is age related
  - Age ≤12 mo: 28 units/kg/h
  - Age >12 mo: 20 units/kg/h (usual max rate 1000 units/h)
- Obtain blood for APTT 4 h after administering UFH loading dose (not earlier), then 4 h after every change in infusion rate; if bolus not given, obtain initial APTT 6 h after infusion starts
- Adjust UFH infusion to maintain APTT of 60–85 s as shown in Table 22.9
- Obtain anti-FXa level (UFH) within 48 h of initiating UFH therapy; if anti-FXa level and APTT do not correspond, adjust UFH to maintain anti-FXa levels at 0.35–0.7 unit/mL (Table 22.9)

Calculation of Heparin Infusions
- Age <12 mo: weight (kg) × 28 × volume of solution (mL) = units of heparin in x mL of solution; 1 mL/h = 28 units/kg/h
- Age >12 mo: weight (kg) × 20 × volume of solution (mL) = units of heparin in x mL of solution; 1 mL/h = 20 units/kg/h
- Use dedicated IV for UFH administration; avoid UFH levels from heparinized lines, and follow "blood-discarding" protocols if line heparinized

Table 22.9	Unfractionated Heparin Dosing				
APTT (s)	Anti-FXa Level (units/mL)	Bolus (units/kg)	Hold (min)	Rate Change	Repeat APTT (h)
<50	<0.1	50	0	Increase 20%	4
50–59	0.1–0.34	0	0	Increase 10%	4
60–85	0.35–0.7	0	0	No change	24
86–95	0.71–0.89	0	0	Decrease 10%	4
96–120	0.90–1.2	0	30	Decrease 10%	4
>120	>1.2	0	60	Decrease 15%	4

© The Hospital for Sick Children. Adapted from *Pediatric Thromboembolism and Stroke Guidelines*. 3rd ed. Hamilton, Ontario, Canada: Hospital for Sick Children; 2006.

PROTOCOL FOR LMWH THERAPY IN CHILDREN AND NEONATES USING ENOXAPARIN

- Note: these dosage guidelines apply to enoxaparin, unless otherwise indicated, and cannot be directly extrapolated to other LMWHs

Indications

- Consider LMWHs in most patients requiring therapeutic or prophylactic anticoagulation

LMWH Doses

- Before initiating LMWH, obtain patient's weight and CBC, INR, APTT, and creatinine; if appropriate, obtain a prothrombotic workup
- Recommended LMWH dose is age dependent (Table 22.10)
- Adjust dose and monitoring of LMWH according to Table 22.11, assuming no active bleeding or decreased renal function
- If major bleeding surgery in preceding 7–10 d (e.g., intraocular, intracranial, retroperitoneal, GI/GU tract, or bleeding requiring blood products), consult hematologist before anticoagulation therapy
- Avoid trauma, contact sports, and anti-PLT medications while receiving anticoagulant therapy

Monitoring of LMWH

- Venipuncture ideal; must be no contamination from UFH (e.g., from CVL)
- On day(s) 1 and/or 2, draw blood sample 4 h after SC LMWH given; if therapeutic, weekly anti-FXa level sufficient if inpatient or monthly if outpatient
- Therapeutic anti-FXa is usually 0.5–1.0 unit/mL (>1.0 unit/mL required in some)
- Consider bone densitometry baseline and q12mo for osteoporosis for patients taking LMWH >3 mo
- LMWH excreted renally; if renal function changes, check creatinine and anti-FXa levels; may need dose reduction if GFR <30 mL/min/1.73 m^2 (see Table 22.11)

Ongoing Follow-Up

- Avoid aspirin and other anti-PLT drugs, avoid IM injections and arterial punctures
- Measure PLT regularly: <100 × 10^9/L or ↓ 50% from baseline, screen for HIT

Duration of LMWH Therapy

- Depends on age, clot location, and underlying conditions
- For DVT, LMWH usually given minimum 5–7 d and up to 3 mo
- When oral anticoagulation is considered, can start warfarin on day 1 or 2 of LMWH therapy
- If DVT is extensive or massive PE, administer LMWH for 7–14 d and begin warfarin therapy on day 5
- LMWH can also be used for 3 to 12 mo (for entire duration of therapy)

Table 22.10 — Dosing of Low Molecular Weight Heparin (Enoxaparin*)

	Age <2 mo	Age 2 mo–18 yr
Initial treatment dose	1.5 mg/kg/dose q12h	1 mg/kg/dose q12h
Prophylactic dose	0.75 mg/kg/dose q12h OR 1.5 mg/kg/dose q24h	0.50 mg/kg/dose q12h OR 1 mg/kg/dose q24h
Recommended upper dose limit	3 mg/kg/dose q12h	2 mg/kg/dose q12h

*Enoxaparin has 110 units of anti-FXa/mg.
© The Hospital for Sick Children. Adapted from *Pediatric Thromboembolism and Stroke Guidelines*. 3rd ed. Hamilton, Ontario, Canada: Hospital for Sick Children; 2006.

Conversion of LMWH to UFH

- UFH should not be initiated until at least 8 h after SC dose of LMWH
- If UFH is started 8–12 h after SC LMWH, do not administer a bolus; start UFH at the appropriate dose for age
- If UFH is started >12 h after SC LMWH, initiate with either IV bolus followed by IV drip or as SC dose q12h

Prophylaxis With LMWH (Once-Daily Dosing)

- Can give as single SC dose per day rather than two doses per day
- For enoxaparin, dose is age dependent
  - Age ≤2 mo, 1.5 mg/kg SC once daily
  - Age >2 mo, 1.0 mg/kg SC once daily
- Monitoring anti-FXa levels not required unless renal failure, in which case, consult thrombosis specialist

Table 22.11 — Nomogram for Low Molecular Weight Heparin Treatment

Anti-FXa Level	Hold Next Dose	Dose Change	Repeat Anti-FXa Level
<0.35 unit/mL	No	↑ by 25%	4 h post next A.M. dose
0.35–0.49 unit/mL	No	↑ by 10%	4 h post next A.M. dose
0.5–1 unit/mL	No	0	4 h post A.M. dose weekly
1.01–1.5 unit/mL	No	↓ by 20%	4 h post next A.M. dose
1.51–2.0 units/mL	3 h	↓ by 30%	Trough level before next dose, then 4 h post next A.M. dose
>2.0 units/mL	Yes, until level <0.5 unit/mL	↓ by 40%	Trough level before next dose and if not <0.5 unit/mL, repeat before each dose is due

© The Hospital for Sick Children. Adapted from *Pediatric Thromboembolism and Stroke Guidelines*. 3rd ed. Hamilton, Ontario, Canada: Hospital for Sick Children; 2006.

Hematology

22

Antidote for LMWH
- If discontinuing anticoagulation with LMWH for clinical reasons, termination usually suffices
- If immediate reversal required, protamine sulfate reverses 60% of anti-FXa activity

WARFARIN THERAPY
- Warfarin is the most commonly used oral anticoagulant
- Consult hematologist for initiating and monitoring warfarin therapy

Reversal of Warfarin Therapy

Low-Dose Warfarin (INR 1.4–1.8)
- If INR ≤1.5, no reversal necessary for most surgeries; use full-dose warfarin reversal for exceptions, which include high-risk surgeries (i.e., eye surgery, neurosurgery)
- Hold warfarin 72 h before procedure

Full-Dose Warfarin (INR 2.0–3.0 or INR 2.5–3.5)
- Reversal required before surgery because risk of significant hemorrhage; consult with hematologist

Antidote for Warfarin
- Vitamin K is antidote if rapid reversal of warfarin needed; dose and concurrent use of FFP or activated prothrombin complex concentrate depend on clinical context
- If warfarin required again in near future, administer vitamin K_1, 0.5–2 mg SC or PO (not IM), depending on patient size
- If patient will not require warfarin again:
  - Administer vitamin K_1, 2–5 mg SC or PO (not IM)
  - Consider giving activated prothrombin complex concentrate (containing FII, FVII, FIX, FX) at 50 units/kg IV or activated recombinant FVII (rFVIIa) (dose to be specified by pediatric hematologist)

ANTITHROMBOTIC THERAPY

Blocked CVLs
- See Tables 22.12 and 22.13 for management

Diagnostic Workup of Persistently Blocked CVLs
- Indication: failure to function after two doses of alteplase (tPA) or second blockage:
  1. Lineogram to determine CVL location, potential retrograde flow, tip occlusion, or leak
  2. Venogram (gold standard)
     - Venogram normal: local CVL occlusion
     - Venogram abnormal: treat as outlined in Extensive DVT from CVL section

Table 22.12	Guidelines for Managing Blocked Central Venous Lines	
	Chemical-Related Occlusion	**Blood-Related Occlusion**
Indication	Infusion running, then sudden unexplained occlusion	Blood sampling Blood administration Blood backup during infusion
Initial action	1. Attempt to aspirate 2. Flush with 0.9% NaCl 3. Follow HCl guidelines below 4. If no blood return, follow guidelines for alteplase 5. If able to flush the line but no blood return, proceed to diagnostic workup, if clinically indicated*	1. Attempt to aspirate 2. Flush with 0.9% NaCl 3. Follow guidelines for alteplase 4. If able to flush the line but unable to get blood return, proceed to diagnostic workup, if clinically indicated*

*Consider CXR to assess for line position and/or breakage.
© The Hospital for Sick Children. Adapted from *Pediatric Thromboembolism and Stroke Guidelines.* 3rd ed. Hamilton, Ontario, Canada:, Hospital for Sick Children; 2006.

3. If venogram cannot be readily obtained:
   - Doppler US of the large vessels near and including the CVL (80% sensitive for neck vessel thrombosis; only 20% sensitive for upper venous system thrombosis)
   - If Doppler US and lineogram are normal but still no blood return from CVL, consider using CVL for instillation only; venogram strongly recommended to rule out large vessel clot
   - If Doppler US abnormal, recommend venogram to rule out proximal clot
   - If CVL removal is considered *and* a new-onset line-related clot is confirmed, anticoagulation should be in place for 2–5 d before line removal (to avoid embolism)

Extensive DVT From CVL
- V/Q scan may help determine if PE has occurred (30% of children with DVT have asymptomatic PE)
- Options for management:
  - Leave CVL in place and attempt systemic thrombolytic therapy if no contraindications
  - Begin anticoagulation as indicated and consult thrombosis specialist

TRANSFUSION MEDICINE

- See Table 22.14

Table 22.13 Guidelines for Instillation of HCl and Alteplase for Blocked Central Venous Lines

Type of Catheter	Chemical Occlusion HCl 0.1 mol/L	Blood-Related Occlusion Patient Weight	Blood-Related Occlusion Alteplase (tPA)
Single lumen (e.g., Hickman, Cook, Roko, PICC)	2 mL	>10 kg	1 mg/mL; use amount required to fill volume of line, to max 2 mL = 2 mg
		≤10 kg	1 mg diluted to 2 mL (1 mL = 0.5 mg)
Double lumen (e.g., Hickman, Cook, Quinton)	2 mL per lumen	>10 kg	1 mg/mL; use amount required to fill volume of line, to max 2 mL = 2 mg per lumen; treat one lumen at a time
		≤10 kg	1 mg diluted to 2 mL per lumen (1 mL = 0.5 mg)
Subcutaneous ports (e.g., Port-A-Cath, PASport)	3 mL	>10 kg	2 mg diluted with 0.9% NaCl to 3 mL (1 mL = 0.65 mg)
		≤10 kg	1.5 mg diluted with 0.9% NaCl to 3 mL (1 mL = 0.5 mg)
Hemodialysis catheters			See guidelines above for single-lumen catheter
Small Quinton, Cook	1 mL	>10 kg	
Large Quinton, Uldall (for nonnephrology patients, use double-lumen guidelines)	1.5 mL	≤10 kg	0.75 mg diluted to 1.5 mL

Note: After a minimum of 2 h instillation of each drug, withdraw drug, and if possible, flush the catheter with 0.9% NaCl to aspirate blood.

HCl, hydochloric acid.

© The Hospital for Sick Children. Adapted from *Pediatric Thromboembolism and Stroke Guidelines*. 3rd ed. Hamilton, Ontario, Canada: Hospital for Sick Children; 2006.

Table 22.14	Common Blood Products		
Blood Product	Indications	Dosage	Special Considerations
pRBCs	· Maintain tissue oxygenation · Hb <70 g/L ± significant symptoms of anemia	10-15 mL/kg (correct Hb by 20-30 g/L)	· May be more aggressive in neonates, congenital heart disease and critically ill · CMV-negative blood for CMV-negative BMT patients or pregnant women; intrauterine transfusions · Irradiated blood for premature infants, BMT, congenital immunodeficiency, malignancy
Random-donor PLT	· Bleeding in thrombocytopenia or PLT dysfunction · Prophylaxis if PLT <10 × 10⁹/L	1 unit/5 kg to max 6 units (5-10 mL/kg to max 300 mL)	· Consider single-donor PLT for aplastic anemia and those refractory to multiple random-donor PLT · Keep PLT >50 × 10⁹/L for procedures with blood loss, >100 × 10⁹/L for neurosurgery
FFP	· DIC · Reversal of warfarin · Severe liver disease or vitamin K deficiency · Exchange transfusion	10 mL/kg	
Cryoprecipitate	Bleeding with hypofibrinogenemia (<1.0 mg/mL)	1 unit/10 kg	· May use for FVIII and vWF deficiency if concentrates not available
Albumin	Volume expansion	0.5-1.0 g/kg	· Available as 5% or 25% · Limited value in protein-losing states

OBTAINING CONSENT FOR TRANSFUSION

- Describe blood product and outline benefits, risks, and alternatives to transfusion
- See Box 22.1 for risks that should be discussed

Box 22.1	Risks of Transfusions

- Urticaria (1:100)
- Fever (1:300)
- Anaphylaxis (1:40,000)
- Infectious
  - Hepatitis B (1:82,000)
  - Hepatitis C (1:3,100,000)
  - HIV (1:4,700,000)
  - Bacterial sepsis
    - PLT (1:10,000)
    - PRBCs (1:100,000)

TRANSFUSION REACTIONS

Immediate Reactions

- See Figure 22.9

Delayed Reactions

1. Hemolysis
   - DAT (Coombs) positive: due to RBC alloantibodies (presents 3–14 d post-transfusion)
   - DAT negative: consider poor integrity of transfused RBCs (if frozen, overheated, outdated) or nontransfusion–related hemolysis
2. Transfusion-associated graft-versus-host disease
   - Can occur in immunocompromised patients
   - Clinical manifestations include a rash, liver dysfunction, diarrhea, pancytopenia
   - Treated with immunosuppression, but mortality >90%
3. Sepsis from bacterial contamination
4. Posttransfusion purpura (5–10 d after transfusion of PLT-containing blood products that are PLT antigen positive when recipient is antigen negative)
5. Alloimmune neutropenia and thrombocytopenia from transfusion are very rare

Figure 22.9 **Management of Immediate Transfusion Reactions**

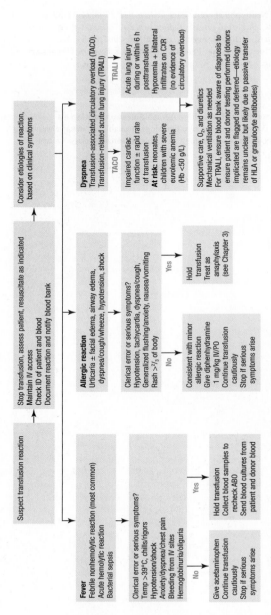

Suspect transfusion reaction

→ Stop transfusion, assess patient, resuscitate as indicated
Maintain IV access
Check ID of patient and blood
Document reaction and notify blood bank

→ Consider etiologies of reaction, based on clinical symptoms

Fever
Febrile nonhemolytic reaction (most common)
Acute hemolytic reaction
Bacterial sepsis

Clerical error or serious symptoms?
Temp >39°C, chills/rigors
Hypotension/shock
Anxiety/dyspnea/chest pain
Bleeding from IV sites
Hemoglobinuria/oliguria

No
Give acetaminophen
Continue transfusion cautiously
Stop if serious symptoms arise

Yes
Hold transfusion
Collect blood samples to recheck ABO
Send blood cultures from patient and donor blood

Allergic reaction
Urticaria ± facial edema, airway edema, dyspnea/cough/wheeze, hypotension, shock

Clerical error or serious symptoms?
Hypotension, tachycardia, dyspnea/cough,
Generalized flushing/anxiety, nausea/vomiting
Rash >2/3 of body

No
Consistent with minor allergic reaction
Give diphenhydramine
1 mg/kg IV/PO
Continue transfusion cautiously
Stop if serious symptoms arise

Yes
Hold transfusion
Treat as anaphylaxis (see Chapter 3)

Dyspnea
Transfusion-associated circulatory overload (TACO).
Transfusion-related acute lung injury (TRALI)

TACO
Impaired cardiac function ± rapid rate of transfusion
At risk: neonates, children with severe euvolemic anemia (Hb <50 g/L)

TRALI
Acute lung injury during or within 6 h posttransfusion
Hypoxemia + bilateral infiltrates on CXR (no evidence of circulatory overload)

Supportive care, O₂, and diuretics
Mechanical ventilation as needed
For TRALI, ensure blood bank aware of diagnosis to ensure patient and donor testing performed (donors implicated are flagged and deferred—etiology remains unclear but likely due to passive transfer of HLA or granulocyte antibodies)

Adapted from Callum JL, Pinkerton PH. *Bloody Easy 2: Blood Transfusions, Blood Alternative and Transfusion Reactions.* 2nd ed. Toronto, Ontario, Canada: Sunnybrook and Women's College Health Sciences Centre; 2005:36, 43, 49. Reprinted by permission of Dr. Jeannie Callum.

FURTHER READING

Boxer LA. Neutrophil abnormalities. *Pediatr Rev.* 2003;24:52–62.

Driscoll MC. Sickle cell disease. *Pediatr Rev.* 2007;28:259–268.

Richardson M. Microcytic anemia. *Pediatr Rev.* 2007;28:5–14.

Sills RH, Hochberg Z, eds. *Practical Algorithms in Pediatric Hematology and Oncology.* Albany, NY: Karger; 2003.

USEFUL WEB SITES

American Society of Hematology. Available at: www.hematology.org

Journal of Pediatric Hematology/Oncology. Available at: www.jpho-online.com/

Medeiros N. Atlas of hematology. Available at: www.hematologyatlas.com/

Hematology

22

Chapter 23 Immunoprophylaxis

Melanie M. Makhija
Dat J. Tran

Chapter 23 Immunoprophylaxis

COMMON ABBREVIATIONS

BCG	bacille Calmette-Guérin
CMV	cytomegalovirus
DTaP-IPV	diptheria, tetanus, acellular pertussis, and inactivated polio vaccine
GA	gestational age
HBV	hepatitis B virus
HCV	hepatitis C virus
HBIG	hepatitis B immune globulin
Hep A	hepatitis A
Hep B	hepatitis B
Hib	*Haemophilus influenzae* type B
HIV	human immunodeficiency virus
HPV	human papillomavirus
HTLV	human T-lymphotropic virus
Inf	influenza
IVIG	intravenous immunoglobulin
Men-C	Menjugate C
MMR	measles, mumps, and rubella
OPV	oral polio vaccine
Pneu-C-7	pneumococcal-7-valent conjugate vaccine
RIG	rabies immunoglobulin
RSV	respiratory syncytial virus
Tdap	tetanus, diphtheria, acellular pertussis
Var	varicella
VZIG	varicella zoster immunoglobulin

IMMUNIZATIONS

- See Table 23.1 for selected common immunizations
- See Tables 23.2, 23.3, and 23.4 for routine immunization schedules
- See Table 23.5 for common myths about immunization
- See Box 23.1 for conditions that are not contraindications to immunization

GENERAL SAFETY AND CONTRAINDICATIONS

Absolute Contraindications

- Anaphylaxis to vaccine component (refer to allergist to determine cause of reaction, which vaccines should be avoided, and for how long)
- Significant immunosuppression (avoid live vaccines only)
- Pregnancy (avoid live vaccines only)

Table 23.1	Selected Common Immunizations/Vaccinations		
Vaccine	Indications for Use	Dosing and Administration	Adverse Reactions
DTaP-IPV + Hib	Routine immunization	0.5 mL IM	Swelling, redness and pain (up to 40%) Fever (5%) Irritability, vomiting uncommon
Hepatitis A	See Hepatitis A section	0.5 mL IM	Pain, erythema, swelling (<5%) Malaise, fever, GI symptoms (10%)
Hepatitis B	Routine immunization	See Hepatitis B section	Pain, erythema, swelling (<5%) Fever (10%)
HPV	Females 9–26 yr	0.5 mL IM	Pain, erythema, swelling (up to 80%) Fever (10%)
Influenza	Varies by province/state	<3 yr: 0.25 mL IM >3 yr: 0.5 mL IM	Pain (10–72%) Fever (<12%) Myalgias, abdominal pain, oculorespiratory syndrome uncommon
MMR*	Routine immunization	0.5 mL SC	Fever (17%), rash (5%) Lymphadenopathy uncommon Febrile seizure (1/3000) Arthralgias (25% adolescents) Thrombocytopenia (1/30,000)
Men-C	Routine immunization	0.5 mL IM	Pain, erythema, swelling (up to 50%) Fever (5%)
Pneu-C-7	Routine immunization of children ≤23 mo Use in 24–59 mo, if at risk	0.5 mL IM	Pain, erythema, swelling (up to 30%) Fever (10%) Irritability, diarrhea, restless sleep, rash/hives uncommon
Rotavirus*	No current routine immunization in Canada	2 mL PO	Fever (20%) Diarrhea and vomiting (<10%)
Varicella*	Routine immunization	0.5 mL SC	Mild local reactions common Rash (<1/100,000)

*Live-attenuated vaccine.

Relative Contraindications

- Chronic illness or immunocompromised state with possible reduced response to vaccines
- History of Guillain-Barré syndrome with onset within 8 wk of a previous immunization
- Immunocompromised patient: vaccines generally deferred but should still be considered if benefits outweigh potential harms or if reduced vaccine immunogenicity still results in benefit

Table 23.2 — Routine Immunization Schedule for Infants and Children

Age at Vaccination	DTaP-IPV	Hib	MMR	Var	Hep B	Pneu-C-7	Men-C	Tdap	Inf	HPV
Birth					★					
2 mo	×	◆			Infant	✓	⊙			
4 mo	×	◆			3 doses	✓	(⊙)			
6 mo	×	◆				✓	⊙		6–23 mo*	
12 mo			■	●	OR	✓ 12–15 mo	OR ⊙ if not yet given		OR 6 mo– 18 yr† 1–2 doses	
18 mo	×	◆	■						yearly	
4–6 yr	×		OR ■	(●)	Preteen/ teen					
14–16 yr					2–3 doses		⊙ if not yet given	▲		3 doses 9–26 yr

Note: Parentheses around symbols indicate that these doses may not be required, depending on the guidelines for the province/state or the age of the child.

*National Advisory Committee on Immunization, Public Health Agency of Canada.

†Advisory Committee on Immunization Practices, Centers for Disease Control and Prevention.

×DTaP-IPV (± Hib): preferred vaccine in this series, including completion of the series in children who received one or more doses of whole-cell pertussis (DTP) vaccine (i.e., recent immigrants). The 4–6-yr dose can be omitted if fourth dose was given after child's fourth birthday.

◆ Hib: for catch-up schedule, the number of doses depends on the age at which first dose was given (Table 23.3). Not usually required past age 5 yr.

■MMR: in the catch-up schedules (Tables 23.3 and 23.4), the first dose should not be given until after 12 mo of age, and the second dose is to be given at least 1 mo after first dose for better measles protection. MMR should be given to all susceptible adolescents and adults.

●Var: children aged 12 mo–12 yr should receive one dose of varicella vaccine (2 doses recommended by CDC in United States). Susceptible individuals ≥13 yr should receive two doses at least 28 d apart.

★Hep B: see section on Hepatitis B vaccine for detailed scheduling and dosage.

✓Pneu-C-7: recommended for all children < 2 yr of age. Schedule depends on age of child when vaccination began. Older children and adults with risk factors may receive the polysaccharide pneumococcal vaccine.

⊙Men-C: recommended for children <5 yr of age, adolescents, and young adults. Schedule depends on age and conjugate vaccine used. At least one dose in the primary infant series should be given after 5 mo of age. If provincial/state policy is to give Men-C to persons ≥12 mo of age, one dose is sufficient. Older than 5 yr, may use quadrivalent conjugate or polysaccharide vaccine.

▲Tdap: combined adsorbed adult-type preparation for persons >7 yr.

Table 23.3	Routine Immunization Schedule for Children <7 Years of Age Not Immunized in Early Infancy							
Timing	DTaP-IPV	Hib	MMR	Var	Hep B	Pneu-C-7	Men-C	Tdap
First visit	×	◆	■	●	★	✓	⊙	
2 mo later	×	(◆)	■		★	(✓)	⊙	
4 mo later	×					(✓)		
6–12 mo later	×	(◆)			★			
4–6 yr of age	(×)							
14–16 yr of age								▲

See Table 23.2 for key of symbols.

Table 23.4	Routine Immunization Schedule for Children 7 to 17 Years of Age Not Immunized in Early Infancy					
Timing	Tdap	IPV	MMR	Var	Hep B	Men-C
First visit	▲	◆	■	●	★	⊙
2 mo later	▲	◆	■	(●)	(★)	
6–12 mo later	▲	◆			★	
10 yr later	▲					

See Table 23.2 for key of symbols.

Table 23.5	Common Myths of Events Linked to Vaccine Exposure	
Exposure	Events Judged Not to Be Causally Linked With Exposure	Year Reviewed and National Academies Press Site Address for Each Citation
Multiple immunizations	· Infection susceptibility · Type I diabetes mellitus · SIDS	2002-http://fermat.nap.edu/catalog/10306.html 2003-http://fermat.nap.edu/catalog/10649.html
MMR and other vaccines with thimerosal	· Autism	2004-http://fermat.nap.edu/catalog/10997.html
Influenza vaccine	· Relapses of multiple sclerosis	2004-http://fermat.nap.edu/catalog/10822.html
Diphtheria and/ or tetanus toxoid– containing vaccines	· SIDS · Infantile spasms · Encephalopathy	2003-http://fermat.nap.edu/catalog/10649.html 1994-http://fermat.nap.edu/catalog/2138.html
Whole-cell pertussis vaccines	· SIDS	2003-http://fermat.nap.edu/catalog/10649.html

Box 23.1	Conditions That Are Not Contraindications to Immunization

- Premature infants
- Pregnancy (inactivated vaccines)
- Neurologic disorder
- Cancer (inactivated vaccines)
- Minor acute illness regardless of fever
- Antimicrobial therapy, except:
  1. Live oral typhoid: delay until 48 h after last dose of antibiotics
  2. Live-attenuated varicella vaccine: reduced effectiveness if given concurrently with antivirals active against herpes group viruses
- Tuberculin skin testing

Egg Allergy

- Influenza and yellow fever vaccines prepared in embryonated eggs should not be given unless risk of disease outweighs small risk of hypersensitivity
- See Chapter 8 for evaluation and graded challenge or desensitization
- Allergies/atopy not a contraindication to immunization with egg-containing vaccine
- Egg allergy not a contraindication to MMR immunization

Adverse Event Reporting

- All adverse events should be reported to the local public health unit; severe adverse events should also be reported to national monitoring programs: Canadian Adverse Events Following Immunization Surveillance System (CAEFISS) in Canada and Vaccine Adverse Events Reporting System (VAERS) in the United States

IMMUNIZATION IN IMMUNOCOMPROMISED PATIENTS

PRIMARY IMMUNODEFICIENCIES

- Live vaccines generally contraindicated (see Table 23.1)
- Inactivated vaccines as per routine schedule, although response may be inadequate
- For specific immunodeficiencies, see *Canadian Immunization Guide*, 7th ed., or *American Academy of Pediatrics Redbook*, 27th ed.
- Household contacts may receive all routine vaccines as per schedule

PATIENTS WITH HIV INFECTION

- All vaccines indicated except BCG, OPV, smallpox
- Consider withholding MMR, varicella, and rotavirus vaccines if severely immunocompromised
- Varicella vaccine: children ≥12 mo with asymptomatic or mildly symptomatic HIV infection and CD4 ≥25% may be vaccinated with two doses 3 mo apart

PATIENTS TAKING CORTICOSTEROIDS

- Live-virus vaccines are not contraindicated for:
  - Topical therapy/local injections/inhaled steroids
  - Physiologic maintenance doses of steroids or low-dose steroids (<2 mg/kg/d prednisone equivalent)
- High-dose steroids (greater than physiologic; >2 mg/kg/d prednisone equivalent):
  - <14 d therapy: delay giving live vaccines by 2 wk if patient's condition allows, but may give immediately, if necessary
  - >14 d therapy: wait at least 1 mo after discontinuation of steroids

PATIENTS TAKING OTHER IMMUNOSUPPRESSIVE THERAPY

- Immunosuppressants other than corticosteroids include cytostatics (cyclophosphamide, methotrexate, azathioprine, dactinomycin), antibodies (antilymphocyte and antithymocyte antibodies, OKT3, anti-CD25), cyclosporine, tacrolimus
- Inactivated vaccines are indicated: attempt to give all appropriate vaccines at least 14 d before or 3 mo after therapy
- Live vaccines generally contraindicated; however, consider risk–benefit ratios
- Children with lymphoblastic leukemia should receive varicella vaccine if in remission for >12 mo, total lymphocyte count >1.2×10^9/L, and patient not receiving radiation; maintenance therapy should be withheld for 1 wk before and 1 wk after immunization; two doses 1–3 mo apart recommended

Immunoprophylaxis

23

SELECTED INFECTIONS AND PROPHYLAXIS

HEPATITIS A

Pre-exposure Prophylaxis

- Hepatitis A vaccine recommended for those at increased risk of infection
  - Travelers to endemic countries
  - Residents of endemic areas or areas at risk of outbreaks
  - Chronic liver disease (including hepatitis C), recipients (or likely recipients) of hepatotoxic medications
  - Hemophilia A or B patients receiving plasma-derived replacement clotting factors

Postexposure Prophylaxis

- Hepatitis A vaccine highly effective in first wk postexposure; give to close contacts of proven or suspected cases (household, school, day care)
- Protection occurs within 2 wk of immunization so can elicit adequate immune response given long hepatitis A incubation (2–7 wk)

- Immunoglobulin (nonspecific Ig) should be used if vaccine unavailable; in infants <1 yr; for immunocompromised or other vaccine contraindications (see General Safety and Contraindications section)
- Dose varies according to duration of protection needed and according to manufacturer
- IVIG 5% (50 g/L protein): for protection lasting <3 mo, 0.02 mL/kg; for 3–5 mo, 0.06 mL/kg; >5 mo, 0.06 mL/kg every 5 mo
- Usual postexposure prophylaxis dose: 0.02 mL/kg as soon as possible after exposure

HEPATITIS B

- See Table 23.6

Postexposure Prophylaxis

- Infants born to infected mothers
  - Give initial dose of vaccine within 12 h of birth
  - Give IM dose 0.5 mL HBIG immediately after birth; efficacy decreases sharply after 48 h
- Response to HBV is diminished if birth weight <2 kg
  - If mother known negative, delay immunization until infant weight >2000 g or >1 mo
  - If mother positive, give HBV/HBIG (3 doses per Table 23.6) plus fourth dose of HBV and assess response (HBsAb)
  - If maternal status unknown, do serologic testing at birth, and consider HBV and HBIG administration while results pending

HIV

- See Table 23.7

Table 23.6	Dosing and Schedule for Hepatitis B Vaccines					
	Recombivax HB			Engerix B		
Recipients	mcg	mL	Schedule (mo)	mcg	mL	Schedule (mo)
Infants of HBV-negative mothers or children <11 yr†	2.5	0.25	0, 1, 6*	10	0.5	1, 2, 6 OR 0, 1, 2, 12
Infants of HBV-positive mothers†	5.0	0.5	0, 1, 6*	10	0.5	0, 1, 6 OR 0, 1, 2, 12
11–15 yr	10.0	1.0	0, 4–6	20	0.5	0, 6
11–19 yr	10.0	1.0	0, 1, 6*	10	0.5	0, 1, 6 OR 0, 1, 2, 12

*Although schedule of 0, 1, and >2 mo is approved, preferred schedule is 0, 1, and 6 mo.
†Thimerosal preservative-free preparation recommended.

Table 23.7

Table 23.7	Prevention of Selected Opportunistic Infections in HIV	
Pathogen	Indications	Antimicrobial Options
Pneumocystis jiroveci	All infants 1–12 mo; children >12 mo with CD4% <15%	Trimethoprim-sulfamethoxazole Alternatives: dapsone, pentamidine (aerosolized), atovaquone
Mycobacterium avium complex (MAC)	≥6 yr: CD4 <50; 2–6 yr: CD4 <75; 1–2 yr: CD4 <500; <1 yr: CD4 <750	Azithromycin or clarithromycin
Mycobacterium tuberculosis	Tuberculin skin test ≥5 mm or prior untreated positive result; contact with active TB case	Isoniazid Alternatives: rifampin if known isoniazid resistance; consult local tuberculosis expert if known multidrug resistance
Toxoplasma gondii	IgG positive and severe immune suppression	Trimethoprim-sulfamethoxazole Alternatives: dapsone + pyrimethamine; atovaquone

INFLUENZA

- Any healthy child or adolescent may receive influenza vaccine
- Strongly recommended for children at high risk of influenza complications:
  - Chronic illnesses
  - Increased aspiration risk
  - Taking ASA (increased risk of Reye syndrome with influenza)
  - Age 6–23 mo (National Advisory Committee on Immunization [NACI], Canada); age 6 mo–18 yr (Advisory Committee on Immunization Practices [ACIP], United States)
  - Close contact with high-risk individuals (e.g., health care workers, household contacts, child care workers)
- Previously unvaccinated children <9 yr require two doses at least 4 wk apart; a second dose within the same season is not required if the child received a dose during the previous influenza season

MENINGOCOCCAL DISEASE

Postexposure Prophylaxis

- Chemoprophylaxis with rifampin, ceftriaxone, or alternatives for close contacts of a patient with invasive meningococcal disease, health care workers with intense unprotected contact (not wearing mask) with patient (e.g., intubating, resuscitating), airline passengers on either side of the patient
- Close contacts should be vaccinated: increased risk of disease for 1 yr; for patients older than 2 yr, quadrivalent polysaccharide or conjugate vaccines available against strains A, C, Y, and W-135

Immunoprophylaxis

23

- Close contacts include:
  - Household contacts
  - Persons who sleep in same room as patient
  - Persons in contact with oral/nasal secretions of patient
  - Children and staff in child care or nursery school attended by patient

PERTUSSIS

- Postexposure prophylaxis:
  - Vaccinate all unimmunized or partially immunized close contacts <7 yr
  - Fourth dose of DTaP if third dose was given >6 mo before
  - Booster dose of DTaP if last dose >3 yr before and child <7 yr old
  - Chemoprophylaxis for all close contacts (household, child care): azithromycin (5 d), erythromycin (14 d), or clarithromycin (7 d)

RABIES

Pre-exposure Management

- Offer rabies vaccination if high risk of contact with rabid animals
  - Travelers to endemic areas with poor access to postexposure management
  - Children too young to avoid animals or report traumatic contact traveling to endemic areas
- Three doses of vaccine required; give on days 0, 7, and 21

Postexposure Management

- Treatment with vaccine and RIG highly effective in preventing rabies in exposed individuals
- Consider in every potential animal exposure
- See Table 23.8

Dosing, Schedule, and Administration

Postexposure Prophylaxis of
Previously Unimmunized Individual

- Give five doses of vaccine IM: first dose as soon as possible after exposure and then on days 3, 7, 14, and 28 after the first dose
- 20 IU/kg RIG should also be given on day 0; do not exceed recommended dose
  - Infiltrate into wound and surrounding area; if not anatomically feasible, inject remaining volume IM at site distant from vaccine site
  - If >1 wound, infiltrate each with part of RIG using separate needle and syringe
  - If site unknown, give all RIG IM at site distant from vaccine site
- *Do not* administer vaccine in same syringe or at same site as RIG

Table 23.8	Postexposure Prophylaxis When Not Previously Immunized Against Rabies	
Animal Species	**Condition of Animal at Time of Exposure**	**Management of Exposed Person**
Dog, cat, or ferret	· Healthy and available for 10 d observation	· Local wound treatment · At first sign of rabies in animal, give RIG (local and IM) and vaccine, unless bite wound to the head or neck (begin immediately)
	· Rabid or suspected* · Unknown or escaped	· Local wound treatment · RIG (wound site and IM) and vaccine
Skunk, bat, fox, raccoon/other carnivores (includes bat found in room when a person is sleeping)	· Regard as rabid* unless geographic area is known to be rabies free	· Local treatment of wound · RIG (local and IM) and vaccine
Livestock, rodents, hares, rabbits	· Consider individually; consult appropriate public health officials; consider prophylaxis if animal behavior unusual	

*If possible, animal should be humanely killed and brain tested for rabies; holding for observation not recommended. Discontinue vaccine if fluorescent antibody test of animal brain negative.

Adverse Reactions
- Common reactions include local pain, erythema, swelling; serious side effects rare
- Mild systemic reactions include headache, nausea, muscle aches, dizziness
- Systemic allergic reactions uncommon in primary immunization but occur in up to 7% receiving booster dose with onset after 2 to 21 d

Precautions
- For postexposure vaccination in patients with egg allergies with RabAvert vaccine when no other rabies vaccine options available, vaccinate in centers where anaphylaxis management is readily available

RSV
- See Box 23.2
- No available vaccine; palivizumab immunoglobulin (RSV-Ig) used
- Note: palivizumab *not* indicated for treatment of active RSV infection

VARICELLA

Indications

- See Table 23.2 for routine immunization schedule
- Children with history of varicella infection at <1 yr of age may not develop long-term immunity; should receive vaccine as per regular schedule
- Older children who are close contacts of immunocompromised patients
- Older children at high risk of severe varicella:
  - Chronic salicylic acid therapy (associated risk of Reye syndrome)
  - Cystic fibrosis
  - Immunocompromised children, depending on type and severity (see Immunization in Immunocompromised Patients section)

Postexposure Immunization

- Give varicella vaccine within 3–5 d of exposure to prevent infection or reduce severity
- See Box 23.3 for indications for use of VZIG
- VZIG dosing: 125 IU/10 kg to max 625 IU; min. dose 125 IU
- Maximal benefit if administered within 96 h after first exposure, lasting approximately 3 wk

Precautions

- For children receiving long-term salicylic acid therapy, avoid ASA for 6 wk after varicella immunization (increased risk of Reye syndrome)
- Concurrent antivirals used against Herpesviridae may reduce efficacy of vaccine; discontinue, if possible, for at least 24 h before and 4 wk after vaccination

Box 23.3   Indications for Use of Varicella Zoster Immunoglobulin

Significant Exposure to Varicella
- Continuous household contact
- Being indoors for more than 1 h with a person with varicella
- Having more than 15 min of face-to-face contact with a patient with varicella
- Touching the lesions of a person with active varicella or zoster

Increased Risk of Severe Varicella
- Immunocompromised patients
- Newborns of mothers who develop varicella 5 d before or 48 h after delivery
- Pregnancy (to protect mother; no protection against varicella embryopathy)
- Hospitalized premature infant (<28 wk or ≤1000 g) with exposure, regardless of maternal history
- Hospitalized premature infant (≥28 wk) if mother susceptible
- Postallogeneic hematopoietic stem cell transplant recipients, regardless of varicella history or serologic test result

INTRAVENOUS IMMUNOGLOBULIN PREPARATIONS

IVIG

- Concentrated solution derived from human plasma containing mainly IgG and small amounts of IgA and IgM; contains between 100 g/L and 180 g/L protein. Used for treatment of immunodeficiencies, Kawasaki disease, immune thrombocytopenia purpura and prevention of infections in HIV, leukemia, and after bone marrow transplant
- Maximum plasma levels 2 d after injection; half-life 21–27 d

Adverse Effects

- Minor: headache, rhinitis, fever, malaise, vomiting, nausea, asthma, abdominal or back pain, myalgias, tremors
- Severe: anaphylaxis, Stevens-Johnson syndrome, hypotension, MI, stroke, seizure, pulmonary embolism, transfusion-induced lung injury, acute renal failure, thrombosis, cytopenia

Relative Contraindications

- Hypersensitivity to IVIG, blood products, or components: may be avoided by pretreatment with hydrocortisone, diphenhydramine, aspirin/ibuprofen, and IV hydration. Anaphylaxis to IVIG is an absolute contraindication
- IgA deficiency

CMV HYPERIMMUNOGLOBULIN

- Indicated for prophylaxis (with ganciclovir) in solid-organ transplant patients at greatest risk of primary CMV disease (e.g., seropositive donor to seronegative recipient)
- Use in seropositive recipients to reduce disease severity
- Use in prophylaxis for allogeneic hematopoietic stem cell transplant recipients remains controversial

RISK OF SEROCONVERSION AFTER PERCUTANEOUS NEEDLE-STICK INJURY FROM DOCUMENTED INFECTED SOURCE/PATIENT

- HBV: 5% from HBeAg negative; 19–30% from HBeAg positive
- HCV: 1.8%
- HIV: 0.31%

MANAGEMENT

- Local wound care: immediately cleanse site, allow wound to bleed freely
- Assess hepatitis B and tetanus immunization status and update, if needed
- Baseline blood tests:
  - Source patient: serology for HBV, HCV, and HIV (requires consent)
  - Health care worker: serology for HBV, HCV, and HIV; CBC and liver enzymes, if initiating postexposure prophylaxis with antiretroviral medications
- Counseling of health care worker as to whether HIV prophylaxis indicated in consultation with infectious disease consultant
- HIV postexposure prophylaxis regimens may involve two or three antiretrovirals
- Follow-up counseling and testing in 6 wk, 3 mo, and 6 mo
- Management of community needle-stick injuries (e.g., child playing with discarded needle) generally similar with few modifications:
  - HIV, HBV, and HCV status of source unknown in vast majority of cases
  - If child did not receive complete HBV immunization series, give HBIG and first HBV dose immediately; continue vaccination series if no antibodies present and hepatitis B surface Ag (HBsAg) negative
  - If child received complete HBV immunization and is hepatitis B surface antibody (HBsAb) positive or HBsAg positive, no prophylaxis indicated; if HBsAg positive, refer to infectious disease and/or gastroenterology (hepatology) consultant
  - Risk of acquiring HIV from discarded needles extremely remote; infectious disease consultation for risk–benefit counseling required
  - Postexposure HIV prophylaxis not indicated >72 h after exposure

EXPRESSED BREAST MILK: ERRORS IN ADMINISTRATION

- Main pathogens of concern: HBV, HCV, HIV, HTLV-I, HTLV-II, and CMV (Table 23.9)

Table 23.9	Pathogens Potentially Transmissible by Breast Milk
HIV	Estimated overall risk of transmission 0.00064/L of breast milk
HTLV I/II	Breast milk transmission is the primary mode of transmission; the risk from a single exposure is unknown
HBV	Not considered a significant mode of transmission, but theoretical risk present
HCV	Transmission theoretically possible but has not been documented
CMV	Excreted in breast milk; main risk in premature newborns who lack protective antibody (<28 wk gestation or seronegative mother)

LABORATORY TESTING

- Laboratory testing of donor mother and recipient patient's mother (informed consent is required):
  - HBsAg
  - Hepatitis C serology
  - HIV serology
  - HTLV I and II serology
  - CMV serology
- Laboratory testing of recipient infant only advised if infant received blood products
- HIV serology and HBsAg are ordered *stat* as the results may affect prophylaxis administration

POSTEXPOSURE PROPHYLAXIS

- Where indicated, HBIG and vaccine must be given within 48 h of the incident
- Counsel in regard to HIV postexposure prophylaxis as soon as possible
- Decision to prescribe HIV postexposure prophylaxis individualized based on donor's HIV status and HIV risk factors in consultation with infectious disease consultant and the child's caregivers
- Postexposure prophylaxis not available for HCV, HTLV-I, or HTLV-II, and not usually indicated for CMV

FURTHER READING

Canadian Immunization Guide. 7th ed. National Advisory Committee on Immunizations; 2006.

Pickering LK, Baker CJ, Long SS, McMillan JA, eds. *Red Book: 2006 Report of the Committee on Infectious Diseases*. 27th ed. Elk Grove Village, Ill: American Academy of Pediatrics; 2006.

Immunoprophylaxis

23

USEFUL WEB SITES

American Academy of Pediatrics immunization Web site. Available at: www.cispimmunize.org/

American Academy of Pediatrics *Redbook* online. Available at: aapredbook.aappublications.org/

Centers for Disease Control and Prevention information for parents and health care providers. Available at: www.cdc.gov/vaccines/

Centers for Disease Control and Prevention, National Immunization Program. Available at: http://www.cdc.gov/vaccines/

Children's Hospital of Philadelphia education center Web site for parents and health care providers. Available at: www.chop.edu/consumer/jsp/microsite/microsite.jsp?id=75918

Public Health Agency of Canada. *Canadian Immunization Guide*. Available at: www.phac-aspc.gc.ca/im/index.html

Public Health Agency of Canada. Immunizations related to travel outside of Canada. Available at: www.phac-aspc.gc.ca/tmp-pmv/236_e.html

World Health Organization immunization Web site. Available at: www.who.int/immunization/en/

Chapter 24 Infectious Diseases

Michelle Bridge

Sloane J. Freeman

Ari Bitnun

COMMON ABBREVIATIONS

ADEM	acute disseminated encephalomyelitis
CMV	cytomegalovirus
CSF	cerebrospinal fluid
EBV	Epstein-Barr virus
EM	electron microscopy
FSWU	full septic workup
GAS	group A streptococcus
HCV	hepatitis C virus
HHV	human herpes virus
HIV	human immunodeficiency virus
HSV	herpes simplex virus
ICP	intracranial pressure
INH	isoniazid
LIP	lymphoid interstitial pneumonitis
LP	lumbar puncture
LTBI	latent tuberculosis infection
PCR	polymerase chain reaction
PJP	*Pneumocystis jiroveci* pneumonia
PMN	polymorphonuclear cells (neutrophils)
PPD	purified protein derivative
SBI	serious bacterial infection
SCID	severe combined immunodeficiency
SNHL	sensorineural hearing loss
STI	sexually transmitted infection
TB	tuberculosis
TMP/SMX	trimethoprim/sulfamethoxazole
TST	tuberculin skin test
UTI	urinary tract infection
VZV	varicella zoster virus

FEVER WITHOUT A SOURCE

DEFINITIONS

- Fever: rectal temperature ≥38°C
- Fever without source: acute febrile illness with no apparent etiology after careful history and physical examination

- SBI: include meningitis, sepsis, bone and joint infections, UTI, pneumonia, enteritis
- Occult bacteremia: presence of pathogenic bacteria in blood without appearance of toxicity
- Toxic: clinical picture consistent with sepsis (i.e., lethargy with signs of poor perfusion, marked hypoventilation or hyperventilation, cyanosis)
- FSWU: CBC, cultures of blood, catheter urine and CSF; CXR, and stool cultures if indicated

GENERAL PRINCIPLES

- All *toxic* patients should undergo resuscitation (see Chapter 1), FSWU, admission, and empiric IV antibiotics according to child's age

MANAGEMENT OF NONTOXIC FEBRILE NEONATES 0–1 MO

- Febrile neonates are at high risk of SBI (12–13%): require admission, FSWU, and empiric antibiotic therapy
- Neonatal HSV and enteroviral infections can mimic bacterial sepsis; consider in differential diagnosis
- If concern over HSV, send CSF for HSV PCR and look for disseminated disease (blood HSV PCR, liver enzymes, HSV swabs of conjunctiva, nose, mouth, and rectum)

Treatment

- Broad-spectrum parenteral antimicrobial therapy (e.g., ampicillin and tobramycin; ampicillin and cefotaxime, if meningitis suspected) pending culture results
- If HSV is a significant concern, consider empiric therapy with acyclovir pending PCR results

MANAGEMENT OF NONTOXIC FEBRILE INFANTS 1–3 MO

- See Table 24.1 for criteria to identify low-risk patients
- Close follow-up essential if outpatient management
- Antibiotic choice for admitted infants: ampicillin and cefotaxime, or consult local institutional guidelines; vancomycin should be added if penicillin-nonsusceptible *S. pneumoniae* is a concern
- See Figure 24.1 for management of febrile infants 1–3 mo of age

MANAGEMENT OF NONTOXIC FEBRILE INFANTS 3–36 MO

- Overall risk of bacteremia: approximately 1.6%
- Elevated WBC more predictive of bacteremia than height of fever in this population; WBC >30,000 carries 18.3% risk, whereas temperature >41.0°C carries 2.8% risk

Table 24.1	Criteria for Determining Febrile Infants at Low Risk (1%) of Having a Serious Bacterial Infection*	
	"Rochester Criteria"	Baker et al.
Age group	Up to 60 d	29–56 d
Past health	Born at >37 wk gestation Home with or before mother No subsequent hospitalizations No perinatal, postnatal, or current antibiotics No treatment for unexplained hyperbilirubinemia No chronic disease	No known immune deficiency
Physical examination	Rectal temperature >38.0°C Appears generally well with no evidence of skin, soft tissue, bone, joint, or ear infection	Rectal temperature >38.2°C Infant observation score ≤10 (see reference for score)
Laboratory: Total WBC Bands Band/mature PMN	$5.0–15.0 \times 10^9$/L $<1.5 \times 10^9$/L †	$<15.0 \times 10^9$/L † Ratio <0.2
Urine	<10 WBC/HPF‡	<10 WBC/HPF‡
CSF	†	Nonbloody; $<8 \times 10^6$ WBC/L Negative Gram stain
Stool (if diarrhea)	<5 WBC/HPF§	†
Chest X-ray	†	No evidence of discrete infiltrate

*Both sets of criteria assume that the minimal investigative workup includes a culture of blood and urine (obtained by bladder catheterization or puncture).
†Indicates that a particular item was not part of the stated criteria.
‡Refers to examination of centrifuged urine sediment, examined under 40× microscopy.
§Refers to a fecal smear, stained for WBC, examined under 40× microscopy.
WBC, white blood cells; HPF, high-power field.
Adapted from Pusic MV. Clinical management of fever in children younger than three years of age. Pediatr Child Health, 2007; 12: 469–472, and Baraff LJ. Management of fever without source in infants and children. Ann Emerg Med, 2000; 36: 602–614.

Recommendations

- Strongly consider urinalysis for males <6 mo and females <2 yr; if suggestive of UTI, obtain culture by catheter
- CBC and blood cultures at discretion of physician; depends on age, fever duration, clinical appearance, previous medical history, immunization status (especially against pneumococcus), and parental reliability
- Some evidence supports selective administration of empiric antibiotics to patients with high WBC counts
- Judicious use of empiric antibiotics in selected circumstances (poor clinical appearance, previous medical history, lack of immunization, unreliable parents) may be reasonable

Figure 24.1 **Management of Febrile Infants 1–3 Months**

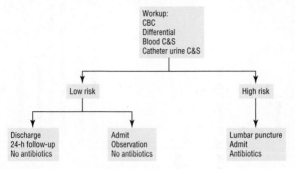

Some centers still use Baker's modified criteria, which include LP for all infants <3 mo.

Infectious Diseases

24

BACTERIAL INFECTIONS

- See Table 24.2 for initial empiric antibiotic therapy
- See Table 24.3 for empiric antibiotic therapy for human and animal bites

TUBERCULOSIS

- Children less able to contain infection than adults; more susceptible to extrapulmonary complications (miliary disease, meningitis, osteomyelitis)

Investigations

- History of exposure (duration, proximity); disease site and severity of source patient, duration of symptoms, antituberculous therapy given, culture results, and susceptibilities of isolate
- TST: 5 tuberculin units (5 TU), 0.1 mL PPD intradermal on volar aspect of forearm, using 27-gauge needle and tuberculin syringe (Mantoux test)
- CXR
- Stains for acid-fast bacilli and TB cultures
  - Sputum if possible (>8 yr old, cavitary disease)
  - Gastric aspirate ×3 in early morning before ambulation or feeding (if respiratory symptoms or positive CXR)
  - Urine first morning void ×3 (if suspected renal involvement)
  - CSF (if suspected meningitis)
- Histology and TB culture when indicated: lymph nodes, liver, spleen, bone marrow; the Amplified Mycobacterium Tuberculosis Direct Test (AMTD) or PCR may be considered on a selective basis
- Caregivers of hospitalized child should be screened for pulmonary TB by CXR, irrespective of symptoms

Table 24.2 Initial Empiric Antibiotic Therapy

System	Suspected Microbial Agent	Antimicrobial	Duration	Comments
CNS				
Meningitis				
Up to 6 wk	GBS, gram-negative enteric bacilli (Escherichia coli), Listeria	Ampicillin + cefotaxime ± vancomycin	GBS, Listeria: 14–21 d; E. coli: 21 d	See Meningitis section
6 wk–3 mo	Organisms from both neonatal and older age range	Ampicillin + cefotaxime + vancomycin	S. pneumoniae: 10–14 d; N. meningitidis: 7 d; gram-negative enteric bacilli: 21 d (min.); Staphylococcus aureus: 21 d (min.); H. influenzae: 7 d	
>3 mo	S. pneumoniae, N. meningitidis, H. influenzae	Ceftriaxone + vancomycin; penicillin allergic: rifampin + vancomycin	—	
VP shunt	Coagulase-negative staphylococci, enteric gram-negative organisms	Vancomycin + cefotaxime (or ceftriaxone)	21 d	Use ceftazidime if concerned about P. aeruginosa
Brain abscess	Streptococci, staphylococci, enterobacteriaceae, anaerobes	Ceftriaxone + cloxacillin + metronidazole	6 wk	Treatment should take into account source of infection; treatment duration depends on response to therapy
Encephalitis	HSV, enterovirus, arboviruses, M. pneumoniae	HSV, VZV: acyclovir	14–21 d	See Encephalitis section

(continued)

Table 24.2 Initial Empiric Antibiotic Therapy (continued)

System	Suspected Microbial Agent	Antimicrobial	Duration	Comments
Respiratory				
Epiglottitis	H. influenzae type b, GAS, S. aureus	Cefuroxime	–	–
Bacterial tracheitis	S. aureus, GAS, H. influenzae	Cefuroxime	–	–
Bacterial pneumonia, community-acquired				
Neonate	GBS, gram-negative enteric bacilli (E. coli), Chlamydia trachomatis, S. aureus, Listeria	Ampicillin + gentamicin ± erythromycin	10–21 d	Add erythromycin if Chlamydia suspected
1–3 mo	S. pneumoniae, C. trachomatis, Bordetella pertussis, S. aureus, H. influenzae	Cefuroxime (IV) ± erythromycin (IV) or clarithromycin (PO)	10 d	Admission recommended Consider cefotaxime + erythromycin or clarithromycin ± cloxacillin (if suspect S. aureus and critically ill)
3 mo–5 yr	S. pneumoniae, S. aureus, H. influenzae, M. pneumoniae, Chlamydia pneumoniae	Ampicillin (IV) (amoxicillin if PO) CCU: cefuroxime + erythromycin or clarithromycin	–	Penicillin allergic: clindamycin, or erythromycin, or clarithromycin
>5 yr	S. pneumoniae, H. influenzae, S. aureus, Chlamydia pneumoniae, M. pneumoniae	Ampicillin (amoxicillin if PO) + erythromycin (IV) or clarithromycin (PO); CCU: cefuroxime + erythromycin (IV) or clarithromycin (PO)	–	If outpatient, consider clarithromycin, or erythromycin or amoxicillin monotherapy

(continued)

Infectious Diseases

24

499

Table 24.2 Initial Empiric Antibiotic Therapy (continued)

System	Suspected Microbial Agent	Antimicrobial	Duration	Comments
Atypical pneumonia	M. pneumoniae, Chlamydia pneumoniae	Erythromycin or clarithromycin	10 d	Respiratory quinolone is reasonable alternative in older children
Non–community-acquired pneumonia				
Immunocompromised	PJP, gram-negative enteric bacilli (E. coli), P. aeruginosa, S. aureus, CMV, respiratory viruses	Piperacillin/tazobactam + tobramycin ± cotrimoxazole (for PJP)	–	Consider type and degree of immunocompromise and clinical status when selecting empiric therapy
Aspiration	Oral anaerobes, gram-negative enteric bacilli (E. coli)	Mild-moderate: none Moderately severe: penicillin Hospital acquired: add gentamicin Severe: clindamycin + gentamicin	–	–
Sickle cell disease	S. pneumoniae, M. pneumoniae, H. influenzae	Cefotaxime ± erythromycin (IV) or clarithromycin (PO) ± vancomycin	–	Vancomycin should be added if patient seriously ill
Pertussis	B. pertussis	Erythromycin (to prevent transmission)	14 d	Peripheral lymphocytosis; admit if severe or if apnea; treat secondary bacterial infections (especially S. pneumoniae)

(continued)

Table 24.2 Initial Empiric Antibiotic Therapy (continued)

System	Suspected Microbial Agent	Antimicrobial	Duration	Comments
Septicemia/Bacteremia (Without Meningitis)				
Neonate	GBS, gram-negative enteric bacilli (E. coli), Enterococcus, Listeria	Ampicillin + tobramycin	–	Gentamicin acceptable depending on susceptibility data in particular area
1–3 mo	Organisms from both neonatal and older age range	Ampicillin + cefotaxime	–	–
>3 mo	S. pneumoniae, N. meningitidis, S. aureus, H. Influenzae	Cefotaxime + vancomycin	–	Add gentamicin if urinary or abdominal source suspected
Fever with neutropenia				
Stable	–	Piperacillin/tazobactam + gentamicin	–	–
Unstable	–	Meropenem + gentamicin + vancomycin	–	–
Sickle cell disease with fever	S. pneumoniae, H. influenzae	Cefotaxime ± vancomycin	–	–
Typhoid fever	Salmonella typhi	Cefotaxime	–	Can narrow therapy, based on antibiotic susceptibilities
Suspected abdominal source	Gram-negative enteric bacilli (E. coli)	Ampicillin + gentamicin + metronidazole	–	–

(continued)

Infectious Diseases

24

Table 24.2 Initial Empiric Antibiotic Therapy (continued)

System	Suspected Microbial Agent	Antimicrobial	Duration	Comments
Asplenia	Encapsulated organisms: *S. pneumoniae, H. influenzae, N. meningitidis*	Cefuroxime ± vancomycin	–	–
Skin and Soft Tissue				
Cellulitis	Neonates: gram-negative bacilli, *S. aureus*	IV cloxacillin + aminoglycoside	7–10 d	–
Cellulitis	Infants and children: *S. aureus*, GAS	Mild: PO cephalexin or cloxacillin Moderate to severe: IV cefazolin or clindamycin + cloxacillin	7–10 d	If invasive GAS disease suspected (chickenpox, immunocompromised, trauma): IV penicillin + clindamycin Selected severe cases of invasive GAS: IVIG
Periorbital cellulitis Traumatic	*S. aureus*, GAS	Cefazolin or cloxacillin	10–14 d	Mild disease: cephalexin
Nontraumatic	*S. pneumoniae*, GAS, *S. aureus*, *H. influenzae, Moraxella catarrhalis*	Cefotaxime or ceftriaxone	10–14 d	If no associated bacteremia and mild disease, step-down to oral therapy with cefuroxime, cefprozil or amoxicillin/clavulanate
Orbital cellulitis	*S. pneumoniae, S. aureus*, GAS, *H. influenzae, M. catarrhalis*, anaerobes	Cloxacillin + ceftriaxone, ± clindamycin or metronidazole	–	Risk: vision loss, cavernous sinus thrombosis; epidural, subdural, or brain abscess

(continued)

Table 24.2   Initial Empiric Antibiotic Therapy (continued)

System	Suspected Microbial Agent	Antimicrobial	Duration	Comments
Necrotizing fasciitis	Invasive GAS, polymicrobial	Clindamycin + cloxacillin	—	Consider IVIG
Cervical adenitis	S. aureus, GAS; neonates: GBS	IV: cefazolin or cloxacillin; PO: cephalexin or cloxacillin; dental source: penicillin V or clindamycin	10 d	Differential diagnosis for chronic adenitis: (a) Focal adenitis: B. henselae, atypical mycobacteria, TB (b) Generalized: EBV, CMV, toxoplasmosis, histoplasmosis, HIV (c) Noninfectious: malignancy, drugs (phenytoin, INH), Kawasaki disease, congenital anomalies (cystic hygroma, branchial cleft cyst, thyroglossal duct cyst)
Impetigo	GAS, S. aureus	Mild: topical mupirocin; severe: cephalexin	—	—
Musculoskeletal				
Septic arthritis				
Neonate	GBS, S. aureus, gram-negative enteric bacilli (E. coli)	Cloxacillin + gentamicin (or cefotaxime)	3–4 wk	Emergent drainage; consult orthopedic surgeon
1–3 mo	H. influenzae type b, Streptococcus spp., Staphylococcus spp., neonatal pathogens (see above)	Cefotaxime + cloxacillin	3–4 wk	Consider clindamycin if significant β-lactam allergy

(continued)

Table 24.2 Initial Empiric Antibiotic Therapy *(continued)*

System	Suspected Microbial Agent	Antimicrobial	Duration	Comments
>3 mo	GAS, S. aureus, S. pneumoniae	Cefazolin	–	Consider clindamycin if significant β-lactam allergy
Adolescent	As above; also consider *Neisseria gonorrhoeae*	Cloxacillin or cefazolin ± ceftriaxone	–	Consider clindamycin + ciprofloxacin (for *N. gonorrhoeae*) if significant β-lactam allergy
Acute osteomyelitis			4–6 wk	IV antibiotics until afebrile and improved; monitor clinical improvement using serial examinations, CBC and ESR or CRP
Neonate	S. aureus, GBS, gram-negative enteric bacilli (E. coli)	Cloxacillin + gentamicin	–	–
1–3 mo	H. influenzae, Streptococcus spp., Staphylococcus spp., neonatal pathogens (see above)	Cefotaxime + cloxacillin	–	Consider clindamycin if significant β-lactam allergy
>3 mo	S. aureus, S. pneumoniae, GAS	Cefazolin	–	Consider clindamycin if significant β-lactam allergy
Sickle cell disease	S. aureus, Salmonella, S. pneumoniae	Cefotaxime + cloxacillin	–	Consider clindamycin if significant β-lactam allergy

(continued)

Table 24.2 Initial Empiric Antibiotic Therapy (continued)

System	Suspected Microbial Agent	Antimicrobial	Duration	Comments
Puncture wound of foot				
Through shoes	*Pseudomonas aeruginosa*	Piperacillin + gentamicin	—	Significant β-lactam allergy: ciprofloxacin + gentamicin
Not through shoes	*S. aureus*	PO: cephalexin IV: cefazolin	—	—
Ear, Nose, and Throat				
Otitis media (acute)	*S. pneumoniae*, *M. catarrhalis*, nontypeable *H. influenzae*, GAS	Initial: amoxicillin or high-dose amoxicillin (90 mg/kg/d); empiric high-dose indicated if child received antibiotics during the preceding mo or has history of recurrent AOM	<2 yr: 10 d; >2 yr: 5–7 d	Other agents: cefprozil, cefuroxime, erythromycin, clarithromycin, azithromycin Failure day 3: high-dose amoxicillin/clavulanate or IM ceftriaxone Consider watchful waiting for 48–72 h before initiating antibiotics in otherwise healthy children >2 yr with mild disease and good follow-up
Mastoiditis	*S. pneumoniae*, GAS, *S. aureus*, nontypeable *H. influenzae*, *M. catarrhalis*	Cefuroxime IV	10 d	Consider oral therapy, when clinically indicated, with cefuroxime or amoxicillin/clavulanate

(continued)

Infectious Diseases

Table 24.2 Initial Empiric Antibiotic Therapy *(continued)*

System	Suspected Microbial Agent	Antimicrobial	Duration	Comments
Sinusitis	Acute: *S. pneumoniae*, GAS, *S. aureus*, nontypeable *H. influenzae*, *M. catarrhalis*	Mild: amoxicillin; Moderate-severe: cefuroxime IV	10–21 d	–
	Chronic: aerobic and anaerobic streptococci, *S. aureus*, nontypeable *H. influenzae*, anaerobes (including *Bacteroides* spp.), fungi	Amoxicillin-clavulanate	>21 d	If persistent, consult otolaryngologist
Pharyngitis	GAS	Penicillin V; penicillin allergic: erythromycin or clarithromycin	10 d	For carrier state eradication, penicillin and clindamycin × 10 d; add rifampin last 4 d Complications: rheumatic fever, poststreptococcal glomerulonephritis Consider viral differentials: EBV pharyngitis, coxsackie (herpangina, hand-foot-and-mouth disease)
Otitis externa	*P. aeruginosa*, Enterobacteriaceae, *S. aureus*	Ciprodex ear drops	7 d	Systemic antibiotics may be required in severe disease; mild disease may be treated with acetic acid/steroid and aural toilet
Conjunctivitis				
Neonate	*N. gonorrhoeae* *C. trachomatis* HSV	Cefotaxime Erythromycin (PO) Acyclovir (IV)	–	–

(continued)

Table 24.2	Initial Empiric Antibiotic Therapy (continued)			
System	Suspected Microbial Agent	Antimicrobial	Duration	Comments
	P. aeruginosa	Piperacillin + aminoglycoside + gentamicin ophthalmic solution		
	Other	Polytrim ophthalmic solution		
Older infants and children	Nontypeable H. influenzae, S. pneumoniae, S. aureus	Polysporin ophthalmic solution or ointment, Polytrim ophthalmic solution Alternatives: gentamicin ophthalmic solution or ointment, bacitracin ointment, sulfacetamide ointment, moxifloxacin (Vigamox)	–	–
	N. gonorrhoeae	Ceftriaxone (IV)		
Genitourinary				
UTI				
Neonate	E. coli, Proteus spp., Klebsiella spp., Enterococcus spp., P. aeruginosa	Ampicillin + aminoglycoside	–	Culture only catheter or suprapubic specimens
Infants and older children	E. coli, Proteus spp., Klebsiella spp., Enterococcus spp., P. aeruginosa	Oral: cephalexin IV: ampicillin + gentamicin	–	Oral antibiotics may be initiated if child not toxic; cefixime is an alternative oral agent; consider step-down to oral sequential therapy, when clinically indicated

(continued)

Infectious Diseases

24

Table 24.2 Initial Empiric Antibiotic Therapy (continued)

System	Suspected Microbial Agent	Antimicrobial	Duration	Comments
Pyelonephritis	E. coli, Proteus spp., Klebsiella spp., P. aeruginosa	Oral: cephalexin IV: ampicillin + gentamicin	–	Cefixime is an alternative oral agent Oral antibiotics may be initiated if child not toxic
Gastrointestinal				
Nosocomial	C. difficile	Metronidazole (PO or IV); vancomycin (PO)	14 d	History of antibiotic use; treat if symptomatic or if fever/neutropenia Stop antibiotics if possible; relapse 10-20%
Bloody diarrhea	Salmonella spp., Shigella spp., Campylobacter jejuni/coli, verotoxin-producing E. coli (including 0157:H7), Yersinia enterocolitica, toxin-producing C. difficile, Entamoeba histolytica	See comments	–	Empiric antibiotics indicated for all Shigella and E. histolytica infections; Salmonella in severe infections or at-risk patients including immunocompromised or <3 mo old; Yersinia infections in presence of terminal ileitis or mesenteric lymphadenitis; toxin-producing C. difficile; enteric infections with sepsis Antibiotics not indicated for verotoxin E. coli infections, uncomplicated Yersinia, Salmonella, Campylobacter infections

Table 24.3 Antibiotic Agents for Human or Animal Bite Wound Infections

Source of Bite	Organism(s) Likely to Cause Infection	Antimicrobial Agent			
		Oral Route	Oral Alternatives for Penicillin-Allergic Patients*	IV Route	IV Alternative for Penicillin-Allergic Patients
Dog/cat†	Pasteurella spp., S. aureus, streptococci, anaerobes, Capnocytophaga canimorsus, Moraxella, Corynebacterium spp., Neisseria spp.	Amoxicillin-clavulanate	1. Doxycycline + clindamycin (>8 yr) OR 2. TMP/SMX + clindamycin (≤8 yr)	1. Penicillin + cloxacillin OR 2. Piperacillin-tazobactam	TMP/SMX + clindamycin
Human†	Streptococci, S. aureus, Eikenella corrodens, anaerobes	Amoxicillin-clavulanate	1. Doxycycline + clindamycin (>8 yr) OR 2. TMP/SMX + clindamycin (≤8 yr)	1. Penicillin + cloxacillin OR 2. Piperacillin-tazobactam	TMP/SMX + clindamycin

*For patients with history of allergy to penicillin, alternative drugs recommended. In some circumstances, cephalosporin or other β-lactam class drugs may be acceptable. However, these drugs should not be used for patients with immediate hypersensitivity (anaphylaxis) to penicillin.

†Assess need for testing and prophylaxis for tetanus, rabies, HIV, HBV, HCV; irrigate and debride but do not suture; signs of infection: admit for IV antibiotics; joint involvement: urgent surgical consultation.

Definition of Positive TST in Children

- Must read largest diameter of induration (not erythema) 48–72 h after placement (Table 24.4).
- History of BCG vaccine should not change interpretation of TST

Clinical Classification of a Child With a "Positive" TST

- LTBI: asymptomatic with normal CXR findings
- Tuberculosis disease: symptoms or signs of active tuberculosis OR suggestive CXR findings OR microbiologic or pathologic proof of active tuberculosis

Treatment

- Teens, patients who are pregnant, malnourished, or with CNS disease should be supplemented with pyridoxine if treated with INH because of risk of peripheral neuritis or seizures
- Expert consultation
- LTBI (TST positive):
  - Daily INH for 9 mo (twice weekly directly observed therapy if poor compliance)
  - Rifampin should be used if the source isolate is INH resistant
- Active pulmonary TB:
  - 6 mo of combination therapy
    - In absence of susceptibility results, start with four drugs (INH, rifampin, pyridoxine, and ethambutol)
    - Step down to three drugs if fully sensitive strain
    - Treat for 2 mo with three or four drugs, then INH and rifampin to complete course
- Extrapulmonary TB:
  - 6–12 mo therapy with multiple drugs (variable duration depending on site of infection)
  - Adjunctive corticosteroid therapy warranted in some cases

Table 24.4	Definition of Positive Tuberculin Skin Test*
Induration	**Group**
≥5 mm	Documented contact with known infectious case Clinical or radiographic evidence of TB Immunocompromised (HIV or immunosuppressive therapy)
≥10 mm	Increased exposure risk: recent immigrants or travel to endemic areas, injection drug users, residents of prisons or institutions, health care workers, Aboriginal North Americans Increased risk of disseminated disease: <4 yr, chronic medical conditions (lymphoma, Hodgkin disease, diabetes mellitus, chronic renal failure, malnutrition)
≥15 mm	≥4 yr with no risk factors

*Adapted from 2006 Red Book.

HSV: CHILDREN AND INFANTS BEYOND THE NEONATAL PERIOD

- Two serotypes: HSV 1 and HSV 2
- Transmission via direct contact with infected oral or genital secretions or lesions
- Patients with primary infection shed virus for at least 1 wk; patients with recurrent infection for 3–4 d

Clinical Syndromes

- Asymptomatic primary infection most common
- Disseminated infection in immunocompromised host; generalized skin or mucosal lesions with visceral involvement

Mucocutaneous Disease

- Gingivostomatitis: ulcerative exanthema of gingival and oral mucous membranes (often anterior), fever, irritability, and submandibular adenopathy
- Herpes labialis: vesicles, usually on vermilion border of the lips
- Eczema herpeticum: emergency; widespread vesicular eruption starting in areas of skin breakdown and spreading rapidly
- Herpetic whitlow: single or multiple vesicular lesions on distal finger
- Genital herpes: usually caused by HSV 2

Ocular Involvement

- Conjunctivitis, keratitis usually secondary to autoinoculation

CNS Disease

- Encephalitis (primary or recurrent infection): fever, altered level of consciousness, personality changes, seizures, focal neurologic findings, coma, death
- Meningitis: nonspecific clinical signs, usually mild and self-limited

Diagnosis

- EM/direct fluorescent antibody staining/PCR or culture of vesicular fluid from skin lesions, mucosal lesions, CSF, or blood
- Repeat LP should be considered if strongly suspect HSV and initial LP negative or if ongoing active viral replication a concern

Treatment

- Urgent ophthalmology consultation if any ocular involvement

Mucocutaneous Disease

- IV acyclovir necessary for severe or complicated infections, all neonatal infections
- Oral acyclovir may be effective if initiated early in primary gingivostomatitis or genital herpes
- Prophylactic oral acyclovir may be of benefit in those with frequent recurrence

Infectious Diseases

24

CNS Disease
- Encephalitis: IV acyclovir for 21 d
- Meningitis: usually no treatment necessary

EBV

Clinical Manifestations
- Wide spectrum: asymptomatic (infants and young children) to fulminant infection (immunocompromised)
- Infectious mononucleosis: fever, exudative pharyngitis, lymphadenopathy, hepatosplenomegaly, atypical lymphocytosis, morbilliform rash (most frequent in those treated with ampicillin or penicillin)
- EBV pharyngitis—typically exudative with extensive false membranes (less in young children)

Diagnosis
- Serology (Table 24.5)
- Nonspecific tests for heterophile antibody (e.g., monospot) often negative in children <4 yr
- >10% atypical lymphocytes and positive monospot highly suggestive of acute infection

Treatment
- Supportive; rest during acute phase
- Avoid contact sports if splenomegaly present
- Corticosteroids considered in select cases (impending airway obstruction, massive splenomegaly, myocarditis, hemolytic anemia, hemophagocytic syndrome)
- Antiviral treatment required in immunocompromised host or in presence of severe disease (encephalitis)
- Amoxicillin associated with rash in approximately 80% of patients with primary EBV

Complications
- Hematologic: thrombocytopenia, agranulocytosis, hemolytic anemia, hemophagocytic syndrome

Table 24.5	Serum EBV Antibodies in EBV Infection			
Anti-EA IgG	Anti-VCA IgG	Anti-EBNA IgG	Anti-VCA IgM	Interpretation
–	–	–	–	No prior exposure to EBV
±	±	–	+	Acute infection
±	+	±	±	Recent infection
–	+	+	–	Past infection (at least 2–6 mo ago)

EA, early antigen; EBNA, Epstein-Barr nuclear antigen; VCA, viral capsid antigen.

- CNS: aseptic meningitis, encephalitis, Guillain-Barré syndrome, transverse myelitis, optic neuritis, cranial nerve palsies
- Others: orchitis, pneumonia, myocarditis, splenic rupture

VZV

- Transmission: airborne from respiratory secretions, direct contact of chickenpox or zoster lesions, transplacental
- Most contagious 2 d before onset of rash until vesicles have crusted over
- Incubation period: 10–21 d (28 d if varicella zoster immune globulin given)

Clinical Manifestations

- Primary infection (chickenpox): generalized pruritic vesicular rash, mild fever, pharyngitis
- Complications: bacterial superinfection of skin lesions including invasive GAS, thrombocytopenia, arthritis, hepatitis, cerebellar ataxia, encephalitis, meningitis, glomerulonephritis, pneumonia
- Reactivation (zoster) of latent virus in dorsal root ganglion: grouped vesicular lesions in distribution of one to three dermatomes, sometimes with localized pain

Diagnosis

- Clinical diagnosis usually sufficient; direct fluorescent antigen/EM/PCR of vesicular scrapings

Treatment

- Acyclovir therapy not routinely recommended in healthy children <12 yr
- Acyclovir may be considered in patients at risk of moderate to severe varicella:
  - Children >12 yr of age
  - Chronic cutaneous or pulmonary disorders
  - Long-term salicylate therapy
  - Recent corticosteroid use
  - Immunocompromised patients
- Avoid ASA due to risk of Reye syndrome; avoid use of other NSAIDs; acetaminophen recommended for control of fever
- Postexposure prophylaxis: see Chapter 23

HIV

Epidemiology

- Mother-to-child transmission (in utero 5%, intrapartum 20%, breast milk transmission 14%)
- Factors affecting the risk of vertical transmission of HIV (Table 24.6) include maternal factors (viral load before delivery, advanced HIV disease, low CD4 count, acute HIV, poor adherence to antiretroviral therapy), obstetric factors (prolonged rupture of membranes [>4 h], chorioamnionitis, other STIs [such as HSV-2], vaginal delivery), and fetal factors (prematurity, breastfeeding)

Table 24.6	Effect of Various Interventions on Vertical Transmission of HIV	
Intervention		**Approximate Risk of Transmission**
No interventions, breastfed		40%
No interventions, exclusively formula fed		25%
Elective cesarean section with zidovudine monotherapy or no antiretroviral therapy to mother and zidovudine or no therapy to infant		12%
Single-dose nevirapine to mother and child		12%
Three-part zidovudine (mother, intrapartum, baby)		8%
Maternal highly active antiretroviral therapy (two nucleoside analogues + protease inhibitor or nevirapine) + zidovudine to infant		≤1%

Manifestations of HIV Infection

- Natural history of untreated, perinatally HIV-infected children: 30–40% develop AIDS-defining conditions in <1 yr, many have relatively mild symptoms, some remain asymptomatic during early childhood

Clinical Manifestations

- Mild symptoms (category A): generalized lymphadenopathy, hepato-splenomegaly, parotitis, dermatitis, recurrent sinusitis or otitis media
- Moderate symptoms (category B): bacterial meningitis, sepsis or pneumonia, recurrent or chronic diarrhea, cardiomyopathy, nephropathy, CMV or toxoplasmosis with onset prior to 1 mo of age, complicated chickenpox, persistent fever (>1 mo), LIP, nocardiosis
- Severe symptoms (category C): opportunistic infections (PJP, esophageal candidiasis, disseminated CMV, cryptococcal meningitis, CNS toxoplasmosis, *Mycobacterium tuberculosis* disease, *Mycobacterium avium* complex infection, chronic enteritis [*Cryptosporidium, Isospora*]), malignancies (Kaposi sarcoma, lymphomas, smooth-muscle tumors), HIV encephalopathy (global developmental delay), HIV-associated wasting (failure to thrive)
- See Table 24.7 for age-specific CD4 counts and immunologic category

General Indications for Initiating Antiretroviral Therapy

- Age <12 mo (regardless of clinical symptoms, immune status, viral load)
- AIDS or other significant HIV-related symptoms, irrespective of CD4 count or viral load
- Severe immune suppression (CD4 <15%), irrespective of symptoms or viral load
- In children who do not meet the above criteria, treatment may be considered (or deferred) depending on their overall health, viral load, and CD4 count

Table 24.7	Age-Specific CD4 Counts and Immunologic Category		
Degree of Suppression	Age <12 mo	Age 1–5 yr	Age 6–12 yr
Normal range (immune category 1)	>1500 (≥25%)	>1000 (≥25%)	>500 (≥25%)
Moderate (immune category 2)	750–1499 (15–24%)	500–749 (15–24%)	200–499 (15–24%)
Severe (immune category 3)	<750 (<15%)	<500 (<15%)	<200 (<15%)

CD4% = CD4 T cells/100 lymphocytes.

Other Therapeutic Considerations

- For opportunistic infection prophylaxis and immunization guidelines, see Chapter 23
- IVIG may be of benefit in selected children with poorly controlled HIV disease
- CMV-negative blood transfusions

Care of the Infant Vertically Exposed to HIV

- See Table 24.8

Table 24.8	Timetable for Care of the Infant Vertically Exposed to HIV*
Timeline	Management
For the Infant Vertically Exposed to HIV	
Pregnancy	Ensure appropriate maternal care including antiretroviral therapy starting in second trimester or earlier Offer counseling services Elective cesarean section to reduce perinatal transmission (if viral load >1000 copies/mL)
During delivery	Zidovudine IV 2 mg/kg/h for first hour, then 1 mg/kg/h Reduce invasive monitoring, such as scalp electrodes
At birth	Breastfeeding contraindicated Start zidovudine syrup 2 mg/kg/dose qid for 6 wk† Encourage hepatitis B vaccine series; if mother is HBsAg positive, give HBIG and vaccine series
Before discharge	Perform CBC, CD4 count, and HIV PCR (culture optional)‡ Consult with pediatric HIV program
At 1 mo	Perform blood test for HIV PCR (culture optional)‡ Perform CBC and differential and T-cell counts Discontinue zidovudine at 6 wk If HBV vaccine series is started, give second dose

(continued)

Table 24.8	Timetable for Care of the Infant Vertically Exposed to HIV* (continued)
Timeline	Management
At 2 mo	Give routine immunizations§ Perform blood for HIV PCR (culture optional)‡ PCP prophylaxis with TMP/SMX as 2.5 mg/kg/dose TMP bid 3 d/wk should be initiated unless mother and infant appropriately managed, maternal viral load <50 copies/mL, and infant clinically well
At 3–4 mo	Review all HIV tests‡ If all PCR and cultures are negative, likely infant not infected; TMP/SMX can be discontinued If more than one HIV PCR (or culture) positive, infant confirmed infected and should be referred to pediatric HIV program
At 4 mo	Give routine immunizations
For the Infant With Negative HIV PCR (and Negative Culture and p24 Antigen if Done)	
At 6 mo	Perform general and developmental assessment Give routine immunizations If HBV vaccine series started, give third dose
At 18 mo	Perform general and developmental assessment Check HIV serology to finalize HIV status
Annually	Perform general and developmental assessment
For the Infant With Positive PCR or Culture, Follow-Up in Conjunction With a Pediatric HIV Program	

*Intended as guideline only.
†Dose modification may be needed for premature infants.
‡If PCR, p24 Ag, or culture test is positive for the first time, repeat immediately for confirmation.
§OPV should not be used (no longer available for routine use in Canada; all provinces switched to IPV); do not give BCG vaccine until child's HIV status established with certainty.
Canadian Paediatric Society Statement, Infectious Diseases and Immunization Committee. Care of the infant born to an HIV positive mother. *Paediatr Child Health*, 2000; 5(3): 161–164 (Table 1).

FUNGAL INFECTIONS

SELECTED FUNGAL INFECTIONS IN THE IMMUNOCOMPETENT HOST

- See Table 24.9

SELECTED INVASIVE FUNGAL INFECTIONS IN THE IMMUNOCOMPROMISED HOST

- See Table 24.10

OVA AND PARASITES

- See Table 24.11

Table 24.9 Selected Fungal Infections in the Immunocompetent Host

Pathogen	Risk Factors	Organ Involvement	Diagnostic Tests	Antifungal Agents
Candida spp.	Neonates, antibiotic therapy	Mucosal surfaces; diaper area	Gram stain, culture	Nystatin, fluconazole, amphotericin B
Dermatophytes	Direct or indirect contact with human or animal cases	Skin, nails	Tissue stain and culture	Terbinafine, itraconazole, fluconazole
Blastomycosis	Travel to northern Ontario, Great Lakes region, St Lawrence River; Midwest, Southeast, and south-central United States	Lung, skin, bone, brain	Serology, tissue stain and culture (BAL, biopsy)	Amphotericin B, itraconazole
Histoplasmosis	Travel to Ohio, Mississippi River basins; spelunking; bird and bat guano; soil upheaval	Lung, disseminates to multiple organs	Serology, tissue stain and culture (BAL, biopsy)	Amphotericin B, itraconazole
Coccidioidomycosis	Travel to southwestern United States, Mexico, Central and South America	Lung, rarely disseminates	Serology, tissue stain and culture (BAL, biopsy)	Fluconazole, itraconazole, amphotericin B
Cryptococcosis	Travel to Vancouver Island, British Columbia lower mainland	Brain, lung, skin	CSF India ink stain; CSF, blood antigen	Amphotericin B, fluconazole

Table 24.10   Selected Invasive Fungal Infections in the Immunocompromised Host

Pathogen	Prevalence	Risk Factors	Organ Involvement	Diagnostic Tests	Potential Antifungal Agents
Candida spp.	++++	Indwelling lines; prematurity; malignancy; transplantation; prolonged antibiotics; HIV	Blood, liver, spleen, CNS	Stains and culture of specimens	Amphotericin B, fluconazole, caspofungin
Aspergillus spp.	++	Malignancy; transplantation; SCID	Lung, sinuses, brain, bone	Stains and culture of aspirates, tissue samples	Voriconazole, amphotericin B, caspofungin
Zygomycosis	+	Malignancy; transplantation; SCID	Sinuses, lung, brain	Stains and culture of aspirates, tissue samples	Posaconazole, amphotericin B
Cryptococcosis	+	HIV, corticosteroids, malignancy, transplantation, diabetes mellitus	Brain, lung, skin	CSF India ink stain; CSF, blood antigen detection	Amphotericin B, fluconazole

Table 24.11 Ova and Parasites

Parasite	Geographic Distribution and Epidemiology*	Common Sources	Common Symptoms	Eosinophilia (Grade: Mild-Moderate-High)	Treatment: Drug of Choice (Alternatives in Brackets)
Helminths					
Roundworm (*Ascaris lumbricoides*)	Worldwide (common in tropics and subtropics)	Fecal-oral (ingestion of infective ascaris eggs)	Most asymptomatic Acute transient pneumonitis with fever (Löffler syndrome) during larva migration May cause bowel or biliary tree obstruction Late: none	Early (during larval migration): moderate-high	Albendazole (mebendazole or ivermectin)
Hookworm (*Ancylostoma duodenale, Necator americanus*)	Worldwide (most common in moist warm climates), S. Europe, N. Africa, N. Asia, S. America, SE United States	Soil (skin contact); walking in bare feet/sandals (filariform larva penetrate skin)	Most asymptomatic Hypochromic normocytic anemia and protein energy malnutrition	Early (during larval migration): moderate-high Late: mild-moderate	Albendazole (mebendazole or pyrantel pamoate)
Pinworm (*Enterobius vermicularis*)	Worldwide	Fecal-oral (human to human)	Pruritis ani or pruritis vulvae	None	Mebendazole (pyrantel pamoate or albendazole); if recurs, consider treating family

(continued)

Table 24.11 Ova and Parasites (continued)

Parasite	Geographic Distribution and Epidemiology*	Common Sources	Common Symptoms	Eosinophilia (Grade: Mild-Moderate-High)	Treatment: Drug of Choice (Alternatives in Brackets)
Strongyloides stercoralis	Tropics/subtropics	Soil (skin contact); walking in bare feet/sandals Direct contact (human-to-human, lab setting) Autoinfection	Most asymptomatic Pneumonitis (Löffler-like syndrome) during larval migration Disseminated hyperinfection in immunocompromise	Early (during larval migration): moderate-high Late: mild-moderate Immunocompromise: may have no eosinophilia despite dissemination	Ivermectin (albendazole)
Whipworm (Trichuris trichiura)	Worldwide Common in tropical regions with poor sanitation	Fecal-oral (ingestion of eggs)	Most asymptomatic Dysentery syndrome: abdominal pain, tenesmus, bloody diarrhea Recurrent rectal prolapse	None-moderate	Mebendazole (albendazole or ivermectin)
Pork tapeworm (Taenia solium)	Worldwide ↑ risk if close contact with pigs High prevalence in Mexico, Central and South America, Africa, India, SE Asia, Philippines, S. Europe	Ingestion of raw/undercooked pork Cysticercosis occurs if ingest T. solium eggs (contaminated food or water)	Asymptomatic or mild GI symptoms; passage (passive) of proglottids Neurocysticercosis usually presents with seizures	Mild or none	Praziquantel (niclosamide) Cysticercosis: consult infectious disease specialist

(continued)

Table 24.11 Ova and Parasites (continued)

Parasite	Geographic Distribution and Epidemiology*	Common Sources	Common Symptoms	Eosinophilia (Grade: Mild-Moderate-High)	Treatment: Drug of Choice (Alternatives in Brackets)
Beef tapeworm (*Taenia saginata*)	Worldwide; cattle-breeding areas High prevalence in central Asia, Near East, central and E. Africa	Ingestion of raw or undercooked beef	Mild GI symptoms, passage (active and passive) of proglottids	Mild or none	Praziquantel (niclosamide)
Fish tapeworm (*Diphyllobothrium latum*)	Siberia, Northern Europe, North America, Japan, Chile	Ingestion of raw or undercooked freshwater fish (smoked or dried fish)	Most asymptomatic; mild GI symptoms; pernicious anemia	Mild or none	Praziquantel (niclosamide)
Protozoa					
E. histolytica (symptomatic)	Worldwide, highest risk in developing countries Risk groups: travel, recent immigrants, institutionalized populations	Fecal-oral	May be asymptomatic Amebic dysentery (bloody diarrhea); liver abscess (rarely at other sites)	No	Metronidazole or tinidazole (followed by lumicidal agent iodoquinol or paromomycin)

(continued)

Table 24.11 Ova and Parasites (continued)

Parasite	Geographic Distribution and Epidemiology*	Common Sources	Common Symptoms	Eosinophilia (Grade: Mild-Moderate-High)	Treatment: Drug of Choice (Alternatives in Brackets)
Blastocystis hominis† (symptomatic)	Worldwide	Fecal-oral	Most asymptomatic Bloating, flatulence, diarrhea, abdominal pain, nausea	No	Metronidazole (iodoquinol or TMP/SMX)
Dientamoeba fragilis (symptomatic)	Worldwide; associated with pinworm infections	Fecal-oral	Most asymptomatic Mild-moderate GI symptoms (cramping, diarrhea, weight loss, nausea)	No	Iodoquinol (consider treating for pinworm as well)
Giardia lamblia (symptomatic)	Worldwide, more prevalent in warm climates	Fecal-oral	GI tract symptoms: abdominal pain, diarrhea, flatulence	No	Metronidazole (nitazoxanide or tinidazole)
Malaria	S. Africa, tropics/subtropics	Anopheles species mosquito	High fever with chills, sweats, headache	No	Depends on species, geographic origin; consult infectious disease specialist

*For more detailed geographic distribution, visit the Center for Disease Control and Prevention Web site (http://www.cdc.gov).
†Role as pathogen controversial.

CNS INFECTIONS

MENINGITIS

Background

- Aseptic meningitis (i.e., routine bacterial cultures are negative); common causes include prior antibiotic therapy, viruses, unusual or slow-growing pathogens (*Mycobacterium tuberculosis*, *Cryptococcus neoformans*), or noninfectious causes (ruptured dermoid cyst, drugs such as cotrimoxazole, IVIG)

Diagnosis

- LP for cell count, chemistry (protein, glucose), Gram stain, culture (Table 24.12)
- Gram stain helpful for etiology: gram-positive diplococci (*Streptococcus pneumoniae*), gram-negative diplococci (*Neisseria meningitidis*), small pleomorphic gram-negative coccobacilli (*H. influenzae*)
- Focal neurologic findings mandate neuroimaging before LP

Management

- Monitor ABCs, neurologic status, fluids (see pp. 5–9)
- Daily assessment of hydration, weight, electrolytes (risk of SIADH), head circumference, metastatic foci of infection

Empiric Antibiotic Therapy

- See Table 24.2
- Antibiotics should not be delayed for LP if clinical suspicion is high
- Empiric antibiotic therapy should not be altered on the basis of Gram stain results but on the basis of culture and antibiotic susceptibility results

Table 24.12	Cerebrospinal Fluid Findings Based on Infection Type				
	Normal Values		**Abnormal Values**		
Component	Neonate	>1 mo	Bacterial	Viral	TB
WBC ($\times 10^6$/L)*	0–30	<5	50–5000	20–2000	100–500
%PMN	<60	0	95	<30[†]	<30[†]
Protein (g/L)[‡]	<1.7	<0.3	>0.6	0.3–0.8	0.5–0.8
Glucose (mmol/L)	1.7–6.4	>2.8	<2.8	<3.3	<2.8
Glucose (% of serum glucose)	45–125	>50	<40	<50	<40

*WBC to RBC ratios in CSF specimens contaminated with blood must be interpreted with caution. Rough estimate of WBC:RBC from "bloody tap" alone is 1:1000 (can corroborate by doing the calculation on the peripheral blood). Do not withhold treatment if clinical picture is suggestive of meningitis. Seizures alone do not increase CSF WBC count.
[†]Early in course, PMN predominance may be seen.
[‡]Increased protein seen in meningitis, encephalitis, abscess, leukemia, or other intracranial malignancy.
From Crain EF, Gershel JC. *Clinical Manual of Emergency Pediatrics*. 3rd ed. New York, NY: McGraw-Hill; 1997.

- Corticosteroid therapy controversial
  - Benefit clearly demonstrated for *H. influenzae* meningitis
  - Adult studies indicate potential benefit in pneumococcal meningitis
  - If given, administer before or within 1 h of starting antibiotics
- Hearing assessment; neurologic assessment, and follow-up
- If prolonged or recurrent fever, consider
  - Nosocomial illness (gastroenteritis, respiratory infection)
  - Phlebitis
  - Secondary focus (arthritis, pneumonia, pleural or pericardial effusion, pericarditis, sinusitis, mastoiditis, brain abscess)
  - Subdural effusions (common) or subdural empyema
  - Drug fever
  - Failure of conventional management
  - Persistent fever may occasionally occur as part of the clinical course in the absence of complications
- Prophylactic antibiotic therapy for family and index case if meningitis due to *H. influenzae* or *N. meningitidis* (rifampin generally first choice in children)

ENCEPHALITIS

Background

- Encephalopathy (altered state of consciousness persisting for >24 h) plus two or more of the following:
  - Fever
  - Seizure
  - Focal neurologic findings
  - CSF pleocytosis (five or more cells)
  - Compatible EEG
  - Abnormal diagnostic imaging (CT, MRI)
- No organism identified in >50% of cases
- History: season, travel, camping, insect bites, animal contact (cats, horses, mice, hamsters), unpasteurized milk, TB exposures, history of flu-like illness, varicella, rash, seizures, vomiting, diarrhea, lymphadenopathy, mononucleosis-like illness, neurologic defects, recent immunizations

Diagnosis

- Paired serology (initial and then convalescent in 2–4 wk):
  - Arboviruses (West Nile virus, eastern equine encephalitis virus, western equine encephalitis virus, St Louis encephalitis virus, California encephalitis virus, Powassan virus), herpes group viruses (HSV, EBV, VZV, CMV, HHV-6), influenza A and B, *Mycoplasma pneumoniae*, *Bartonella henselae*, measles, mumps, parvovirus B19, syphilis, Lyme disease
  - CSF examination:
    – Typically see elevated levels of protein, normal glucose, pleocytosis with predominant monocytosis

- Bacterial culture
- PCR for enteroviruses, HSV 1/2, EBV, CMV, VZV, HHV-6, HHV-7, *M. pneumoniae*
- NP swab (influenza A and B, parainfluenza, adenovirus)
- Throat swab for *M. pneumoniae* PCR (viral culture medium needed)
- Stool for EM and viral culture (adenovirus and *Enterovirus*)
- Other microbiologic investigations may be considered on a selective basis (rabies, etc.)
- EEG, CT, or MRI, as indicated clinically

Treatment

- Empiric IV acyclovir warranted for all children with encephalitis
- Other specific treatment considerations:
  - Acyclovir for varicella encephalitis
  - Ceftriaxone for Lyme disease
  - Azithromycin for *B. henselae*
  - Quinolones or macrolides for *M. pneumoniae*
- Steroid treatment for ADEM or vasculitis

CONGENITAL INFECTIONS

- See Box 24.1 and Table 24.13 for differential diagnosis and selected clinical features
- See Box 24.2 and Table 24.14 for investigations and treatment

NEONATAL HSV

Transmission

- Maternal primary genital infection: 33–50%
- Maternal recurrent genital infection: 0–5%
- Increased risk: PROM >6 h, fetal scalp monitoring, forceps, prematurity

Box 24.1	CHEAP TORCHES Congenital Infection Acronym
C	Chickenpox
H	Hepatitis viruses (hepatitis B, hepatitis C)
E	Enteroviruses
A	AIDS (HIV)
P	Parvovirus B19
T	Toxoplasmosis
O	Other (lymphocytic choriomeningitis virus, malaria, TB)
R	Rubella
C	CMV
H	HSV
E	Every other STI (human papillomavirus)
S	Syphilis

Table 24.13   Selected Clinical Features of Common Congenital Infections

Infection	General	CNS	Eye	Ear	Cardiac	Hematologic	Reticuloendothelial System	Skin	Musculoskeletal
CMV	IUGR	Microcephaly, periventricular calcifications Late: speech and language delay, mental retardation	Chorioretinitis	SNHL	Hydrops	Cytopenias	Hepatosplenomegaly	Petechiae, blueberry muffin rash	–
Toxoplasmosis	IUGR	Hydrocephalus, macrocephaly (or microcephaly), parenchymal calcifications Late: seizures, psychomotor delay	Chorioretinitis	SNHL	Hydrops	Cytopenias	Hepatosplenomegaly	Maculopapular rash	–
Syphilis	IUGR, snuffles Late: frontal bossing, saddle nose, Hutchinson teeth, mulberry molars	Aseptic meningitis, cranial nerve palsies Late: mental retardation, cranial nerve palsies, hydrocephalus	Chorioretinitis, cataracts Late: interstitial keratitis	SNHL	Hydrops	Hemolytic anemia, thrombocytopenia	Hepatosplenomegaly	Desquamating or maculopapular rash involving palms and soles	Pseudoparalysis, osteitis Late: saber shins, Clutton joints

(continued)

Table 24.1.3 Selected Clinical Features of Common Congenital Infections *(continued)*

Infection	General	CNS	Eye	Ear	Cardiac	Hematologic	Reticuloendothelial System	Skin	Musculoskeletal
Rubella	IUGR Late: endocrinopathies (diabetes mellitus, thyroid disorders)	Microcephaly, meningoencephalitis Late: mental retardation, panencephalitis	Cataracts Late: salt and pepper retinitis	SNHL	PDA, pulmonary stenosis	–	Hepatosplenomegaly	Blueberry muffin rash	Bony lucencies
HSV	IUGR	Microcephaly, hydranencephaly, cerebral calcifications	Chorioretinitis, microphthalmia	–	Hydrops	Cytopenias	Hepatosplenomegaly	Skin lesions and scars	–
VZV	Esophageal dilatation and reflux, hydronephrosis, hydroureter	–	Microphthalmia, chorioretinitis	–	–	–	Cicatricial scars	Limb hypoplasia

Clinical Manifestations

- Disseminated disease: earliest onset, first week of life (25%)
- Localized CNS disease: latest onset, second to third week of life (35%)
- Localized to skin, eyes, mouth (40%)
- Initial symptoms may occur up to 4 wk of age
- Suspect disseminated disease in neonates with clinical sepsis, negative bacterial cultures, and liver dysfunction
- High morbidity and mortality rates, even when appropriately treated
- Recurrent skin lesions frequent; may be associated with CNS sequelae if occur <6 mo

Diagnostic Approach

- Infants born to mothers with active lesions at delivery should have oropharyngeal, eye, stool or rectum, and urine cultures/PCR at 48 h of age
- Symptomatic infants should have culture/PCR of skin/mucosal lesions, blood, CSF
- All infants with suspected HSV disease must have an LP and HSV culture/PCR of CSF
- Treatment: IV acyclovir × 14 d if disease limited to skin, eyes, and mouth; 21 d if CNS involvement or dissemination
- Prevention: C-section recommended in mothers with active lesions if rupture of membranes <6 h; may consider if rupture of membranes >6 h

Table 24.14

Table 24.14 Transmission, Diagnosis, and Treatment of Common Congenital Infections

Congenital Infection	Transmission and Key Points	Diagnosis	Treatment
Toxoplasmosis	· Risk of transmission · 1st trimester: 15% (40% severe) · 2nd trimester: 30% (8% severe) · 3rd trimester: 60% (0% severe) · 70–90% asymptomatic at birth · Prevention: maternal avoidance of undercooked meat and cat feces	· Serology: IgM or IgA antibodies in first 6 mo of life or persistence of IgG antibody beyond 12–18 mo of life · Detection of organism by PCR in amniotic fluid, CSF, vitreous fluid, tissue samples · Histologic demonstration of organism	Pyrimethamine + sulfadiazine (or clindamycin) and leucovorin if congenital infection is confirmed
Syphilis (*Treponema pallidum*)	· Transplacental transmission at any time during pregnancy/delivery, any stage of disease (highest risk during secondary syphilis: 60–100%) · Most asymptomatic at birth · Indications for evaluation for congenital syphilis: · Signs and symptoms in infant · Mother's treatment not documented or inadequate (i.e., not with penicillin) · Less than fourfold drop in mother's nontreponemal titer · Mother treated <1 mo before delivery · Maternal relapse or reinfection after treatment	· Serologic diagnosis: infant nontreponemal titer 4× higher than mother's at birth, infant nontreponemal titer increases after birth, infant treponemal test remains positive at 12–18 mo · Direct detection (dark-field microscopy, direct fluorescent antibody) of organism in samples from active lesions (snuffles, ulcers) · Consider testing for other associated STIs (gonorrhea, chlamydia, HIV, hepatitis B and C)	Parenteral penicillin G for 10–14 d
Rubella	Risk of congenital defects varies with transmission timing: · 1st mo gestation: >50% · 2nd mo gestation: 20–30% · 3rd or 4th mo gestation: 5%	· Isolation of virus from throat swab, urine, blood, CSF · IgM indicates recent postnatal or congenital infection · Stable or ↑IgG over few mo confirms diagnosis of congenital rubella	Supportive

(continued)

Infectious Diseases

24

Table 24.14 Transmission, Diagnosis, and Treatment of Common Congenital Infections (continued)

Congenital Infection	Transmission and Key Points	Diagnosis	Treatment
CMV	· Most common congenital infection · 85–90% asymptomatic at birth · Neurologic sequelae develop in 10–15% of cases · Late-onset hearing loss most common manifestation in asymptomatic newborns · Transmission during pregnancy: · 40% for primary infection (95% symptomatic) · 0.5–1% for reactivation or reinfection (rarely symptomatic)	· Isolation of CMV in culture from urine and/or saliva within 2–3 wk of birth · CMV in urine beyond this time cannot distinguish congenital from perinatal acquisition · Presence of CMV-specific IgM suggestive but not diagnostic of congenital CMV infection	Ganciclovir for CNS disease and/or chorioretinitis (shown to decrease progression of hearing impairment)
Parvovirus B19	· Transmission risk: 30% · Potential adverse outcomes include fetal loss and nonimmune hydrops fetalis · 10% risk fetal loss if infection <20 wk gestation; 1% risk if >20 wk gestation	· Serology in the mother; IgM indicates infection within previous 2–4 mo, IgG appears on day 7 of the illness and persists for life · Fetal US may be useful if maternal contact or during aplastic crisis	Supportive Intrauterine blood transfusions for hydrops fetalis
Varicella	· Varicella embryopathy: · Associated with maternal infection in first half of gestation · Prior to wk 13: 0.5%; between 13–20 wk: 2.2% · Unapparent congenital varicella (may manifest as zoster later in life) · Associated with infections after 20 wk gestation	· Vesicular fluid or scab specimen for PCR · Virus can be isolated from vesicle scrapings during first 3–4 d of eruption	Supportive

PERINATAL VARICELLA INFECTION

- High risk of severe neonatal disease if maternal onset of skin lesions 5 d before delivery to 2 d after delivery (mortality approximately 30%)
- Prevention: VZIG in immediate postpartum period
- Treatment: IV acyclovir if baby develops varicella

FEVER IN THE RETURNING TRAVELER

- Differential diagnosis can be narrowed down based on travel itinerary (regions visited), exposure history, and incubation periods
  - Most infections acquired during travel present within first month of return
  - Malaria (most commonly *P. vivax*), tuberculosis, brucellosis, hepatitis viruses, and amebic liver abscess may have incubation periods >4 wk
- Life-threatening travel-related infections include malaria, typhoid fever, meningococcemia, and viral hemorrhagic fevers
- Malaria must be excluded in all people returning from endemic areas, irrespective of clinical impression
- Infection control considerations paramount; some pathogens may pose substantial public health risk

GENERAL APPROACH

History

- See Table 24.15

Table 24.15	Key Points on History for Fever in the Returning Traveler
Travel Itinerary	Exact dates and countries visited; rural vs. urban areas
Immunizations	Routine childhood vaccines plus additional vaccines given pretravel Proof of vaccination insufficient to exclude pathogen; travel-related vaccine efficacy varies (e.g., typhoid vaccines 70% effective)
Malaria prophylaxis	Agent and adherence, use after return, if appropriate Use of bed nets, mosquito repellents
Exposure history	Sick contacts, animal contacts, freshwater exposure (swimming), walking barefoot, consumption of unpasteurized milk products, undercooked meat, fish or seafood or unusual foods; bloodborne pathogen exposure (needles, tattoos, transfusions), sexual contacts, insect bites (ticks)

Investigations

- Recommended in all cases: CBC and differential, liver function tests, urinalysis, blood cultures
- If returning from endemic areas, malaria smears ×3 (thick and thin) every 12–24 h (initial negative smear does not rule out malaria)
- Other investigations (CXR, TST, stool examination for EM, culture, ova and parasites, and *Clostridium difficile* toxin, serology for various pathogens) should be considered on selective basis

Management

- High suspicion of malaria should prompt admission for observation, irrespective of malaria smear results; empiric therapy considered selectively
- Empiric therapy for typhoid fever should be considered if returning from high-prevalence regions (e.g., South Asia) and no cause of fever identified after initial investigations

IMMIGRANT AND REFUGEE CHILDREN

- See Table 24.16

Table 24.16	Common Health Issues Encountered in Immigrant/Refugee Children	
	Health Issue	**General Approach**
General	Estimated age, dental caries, vision and hearing problems, genetic conditions, congenital anomalies, developmental delay	Routine well-child screening Screen for underlying medical conditions Vision and hearing assessment Assess dental health
Nutritional	Anemia, malnutrition, rickets, iodine deficiency	Evaluate nutritional status: weight and height, assess for signs of vitamin/mineral deficiency (e.g., rickets)
Infectious	Inadequate immunizations, TB, gastrointestinal parasites, hepatitis B, syphilis, malaria, HIV	Review and update immunization status
Toxin exposure	Lead, environmental pollution, prenatal exposures including alcohol, radioactivity	Review environmental exposures: lead poisoning, heavy metals, chemical pollution
Mental health	Depression, anxiety, post-traumatic stress disorder, hyperactivity/attention deficit	Assess development status, school placement and mental health

INVESTIGATIONS

- Done selectively based on geographic origin, clinical history, and physical examination findings

Selected Screening Tests

- CBC + differential (anemia and eosinophilia)
- Urinalysis (proteinuria, hematuria)
- TST
- CXR
- HBsAg, HCV serology (with counseling), HIV (with counseling and informed consent)
- Syphilis serology (if sexually active, suspected sexual assault, suspected congenital syphilis)
- Sickle cell preparation (in children of African descent)
- G6PD screen and Hb electrophoresis (African, Asian, Mediterranean descent)

Microbiologic Tests

- Stool for ova and parasites ×2 (asymptomatic infection with intestinal protozoa and roundworms is common)
- Stool for C&S (if symptomatic)
- Screening for STIs (see p. 433)

ANTIMICROBIALS

- See Tables 24.17 through 24.20

Table 24.17 Antibiotic Guidelines*

Antibiotic	Route	S. aureus (MSSA)	S. aureus (MRSA)	S. aureus (CA-MRSA)	S. pneumoniae	Streptococcus spp.—Groups A, B, C, G	Gram-Negative Enterics	H. influenzae	N. gonorrhoeae	N. meningitidis	Pseudomonas aeruginosa	B. fragilis	CSF Activity
Penicillin G	IV	–	–	–	+	+	–	–	–	+	–	–	+ (high dose)
Ampicillin/amoxicillin	IV/PO	–	–	–	+	+	±	±	–	+	–	–	+ (high dose)
Amoxicillin-clavulanate	PO	+	–	–	+	+	±	+	+	+	–	+	NA
Cloxacillin	PO/IV	+	–	–	+	+	–	–	–	–	–	–	+ (high dose)
Piperacillin	IV	–	–	–	+	+	+	±	+	+	+	–	+ (high dose)
Piperacillin/tazobactam	IV	+	–	–	+	+	+	+	+	+	+	+	NA
Ticarcillin/clavulanate	IV	+	–	–	+	+	+	+	+	+	+	+	–
Imipenem/meropenem	IV	+	–	–	+	+	+	+	+	+	+	+	+
Vancomycin	IV	+	+	+	+	+	–	–	–	–	–	–	+
Erythromycin	PO/IV	±	±	±	+	±	–	±	±	+	–	–	–
Clarithromycin	PO	+	±	±	+	±	–	+	±	NA	–	–	–
Azithromycin	PO	+	±	±	+	±	–	+	±	+	–	–	–

(continued)

Table 24.17 Antibiotic Guidelines* (continued)

Antibiotic	Route	S. aureus (MSSA)	S. aureus (MRSA)	S. aureus (CA-MRSA)	S. pneumoniae	Streptococcus spp.—Groups A, B, C, G	Gram-Negative Enterics	H. influenzae	N. gonorrhoeae	N. meningitidis	Pseudomonas aeruginosa	B. fragilis	CSF Activity
Clindamycin	PO/IV	+	±	+	+	+	-	-	-	-	-	±	NA
Doxycycline	PO	±	±	+	±	±	±	+	±	+	-	-	-
Cotrimoxazole	PO/IV	+	±	+	+	±	+	±	±	+	-	-	+
Ciprofloxacin	PO/IV	+	±	±	±	±	+	+	+	+	+	-	+
Moxifloxacin	PO/IV	+	±	±	+	+	+	+	+	+	±	+	+
Gentamicin	IV/IM	+	-		-	-	+	+	-	-	+	-	-
Tobramycin	IV/IM	+	-		-	-	+	+	-	-	+	-	-
Amikacin	IV	+	-		-	-	+	+	+	-	+	-	-
Chloramphenicol	PO/IV	±	-		+	+	±	+	+	+	-	+	+
Metronidazole	PO/IV	-	-	-	-	-	-	-	-	-	-	+	+
Rifampin†	PO	+	+	+	-	+	-	Proph.	Proph.	Proph.	-	-	+
Linezolid	PO/IV	+	+	+	+	+	-	±	NA	-	-	±	+

*Meant as guideline only; individual susceptibilities will vary.

†Rifampin monotherapy should not be used for treatment of active infections because of tendency for rapid emergence of resistance.

+ Effective. — Ineffective. ± May cover some strains.

NA, not applicable; MSSA, methicillin-sensitive S. aureus; MRSA, methicillin-resistant S. aureus; CA-MRSA, community-associated MRSA; Proph., prophylaxis.

Adapted from Gilbert DN, Moellering RC, Eliopoulos GM, Sande MA, eds. The Sanford Guide to Antimicrobial Therapy 2007. 37th ed. Sperryville, Va: Antimicrobial Therapy, Inc; 2007:65–70.

Infectious Diseases

24

Table 24.18 Cephalosporins*†

Generic Name	Trade Name	Route	S. aureus‡	Streptococcus spp.	Gram-Negative Enterics	H. influenzae	N. gonorrhoeae	N. meningitidis	P. aeruginosa	Bacteroides fragilis	CSF Activity
1st generation											
Cefazolin	Ancef	IV	+	+	UTI only	–	+	–	–	–	–
Cephalexin	Keflex	PO	+	+	UTI only	–	–	–	–	–	–
Cefadroxil	Duricef	PO	+	+	UTI only	–	–	–	–	–	–
2nd generation											
Cefuroxime	Zinacef	IV	+	+	UTI only	+	±	+	–	–	+
Cefuroxime	Ceftin	PO	+	+	UTI only	+	±	±	–	–	–
Cefaclor	Ceclor	PO	+	+	UTI only	+	±	±	–	–	–
Cefprozil	Cefzil	PO	+	+	UTI only	+	±	±	–	–	–
Cefoxitin	Mefoxin	IV	+	+	±	+	±	±	–	+	±
Cefotetan	Cefotan	IV	+	+	±	+	±	±	–	+	–

(continued)

Table 24.18 Cephalosporins*† (continued)

Generic Name	Trade Name	Route	S. aureus‡	Streptococcus spp.	Gram-Negative Enterics	H. influenzae	N. gonorrhoeae	N. meningitidis	P. aeruginosa	Bacteroides fragilis	CSF Activity
3rd generation											
Cefotaxime	Claforan	IV	+	+	+	+	±	+	–	–	+
Ceftriaxone	Rocephin	IV/IM	+	+	+	+	±	+	–	–	+
Ceftizoxime	Cefizox	IV	+	+	+	+	±	±	–	±	+
Ceftazidime	Fortaz	IV	±	+	+	+	±	±	+	–	+
Cefoperazone	Cefobid	IV	+	+	+	+	±	±	+	–	+
Cefixime	Suprax	PO	–	+	+	+	+	±	–	–	–
4th generation											
Cefepime§	Maxipime	IV	+	+	+	+	+	+	+	–	+

*Meant as guideline only; individual susceptibilities will vary.
†Cephalosporins are inactive against *Enterococcus* (use ampicillin ± gentamicin or vancomycin ± gentamicin), *Listeria* (use ampicillin + gentamicin), methicillin-resistant coagulase-negative *Staphylococcus*, and MRSA (use vancomycin). First-generation cephalosporins are the cephalosporins of choice for susceptible *S. aureus* and *Streptococcus* spp.
‡MRSA is resistant to all currently available cephalosporins.
§Cefepime has better gram-positive coverage than third-generation cephalosporins.
Adapted from Gilbert DN, Moellering RC, Eliopoulos GM, Sande MA, eds. *The Sanford Guide to Antimicrobial Therapy 2007.* 37th ed. Sperryville, VA: Antimicrobial Therapy, Inc, 2007:65–70.

Table 24.19	In Vitro Activity of Selected Antifungal Agents*				
	Antifungal				
Microorganism	**Fluconazole**	**Voriconazole**	**Posaconazole**	**Echinocandins[†]**	**Polyenes[‡]**
Candida albicans	+++	+++	+++	+++	+++
Candida glabrata	±	+	+	+++	++
Candida tropicalis	+++	+++	+++	+++	+++
Candida parapsilosis	+++	+++	+++	++ [§]	+++
Candida krusei	-	++	++	+++	++
Candida lusitaniae	+++	+++	+++	+++	+
Aspergillus spp.	-	+++	+++	++	++
Fusarium spp.	-	++	++	-	++[‖]
Zygomycetes	-	-	+++	-	+++[‖]
Blastomyces dermatitidis[#]	+	++	++	-	+++
Histoplasma capsulatum[#]	+	++	++	-	+++
Coccidioides immitis[#]	+++	++	++	-	+++

*Meant as guideline only; individual susceptibilities will vary; -, no activity; ±, possible activity; +, active but third-line agent (least active clinically); ++, active but second-line agent (less active clinically); +++, active, first-line agent (usually active clinically).

[†]Includes caspofungin, micafungin, and anidulafungin.

[‡]Amphotericin B deoxycholate, amphotericin B lipid complex (ABLC), liposomal amphotericin B (AmBisome).

[§]Reduced efficacy has been noted in clinical practice.

[‖]Lipid preparations are preferred.

[#]Itraconazole is active against these dimorphic fungi and can be used as a first-line agent (+++).

Adapted from Gilbert DN, Moellering RC, Eliopoulos GM, Sande MA, eds. *The Sanford Guide to Antimicrobial Therapy 2007.* 37th ed. Sperryville, Va: Antimicrobial Therapy, Inc, 2007:109.

Table 24.20

In Vitro Activity of Selected Antiviral Agents*

Virus	Acyclovir[†]	Ganciclovir[‡]	Foscarnet	Cidofovir	Ribavirin	Amantadine	Oseltamivir
HSV	+++	++	++	++	-	-	-
EBV	++	+++	++	++	-	-	-
CMV	±	+++	+++	+++	-	-	-
HHV-6	+	+++	+++	++	-	-	-
VZV	++	+	++	+	-	-	-
BK virus	-	-	-	+	-	-	-
Adenovirus	-	±	-	+	±	-	-
RSV	-	-	-	-	+	-	-
Influenza A	-	-	-	-	-	++	+++
Influenza B	-	-	-	-	-	-	++

*Meant as guideline only; individual susceptibilities will vary; -, no activity; ±, possible activity; +, active but third-line agent (least active clinically); ++, active but second-line agent (less active clinically); +++, active, first-line agent (usually active clinically).
[†]Valacyclovir has the same spectrum of activity.
[‡]Valganciclovir has the same spectrum of activity.
Adapted from Gilbert DN, Moellering RC, Eliopoulos GM, Sande MA, eds. *The Sanford Guide to Antimicrobial Therapy 2007*. 37th ed. Sperryville, Va: Antimicrobial Therapy, Inc, 2007:150.

FURTHER READING

Baraff LJ. Management of fever without a source in infants and children. *Ann Emerg Med.* 2000;36:602–614.

Ford-Jones EL. An approach to the diagnosis of congenital infections. *Paediatr Child Health.* 1999;4:109–112.

Pickering LK, Baker CJ, Long SS, McMillan JA, eds. *Red Book: 2006 Report of the Committee on Infectious Diseases.* 27th ed. Elk Grove Village, Ill: American Academy of Pediatrics; 2006.

Pusic MA. Clinical management of fever in children younger than three years of age. *Paediatr Child Health.* 2007;12:469–472.

USEFUL WEB SITES

HIV AIDS information (e.g., perinatal treatment guidelines, antiretroviral information). Available at: **www.aidsinfo.nih.gov**

Canadian Immunization Awareness Program. Available at: **www.immunize.cpha.ca**

Canadian STD treatment guidelines. Available at: **www.phac-aspc.gc.ca/std-mts/publications_e.html**

National Advisory Committee on Immunization (Canadian guidelines). Available at: **www.phac-aspc.gc.ca/naci-ccni/**

Travel medicine information. Available at: **www.cdc.gov/travel** and **www.travelhealth.gc.ca**

Chapter 25 Metabolic Disease

Fatma Al-Jasmi
Julian A.J. Raiman

COMMON ABBREVIATIONS

ADHD	attention deficit/hyperactivity disorder
AD	autosomal dominant
AG	anion gap
AR	autosomal recessive
BMT	bone marrow transplant
CDG	congenital disorders of glycosylation
CPS	carbamoyl phosphate synthetase
ERT	enzyme replacement therapy
FAOD	fatty acid oxidation defect
FDPase	fructose 1,6-diphosphatase
FFA	free fatty acid
FTT	failure to thrive
GALT	galactose 1-phosphate uridyltransferase
G6PD	glucose-6-phosphate dehydrogenase
GSD	glycogen storage disease
HCC	hepatocellular carcinoma
HELLP	hemolytic anemia, elevated liver enzymes, and low platelet count
HFI	hereditary fructose intolerance
HSM	hepatosplenomegaly
IEM	inborn error of metabolism
LCHAD	long chain 3-hydroxyacyl-coenzyme A dehydrogenase
LFTs	liver function tests
MCAD	medium chain acyl-coenzyme A dehydrogenase
MELAS	*m*itochondrial *e*ncephalomyopathy, *l*actic *a*cidosis, *s*troke-like episodes
MMA	methylmalonic acidemia
MPS	mucopolysaccharidosis
MR	mental retardation
MRS	magnetic resonance spectroscopy
MSUD	maple syrup urine disease
NAGS	*N*-acetylglutamate synthase
NH_4	ammonia
NTBC	2-(2-nitro-4-trifluoromethylbenzoyl)-1,3-cyclohexanedione
OTC	ornithine transcarbamylase
PA	propionic acidemia

PDH	pyruvate dehydrogenase
Phe	phenylalanine
PKU	phenylketonuria
qAA	quantitative amino acid
RTA	renal tubular acidosis
SLO	Smith-Lemli-Opitz syndrome
UCD	urea cycle defect
UOA	urine organic acids
VLCAD	very long chain acyl-coenzyme A dehydrogenase
VLCFA	very long chain fatty acid
XL-ALD	X-linked adrenoleukodystrophy

GENERAL METABOLIC CONCEPTS

- Inherited metabolic diseases caused by defects in one or more steps of metabolic pathways (IEM)
- Most are AR disorders, although AD, X-linked, or mitochondrial inheritance occurs
- Rare individually (some <1 in 500,000 live births); relatively common collectively (1 in 4–5000)
- May present from fetal life to old age, affecting any or all body systems
- Vast majority of metabolic disorders occur because of enzyme defects resulting in
  1. Substrate accumulation (e.g., ↑Phe in PKU and ↑NH_4 in UCD)
  2. Lack of product (e.g., ↓ glucose in GSD type I)
  3. Accumulation of alternative product (e.g., ↑ galactitol in galactosemia)
  4. Secondary metabolic phenomena (e.g., in PA, the organic acid inhibits the urea cycle, resulting in hyperammonemia)

CLASSIFICATION OF INBORN ERRORS OF METABOLISM

- Two main groups: small molecule disorders and organelle disorders (Figure 25.1, Table 25.1)

SMALL-MOLECULE DISORDERS

- Classified into disorders of protein, carbohydrate, or fat (see Figure 25.1)
- Usually present as intoxication when toxic metabolites build up (e.g., aminoacidopathies, organic acidemia, UCD) or if delay in fuel provision (e.g., MCAD deficiency, GSD)
- See Tables 25.2, 25.3, and 25.4

Figure 25.1 Classification of Inborn Errors of Metabolism

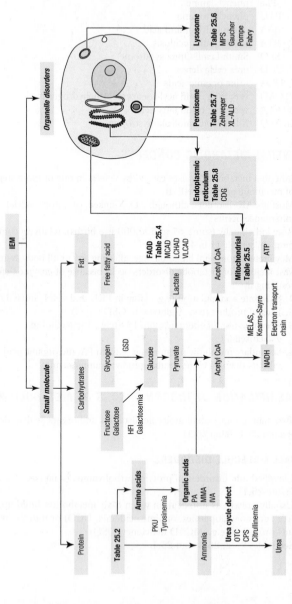

© The Hospital for Sick Children, 2009. New artwork created by The Hospital for Sick Children, for *The Hospital for Sick Children Handbook of Pediatrics*, 11th edition.

Table 25.1	Clinical Differentiation of Organelle Disorders and Small Molecule Disorders	
Feature	**Organelle Disorder**	**Small Molecule Disorder**
Definition	Disorders within specific subcellular organelles (e.g., lysosomes, peroxisomes, mitochondria)	Disorders of intermediary metabolism (fat, protein, carbohydrates)
Onset	Gradual	Often sudden, even catastrophic
Course	Slowly progressive	Relapses and remissions
Physical findings	Characteristic features	Nonspecific
Histopathology	Often characteristic changes	Generally nonspecific changes
Response to supportive therapy	Poor	Brisk

Adapted from Clarke JTR. *A Clinical Guide to Inherited Metabolic Diseases*. 3rd ed. Cambridge, England: Cambridge University Press; 2006:243. Reprinted with the permission of Cambridge University Press.

ORGANELLE DISORDERS

- Classified into lysosomal, peroxisomal, and mitochondrial disorders (see Table 25.1 and Figure 25.1)
- Mitochondrial disorders present similar to small molecule disorders
- Patients with organelle disorders are usually dysmorphic
- Lysosomal storage disorders: appearance normal at birth; features progressively coarser as storage accumulates
- See Tables 25.5, 25.6, and 25.7

Table 25.2 Selected Disorders of Amino Acid Metabolism

Disorder (Enzyme)	Clinical Features	Investigation/Diagnosis*	Treatment
Phenylketonuria (phenylalanine hydroxylase) Classic/mild PKU and mild hyperphenylalaninemia	· Poor control: risk of IQ loss, late neurologic signs · Untreated patients: severe MR, hypopigmentation, eczema, musty smell	· Plasma amino acids: ↑Phe · Urine: pterins for exclusion of biopterin defects (atypical PKU)	· Diet therapy · Intake titrated to plasma levels
Tyrosinemia type I (fumarylacetoacetate hydrolase)	· Untreated patients: hepatic dysfunction, coagulopathy, RTA, boiled cabbage odor · Secondary porphyria · Risk of HCC · Common in French Canadians	· Plasma amino acid: ↑ tyrosine · Urine: ↑ urinary succinylacetone · Other: high alpha fetoprotein	· NTBC (substrate inhibitor) · Diet therapy · Liver transplantation: NTBC nonresponders, HCC
Homocystinuria (cystathionine β-synthase)	Marfanoid habitus, MR, osteoporosis, lens dislocation, myopia, thrombosis	· Total plasma homocysteine level · Plasma amino acid: ↑ methionine	· Vitamin B₆ (cofactor/50% responsive) · B₆ nonresponsive: folate; betaine (alternative pathway) · Diet therapy · Aspirin (post-thrombosis)
MSUD (branched-chain keto acid dehydrogenase complex)	· Severe/neonatal: acute neonatal encephalopathy + seizures; maple syrup odor · Mild/intermittent form: ketoacidosis during episodes of catabolic stress	· Normal blood gas, NH₄, lactate · Ketonuria · Plasma amino acid:↑ branched-chain amino acids · UOA: ↑ keto acids	· Diet therapy: branched-chain amino acid-restricted diet
Nonketotic hyperglycinemia (glycine cleavage enzyme)	· ↑Fetal movements (in utero seizures), intractable seizures, hypotonia, severe developmental delay	· CSF amino acid: ↑ glycine · Plasma amino acid: ↑ glycine · CSF:plasma (glycine) >0.06.	· Supportive

(continued)

Table 25.2   Selected Disorders of Amino Acid Metabolism (continued)

Disorder (Enzyme)	Clinical Features	Investigation/Diagnosis*	Treatment
Canavan disease (aspartoacylase)	· Macrocephaly, hypotonia, developmental delay, spasticity, seizures	· UOA: ↑ N-acetylaspartic acid · Characteristic MRI/MRS	· Supportive
Organic Acidopathies			
PA (propionyl-CoA carboxylase)	· Hepatomegaly, seizures, vomiting, FTT, protein intolerance, developmental delay, hypotonia, acidosis/↑NH₄ with decompensation · Complications: cardiomyopathy, bone marrow suppression, renal disease, pancreatitis	· Metabolic acidosis with ↑AG, ↑NH₄ · UOA: metabolites of propionyl-CoA (PA); · UOA: large methylmalonic acid (MMA) · Plasma acylcarnitine: ↑ propionylcarnitine · ↓ Free carnitine level	· Diet therapy: low protein · L-carnitine, metronidazole (gut sterilization) · As above
MMA (methylmalonyl-CoA mutase)			
Glutaric aciduria type I (glutaryl-CoA dehydrogenase)	· Encephalopathy, dystonia, macrocephaly, subdural hemorrhages · ↑ Frequency in Ojibway-Cree	· Ketoacidosis, ↑NH₄, ↓ glucose · UOA: glutaric acid, 3-OH glutaric · Plasma acylcarnitine: ↑ glutarylcarnitine · ↓ Free carnitine level	· Diet therapy: low protein · Riboflavin, carnitine
Urea Cycle Defect			
OTC deficiency (OTC) X-linked	· Neonatal onset: 24–48 h with sepsis-like presentation; ↓ feeding, vomiting, lethargy, coma · Males usually do not survive · Female carriers/late-onset males (~20%): present later with recurrent metabolic decompensations associated with catabolic stress	· Respiratory alkalosis, ↑NH₄, ↑AST/ALT, ↑INR · Plasma amino acid: ↓ citrulline, ↑ glutamine · UOA: ↑ urine orotic acid	· Low protein diet · Sodium benzoate/sodium phenylbutyrate and citrulline · Liver transplantation

*Final diagnosis requires specific enzyme assay/molecular testing.

Table 25.3   Selected Disorders of Carbohydrate Metabolism

Disease	Clinical Features	Investigation/Diagnosis*	Treatment
Galactosemia (GALT)	· Hepatomegaly, jaundice, FTT, cataracts · Risk of *Escherichia coli* infection · Neurocognitive problems · Ovarian problems	· ↑ Conjugated bilirubin, ↑INR, RTA, hemolytic anemia · Positive urine-reducing substances · RBC GALT before blood transfusion	· Diet therapy: restriction of galactose and lactose · Calcium supplements
HFI (aldolase B)	· On ingestion of fructose, sucrose, sorbitol: variable symptoms; seizures, colic, vomiting, diarrhea, jaundice	· Positive urine-reducing substances · Blood: ↓ glucose, lactic acidosis, ↑ uric acid, RTA: generalized aminoaciduria · Response to diet therapy	· Diet therapy: restriction of fructose, sucrose, sorbitol
GSD			
GSD I (glucose-6-phosphatase)	· Characteristic facies, massive hepatomegaly, seizures, short stature, bleeding diathesis, nephromegaly · Recurrent infection (Ib) · Crohn-like bowel disease	· ↓ Glucose, ↑ lactate, ↑ uric acid, ↑ triglycerides, · ↓ Response to glucagon, type Ib: neutropenia	· Frequent daytime feedings · Overnight glucose, uncooked cornstarch, allopurinol · G-CSF for GSD Ib
GSD III (debranching enzyme)	· Similar to type I but milder ± muscle (skeletal/cardiac) involvement	· ↓ Glucose, ↑AST, ↑ALT, ↑CK · ↑ Urine myoglobin	
Disorders of Gluconeogenesis			
FDPase deficiency	· Episodic hypoglycemia, lactic acidosis, hepatomegaly, seizures	· ↑ Lactate, ketones, marked hypoglycemia, metabolic acidosis, RTA	· Treat hypoglycemia (D10W) · Treat acidosis (saline ± bicarbonate)

*Final diagnosis requires specific enzyme assay/molecular testing.

Table 25.4	**Selected Fatty Acid Oxidation Defects**		
Defect	Clinical Features	Investigation/Diagnosis	Treatment
MCAD deficiency	· Encephalopathy, Reye-like syndrome, hepatomegaly, hypoketotic hypoglycemia	· ↓ Blood glucose, ↓ urine ketones · Plasma acylcarnitine ↑C8 · ↑ Plasma FFA:3-hydroxybutyrate · UOA: dicarboxylic aciduria	· Avoid fasting · Supportive management during intercurrent illness
VLCAD, LCHAD deficiency	· Cardiac/skeletal myopathy, liver dysfunction, retinopathy (LCHAD)	· Abnormal LFTs, ↑CPK · Abnormal echocardiography · Plasma acylcarnitine profile · Plasma free carnitine level	· (± Carnitine) · Fat-restricted diet, MCT/essential fatty acid supplementation

*Final diagnosis requires specific enzyme assay/molecular testing.

Table 25.5	**Selected Mitochondrial Disorders**		
Disorder	Clinical Features	Investigation/Diagnosis*	Treatment
MELAS	· Encephalomyopathy, lactic acidosis, strokelike episodes	· Blood: ↑ lactate · CSF: ↑ lactate · UOA: ↑ lactate, ketones · MRI/MRS: lactate peak, hyperintense lesion in basal ganglia, brainstem · Skin and muscle biopsy · DNA depletion studies	· Supportive therapy · Avoid mitochondrial toxins: sodium valproate, barbiturates, tetracyclines, and chloramphenicol · Diet therapy: high-lipid, low-carbohydrate diet · Consider L-arginine in MELAS (acute attack)
Kearns-Sayre syndrome	· Triad (onset <20 yr, ophthalmoplegia, retinopathy) ± ataxia, heart block, ↑CSF protein		
Leigh	· Subacute necrotizing encephalomyopathy, extrapyramidal symptoms, leukodystrophy, necrotic lesions in thalamus, brainstem		

*Final diagnosis requires specific enzyme assay/molecular testing.

Table 25.6 Selected Lysosomal Storage Disorders

Disease (Enzyme)	Clinical Features	Investigation/Diagnosis*	Treatment
Pompe disease/GSD II (*α-glucosidase*)	· Cardiomyopathy, profound hypotonia, hyporeflexia, large tongue	· Blood: ↑ALT, AST, CK · ECG changes: ↓PR, ↑QRS · EMG: myopathic features · Atypical oligosaccharides	· Supportive · ERT
Mucopolysaccharidoses			
Hurler/MPS I (*α-L-iduronidase*)	· Attenuated: coarse facial features, HSM, macrocephaly, cardiac disease, recurrent ear infections, joint restriction · Severe MR	· Urine MPS · Blood film (vacuolation) · Skeletal survey (dysostosis multiplex) · Enzyme testing	· Severe type: BMT for patient <18 mo · Attenuated type: ERT
Hunter/MPS II (*iduronate-2-sulfatase*)	· Corneal clouding only in Hurler		· Attenuated type: ERT · Supportive
Sphingolipidoses			
Gaucher (*glucocerebrosidase*)	· Type 1: HSM, bleeding tendency, ↓ platelets, osteopenia, pain · Type 2: with CNS involvement, ophthalmoplegia, spasticity	· Gaucher cells in bone marrow · Enzyme testing	· ERT for type 1 only
Fabry (*α-galactosidase A*)	· Pain/paresthesia in limbs, angiokeratoma, renal failure, cardiomyopathy	· Urine glycolipid (↑Gb3) · Enzyme analysis · Mutation analysis	· ERT
GM₂ gangliosidosis **Tay-Sachs/Sandhoff** (*β-hexosaminidase*)	· Macrocephaly, hypotonia, developmental regression, cherry-red spot	· Enzyme testing on WBC	· Supportive

*Final diagnosis requires specific enzyme assay/molecular testing.

Table 25.7	Selected Peroxisomal Disorders		
Disorder (Enzyme/Protein)	Clinical Features	Investigation/ Diagnosis*	Treatment
XL-ALD (ALD protein)	· ADHD, adrenal insufficiency, developmental regression	· Blood: ↑VLCFA · Brain MRI (leukodystrophy)	· Presymptomatic: Lorenzo's oil/diet · Symptomatic: early BMT · Steroids for adrenal insufficiency
Zellweger (peroxins)	· Severe hypotonia, seizures, cataracts, dysmorphic features, epiphyseal stippling, renal cysts, liver dysfunction	· Blood: liver dysfunction, ↑ conjugated bilirubin, ↑VLCFA · X-ray of long bones, renal US	· Supportive

*Final diagnosis requires specific enzyme assay/molecular testing.

PRACTICAL APPROACH TO INBORN ERRORS OF METABOLISM

HISTORY AND PHYSICAL EXAMINATION

Family History

- Draw three-generation pedigree
- Determine consanguinity, ethnic/geographic background, sibling death from unexplained disease, previous multiple miscarriages

Prenatal History

- Maternal disease (e.g., maternal PKU)
- Maternal acute fatty liver of pregnancy or HELLP syndrome (mothers carrying a fetus affected by LCHAD or other FAOD)
- Abnormal or increased fetal movement or hiccups (may indicate seizures in utero)
- Prenatal screening tests (e.g., Ashkenazi Jews)
- Newborn screening

Diet

- Relationship between introduction of new foods and development of symptoms (e.g., galactosemia after introduction of milk; HFI after weaning)
- FAOD presents when children lengthen interval between feedings (e.g., overnight fasting around 6–8 mo)
- Aversion to protein diet in case of UCDs

Development

- Global developmental delay
- Developmental regression
- Behavioral problems: aggressive and destructive behavior (e.g., Sanfilippo disease [MPS III], self-mutilation (e.g., Lesch–Nyhan), irritability, hyperactivity, and nocturnal restlessness

Drug History

- Adverse response to drug exposure:
  - Rifampin, progesterone, and barbiturates in porphyria
  - Chloroquine in G6PD deficiency

History of Presenting Illness

- Age of presentation: "intoxication defects" display no symptoms in first hours of life; present with nonspecific, progressive symptoms day 2–5
- Response to metabolic stress (intercurrent illnesses, fasting, fever, surgery, puberty)

Physical Examination

- See Box 25.1

LABORATORY EVALUATION

- See Table 25.8

Table 25.8	Laboratory Evaluation if Acute Metabolic Disease Suspected	
Basic Metabolic Investigations*	**Special Metabolic Investigations**	
Blood gas and plasma electrolytes	Acylcarnitines, total and free carnitine	
Plasma glucose	Plasma amino acids	
Plasma lactate	Urinary organic acids	
Plasma ammonium	Plasma (5 mL) and urine (5–20 mL) stored frozen, and dried blood spots stored at 4°C, for further investigation (e.g., in the event of death)	
Urinary ketones (Ketostix) and urine-reducing substances		

*In addition to CBC, LFTs (bilirubin, ALT, AST, INR), CK, creatinine, urea, urate.
Adapted from Blau N, Hoffman GF, Leonard J, Clarke JTR. *Physician's Guide to the Treatment and Follow-Up of Metabolic Diseases*. Berlin, Germany: Springer-Verlag; 2006. With the kind permission of Springer Science & Business Media.

Growth Variables
- FTT (e.g., small molecule disorder)
- Macrocephaly (e.g., GA1, Canavan, Alexander, Hunter disease)

Dysmorphic Features
- Coarse facial features (e.g., MPS)
- Inverted nipples and abnormal fat distribution (e.g., CDG)
- Syndactyly of second and third toes, genital abnormalities (e.g., SLO)

Eye Examination
- Cataracts (e.g., galactosemia, peroxisomal disorders)
- Corneal clouding (e.g., Hurler syndrome)
- Dislocation of lens (e.g., homocystinuria)
- Macular cherry-red spot (e.g., GM_1 and GM_2 gangliosidosis, sialidosis, Niemann–Pick disease)
- Pigmentary retinopathy (e.g., FAOD, mitochondrial, peroxisomal disorders)

Cardiovascular Disease
- Signs of heart failure (e.g., Pompe disease)
- Valvular heart diseases (e.g., MPS)

Abdominal Examination
- HSM (e.g., MPS, GSD, GM_1, Niemann–Pick, Wolman, tyrosinemia)
- Splenomegaly (e.g., Gaucher disease)
- Hepatomegaly (e.g., GSD, FDPase, CDG)
- Inguinal and umbilical hernia (e.g., MPS)

Neurologic Examination
- Supranuclear paralysis (e.g., Gaucher, Niemann–Pick type C)
- Hypotonia (e.g., Pompe, Zellweger)
- Spasticity (e.g., nonketotic hyperglycinemia, Menkes)
- Ataxia, peripheral neuropathy and dystonia (e.g., GA1, neurotransmitter defects, PDH deficiency)

Skeletal Examination
- Limitation in joint movements (e.g., MPS I, II, IV, VI)
- Scoliosis (e.g., homocystinuria)

Skin and Hair
- Alopecia or kinky hair (e.g., Menkes, arginosuccinic aciduria)
- Fair coloring (e.g., PKU, albinism)
- Hirsutism (e.g., Hurler, Hunter)
- Ichthyosis (e.g., Sjögren-Larsson)

Unusual Odor
- Burnt sugar (MSUD), sweaty feet (isovaleric acidemia), musty (PKU), and cabbage smell (tyrosinemia type I)

MANAGEMENT OF IEM

Control of Accumulated Substrate

Restrict Dietary Intake
- UCD and organic acidopathies: stop/restrict exogenous protein intake
- Amino acid disorders: restriction of specific amino acids (e.g., Phe in PKU, tyrosine in tyrosinemia)
- Galactosemia: limit galactose intake

Control Endogenous Production of Substrate
- UCD and organic acidopathies: provide sufficient calories using IV D10W and Intralipid for reversal of breakdown of endogenous protein; protein reintroduced into diet after 24–48 h exclusion

Clear Toxic Metabolites
- Severe hyperammonemia, ↑ leucine (MSUD) and lactic acidosis: hemodialysis
- Organic acidopathies: carnitine for elimination of toxic metabolites and restoration of intramitochondrial free acyl-CoA
- UCD: sodium benzoate and sodium phenylacetate/butyrate allow metabolism and excretion of waste nitrogen through alternative pathway

Supply Deficient Product
- FAOD, GSD: give glucose

Enzyme Replacement Therapy
- Gaucher disease, Fabry disease, attenuated form of MPS I, MPS II, MPS VI, Pompe disease

Cofactor Replacement Therapy
- Multiple carboxylase deficiency: biotin
- Pyridoxine-responsive homocystinuria and pyridoxine-dependent seizures: pyridoxine
- Vitamin B_{12}–responsive MMA: vitamin B_{12}
- PDH deficiency: thiamine

Organ Transplantation
- MPS I and XL-ALD: BMT
- UCD: liver transplantation

Supportive Management
- Control seizures and relieve spasticity, facilitate feeding, prevent constipation

Genetic Counseling
- Recurrence risk, prenatal diagnosis for future pregnancies, sibling screening

HYPERAMMONEMIA

- May present at any age
- Investigation of encephalopathy of unclear cause must include plasma NH₄ levels
- Severe hyperammonemia is a medical emergency because of risk of cerebral edema
- See Figure 25.2 for an approach to hyperammonemia

Figure 25.2 **Approach to Hyperammonemia**

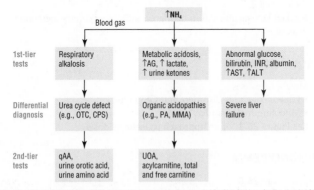

© The Hospital for Sick Children, 2009. New artwork created by The Hospital for Sick Children, for *The Hospital for Sick Children Handbook of Pediatrics*, 11th edition.

MANAGEMENT

- Supportive: antiseizure medication, antibiotics for sepsis, ventilation
- No protein intake; NPO
- Start D10W 0.45% NaCl with 20 mmol of KCl/L at 1.5 × maintenance (150 mL/kg/d), aiming for 8–10 mg/kg/min glucose intake (watch sodium intake from benzoate/butyrate)
- Consult metabolic specialist
- Consider IV Intralipid 0.5–2 g/kg/d
- Alternative pathway for nitrogen excretion: sodium benzoate 250 mg/kg IV bolus over 2 h, then continuous infusion of 250 mg/kg/d; consider sodium phenylbutyrate 250 mg/kg IV bolus, then continuous infusion with 250 mg/kg/d
- Replenish urea cycle intermediates with arginine hydrochloride IV/PO up to 300 mg/kg/d or citrulline PO 170 mg/kg/d (especially OTC)
- Start hemodialysis immediately if NH₄ level >500 μmol/L or if patient deteriorating (e.g., encephalopathy)
- L-Carnitine 100–200 mg/kg/d in case of suspected or confirmed organic acidopathies
- Consider carbamyl glutamate 100 mg/kg/d divided into 3 doses in cases of CPS deficiency, NAGS deficiency, or organic acidopathies

- Consider antiemetics in noncomatose children (sodium benzoate causes nausea and vomiting)
- Monitor NH_4 level, blood gas, and electrolytes on regular basis
- Neurovitals q2–4h; if patient deteriorates (↓LOC), NH_4 level stat
- Accurate ins/outs, daily weight (look for signs of fluid overload)

METABOLIC ACIDOSIS

- See Figure 25.3 for approach
- First step: calculate $AG = Na^+ + K^+ - (Cl^- + HCO_3^-)$ (normal, <16 mmol/L)
- Marked ketosis unusual in neonates: indicates primary metabolic disease

LACTIC ACIDOSIS

- Metabolic causes
  - Gluconeogenesis disorders and GSD type I
  - Mitochondrial disorders
- See Figure 25.4 for an approach to lactic acidosis

HYPOGLYCEMIA

- See Figure 25.5
- Definition: blood glucose ≤2.6 mmol/L
- Metabolic causes of hypoglycemia:
  - Ketotic: deficiency of glucose supply (GSD, gluconeogenesis defect)
  - Hypoketotic: overutilization of glucose (as a result of defects in fatty acid or ketone oxidation, hyperinsulinism)

MANAGEMENT

- Critical blood work (glucose, FFAs, ketone bodies [3-hydroxybutyrate], insulin, growth hormone, cortisol, TSH, T_4, acylcarnitine, qAA, NH_4, lactate, UOAs); urine dip for ketones
- Glucose bolus (5–10 mL/kg D10W) followed by continuous infusion 7–10 mg/kg/min (D10W + variable NaCl concentration: 100–150 mL/kg/d); keep blood glucose >5 mmol/L (avoid rebound hypoglycemia)
- Rule out severe systemic illness, liver disease, sepsis, infant of diabetic mother
- Timing of hypoglycemia helpful: within minutes of feeding (hyperinsulinism), within 1–6 h (GSD), after 8–24 h fasting (FAOD)
- Other clues to diagnosis:
  - Response to glucagon administration: absent in GSD type I
  - Glucose requirement (mL/h × %dextrose/6 × weight [kg]); if >10 mg/kg/min, indicates endocrine cause—usually hyperinsulinism

Figure 25.3 Approach to Metabolic Acidosis

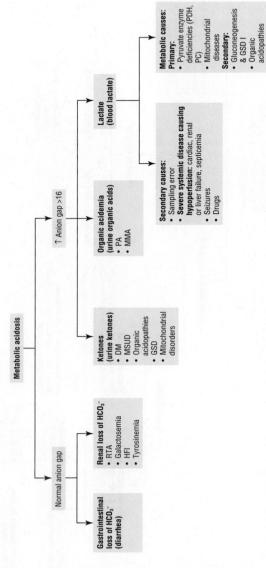

Metabolic acidosis

Normal anion gap

Gastrointestinal loss of HCO₃⁻ (diarrhea)

Renal loss of HCO₃⁻
• RTA
• Galactosemia
• HFI
• Tyrosinemia

↑ Anion gap >16

Ketones (urine ketones)
• DM
• MSUD
• Organic acidopathies
• GSD
• Mitochondrial disorders

Organic acidemia (urine organic acids)
• PA
• MMA

Lactate (blood lactate)

Metabolic causes:
Primary:
• Pyruvate enzyme deficiencies (PDH, PC)
• Mitochondrial diseases
Secondary:
• Gluconeogenesis & GSD I
• Organic acidopathies

Secondary causes:
• Sampling error
• **Severe systemic disease causing hypoperfusion:** cardiac, renal or liver failure, septicemia
• Seizures
• Drugs

Adapted from Clarke JTR. A Clinical Guide to Inherited Metabolic Diseases (3rd ed.). Cambridge: Cambridge University Press, 2006. © Joe T.R. Clarke, 2006.

Metabolic Disease

25

Figure 25.4 Approach to Lactic Acidosis

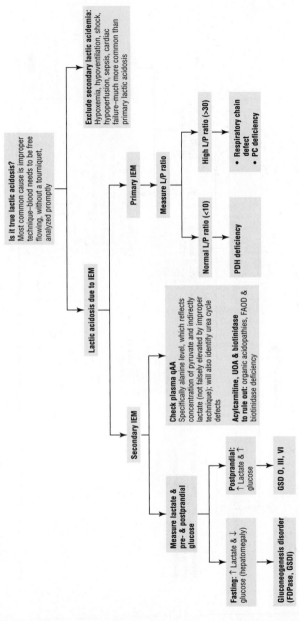

Is it true lactic acidosis?
Most common cause is improper technique–blood needs to be free flowing, without a tourniquet, analyzed promptly

Exclude secondary lactic acidemia: Hypoxemia, hypoventilation, shock, hypoperfusion, sepsis, cardiac failure–much more common than primary lactic acidosis

Lactic acidosis due to IEM

Primary IEM

Measure L/P ratio

Normal L/P ratio (<10)

PDH deficiency

High L/P ratio (>30)

• Respiratory chain defect
• PC deficiency

Secondary IEM

Check plasma qAA
Specifically alanine level, which reflects concentration of pyruvate and indirectly lactate (not falsely elevated by improper technique); will also identify urea cycle defects

Acylcarnitine, UOA & biotinidase to rule out: organic acidopathies, FAOD & biotinidase deficiency

Measure lactate & pre- & postprandial glucose

Postprandial: ↑ Lactate & ↑ glucose

GSD 0, III, VI

Fasting: ↑ Lactate & ↓ glucose (hepatomegaly)

Gluconeogenesis disorder (FDPase, GSDI)

Figure 25.5 **Hypoglycemia**

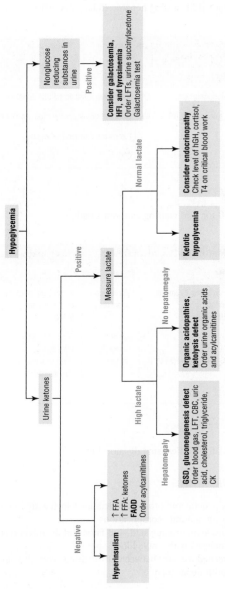

© The Hospital for Sick Children, 2009. New artwork created by The Hospital for Sick Children, for *The Hospital for Sick Children Handbook of Pediatrics*, 11th edition.

HEPATOCELLULAR DYSFUNCTION

- See Table 25.9 for IEM causing hepatocellular dysfunction

Table 25.9	Metabolic Disorders Causing Hepatocellular Dysfunction	
Small-Molecule Disorder	**Organelle Disorder**
Amino acid disorders (Tyrosinemia type I)	Mitochondrial disorder (MtDNA depletion)
Carbohydrate disorders (galactosemia, HFI, GSD IV)	Lysosomal storage disorder (Niemann–Pick type C)
UCD	Peroxisomal disorders (Zellweger)
FAODs (CPTII, LCHAD)	CDG

CARDIOMYOPATHY

- See Table 25.10 for IEM causing cardiomyopathy

Table 25.10	Metabolic Disorders Causing Cardiomyopathy		
Small-Molecule Disorder		**Organelle Disorder**	
FAOD	· Primary systemic carnitine deficiency · LCHAD	Mitochondrial syndromes	· Kearns-Sayre syndrome · Barth syndrome · MELAS
Organic acidopathies	· PA · MMA · HMG-CoA lyase deficiency	Lysosomal storage disorder	· Pompe disease · Fabry disease · Hurler syndrome · Hunter syndrome
Carbohydrate	· GSD III		

DYSMORPHIC FEATURES

- See Table 25.11 for IEM causing dysmorphism

NEWBORN SCREENING

- Aim to identify genetic and other disorders for which early treatment could prevent or ameliorate complications
- Screen for amino acid, organic acid, and fatty acid disorders (via acylcarnitine analysis) with single blood spot
- Conditions screened for vary between jurisdictions; consult your local public health department

Table 25.11	Metabolic Disorders Causing Dysmorphism
Organelle Metabolism	**Investigations**
Lysosomal disorders (e.g., MPS, I-cell disease, mannosidosis)	Urine MPS screening Urine oligosaccharide screening
Peroxisomal disorders (e.g., Zellweger, rhizomelic chondrodysplasia punctata)	Plasma VLCFA Plasma phytanic acid
Mitochondrial disorders (e.g., glutaric aciduria type II, PDH)	Plasma lactate and pyruvate Plasma acylcarnitine profile, UOA
Biosynthetic Defects	
SLO	Serum 7-dehydrocholesterol
CDG	Isoelectric focusing plasma transferrin
Menkes	Copper, ceruloplasmin
Homocystinuria	Plasma qAA, plasma total homocystein
Fetal Intoxication	
Maternal PKU	Plasma qAA

PERIMORTEM/POSTMORTEM INVESTIGATIONS

- In cases of death without known etiology, helpful to collect samples to investigate for IEM (to establish or confirm diagnosis for future genetic counseling)
- Try to collect blood and urine samples before expected death
- Parents may consider postmortem biopsy if autopsy not acceptable to them
  - Liver and muscle biopsy should be done within 1 h
  - Skin fibroblasts may remain viable for 2 d (but the earlier, the better)
- If IEM suspected, immediately (within first hour postmortem) collect:
  - Plasma: heparinized 5 mL and store at −80°C
  - Blood spots on Guthrie card (acylcarnitine analysis, DNA extraction)
  - Blood with EDTA: 5–10 mL; store at 4°C (DNA extraction)
  - Urine: 10–15 mL in different tubes and should be deep frozen
  - Vitreous humor, only if urine not available; store at −20°C
  - Skin biopsy (0.5 cm) for fibroblast culture
  - Liver: three or more samples of 1 cm³ (snap-frozen in liquid nitrogen; stored on dry ice at −80°C for histochemical and enzymologic analysis)
  - Muscle (skeletal or heart), as clinically indicated

FURTHER READING

Clarke JTR. *A Clinical Guide to Inherited Metabolic Diseases.* 3rd ed. Cambridge, England: Cambridge University Press; 2006.

USEFUL WEB SITES

eMedicine. Available at: www.emedicine.com/
GeneTests Web site. Available at: www.genetests.org
The Ontario Newborn Screening Program. Available at:
www.health.gov.on.ca/english/providers/program/child/screening/screen_sum.html
UpToDate. Available at: www.uptodate.com

Metabolic Disease

25

Chapter 26 Neonatology

Gagan Saund
Constance Williams
Aideen Moore

Chapter 26 Neonatology

COMMON ABBREVIATIONS

AXR	abdominal X-ray
BE	base excess
BW	birth weight
CAH	congenital adrenal hyperplasia
CHF	congestive heart failure
CPAP	continuous positive airway pressure
EBM	expressed breast milk
ECMO	extracorporeal membrane oxygenation
ELBW	extremely low birth weight
ETT	endotracheal tube
FiO_2	fraction of inspired oxygen
FSWU	full septic workup
GA	gestational age
GBS	group B streptococcus
GIR	glucose infusion rate
HBR	hyperbilirubinemia
HFO	high-frequency oscillation
HIE	hypoxic ischemic encephalopathy
HMF	human milk fortifier
IDM	infant of diabetic mother
IPPV	intermittent positive pressure ventilation
IUGR	intrauterine growth restriction (BW <10th percentile for GA)
IVH	intraventricular hemorrhage
LBW	low birth weight
LGA	large for gestational age (BW >90th percentile for GA)
MAP	mean airway pressure
NEC	necrotizing enterocolitis
NPT	nasopharyngeal tube
OI	oxygenation index
$PaCO_2$	arterial partial pressure of carbon dioxide
PaO_2	arterial partial pressure of oxygen
PDA	patent ductus arteriosus
PFO	patient foramen ovale
PPHN	persistent pulmonary hypertension of the newborn
PROM	premature rupture of membranes
PVL	periventricular leukomalacia
RDS	respiratory distress syndrome
ROP	retinopathy of prematurity
SEH	subependymal hemorrhage

SGA	small for gestational age (BW <10th percentile for GA)
(T)PN	(total) parenteral nutrition
TR	tricuspid regurgitation
TSB	total serum bilirubin
TTN	transient tachypnea of the newborn
UAC	umbilical artery catheter
UVC	umbilical vein catheter
VLBW	very low birth weight

CLASSIFICATION OF THE NEONATE

- Term: 37 completed wk to 41 wk and 6 d
- Premature: <37 wk
- LBW: <2500 g
- VLBW: <1500 g
- ELBW: <1000 g

NEWBORN RESUSCITATION

- Normal sequence of response to resuscitation: increased HR → reflex activity → improved color → spontaneous breathing → improved tone and responsiveness
- See Figure 26.1 and Box 26.1 for management and resuscitation
- See Table 26.1 for APGAR score

EQUIPMENT IN CASE ROOM

- Radiant warmer turned on
- Clean warm towels
- Gloves, barrier precautions
- Stethoscope
- O_2 bagging equipment with masks (sizes 0, 1, 2)
- Suction equipment turned on
- Meconium aspirator (Figure 26.2)
- Laryngoscope
- ETTs (sizes 2.5, 3.0, 3.5, 4.0) (Tables 26.2 and 26.3)
- Magill forceps
- Gastric tubes (size 5, 8F)
- Umbilical catheterization tray (catheter sizes 3.5, 5.0F) (Box 26.2)
- Emergency drugs: epinephrine 1:10,000; 0.9% NaCl; D10W; naloxone 0.4 mg/mL; $NaHCO_3$ 4.2% concentration (0.5 mEq/mL)
- Additional factors in initial management:
  - SGA infant: hypothermia, hypoglycemia, hyperviscosity syndrome (polycythemia)
  - LGA infant: birth trauma, asphyxia, hypoglycemia, HBR

Figure 26.1 Guide to the Assessment and Management of a Neonate at Delivery

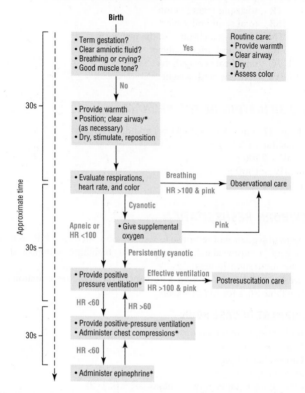

*Endotracheal intubation may be considered at several steps.

Used with permission of the American Academy of Pediatrics, *Textbook of Neonatal Resuscitation*, 5th ed. Elk Grove Village, Ill.: American Academy of Pediatrics; 2006.

- Premature infants: avoid hypothermia at <28 wk GA; do not dry (wrapping body in clear plastic wrap may reduce heat loss/ evaporation in ELBW infants); low threshold for intubation at <32 wk GA; early use of surfactant beneficial; avoid hyperoxia (i.e., saturation >95%); may initiate PPV with air (FiO2, 0.21), and supplemental O2 should be used if HR <100 beats/min or remains cyanotic; provide PEEP of minimum 3–6 cm H2O during resuscitation

Box 26.1	ABCD of Newborn Resuscitation
Airway	• Put baby's head in sniffing position • Suction mouth, then nose
Breathing	• PPV: start in room air, for apnea, gasping, or pulse <100 beats/min • If no response, increase FiO_2 to 100% • Ventilate at rate of 40–60 breaths/min • Assess for rising HR, breath sounds, chest rise • Intubate if no response to maneuvers, use CO_2 detector if intubated
Circulation	• Compressions if HR <60 after 30 s of PPV • Give 3 compressions: 1 breath every 2 s • Compress ⅓ AP diameter of the chest
Drugs	• Epinephrine: if HR <60 after 30 s of compressions and ventilation; 1:10,000 solution 0.1–0.3 mL/kg IV or 0.3–1 mL/kg ETT while IV access being obtained • Volume expanders: 0.9% NaCl recommended 10 mL/kg; others: Ringer's lactate, O Rh-negative blood; give over 5–10 min

- See Table 26.4 for survival rates for premature infants
  - Overall survival for <1000 g infants is 70%; 15% have severe neurodevelopmental impairment at 20 mo
- Parkin assessment of GA: scores GA from 27 to 41 wk based on
  - Soft tissue assessment (skin texture, skin color, breast size)
  - Ear firmness: palpation and folding of upper pinna

Table 26.1	Apgar Score*		
Sign†	0	1	2
Heart rate	Absent	<100 beats/min	>100 beats/min
Respiratory effort	Absent	Gasping; slow, irregular	Regular, good cry
Reflex **I**rritability	No response	Grimace	Cry
Muscle **T**one	Limp, flaccid	Some flexion of extremities	Active, well flexed
Color	Blue, pale	Body pink; extremities blue	Completely pink

*Apgar scoring system should not be used to determine need for resuscitation; should be done at 1 and 5 min and thereafter at 5-min intervals until score of 7 is achieved.
†Sign components of Apgar score can be remembered by mnemonic: **H**ow **R**eady **I**s **T**his **C**hild
Adapted from Ostheimer GW. Resuscitation of newborn infant. *Clin Perinatol.* 1982;9:183.

Figure 26.2 Management of Meconium-Stained Delivery

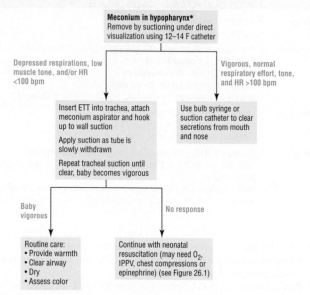

Meconium in hypopharynx*
Remove by suctioning under direct visualization using 12–14 F catheter

Depressed respirations, low muscle tone, and/or HR <100 bpm

Vigorous, normal respiratory effort, tone, and HR >100 bpm

Insert ETT into trachea, attach meconium aspirator and hook up to wall suction

Apply suction as tube is slowly withdrawn

Repeat tracheal suction until clear, baby becomes vigorous

Use bulb syringe or suction catheter to clear secretions from mouth and nose

Baby vigorous

No response

Routine care:
• Provide warmth
• Clear airway
• Dry
• Assess color

Continue with neonatal resuscitation (may need O$_2$, IPPV, chest compressions or epinephrine) (see Figure 26.1)

*Note: Aspirate stomach early to avoid further aspiration of swallowed meconium; presence of meconium in premature delivery may indicate *Listeria* infection.
Used with permission of the American Academy of Pediatrics, *Textbook of Neonatal Resuscitation*, 5th ed. Elk Grove Village, Ill.: American Academy of Pediatrics; 2006.

Table 26.2	Endotracheal Tube Size		
GA (wk)	**Weight (kg)**	**ETT Size (mm)**	**Depth of Insertion* (cm)**
<28	<1.0	2.5	6–7
28–34	1.0–2.0	3.0	7–8
34–38	2.0–3.0	3.5	8–9
>38	>3.0	3.5–4.0	9–10

*Depth of insertion (cm from lips) for oral tubes: 6 + weight (kg); nasal tubes: 7 + weight (kg).
Used with permission of the American Academy of Pediatrics, *Textbook of Neonatal Resuscitation*, 5th ed. Elk Grove Village, Ill.: American Academy of Pediatrics; 2006.

Table 26.3	Management of Poor Response to Intermittent Positive Pressure Ventilation	
Cause of Nonresponse	**Diagnostic Considerations**	**Action**
ETT not in correct location	Observe chest movement; auscultate for symmetric air entry; CXR	Pull back ETT if in right main stem bronchus; reintubate if uncertain and reassess
Tension pneumothorax	Displaced apex beat ± hemodynamic compromise; decreased or unequal air entry; CXR or transillumination to confirm	Urgent drain with butterfly needle if unstable; insert chest tube
Massive meconium aspiration	History of fetal distress and "pea-soup" liquor staining; CXR; ↑ risk of PPHN; ↑ risk of pneumothorax	See Figure 26.2
Diaphragmatic hernia	Scaphoid abdomen noted at birth ± respiratory distress; bowel sounds heard over chest; CXR diagnostic; ↑ risk of PPHN	Pass NG tube and connect to low Gomco; intubate; IPPV; sedate and paralyze
Hypoplastic lungs	History of oligohydramnios ± PROM ± Potter facies; bell-shaped chest; CXR	Urgent intubation; ventilatory support; requires high peak pressures
Sepsis or congenital pneumonia	History of PROM, GBS, or maternal fever; hemodynamic compromise; CXR (may look like RDS); cultures may be positive	Antibiotics; ventilatory support ± volume expanders ± inotropes
Severe RDS	Prematurity, stiff lungs, "ground glass" CXR	Higher pressures required; early surfactant via ETT
Cyanotic congenital heart disease	Persistent cyanosis despite adequate ventilation	Hyperoxia test, ECG, CXR, consider prostaglandin infusion, echocardiogram; see Chapter 9
Acute blood loss	History of abruption, previa, nuchal chord; asystole, bradycardia, pallor after oxygenation; subgaleal hemorrhage	Volume resuscitation: 0.9% NaCl 10 mL/kg, repeat; transfuse blood if large volume loss
Severe HIE	Agonal respirations, gasping, bradycardia, asystole	Cord and blood gases; discontinuation of resuscitation after 10 min of asystole despite adequate resuscitation

Box 26.2 Calculations for Umbilical Artery Catheter and Umbilical Vein Catheter Placement

- UAC insertion depth: weight (kg) × 3 + 9 (for T6–T10 position)
- UVC insertion depth: ½ UAC depth + 1 (in IVC, T9 above diaphragm)

Table 26.4 Survival Rates for Premature Infants Admitted to the Neonatal Intensive Care Unit

BW (g)	Survival (%)		Gestational Age (wk)	Survival (%)
<500	–		<22	–
500–749	70		23	35
750–999	88		24	71
1000–1249	96		25	78
1250–1499	97		26	85
1500–2499	98		27	94
2500–4499	98		28	94
>4499	99		29	97

Adapted from Canadian Neonatal Network. Survival rates for premature infants admitted to NICU. In: *Annual Report 2007.* Edmonton, Alberta: Canadian Neonatal Network; 2007:13–14. Reprinted by permission of the Canadian Neonatal Network.

FLUIDS AND ELECTROLYTES

- High surface area:weight ratio
- Immature renal function
- Immature skin; higher losses in premature infants
- See Table 26.5 for fluid guidelines

Table 26.5 Guidelines for Neonatal Fluid Therapy

BW (g)	Water Requirements (mL/kg/d) by Age		
	1–2 d	3–7 d	7–30 d
<750	100–200	150–200	160–180
750–1000	80–150	100–150	120–180
1000–1500	60–100	100–150	120–180
>1500	60–80	100–150	120–180

Adapted from Kirpalani HM, Moore AM, Perlman M. *Residents Handbook of Neonatology.* 3rd ed. Hamilton, Ontario, Canada: BC Decker; 2007:85, Table 3.

GOALS OF THERAPY

1. Achieve balance between input and output
   - Weight is most useful indicator of fluid status; weigh q12h for first 5 d, then daily; use BW for fluid calculations until return to BW
2. Meet normal metabolic and growth requirements
   - Premature: 15–20 g/kg/d; term: 10–20 g/kg/d (see p. 388)
3. Replace necessary losses
   - Insensible fluid losses: 70% through skin, 30% through respiratory tract
     - <1500 g: 30–60 mL/kg/d
     - 1500–2500 g: 15–35 mL/kg/d
     - >2500 g: 10–15 mL/kg/d
   - Urinary output: 50–100 mL/kg/d
   - Fecal losses: 5–10 mL/kg/d, usually minimal during first week
   - Assess fluid balance q8–12h for 2–3 d, then as clinically indicated, but minimum every 24 h
     - Prediuretic phase: ~day 1–2 (urine output <1–2 mL/kg/h)
     - Diuretic phase: ~day 2–3 (urine output >1–2 mL/kg/h; negative balance)
     - Postdiuretic phase: after day 2–4 (fluid balance stabilizes, then becomes positive)

APPROACH

- Start with minimum fluid requirements; adjust by monitoring urine output, weight, serum Na^+; in first 2 d, Na^+ and K^+ not usually required (see Table 26.5)
- Glucose concentration of 5–10% to maintain caloric requirement and osmolarity; normal glucose infusion rate (GIR) is 4–6 mg/kg/min, may increase to 10–12 mg/kg/min as tolerated: GIR (mg/kg/min) = carbohydrate (mg/mL) × infusion rate (mL/h) ÷ weight (kg) ÷ 60 min (e.g., 0.8-kg infant infusing D10W at 3 mL/h = 100 mg/mL × 3 mL/h ÷ 0.8 kg ÷ 60 min = 6.2 mg/kg/min)
  Note:

$$DxW = x \times 10 \text{ mg/mL of carbohydrate}$$
$$(e.g., D5W = 50 \text{ mg/mL of carbohydrate})$$

  - Add Na^+ (2–3 mmol/kg/d) and K^+ (1–2 mmol/kg/d) once diuretic phase established
  - Larger doses of Na^+ may be required in postdiuretic phase in infants <750 g because of high urinary Na^+ losses; measure urine Na^+ concentration and urine output before large IV doses given because of risk of hypernatremia
  - In all infants <1000 g BW and infants 1000–1500 g not expected to be taking full oral feeds within 4–7 d, start parenteral nutrition (see Nutrition section); avoid glucose-only regimens beyond 24 h of age

HYPONATREMIA

- Na$^+$ <130 mmol/L
- See Chapter 16 for further details

EXCESS NA$^+$ LOSS

- Renal tubular immaturity: high urinary Na$^+$ losses (up to 10–12 mmol/kg/d in premature infants <30 wk)
- Hypoxic injury
- Diuretics
- GI losses
- CAH, salt-losing 21-hydroxylase deficiency
- "Late hyponatremia of prematurity" (>1 wk): inadequate intake in addition to aforementioned

Treatment

- Calculate deficit:
  - [Na$^+$ (desired) − Na$^+$ (actual)] × 0.6 × weight (kg)
- Replace over 24–48 h in addition to providing maintenance and insensible losses
- Monitor serum and urinary Na$^+$ q6–12h
- Consider oral Na$^+$ supplements in LBW infants

WATER RETENTION

- Iatrogenic overload (excess dextrose solutions)
- SIADH
- CHF
- Renal failure

Treatment

- Fluid restriction (½–⅔ of maintenance requirement)
- If symptomatic: 3% NaCl (with caution) to correct to 125 mmol/L ± diuretics
- Monitor serum Na$^+$ q6–12h

HYPERNATREMIA

- Na$^+$ >150 mmol/L
- See Chapter 16 for details

ETIOLOGY

- Dehydration from ↑ insensible losses (mostly <30 wk GA, under radiant warmer or phototherapy)
- Renal or GI losses
- Iatrogenic (excess Na$^+$ administration [e.g., 0.9% NaCl, NaHCO$_3$])

TREATMENT

- Management based on etiology, severity of symptoms, timing (acute or chronic)
- Dehydration is most common cause; assume fluid deficit of 10–15% (100–150 mL/kg) and aim to correct over 24-48 h to avoid too rapid decrease in Na^+
- Water deficit (L) calculated using the following formula (P_{NA}^+ is current plasma Na^+ concentration):

$$\text{Water deficit} = 0.6 \times \text{body weight} \times \left[1 - \frac{P_{Na}^+}{140} \right]$$

- If patient hypotensive, resuscitate with 10–20 mL/kg 0.9% NaCl, subtracting volume from total deficit to be replaced
- If initial Na^+ >160, use 0.9% NaCl with D5 or D10W to replace water deficit, then 0.45% NaCl with D5 or D10W as maintenance fluid
- If initial Na^+ <160, use 0.45% NaCl or 0.2% NaCl with D5 or D10W for deficit; continue as already discussed
- For infants <1.5 kg, deficits may be 20–25% of body weight; initially use 0.2% NaCl, D5 or D10W for replacement of deficit; monitor and adjust further based on Na^+, weight, urine output, urine Na^+
- In hypervolemic hypernatremia: goal is to remove Na^+
  - Therapy: restrict Na^+; restrict H_2O if CHF present; diuretics (furosemide)

HYPOKALEMIA

- K^+ <3.5 mmol/L
- Most commonly iatrogenic (e.g., inadequate intake, diuretics, respiratory alkalosis)
- See Chapter 16 for differential diagnosis and management

HYPERKALEMIA

- K^+ >7 mmol/L
- See Chapter 16 for differential diagnosis and management

ACID-BASE STATUS

RESPIRATORY ACIDOSIS

- Corrected by adjusting ventilation, not $NaHCO_3$
- "Permissive hypercapnia" accepted to minimize lung damage (pH 7.22–7.25 and PCO_2 55–65 mm Hg) in neonates

RESPIRATORY ALKALOSIS

- Generally in infants receiving ventilation; corrected by adjusting ventilation

METABOLIC ACIDOSIS

- See Chapter 16 for details
- See Box 26.3 for causes
- pH <7.3 with
  - HCO_3^- <19 mmol/L on day 1, <21 mmol/L subsequently
  - BE >−5 on day 1, >−4 subsequently

Box 26.3	Causes of Metabolic Acidosis

- Sepsis (consider septic workup)
- Hypoxia, shock, severe anemia
- PDA with CHF
- HCO_3^- losses (renal tubular acidosis, diarrhea)
- Metabolic (aminoacidemia, organic acidemia, congenital lactic acidosis—see Chapter 16)
- Excess protein load
- SEH, IVH

Management

- Treat underlying cause
- $NaHCO_3$ (4.2%) for pH <7.25 and BE >−10
- Base deficit:

$$[HCO_3^- \text{ (desired)} - HCO_3^- \text{ (actual)}] \times \text{weight (kg)} \times 0.3$$

- Correct half of calculated deficit initially, usually over 1–4 h; do not infuse in Ca^{2+}-containing solutions; rapid infusion may increase risk of IVH
- 2 mmol/kg of $NaHCO_3$ increases pH by 0.1 unit

METABOLIC ALKALOSIS

- Usually secondary to excessive $NaHCO_3$ therapy
- Also with hypokalemia, PO_4^- excess, hypochloremia, postexchange transfusion
- See Chapter 16 for details

HYPOGLYCEMIA

- Specific interventions recommended if blood glucose <2.6 mmol/L (Figure 26.3)
- Clinical signs: lethargy, apnea, cyanosis, tremor, tachypnea, seizures
- Critical sample: in presence of hypoglycemia, take blood for glucose, free fatty acids, ketone bodies (β-hydroxybutyrate), insulin, growth hormone, cortisol, TSH, T_4, acylcarnitine, amino acids, lactate, ammonia, blood gas; urine for organic acids; dip urine for ketones

Figure 26.3 Algorithm for the Screening and Immediate Management of Infants at Risk of Neonatal Hypoglycemia

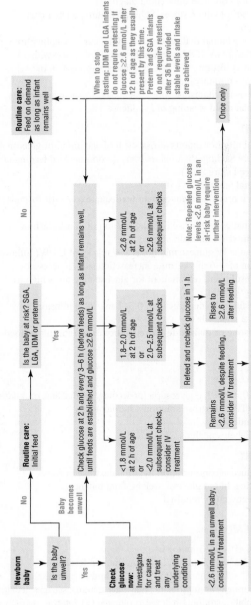

Newborn baby

Is the baby unwell?

No → Is the baby at risk? SGA, LGA, IDM or preterm

Yes →

Check glucose now:
Investigate for cause and treat any underlying condition

<2.6 mmol/L in an unwell baby, consider IV treatment

Routine care:
Initial feed

No → **Routine care:**
Feed on demand as long as infant remains well

Baby becomes unwell

Yes →

Check glucose at 2 h and every 3–6 h (before feeds) as long as infant remains well, until feeds are established and glucose ≥2.6 mmol/L

<1.8 mmol/L at 2 h of age
or
<2.0 mmol/L at subsequent checks, consider IV treatment

1.8–2.0 mmol/L at 2 h of age
or
2.0–2.5 mmol/L at subsequent checks

<2.6 mmol/L at 2 h of age
or
≥2.6 mmol/L at subsequent checks

Refeed and recheck glucose in 1 h

Rises to ≥2.6 mmol/L after feeding

Remains <2.6 mmol/L despite feeding, consider IV treatment

Once only

When to stop testing: IDM and LGA infants do not require retesting if glucose ≥2.6 mmol/L after 12 h of age as they usually present by this time. Preterm and SGA infants do not require retesting after 36 h provided stable levels and intake are achieved

Note: Repeated glucose levels <2.6 mmol/L in an at-risk baby require further intervention

Initiate intravenous infusion of D10W at a rate of 80 mL/kg/d (5.5 mg glucose/kg/min); check glucose 30 min after any change and adjust therapy (up to 100 mL/kg/d and/or D12.5W) in order to maintain glucose level ≥2.6 mmol/L. If rates in excess of 100 mL/kg/d of D12.5W are required, investigation, consultation, and/or pharmacologic intervention are indicated. May start weaning IV 12 h after stable blood glucose is established. Continued breastfeeding is encouraged.

From Fetus and Newborn Committee, Canadian Paediatric Society. CPS position statement. Screening guidelines for newborns at risk for low blood glucose. *Paediatr Child Health*. 2004;9:726. Reprinted by permission of the Canadian Paediatric Society. Also available at http://www.cps.ca

Neonatology

26

575

POTENTIAL CAUSES

- See p. 263 for complete differential diagnosis
- Decreased carbohydrate stores: SGA, premature, RDS, maternal hypertension
- Endocrine: hormonal deficiencies (e.g., GH, cortisol, epinephrine); excess insulin: LGA, IDM, erythroblastosis fetalis, Beckwith-Wiedemann syndrome, islet cell dysplasias, suppression of hypothalamic–pituitary–adrenal axis)
- Miscellaneous mechanisms: shock, asphyxia, sepsis, hypothermia, polycythemia, rapid weaning of IV glucose

MANAGEMENT

- Identify and monitor infants at risk <2 h of age; monitor glucose q3–4h before feeding, then before every second or third feeding after 48–72 h (see Figure 26.3)
- Optimize oral feeds
- IV glucose, if previous management inadequate (see GIR formula, p. xx)
  - Asymptomatic: IV glucose 5–8 mg/kg/min (3–5 mL/kg/h of D10W); increase infusion, if necessary
  - Symptomatic: IV glucose minibolus 2–4 mL/kg of D10W followed by infusion of 4–6 mg/kg/min; increase infusion, if necessary
  - In hyperinsulinism, requirement for glucose may be as high as 10–12 mg/kg/min
- If unsuccessful, consider glucagon 0.5–1 mg/24 h infusion; may increase to 2 mg/24 h
- Hydrocortisone or diazoxide for refractory cases (consult endocrinologist)

HYPERGLYCEMIA

- Glucose >10 mmol/L ± glycosuria (prefeeding, postfeeding, or random)
- Iatrogenic (TPN, dextrose solutions, steroids)
- Stress: exclude sepsis
- Neonatal diabetes mellitus

MANAGEMENT

- Decrease glucose concentration by 2.5% dextrose in stages
- Monitor urine, blood glucose, weight, fluid balance
- Insulin therapy rarely required

HYPOCALCEMIA

- Full term: Ca^{2+} <1.75 mmol/L
- Premature: Ca^{2+} <1.5 mmol/L (lower albumin levels)
- Ionized Ca^{2+} <1.1 mmol/L (preferred method of measurement)
- Symptoms: usually asymptomatic; may have tremors, seizures, lethargy, apnea, irritability, stridor, ↑ reflexes, prolonged QT interval

ETIOLOGY

- Early hypocalcemia (day 1–2): prematurity, IDM, asphyxia, shock, sepsis
- Late hypocalcemia: hypoparathyroidism, hypomagnesemia, maternal hyperparathyroidism, cow's milk–based formula
- Iatrogenic: bicarbonate administration, furosemide

MANAGEMENT

- Identify high-risk infants (premature, SGA, sepsis, cardiovascular compromise)
- Prevent in high-risk infants with maintenance Ca^{2+} as continuous infusion for 48–72 h starting at 6–48 h of age: 0.6–1 mmol/kg/d (25–45 mg/kg/d) elemental Ca^{2+} as Ca^{2+} gluconate (see Chapter 16)
- Acute symptomatic hypocalcemia: slow bolus 1–2 mL of IV 2% Ca^{2+} gluconate over 10 min with ECG monitoring (bradycardias, asystole can occur) followed by maintenance infusion as discussed; observe IV sites closely for extravasation (causes Ca^{2+} burn)
- Asymptomatic infants: variable, may treat when Ca^{2+} <1.8 mmol/L with oral supplementation or IV infusion, as for high-risk infants
- Vitamin D orally in high-risk infants: 400–800 IU/d
- Hypocalcemia may be associated with hypomagnesemia; normal plasma Mg^{2+} levels are 1.2–1.8 mmol/L
- For symptomatic hypomagnesemia, give 0.2 mL/kg of 50% $MgSO_4$ IV, repeat q12h as necessary, and add 3 mmol/L of $MgSO_4$ to maintenance fluid

NUTRITION AND GROWTH

- See Chapter 20 for healthy term infants
- LBW and ELBW infants have unique nutritional requirements (Tables 26.6 and 26.7)
- Nutrition parenteral or enteral or combination
- Aim to supply 70–80 kcal/kg/d during first week of life
- See Figures 26.4 and 26.5 for growth curves between 20-42 weeks' gestation

ENTERAL NUTRITION

- See Table 26.8 for guidelines on advancement of enteral feeds
- Human milk (EBM) preferred source of enteral nutrition
- Trophic feedings (up to 12–24 mL/kg/d) stimulate gut hormones and help with GI adaptation
- Some nutrient needs (e.g., protein, Ca^{2+}, phosphorus, Mg^{2+}, Na^+) not met with exclusive human milk feeding in growing premature infant (see human milk fortification to follow)

Table 26.6	Nutrition Guidelines for Infants <1000 g		
	Parenteral Nutrition*		
Timing	**Protein**	**Lipid**	**Enteral Feeds**
Day 1	1.5 g/kg/d	0.5 g/kg/d	NPO
Day 2	2.5 g/kg/d	1 g/kg/d	Trophic feeds EBM 1 mL q12h
Day 3	3 g/kg/d	2 g/kg/d[†]	Feeds as per enteral feeding protocol once stable (see Table 26.8)
Day 4	3–3.5 g/kg/d	3 g/kg/d	As above
>Day 4	3.5 g/kg/d	3.5 g/kg/d	As above
>Week 3–4	Discontinue PN once full enteral feeds reached		Once at full feeds, increase to 3000 kJ/L, then 3300 kJ/L using HMF if using EBM; if using formula, assess growth and evaluate need for increased calories

*Add electrolytes based on clinical and laboratory assessment. Protein and lipids not to exceed 4 g/kg/d.
[†]Monitor lipid levels when at 2 g fat/kg/d before increasing.

PN

- IV amino acids should be provided as soon as possible after birth to prevent catabolism
- Minimum 1.5 g/kg/d protein necessary to provide neutral/positive nitrogen balance; as much as 4 g/kg/d IV may be necessary to maintain stores, facilitate optimal growth, especially in very premature infants (see Table 26.6)
- Start "electrolyte free" TPN on day 1 (contains amino acid, dextrose. and Ca^{2+} only)

Table 26.7	Nutrition Guidelines for Infants 1001–1500 g		
	Parenteral Nutrition*		
Timing	**Protein**	**Lipid**	**Enteral Feeds**
Day 1	2 g/kg/d	1 g/kg/d	NPO
Day 2	3 g/kg/d	2 g/kg/d[†]	EBM/formula as per institutional feeding protocols
Day 3	3.5 g/kg/d	3 g/kg/d	As above
≥Day 4	3.5 g/kg/d	3.5 g/kg/d	As above
Week 2–4	Discontinue PN once full enteral feeds reached		Evaluate growth and need for increased calorie intake/fortification

*Adjust electrolytes based on clinical and laboratory assessments.
[†]Monitor lipid levels when at 2 g fat/kg/d before increasing.

Figure 26.4 Growth Parameters for Boys (Mean ± 1 and 2 SDs)

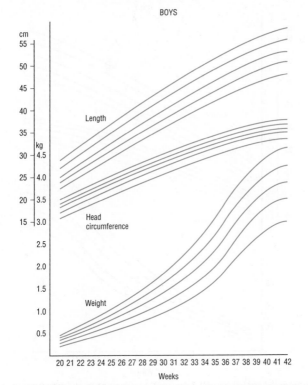

From Kirpalani HM, Moore AM, Perlman M. *Residents Handbook of Neonatology.* 3rd ed. Hamilton, Ontario, Canada: BC Decker; 2007:516, Fig. 2.

Nutritional Supplements

- HMF for premature infants once full feedings established; continue until 2000 g, or beyond, in special circumstances
- Further supplementation may be necessary (e.g., transitional formula, Polycose, Microlipid)
- Preterm formulas are available as either 2800 kJ/L (20 kcal/oz) or 3300 kJ/L (24 kcal/oz)
- Supplemental vitamin D 400 IU/d is given to premature infants receiving fortified human milk or preterm formula and term infants fed exclusively human milk
- Oral iron supplementation: 3–4 mg/kg/d elemental iron for <1000 g BW, 2–3 mg/kg/d for ≥1000 g BW

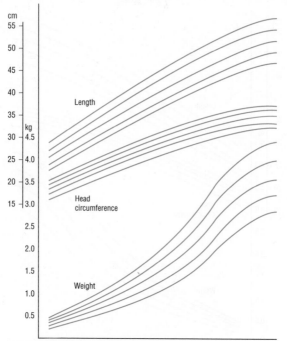

Figure 26.5 Growth Parameters for Girls (Mean ± 1 and 2 SDs)

From Kirpalani HM, Moore AM, Perlman M. *Residents Handbook of Neonatology.* 3rd ed. Hamilton, Ontario, Canada: BC Decker; 2007:517, Fig. 3.

Table 26.8	Guidelines for Initiating and Advancing Enteral Feeds in Relatively Stable Infants			
Weight (g)	Initial Feed Volume* (mL)	Intervals (h)	Volume of Increments (mL)	Frequency of Increments (h)
<750	0.5–1	1–2	0.5–1	≥24
750–1000	1	2	1–2	12–24
1000–1500	1–2	2	1–2	≥24
1500–2000	2–3	2–3	2–4	≥12
2000–2500	4–5	3	3–5	≥8
>2500	10	3–4	7–10	≥6

*Either as a slow bolus or as a continuous drip.
Adapted from Kirpalani HM, Moore AM, Perlman M. *Residents Handbook of Neonatology.* 3rd ed. Hamilton, Ontario, Canada: BC Decker; 2007:109, Table 8.

NEONATAL RESPIRATORY DISTRESS

- See Table 26.9 for differential diagnosis
- See Box 26.4 for goals of therapy
- All term neonates with respiratory distress should be treated with antibiotics (penicillin/ampicillin + aminoglycoside) × 48 h until sepsis ruled out
- See Figure 26.6 for initial management of RDS
- Rapid sequence intubation medications should be used for all non-emergency intubations; atropine 0.02 mg/kg + fentanyl 2 mcg/kg + succinylcholine 2 mg/kg
- See Chapter 2 for intubation procedures

Table 26.9	Differential Diagnosis of Respiratory Distress in Newborn Period	
Pulmonary Disorders		
Common	**Less Common**	
RDS	Pulmonary hypoplasia	
TTN	Upper airway obstruction (e.g., choanal atresia)	
Meconium aspiration	Rib cage anomalies	
Pneumonia	Space-occupying lesions (e.g., diaphragmatic hernia)	
Pneumothorax	Pulmonary hemorrhage	
	Immature lung syndrome	
Extrapulmonary Disorders		
Vascular	**Metabolic**	**Neuromuscular**
PPHN	Acidosis	Cerebral hypertension
Congenital heart disease	Hypoglycemia	Cerebral hemorrhage
Hypovolemia–anemia	Hypothermia	Muscle or NMJ disorders
Polycythemia		Spinal cord problems
		Phrenic nerve palsy
		Drugs: morphine, phenobarbitol

NMJ, neuromuscular junction.
Adapted from Klaus MH, Fanaroff AA, eds. *Care of the High-Risk Neonate.* Philadelphia, Pa: WB Saunders; 2001.

Box 26.4	Goals of Therapy for Neonatal Respiratory Distress

- Maintain arterial values: PCO_2, <50 mm Hg; PO_2, 50–70 mm Hg; pH >7.25
- Maintain O_2 saturation levels: term infants, >94%; premature infants, 88–92%

Figure 26.6 Initial Management of Respiratory Distress Syndrome

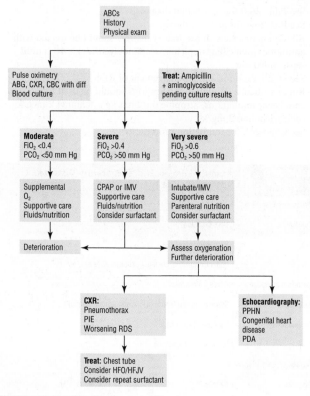

HFJV, high-frequency jet ventilator; PIE, pulmonary interstitial emphysema.

APNEA

- Definition: no respiration for >20 s duration, or >15 s with brady-cardia <100 beats/min or cyanosis
- May be central, obstructive, or mixed
- Do not attribute apnea automatically to prematurity, especially if GA >30 wk; exclude underlying cause
- Immediate resuscitation: surface stimulation, gentle nasopharyngeal suction, ventilation with inflating bag and mask, intubation with IPPV, as needed

- See Table 26.10 for causes and management of apnea
- Continuing management to prevent recurrences:
  - Continuous transcutaneous PO_2 monitoring; adjust FiO_2; target SpO_2 88–92%
  - Minimize handling of small infants
  - Consider altering feeding pattern (i.e., slow continuous, orogastric or IV)
  - Drug therapy: caffeine for apnea of prematurity; loading dose 10 mg/kg IV/PO; maintenance dose 2.5–5 mg/kg/d IV/PO once daily; start 24 h after loading dose
- Persistent apnea: consider short-term assisted ventilation
  - NPT or nasal-prong CPAP
  - ETT CPAP
  - IPPV; often need only slow rate (i.e., ~6–10/min)

Table 26.10	Causes and Management of Apnea	
Cause	**Details**	**Action**
Infection	Neonatal sepsis, meningitis, or NEC	FSWU including LP; antibiotics; NPO for NEC
Thermal instability	Hypo/hyperthermia	Assess body and isolette temperature
Metabolic disorders	Hypoglycemia Hypocalcemia Hypo/hypernatremia Hyperammonemia	See p. 574 Serum Ca^{2+}, ECG Electrolytes, urea; fluid balance, weight Serum NH_4, amino acids, organic acids, LFTs
CNS problems	Asphyxia Intracranial hemorrhage Cerebral malformation Seizures	Observation EEG, head US, CT Head US, CT/MRI EEG; consider anticonvulsants
Decreased O_2 delivery	Hypoxemia Worsening RDS ± complication Anemia/shock Left-to-right shunt (e.g., PDA) Pneumothorax	Check ETT, adjust FiO_2, MAP CXR CBC, electrolytes, urea, ABGs ECG, echocardiography Needle decompression + chest tube
Upper airway	Choanal atresia, macroglossia, Pierre Robin sequence, GERD (vagal stimulation, aspiration)	Attempt passage of NG tube; oropharyngeal airway; CXR for aspiration
Drugs	Maternal prenatal or postnatal exposure	Drug/toxin screen, depending on history and clinical findings

GERD, gastroesophageal reflux disease.
Adapted from Forfar JL, Arneil GC. *Textbook of Paediatrics*. 2nd ed. New York, NY: Churchill Livingstone; 2003.

PERSISTENT PULMONARY HYPERTENSION OF THE NEWBORN

- Definition: severe hypoxemia due to elevated pulmonary vascular resistance and pulmonary artery hypertension
- May be associated with right-to-left shunting through PDA/PFO
- Most often in term or postterm infants
- Secondary causes:
  - Meconium aspiration syndrome
  - TTN
  - Hyaline membrane disease (RDS)
  - GBS pneumonia
  - Pulmonary hypoplasia ± diaphragmatic hernia
  - Severe asphyxia
  - Polycythemia
- Clinical manifestations: marked cyanosis, acidosis, RV heave
- *Must rule out cyanotic congenital heart disease!*

INVESTIGATIONS

- CXR: oligemic lung fields or consistent with underlying disease; cardiomegaly; may look normal
- Pre- and postductal O_2 saturation: difference of >10% suggests PPHN (preductal saturation probe on *right* arm; postductal saturation probe on either *leg*)
- Hyperoxia test to exclude congenital heart disease (see Chapter 9)
- Calculate OI: OI >15 needs aggressive therapy (see following section on management)

$$OI = MAP \times FiO_2 \times 100/PaO_2$$

- ECG: RV strain pattern
- Echocardiogram: cardiac anatomy, function, presence/level of shunt (PFO or PDA)

MANAGEMENT

- Prevention is critical: treat hypothermia, respiratory distress, hypoxia, acidosis
- Goal of treatment: oxygenation and pulmonary vasodilatation
- Conventional ventilation: aim to keep PaO_2 >80 mm Hg, $PaCO_2$ 35–45 mm Hg
- Maintain normal systemic BP to limit right-to-left shunting; use volume priming (10 mL/kg 0.9% NaCl) and inotropes/pulmonary vasodilators (e.g., dobutamine, milrinone)
- Sedate and muscle relax, especially in severe hypoxemia: morphine 0.05–0.1 mg IV bolus, then start at 10 mcg/kg/h (use fentanyl, if systemic hypotension); pancuronium 0.1 mg/kg q2–4h prn
- Consider HFO

- Inhaled nitric oxide (pulmonary vasodilator) for hypoxia, OI >20 (start NO at 5 ppm; titrate up to 20 ppm)
- Correct metabolic acidosis with bicarbonate infusion
- Consider surfactant: 5 mL/kg, repeat q6h prn up to 4 times, if tolerated
- Consider ECMO if multiple OI values >40

PATENT DUCTUS ARTERIOSUS

- Commonly associated with RDS in premature infants; 80% of infants <1000 g, 20% of all premature infants; 50% may be asymptomatic (i.e., "silent ductus")
- Clinical signs: harsh systolic or continuous murmur, hyperactive precordium, bounding pulses, wide pulse pressure >25 mm Hg, hypotension, worsening respiratory status, tachycardia, CHF, pulmonary hemorrhage (*emergency*)
- Echo to confirm presence, size, direction of shunting; institutional definition of a hemodynamically significant PDA in a premature infant is >1.5 mm
- Decision to treat depends on clinical significance: increasing ventilatory and FiO_2 requirements, apnea/bradycardia events, CHF, poor growth, diastolic "steal" causing renal impairment, intestinal ischemia (NEC)

MANAGEMENT

Medical Approach
- Fluid restriction: ⅔ of maintenance fluids

Indomethacin
- Dose: 0.2 mg/kg/dose IV q12h × 3 doses
- Renal impairment: 0.1 mg/kg/dose IV q24h × 5–6 doses
- Adverse effects: platelet dysfunction, decreased renal artery flow leading to decreased GFR and urine output; fluid retention ± hyponatremia; increased creatinine; bowel perforation (rare)
- Contraindications: duct-dependent cardiac lesions, ↑ creatinine (>150 mmol/L), oliguria <0.5 mL/kg/h, NEC, thrombocytopenia <80,000 or clinical bleeding, IVH grade III–IV

Surgical Ligation
- Indication: hemodynamically significant PDA, despite two courses of indomethacin
- Complications: thrombus, interruption of thoracic duct with chylothorax, damage to recurrent laryngeal nerve, ligation of wrong vessel

HEART FAILURE

- See Table 26.11
- See Chapter 9

Table 26.11	Causes of Heart Failure in the Newborn	
Birth	**1-2 Wk**	**>2 Wk**

Decreased cardiac function:
  Asphyxia
  Sepsis
  Electrolyte disorders
	Congenital heart disease:
	  Critical AS
	  Coarctation
	  HLHS
	  TAPVD
		Congenital heart disease:
		  Systemic outflow tract
		    obstruction
		  PDA
		  AVSD
		  TAPVD

Hematologic disorders:
  Anemia
  Hyperviscosity disorders
	Decreased cardiac function:
	  Asphyxia
	  Sepsis
	  Arrhythmias
		Decreased cardiac function:
		  Myocarditis
		  Cardiomyopathy
		  Anomalous coronary artery

Heart rhythm disorders:
  SVT
  Complete AV block
	Renal disorders:
	  Renal failure
	  Systemic hypertension
		Renal/endocrine:
		  Renal failure
		  Thyroid/adrenal disease

Congenital heart disease:
  Severe TR (Ebstein)
  AV malformation
	Endocrine disorders:
	  Hyperthyroidism
	  Adrenal insufficiency
		Pulmonary:
		  Bronchopulmonary dysplasia
		  Hypoventilation syndrome

AS, aortic stenosis; AVSD, atrioventricular septal defect; HLHS, hypoplastic left heart syndrome; TAPVD, total anomalous pulmonary venous drainage.

INFECTION

- High-risk infants: <37 wk GA, prolonged membrane rupture (>24 h), maternal fever, instrumented vaginal delivery, indwelling catheters, maternal UTI, use of broad-spectrum antibiotics
- See Box 26.5 for signs and symptoms

INVESTIGATIONS

- CBC + differential
- Blood culture
- Urinalysis, microscopy, urine culture: suprapubic or catheter sample
- CSF: Gram stain, protein, glucose, culture (defer if cardiorespiratory instability)
- CXR

Box 26.5	Signs and Symptoms of Infection

- Apnea
- Respiratory distress, increasing O_2 or ventilation requirements
- Feeding intolerance, abdominal distension, or ileus
- Temperature instability
- Jaundice
- Lethargy
- Seizures
- Metabolic: hyperglycemia, hypoglycemia, acidosis
- Obvious focus: skin, bones, joints, omphalitis

- "Surface" and ETT cultures may be of little value
- Urine, CSF antigen detection (latex agglutination); useful if antibiotics already initiated

ANTIBIOTIC THERAPY

- Organisms: GBS, coliforms, *Listeria*, coagulase-negative *Staphylococcus* (in infants >7 d with IV catheters)
- Consider *S. aureus* in skin, bone, and joint disease; *Shigella* or *Salmonella* in gastroenteritis
- Consider superinfection with *Candida*, other fungi in prolonged or recurrent illness, high WBCs, indwelling shunt or IV catheter, congenital heart disease (bacterial endocarditis)
- *Ureaplasma urealyticum* sometimes implicated in chronic lung disease
- Initial coverage depends on clinical presentation and local sensitivity/resistance patterns:
  - Ampicillin + aminoglycoside, if sepsis is suspected, OR
  - Ampicillin + cefotaxime, if meningitis is suspected
- Consider cloxacillin if *Staphylococcus* is suspected
- Vancomycin used in late-onset sepsis (>7 d), recurrent illness, especially if indwelling shunt or catheter—for coagulase-negative *S. aureus*
- *Pseudomonas* requires coverage with ceftazidime or ticarcillin
- For NEC, use ampicillin + aminoglycoside + metronidazole
- For *Candida* sepsis, treat with amphotericin B
- See Figure 26.7 for GBS algorithm

Figure 26.7 Algorithm for Neonatal Management of Group B Streptococcus

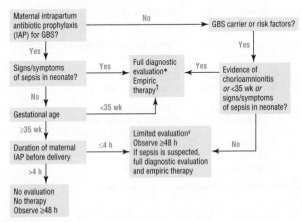

*Includes CBC, differential, blood culture, and CXR if neonate has respiratory symptoms; LP performed at discretion of physician.
†Duration of therapy varies depending on blood culture and CSF results and clinical course of infant.
‡CBC and differential and blood culture.

- Risk factors: prematurity, sibling with severe hyperbilirubinemia (HBR), bruising, cephalohematoma, dehydration, Asian descent, exclusive breastfeeding, IDM, G6PD deficiency, maternal blood group O or Rh negative
- Physiologic jaundice peaks day 3–5, recedes by day 10; persists in some breastfed infants
- Jaundice in first 24 h is pathologic until proven otherwise
- See Table 26.12 for differential diagnosis
- Visual assessment often misleading
- Untreated severe HBR may result in acute bilirubin encephalopathy (lethargy, hypotonia, high-pitched cry, seizures); may lead to hearing deficits, oculomotor disturbances, developmental delay, athetoid CP, and dental dysplasia
- Kernicterus: pathologic finding of deep yellow staining and neuronal necrosis of basal ganglia and brainstem nuclei
- TSB measurements are generally used in the neonate, but the majority of neonatal HBR involves the unconjugated component

Table 26.12	Differential Diagnosis of Jaundice	
Timing of Onset of HBR*	**Diagnosis**	**Tests to Consider**
First 24 h	Hemolytic disease	Check blood group compatibility ± positive direct Coombs test (DAT) ± spherocytosis on blood smear, G6PD assay
1–10 d	Enclosed hemorrhage Polycythemia	Head/abdomen US Venous hematocrit, predisposing causes present
1–10+ d	Infections	± Increased conjugated bilirubin, septic workup, virology, serology for TORCH
3–10+ d	Breast milk icterus Crigler-Najjar syndrome	Diagnosed by exclusion By exclusion, liver biopsy
>7–10 d	Hypothyroidism Galactosemia	Thyroid function tests Check urine for reducing substances Assay urine and blood (see Chapter 25)
	Cystic fibrosis Neonatal hepatitis, biliary atresia, etc.	Sweat test Conjugated HBR Case-specific tests

*Timing of onset of HBR suggests possible diagnoses, but exceptions occur.

MANAGEMENT

- Nomogram (Figure 26.8) shows how TSB can predict risk of developing significant HBR
- Table 26.13 describes management according to risk level

Figure 26.8 Nomogram for Evaluation of Screening Total Serum Bilirubin Concentration in Term and Later Premature Infants

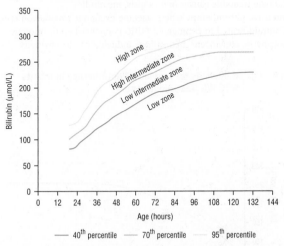

— 40th percentile — 70th percentile — 95th percentile

From Canadian Paediatric Society. CPS Position Statement: guidelines for detection, management and prevention of hyperbilirubinemia in term and late preterm newborn infants (35 or more weeks' gestation). *Paediatr Child Health.* 2007;12(suppl B):4B. Reprinted by permission of the Canadian Paediatric Society. Also available at http://www.cps.ca

Table 26.13	Response to Results of Bilirubin Screening		
Zone	>37 Wk GA and DAT Negative	35–38 Wk or DAT Positive	35–38 Wk and DAT Positive
High	Further testing/treatment*	Further testing/treatment	Phototherapy required
High-intermediate	Routine care	Follow up in 24–48 h	Further testing/treatment
Low-intermediate	Routine care	Routine care	Further testing/treatment
Low	Routine care	Routine care	Routine care

*Arrangements must be made for a timely re-evaluation of bilirubin level. Depending on the level, treatment with phototherapy may be indicated.
From Canadian Paediatric Society. CPS position statement: guidelines for detection, management and prevention of hyperbilirubinemia in term and late preterm newborn infants (35 or more weeks' gestation). *Paediatr Child Health.* 2007;12(suppl B):5B, Table 4.

PHOTOTHERAPY

- Phototherapy is first line of therapy, independent of etiology
- See Figure 26.9 for phototherapy guidelines
- Breastfeeding should continue; phototherapy more effective when combined with feeding
- Supplemental fluids (oral or IV) with phototherapy if risk of exchange transfusion (correct deficit + maintenance fluids + additional 10% when under lights)
- Exclude treatable causes (e.g., sepsis, metabolic)
- Intensive phototherapy when reaching exchange transfusion criteria
- Contraindicated in conjugated HBR, congenital erythropoietic porphyria, concurrent medications inducing photosensitivity

Figure 26.9   **Guidelines for Intensive Phototherapy in Infants >35 Wk Gestational Age**

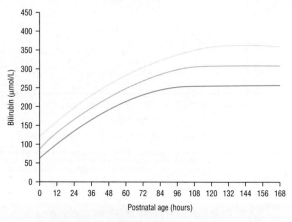

- - - - Infants at lower risk (>38 wk and well)
- - - - Infants at medium risk (>38 wk and risk factors or 35–37 6/7 wk and well)
- - - - Infants at higher risk (35–37 6/7 wk and risk factors)

- It is an option to provide conventional phototherapy in hospital or at home at TSB levels 35–50 μmol/L below those shown, but home phototherapy should not be used in any infant with risk factors.
- Use total bilirubin. Do not subtract direct reacting or conjugated bilirubin.
- Risk factors = isoimmune hemolytic disease, G6PD deficiency, asphyxia, respiratory distress, significant lethargy, temperature instability, sepsis, acidosis.
- For well infants 35–37 6/7 wk can adjust TSB threshold around the medium-risk line: lower levels for infants closer to 35 wk gestation and higher levels for infants closer to 37 6/7 wk.

From Canadian Paediatric Society. CPS position statement: guidelines for detection, management and prevention of hyperbilirubinemia in term and late preterm newborn infants (35 or more weeks' gestation). *Paediatr Child Health.* 2007;12(suppl B):4B. Reprinted by permission of the Canadian Paediatric Society. Also available at http://www.cps.ca

- Can be used prophylactically in high-risk infants (marked bruising of premature infants)
- Infants with positive DAT with predicted severe disease: give IVIG 1 g/kg
- Watch for "delayed" anemia in hemolytic disease of newborn
- Side effects: increased fluid losses (~10 mL/kg/d), skin rash, diarrhea, bronze baby (if conjugated HBR)

EXCHANGE TRANSFUSION

- See Figure 26.10
- In emergencies, use group O Rh-negative blood
- Much controversy exists about safe/critical levels of unconjugated bilirubin; threshold for intervention in "sick" or very premature infants should be low

Figure 26.10   Guidelines for Exchange Transfusion in Infants > 35 Wk Gestational Age

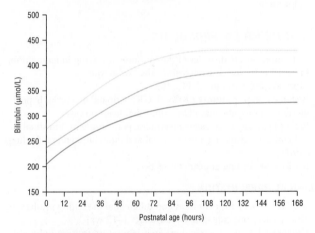

Infants at lower risk (>38 wk and well)
Infants at medium risk (>38 wk and risk factors or 35–37 6/7 wk and well)
Infants at higher risk (35–37 6/7 wk and risk factors)

- Immediate exchange is recommended if infant shows signs of acute bilirubin encephalopathy (hypertonia, arching, retrocollis, opisthotonus, fever, high-pitched cry).
- Risk factors = isoimmune hemolytic disease, G6PD deficiency, asphyxia, respiratory distress, significant lethargy, temperature instability, sepsis, acidosis.
- Use total bilirubin. Do not subtract direct reacting or conjugated bilirubin.
- If infant is well and 35–37 6/7 wk (medium risk), can individualize levels for exchange based on actual gestational age.

From Canadian Paediatric Society. CPS position statement: guidelines for detection, management and prevention of hyperbilirubinemia in term and late preterm newborn infants (35 or more weeks' gestation). *Paediatr Child Health.* 2007;12(suppl B):9B. Reprinted by permission of the Canadian Paediatric Society. Also available at http://www.cps.ca

Neonatology

26

Indications

- Rise of bilirubin above thresholds (see Figure 26.7)
- Hydrops or severe anemia (cord Hb <120 g/L)
- Postnatal rise of unconjugated bilirubin >17 mmol/L/h in Rh incompatibility
- Acute bilirubin encephalopathy

Complications

- Hypotension
- Metabolic abnormalities: hypocalcemia, hypoglycemia, hyperkalemia, hyperthermia, hypothermia, acidosis
- Sepsis
- Hypoxia
- Thrombocytopenia
- Embolization of air bubbles or small thrombi
- Transfusion risks
- Postexchange may develop rebound rise because of redistribution of bilirubin

NECROTIZING ENTEROCOLITIS

- Definition: severe disorder of the intestine, involving inflammation, bacterial overgrowth ± necrosis of the bowel wall
- Mortality for perforated NEC: 40%
- Risk factors: prematurity (90%), IUGR, perinatal asphyxia, hypoglycemia, polycythemia, PDA, congenital heart disease
- Pathophysiology: decreased mesenteric perfusion with intestinal ischemia, infectious agents (bacterial and viral), and enteral feedings (>90%)
- Breast milk feeding appears protective

CLINICAL PRESENTATION

- See Table 26.14 for definition and differential of feeding intolerance
- NEC usually presents at 2–3 wk (range, 1–12 wk)
- Diagnosis based on presenting signs, laboratory tests, radiologic or surgical findings
- GI signs: abdominal distension, abdominal wall tenderness and discoloration, hematochezia, bile-stained gastric aspirates
- Systemic signs: lethargy, temperature instability, apnea and bradycardia, poor perfusion, shock
- Bowel necrosis: persistent thrombocytopenia, metabolic acidosis, shock, GI bleeding, abdominal wall erythema, right lower quadrant mass
- AXR (AP and lateral decubitus): pneumatosis intestinalis (intramural gas) usually in terminal ileum and ascending colon

Table 26.14	Feeding Intolerance
Definition	**Differential Diagnosis**
Gastric aspirate >50% of previous feeding	Immature GI motility
Abdominal girth increase >2 cm	Reflux
Vomiting or diarrhea	Septic ileus
	NEC
	Bowel obstruction (e.g., malrotation with midgut volvulus, intussusception)
	Infectious enterocolitis

MANAGEMENT OF NEC

- FSWU
  - CBC and differential
  - Cultures of blood, urine, stool (bacterial and viral), and CSF (when stable)
- Serial AXRs q6h for 24 h or while clinically unstable
- Monitor blood gas, lactate, glucose, electrolytes, urea, creatinine
- Strictly NPO
- NG tube to straight drainage
- IV fluid resuscitation; correct acidosis and hypoperfusion, anticipate increased fluid requirements because of third spacing
- Blood products, if needed to correct thrombocytopenia, coagulopathy, or anemia
- Ventilatory support may be required for apnea or increasing acidosis
- Broad-spectrum antibiotics initially; then change based on culture results:
  - IV ampicillin + aminoglycoside (vancomycin + aminoglycoside if NEC after 1 wk of age)
  - Include anaerobic coverage (metronidazole) for perforated NEC
  - Consider adding antifungal therapy if patient not responding
- Ensure good vascular access; start PN ASAP
- Surgical consultation for definite NEC
- Duration of NEC treatment based on clinical staging (Table 26.15)

Table 26.15	Duration of Necrotizing Enterocolitis Treatment Regimen According to Modified Bell's Staging Criteria
Manifestation	**Treatment**
Suspected NEC (Stage I)	
"Suspected sepsis" plus mild GI symptoms but no blood in stool or intramural gas	NPO, antibiotics × 3 d, pending cultures
AXR may be normal or show mild ileus	
Definite NEC (Stage II)	
Presence of intramural gas (pneumatosis intestinalis); intestinal dilatation, ileus	NPO, antibiotics × 7–14 d, depending on severity of illness
Advanced NEC (Stage III)	
Definite NEC plus complication (e.g., acidosis, shock, thrombocytopenia, coagulopathy, portal vein gas, evidence of localized or early peritonitis, ascites)	NPO, antibiotics × 10–14 d Likely to require fluid resuscitation, blood products, inotropic and ventilatory support
Perforated NEC	Same as above, minimum 14 d *plus* surgical intervention

Surgical
- Indications: free intraperitoneal air or "fixed loop" on AXR, intractable metabolic acidosis, or abdominal mass
- Intestinal decompression, resection of necrotic bowel, formation of stoma; primary closure may be considered for localized disease
- Insertion of peritoneal drain at the bedside may allow stabilization in critically ill infants

COMPLICATIONS OF NEC
- Strictures (10%), usually large bowel
- Recurrent NEC
- Post-NEC bleeding due to strictures
- Short-bowel syndrome likely if >50–75% of small intestine lost
- Liver cirrhosis secondary to prolonged TPN

NEONATAL ENCEPHALOPATHY

- Definition: brain dysfunction including altered consciousness, irritability or seizures; may be temporary or permanent
- See Table 26.16 for classification of HIE

Table 26.16	Sarnat Classification of Hypoxic Ischemic Encephalopathy		
Signs	Stage 1*	Stage 2†	Stage 3‡
Level of consciousness	Hyperalert	Lethargic	Stuporous, comatose
Tone	Normal	Hypotonic	Flaccid
Posture	Normal	Flexed	Decerebrate
Reflexes	Hyperactive	Hyperactive	Absent
Pupils	Mydriasis	Miosis	Unequal; poor light reflex
Seizures	None	Common	Decerebrate
EEG	Normal	Low voltage with seizures	Burst suppression to isoelectric

*Associated with excellent prognosis and full recovery.
†Associated with variable outcome depending on clinical course.
†Associated with moderate to severe handicap or death.

DIFFERENTIAL DIAGNOSIS

- Perinatal asphyxia/HIE
- Infection: bacterial meningitis or viral encephalitis (e.g., HSV)
- Metabolic: hypoglycemia, inborn errors of metabolism (e.g., hyperammonemia, mitochondrial), HBR (kernicterus)
- Stroke, intracranial hemorrhage (birth trauma, bleeding tendency are risk factors)

CLINICAL FEATURES OF HIE

- Associated with fetal bradycardia, nonreassuring tracing, meconium, uterine rupture, prolapsed cord, metabolic acidosis, APGAR <4 at 5 min
- Multiorgan involvement:
  - Respiratory: PPHN, meconium aspiration, pulmonary hemorrhage
  - Renal: oliguria, acute tubular necrosis, SIADH, urinary retention
  - Cardiovascular: myocardial ischemia, cardiogenic shock, TR
  - Metabolic: acidosis, hypoglycemia, hypocalcemia, hypomagnesemia
  - Hematologic: thrombocytopenia, DIC
  - GI: liver dysfunction, ileus, bowel ischemia, NEC

INVESTIGATIONS

- Neurologic: head US, CT (hemorrhage/trauma), MRI (edema, diffusion restriction, lactate peak); EEG (bedside monitoring, if available); visual-, sensory-, auditory-evoked potentials
- Multiorgan involvement: (as indicated) blood gas, lactate, CBC + differential, glucose, Ca^{2+}, urea/creatinine, urinalysis, LFTs, PTT/INR, ECG; consider FSWU and metabolic screen, depending on presentation

MANAGEMENT

- Supportive care
- Emerging neuroprotective therapies: resuscitation in room air, hypothermia

Long-Term Complications

- Brain damage: spastic, dystonic, athetoid CP; microcephaly; cortical blindness; epilepsy; sensorineural hearing loss; cognitive impairment; behavior problems
- End-organ damage: renal failure, myocardial damage, liver failure (rare)

NEONATAL SEIZURES

- May be difficult to distinguish from normal neonatal movements (e.g., jitteriness, yawning, sucking, chewing) (Table 26.17)
- Causes: perinatal asphyxia (HIE), metabolic (decreased glucose, Ca^{2+}, Mg^{2+}, or Na^+ levels), CNS infections, bleeding, structural brain anomaly, inborn errors of metabolism, drug withdrawal
- Consider inborn error of metabolism in case of intractable seizures plus other neurologic signs

Table 26.17	Clinical Criteria to Distinguish Seizure from Nonseizure Activity		
Criterion		**Seizure**	**Nonseizure**
Elicited by sensory stimuli		No	Yes
Suppressed by gentle restraint/repositioning		No	Yes
Accompanied by autonomic phenomena*		Yes	No
>1 seizure type present		Yes	No
Abnormal neurologic examination		Yes	No
Abnormal EEG in term infant		Yes	No
Abnormal head US/CT/MRI		Yes	No
Abnormal eye movements associated†		Yes	No

*Autonomic signs include changes in HR and blood pressure, apnea, pallor, blotchy or flushed skin, altered pupils, and drooling.
†Tonic horizontal deviation most common in term infants, whereas sustained eye opening with ocular fixation most common in premature infants.
From Kirpalani HM, Moore AM, Perlman M. *Residents Handbook of Neonatology.* 3rd ed. Hamilton, Ontario, Canada: BC Decker; 2007:338, Table 1.

INVESTIGATIONS

- Always check glucose, Ca^{2+}, Mg^{2+}, electrolyte, ABGs
- CBC, differential
- Septic workup (blood, CSF, urine cultures, bacterial and viral), CXR, workup for congenital infection, as indicated (see Congenital Infections, Chapter 24)
- Head US, CT scan, MRI, as indicated
- EEG, evoked potentials
- Metabolic screen, NH_4^+, lactate, LFTs, as indicated
- Consider drug withdrawal

MANAGEMENT

- ABCs (see Chapter 1)
- Seizure control (Chapter 28), treat underlying cause
- Phenobarbital, first-line: hypotension and apnea may occur
- Other anticonvulsants: phenytoin, midazolam, lorazepam, lidocaine, paraldehyde

INTRAVENTRICULAR HEMORRHAGE

- Bleeding from germinal matrix lining ventricles, especially 24–32 wk GA
- See Box 26.6
- Associated with systemic hypertension and hypotension, hypoxia, asphyxia, traumatic birth, acidosis, volume expansion, hypercarbia, hypoglycemia, anemia, seizures, ECMO
- May lead to PVL, communicating hydrocephalus, seizures, developmental delay, CP

INDICATIONS FOR SCREENING HEAD US

- All infants <32 wk and high-risk infants >32 wk
- Routine US at second and sixth week of life to predict long-term outcomes; early US for hemorrhagic lesions; later US for cystic lesions, PVL, or ventriculomegaly
- If IVH, repeat US at regular intervals until ventricular size stabilized
- Consider MRI as well as US at term for ELBW infants

Box 26.6	Grading of Intraventricular Hemorrhage

- Grade 1   Germinal matrix/SEH
- Grade 2   IVH: small (filling <½ of lateral ventricle ± slight dilation) ± SEH
- Grade 3   IVH: large (filling >½ of lateral ventricle with ventricular dilation)
- Grade 4   IVH + intraparenchymal hemorrhage

RETINOPATHY OF PREMATURITY

- See Box 26.7

ZONES

- I: equivalent to posterior pole
- II: extending from edges of zone 1 to equator of globe
- III: crescentic area anterior to zone 2, maximal on temporal side
- See Figure 26.11

EYE EXAMINATION OF PREMATURE INFANTS

- Screening for all infants <1500 g BW OR <30 wk GA
- First examination at 4–6 wk postnatally or 31 wk (whichever is later), then 2–4 wk thereafter if ROP does not exist; more frequently if it does
- Analgesia/sedation for eye examinations

Figure 26.11 Schema Showing Zone Borders and Clock Hours Used to Describe the Location and Extent of Retinopathy of Prematurity

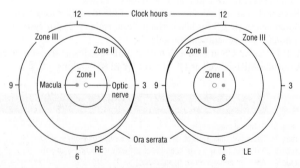

From the International Committee for the Classification of ROP. The international classification of retinopathy of prematurity revisited. *Arch Ophthalmol.* 2005;123:992, Figure 1.

- Opiates, cocaine, alcohol most common; usually incomplete history; high index of suspicion for multiple drug use
- Signs of withdrawal include changes in vital signs, CNS, GI, or vaso-motor manifestations
- Withdrawal symptoms also seen after maternal SSRI use
- Time of onset: usually within 72 h after birth; varies depending on drug (4–5 d for cocaine exposure, 2–4 wk for methadone exposure), timing of use before delivery, labor, presence of other illness
- Duration ranges from 6 d–8 wk; may last up to several months

SCREENING

- Urine (baby): detects recent drug use by mother; many false-negative results
- Meconium: detects longitudinal exposure during last two trimesters; very sensitive
- Hair: indicates drug use in third trimester; most sensitive

MANAGEMENT

- Rule out alternative causes of infant's symptoms
- Continue breastfeeding
- Treat according to severity of symptoms as measured by Neonatal Abstinence Score (Figure 26.12, Table 26.18)

Drug Therapy

- Goal is to reduce symptoms, restore normal sleep and feeding patterns, minimize duration of exposure and dosage of therapeutic agent
- Treatment with same class of drug as that causing the withdrawal
  - Oral morphine: first line in opioid withdrawal; use 0.02 mg/kg q4h
  - Phenobarbital: second line in opioid withdrawal; first line in multi-drug use
  - Diazepam used only as an adjunct to other medications

Neonatology

26

Table 26.18   Neonatal Abstinence Score

Criteria	Score
Metabolic/Vasomotor/Respiratory	
Sweating	1
Fever · 37.2–38.2°C · >38.2°C	1 2
Yawning >3 times	1
Mottling	1
Nasal stuffiness	1
Sneezing >3 times	1
Nasal flaring	2
Tachypnea >60 breaths per min · Plus retractions	1 2
Gastrointestinal	
Excessive sucking	1
Poor feeding	2
Vomiting · Regurgitation · Projectile vomiting	1 2
Diarrhea · Loose · Watery stools	2 3
CNS	
Cry · High pitched · Continuous high pitched	2 3
Sleeps after feeding · <3 h · <2 h · <1 h	1 2 3
Moro reflex · Hyperactive · Very hyperactive	2 3
Tremors when disturbed · Mild · Moderate to severe	3 4
Muscle tone increased	2
Myoclonic jerks	3
Generalized convulsions	5
Total score*	

*Treatment is based on total score: see Figure 26.12.

Figure 26.12 Management Approach for Infant Born to Narcotic-Addicted Mother

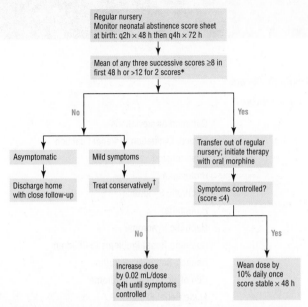

Figure 26.12 Management Approach for Infant Born to Narcotic-Addicted Mother

Regular nursery
Monitor neonatal abstinence score sheet at birth: q2h × 48 h then q4h × 72 h

↓

Mean of any three successive scores ≥8 in first 48 h or >12 for 2 scores*

No ← → Yes

Asymptomatic → Discharge home with close follow-up

Mild symptoms → Treat conservatively[†]

Transfer out of regular nursery; initiate therapy with oral morphine → Symptoms controlled? (score ≤4)

No ← → Yes

Increase dose by 0.02 mL/dose q4h until symptoms controlled

Wean dose by 10% daily once score stable × 48 h

*Initiate pharmacologic therapy for neonatal abstinence score ≥8 if no response to conservative measures or, regardless of score, if symptoms include seizures, vomiting, or severe and persistent diarrhea resulting in weight loss, dehydration, or inability to sleep.
[†]Holding, swaddling, rocking, decrease in environmental stimulation, ad lib feedings, continue scoring system.
Adapted from Besunder JB, et al. Neonatal drug withdrawal syndromes. In: Koren G, ed. *Maternal-Fetal Toxicology. A Clinician's Guide.* New York, NY: Marcel Dekker; 1990:174, Figure 1.

Neonatology

26

FURTHER READING

Klaus MH, Fanaroff AA, eds. *Care of the High Risk Neonate.* Philadelphia, Pa: WB Saunders; 2001.

MacDonald MG, Seshia MMK, Mullett MD, eds. *Avery's Neonatology: Pathophysiology and Management of the Newborn.* Philadelphia, Pa: Lippincott Williams & Wilkins; 2005.

USEFUL WEB SITES

McKusick's Online Mendelian Inheritance in Man (OMIM) database. Available at: www.ncbi.nlm.nih.gov/omim/

Radiology cases in neonatology. Available at: http://www.hawaii.edu/medicine/pediatrics/neoxray/neoxray.html

Chapter 27 Nephrology

Elizabeth Berger
Valerie Langlois

Chapter 27 Nephrology

COMMON ABBREVIATIONS

ABPM	ambulatory blood pressure monitoring
ACE	angiotensin-converting enzyme
APD	automated peritoneal dialysis
ATN	acute tubular necrosis
BMI	body mass index
CAPD	continuous ambulatory peritoneal dialysis
CFU	colony-forming units
Cr	creatinine
CRRT	continuous renal replacement therapy
CVVH	continuous venovenous hemofiltration
CVVHD	continuous venovenous hemodialysis
CVVHDF	continuous venovenous hemodiafiltration
ESRD	end-stage renal disease
FSGS	focal segmental glomerulosclerosis
FTT	failure to thrive
GFR	glomerular filtration rate
GN	glomerulonephritis
GU	genitourinary
HDL	high-density lipoprotein
HSP	Henoch-Schönlein purpura
HTN	hypertension
HUS	hemolytic uremic syndrome
MPGN	membranoproliferative glomerulonephritis
MSK	musculoskeletal
PKD	polycystic kidney disease
PSGN	poststreptococcal glomerulonephritis
PUV	posterior urethral valves
SBE	subacute bacterial endocarditis
TTKG	transtubular potassium gradient
UPJ	ureteropelvic junction
UTI	urinary tract infection
VCUG	voiding cystourethrogram
VUR	vesicoureteral reflux

Nephrology

27

HISTORY

- Urinary symptoms: change in urine color, odor, volume, frequency, pain on urination, incontinence, postvoid dribbling, abdominal or flank pain
- Nephrotoxic medications: antibiotics, antivirals, antifungals, chemotherapy, radiocontrast dye
- Birth: polyhydramnios, oligohydramnios, single umbilical artery, umbilical catheter, prenatal US findings
- Family history: HTN, renal failure/dialysis, renal cystic disease, hematuria, proteinuria, deafness

Systemic Symptoms and Signs

- Renal failure: anorexia, fatigue, nausea, vomiting, FTT
- HTN: headaches, seizures
- Fluid overload: dyspnea, edema
- Renal osteodystrophy: bone pain, skeletal deformities

Symptoms Associated With Underlying Cause of Renal Dysfunction

- Recent infection, fever, bloody diarrhea
- Eye symptoms, rashes, joint pain, mouth sores, hemoptysis, and epistaxis
- Deafness

PHYSICAL EXAMINATION

- General: pallor, fluid overload or volume depletion, evidence of FTT
- Head and neck: fundoscopic findings (e.g., exudates, cotton-wool spots, flame-shaped hemorrhages), jugular venous distension, preauricular pits or tags, deformities of the external ears, branchial fistulae
- Respiratory: signs of pulmonary edema, pleural effusions
- Cardiac: evidence of congestive heart failure, HTN
- Abdominal: bruits, costovertebral angle tenderness, palpable kidney, prune belly
- GU: hypospadias, undescended testes, ambiguous genitalia
- MSK: bony deformities, arthritis

LABORATORY TESTS

Urinalysis

- Evaluate within 1 h of void (ideally first morning void)
- See Table 27.1 for details of dipstick test

Table 27.1	Interpreting Urine Dipsticks	
Test	**Normal Values**	**Comment**
Specific gravity	1.010–1.025	↑ In dehydration, glycosuria; ↓ in diabetes insipidus
pH	4.6–8.0	Influenced by diet, medications
Glucose	Negative	Positive in hyperglycemia, isolated glucosuria, proximal tubular disorder
Protein	≤ Trace	Tests for albumin
Blood	Negative or "trace nonhemolyzed"	Positive from intact RBCs, hemoglobin, myoglobin
Bilirubin	Negative or small amounts	May be due to hepatitis or biliary obstruction
Urobilinogen	Negative or positive	Present in normal urine but may be increased in hepatic dysfunction
Ketones	Negative or trace	Positive in starvation, diabetic ketoacidosis, metabolic disorders
Leukocyte esterase	Negative	Positive in presence of significant leukocytes in urine
Nitrite	Negative	Some bacteria (urea-splitting organisms) convert nitrate to nitrite; a negative result does *not* rule out infection

Tests for Protein

- Dipstick: see Table 27.1
- Protein-to-Cr ratio (mg/mmol) (random spot urine collection)
  - Normal < 50 mg/mmol (6–24 mo) or < 20 mg/mmol (older children)
  - Nephrotic range: > 250 mg/mmol
- 24-h collection:
  - Normal: < 4 mg/m^2/h; abnormal: > 4 mg/m^2/h; nephrotic range: > 40 mg/m^2/h

Urine Microscopy

- See Figure 27.1

Cells

- WBCs: > 2/high-power field may signify infection or inflammation
- RBCs: > 5/high-power field abnormal; normal shape suggests lower urinary tract source; if dysmorphic, likely glomerular source
- Epithelial: may be tubular, squamous, or transitional
- Oval fat bodies: cells with birefringent fat droplets; usually seen in context of heavy proteinuria, but may be normal

Figure 27.1 Findings on Urine Microscopy

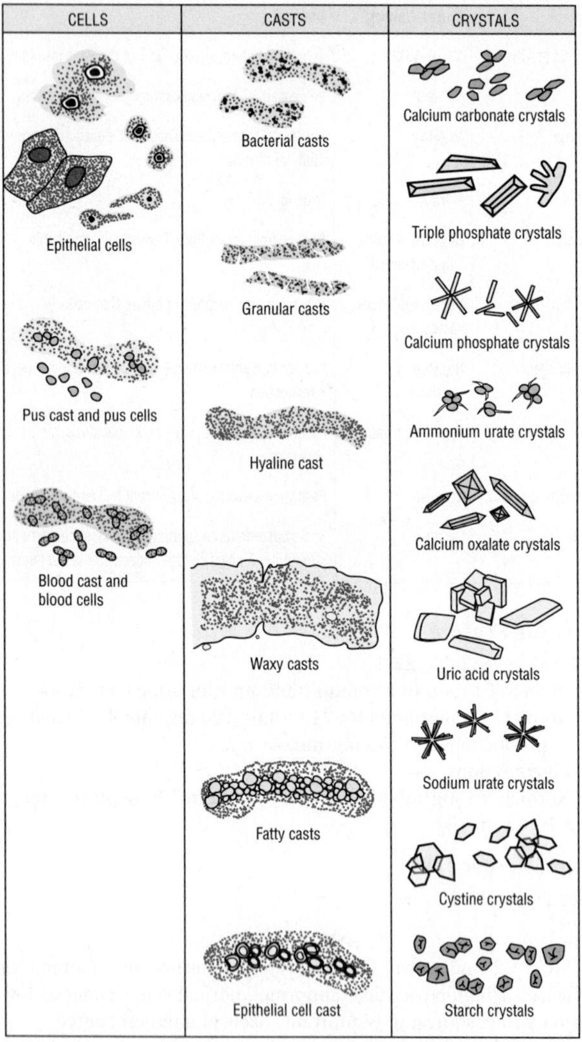

CELLS	CASTS	CRYSTALS
Epithelial cells	Bacterial casts	Calcium carbonate crystals
Pus cast and pus cells	Granular casts	Triple phosphate crystals
Blood cast and blood cells	Hyaline cast	Calcium phosphate crystals
	Waxy casts	Ammonium urate crystals
	Fatty casts	Calcium oxalate crystals
	Epithelial cell cast	Uric acid crystals
		Sodium urate crystals
		Cystine crystals
		Starch crystals

Adapted from Tanagho EA, McAninch JW. *Smith's General Urology*. 15th ed. New York, NY: Lange Medical Books/McGraw-Hill; 2000:54. Reprinted with permission of the McGraw-Hill Companies, Inc.

Nephrology

27

Casts

- Hyaline matrix cast: most frequent; considered physiologic
- RBC cast: appears orange-red at low-power field; indicative of glomerular disease
- Renal tubular epithelial cell cast: found in conditions that primarily affect the tubules
- WBC cast: hyaline matrix cast with neutrophil inclusions seen in inflammatory/infectious conditions
- Fatty casts: frequently seen in nephrotic syndrome
- Granular casts: hyaline matrix casts filled with granules; may be found with proteinuria or under normal conditions

Crystals

- Calcium oxalate: eight-faced bipyramid; oval egg shape
- Uric acid: several shapes (thin rhomboid plates, hexagonal, needle-shaped); yellow-brown
- Calcium phosphate (amorphous phosphate): granular precipitate
- Struvite (magnesium ammonium phosphate): classic pyramid shape, associated with infection; precipitates in alkaline pH
- Cystine: colorless hexagonal plate; rare in alkaline urine; always pathologic
- Calcium carbonate: small spheres alone or grouped in pairs of four
- Drug crystals: sulfamethoxazole, ampicillin, contrast dye

USEFUL CALCULATIONS AND VALUES

Bladder Volume

$$\text{Estimated bladder volume (mL)} = [2 + \text{age (yr)}] \times 30 \text{ (up to a max of 500–700 mL)}$$

Renal Length

- See Figure 27.2

Schwartz Formula for GFR

$$\text{GFR} = K^+ \times \text{length (cm)} \div \text{serum Cr (µmol/L)}$$

- See Table 27.2 for values of K^+
- See Table 27.3 for normal GFR values

Body Surface Area

$$\text{BSA} = \sqrt{\{[\text{height (cm)} \times \text{weight (kg)}] \div 3600\}}$$

Figure 27.2 Renal Length

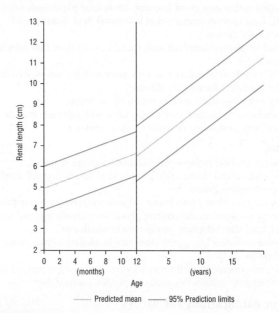

- Predicted mean — 95% Prediction limits

Table 27.2	Normal Value for K⁺ in the Glomerular Filtration Rate Calculation	
Age		**Value for K⁺**
Full-term infant ≤ 1 yr		40
Children 2–12 yr		48
Females 13–21 yr		48
Males 13–21 yr		62

Urinary Calcium/Cr Ratio

- See Table 27.4

Cr Clearance

$$\text{Cr clearance (mL/min/1.73 m}^2) =$$

$$\frac{U_{Cr} \text{ (µmol/L)} \times \text{volume urine (mL)} \times 1.73}{P_{Cr} \text{ (µmol/L)} \times 1440 \text{ min/d (if 24-h urine)} \times \text{BSA (m}^2)}$$

- U_{Cr}: Cr concentration in urine; P_{Cr}: Cr concentration in plasma
- Measures volume of plasma completely cleared of Cr per unit time

- Requires plasma Cr measurement and timed urine collection
- Need to assess completeness of urine collection based on urine Cr
  - Adequate collection in 2-yr-olds to adult females: 130–170 μmol/kg/d
  - Adequate collection in adult males: 170–220 μmol/kg/d

Table 27.3	Normal Glomerular Filtration Rate Values
Age	GFR ± SD (mL/min/1.73 m²)
1 wk	41 ± 15
2–8 wk	66 ± 25
>8 wk	96 ± 22
2–12 yr	133 ± 27
13–21 yr (males)	140 ± 30
13–21 yr (females)	126 ± 22

Table 27.4	Normal Values for Ca²⁺:Cr Ratio
Age	Normal Value (mmol/mmol)
<12 mo	2.2
1–3 yr	1.5
3–5 yr	1.1
5–7 yr	0.8
>7 yr	0.6

TTKG

- See Chapter 16

HYPERTENSION

- Definition: BP ≥95th percentile for age, height, and gender on ≥3 occasions
- See Table 27.5 for BP norms in boys and girls

MEASUREMENT

- Measure BP in right arm of calm patient, held at level of heart
- Correct cuff size: inflatable bladder width at least 40% of arm circumference; bladder length should cover 80–100% of the circumference of the arm (too small cuff will overestimate the BP)

Table 27.5 BP Levels for Boys and Girls by Age and Height Percentile

Boys

Age (yr)	BP Percentile	SBP (mm Hg) Percentile of Height							DBP (mm Hg) Percentile of Height						
		5th	10th	25th	50th	75th	90th	95th	5th	10th	25th	50th	75th	90th	95th
1	50th	80	81	83	85	87	88	89	34	35	36	37	38	39	39
	90th	94	95	97	99	100	102	103	49	50	51	52	53	53	54
	95th	98	99	101	103	104	106	106	54	54	55	56	57	58	58
	99th	105	106	108	110	112	113	114	61	62	63	64	65	66	66
2	50th	84	85	87	88	90	92	92	39	40	41	42	43	44	44
	90th	97	99	100	102	104	105	106	54	55	56	57	58	58	59
	95th	101	102	104	106	108	109	110	59	59	60	61	62	63	63
	99th	109	110	111	113	115	117	117	66	67	68	69	70	71	71
3	50th	86	87	89	91	93	94	95	44	44	45	46	47	48	48
	90th	100	101	103	105	107	108	109	59	59	60	61	62	63	63
	95th	104	105	107	109	110	112	113	63	63	64	65	66	67	67
	99th	111	112	114	116	118	119	120	71	71	72	73	74	75	75
4	50th	88	89	91	93	95	96	97	47	48	49	50	51	51	52
	90th	102	103	105	107	109	110	111	62	63	64	65	66	66	67
	95th	106	107	109	111	112	114	115	66	67	68	69	71	71	71
	99th	113	114	116	118	120	121	122	74	75	76	77	78	78	79
5	50th	90	91	93	95	96	98	98	50	51	52	53	54	55	55
	90th	104	105	106	108	110	111	112	65	66	67	68	69	69	70
	95th	108	109	110	112	114	115	116	69	70	71	72	73	74	74
	99th	115	116	118	120	121	123	123	77	78	79	80	81	81	82

(continued)

Table 27.5 BP Levels for Boys and Girls by Age and Height Percentile (continued)

Boys

Age (yr)	BP Percentile	SBP (mm Hg) Percentile of Height							DBP (mm Hg) Percentile of Height						
		5th	10th	25th	50th	75th	90th	95th	5th	10th	25th	50th	75th	90th	95th
6	50th	91	92	94	96	98	99	100	53	53	54	55	56	57	57
	90th	105	106	108	110	111	113	113	68	68	69	70	71	72	72
	95th	109	110	112	114	115	117	117	72	72	73	74	75	76	76
	99th	116	117	119	121	123	124	125	80	80	81	82	83	84	84
7	50th	92	94	95	97	99	100	101	55	55	56	57	58	59	59
	90th	106	107	109	111	113	114	115	70	70	71	72	73	74	74
	95th	110	111	113	115	117	118	119	74	74	75	76	77	78	78
	99th	117	118	120	122	124	125	126	82	82	83	84	85	86	86
8	50th	94	95	97	99	100	102	102	56	57	58	59	60	60	61
	90th	107	109	110	112	114	115	116	71	72	72	73	74	75	76
	95th	111	112	114	116	118	119	120	75	76	77	78	79	79	80
	99th	119	120	122	123	125	127	127	83	84	85	86	87	87	88
9	50th	95	96	98	100	102	103	104	57	58	59	60	61	61	62
	90th	109	110	112	114	115	117	118	72	73	74	75	76	76	77
	95th	113	114	116	118	119	121	121	76	77	78	79	80	81	81
	99th	120	121	123	125	127	128	129	84	85	86	87	88	88	89
10	50th	97	98	100	102	103	105	106	58	59	60	61	61	62	63
	90th	111	112	114	115	117	119	119	73	73	74	75	76	77	78
	95th	115	116	117	119	121	122	123	77	78	79	80	81	81	82
	99th	122	123	125	127	128	130	130	85	86	86	88	88	89	90

(continued)

27

Table 27.5 BP Levels for Boys and Girls by Age and Height Percentile (continued)

Boys

Age (yr)	BP Percentile	SBP (mm Hg) Percentile of Height							DBP (mm Hg) Percentile of Height						
		5th	10th	25th	50th	75th	90th	95th	5th	10th	25th	50th	75th	90th	95th
11	50th	99	100	102	104	105	107	107	59	59	60	61	62	63	63
	90th	113	114	115	117	119	120	121	74	74	75	76	77	78	78
	95th	117	118	119	121	123	124	125	78	78	79	80	81	82	82
	99th	124	125	127	129	130	132	132	86	86	87	88	89	90	90
12	50th	101	102	104	106	108	109	110	59	60	61	62	63	63	64
	90th	115	116	118	120	121	123	123	74	75	75	76	77	78	79
	95th	119	120	122	123	125	127	127	78	79	80	81	82	82	83
	99th	126	127	129	131	133	134	135	86	87	88	89	90	90	91
13	50th	104	105	106	108	110	111	112	60	60	61	62	63	64	64
	90th	117	118	120	122	124	125	126	75	75	76	77	78	79	79
	95th	121	122	124	126	128	129	130	79	79	80	81	82	83	83
	99th	128	130	131	133	135	136	137	87	87	88	89	90	91	91
14	50th	106	107	109	111	113	114	115	60	61	62	63	64	65	65
	90th	120	121	123	125	126	128	128	75	76	77	78	79	79	80
	95th	124	125	127	128	130	132	132	80	80	81	82	83	84	84
	99th	131	132	134	136	138	139	140	87	88	89	90	91	92	92
15	50th	109	110	112	113	115	117	117	61	62	63	64	65	66	66
	90th	122	124	125	127	129	130	131	76	77	78	79	80	80	81
	95th	126	127	129	131	133	134	135	81	81	82	83	84	85	85
	99th	134	135	136	138	140	142	142	88	89	90	91	92	93	93

(continued)

Table 27.5 BP Levels for Boys and Girls by Age and Height Percentile (continued)

Boys

Age (yr)	BP Percentile	SBP (mm Hg) Percentile of Height							DBP (mm Hg) Percentile of Height						
		5th	10th	25th	50th	75th	90th	95th	5th	10th	25th	50th	75th	90th	95th
16	50th	111	112	114	116	118	119	120	63	63	64	65	66	67	67
	90th	125	126	128	130	131	133	134	78	78	79	80	81	82	82
	95th	129	130	132	134	135	137	137	82	83	83	84	85	86	87
	99th	136	137	139	141	143	144	145	90	90	91	92	93	94	94
17	50th	114	115	116	118	120	121	122	65	65	66	67	68	69	70
	90th	127	128	130	132	134	135	136	80	80	81	82	83	84	84
	95th	131	132	134	136	138	139	140	84	85	86	87	88	88	89
	99th	139	140	141	143	145	146	147	92	93	93	94	95	96	97

(continued)

Nephrology

27

Table 27.5 BP Levels for Boys and Girls by Age and Height Percentile (continued)

Girls

Age (yr)	BP Percentile	SBP (mm Hg) Percentile of Height							DBP (mm Hg) Percentile of Height						
		5th	10th	25th	50th	75th	90th	95th	5th	10th	25th	50th	75th	90th	95th
1	50th	83	84	85	86	88	89	90	38	39	39	40	41	41	42
	90th	97	97	98	100	101	102	103	52	53	53	54	55	55	56
	95th	100	101	102	104	105	106	107	56	57	57	58	59	59	60
	99th	108	108	109	111	112	113	114	64	64	68	68	66	67	67
2	50th	85	85	87	88	89	91	91	43	44	44	45	46	46	47
	90th	98	99	100	101	103	104	105	57	58	58	59	60	61	61
	95th	102	103	104	105	107	108	109	61	62	62	636	64	65	65
	99th	109	110	111	112	114	115	116	69	68	70	70	71	72	72
3	50th	86	87	88	89	91	92	93	47	48	48	49	50	50	51
	90th	100	100	102	103	104	106	106	61	62	62	63	64	64	65
	95th	104	104	105	107	108	109	110	65	66	66	67	68	68	69
	99th	111	111	113	114	115	116	117	73	73	74	74	75	76	76
4	50th	88	88	90	91	92	94	94	50	50	51	52	52	53	54
	90th	101	102	103	104	106	107	108	64	64	65	66	67	67	68
	95th	105	106	107	108	110	111	112	68	68	69	70	71	71	72
	99th	112	113	114	115	117	118	119	76	76	76	77	78	79	79
5	50th	89	90	91	93	94	95	96	52	53	53	54	55	55	56
	90th	103	103	105	106	107	109	109	66	67	67	68	69	69	70
	95th	107	107	108	110	111	112	113	70	71	71	72	73	73	74
	99th	114	114	116	117	118	120	120	78	78	79	79	80	81	81

(continued)

Girls

Age (yr)	BP Percentile	SBP (mm Hg) Percentile of Height							DBP (mm Hg) Percentile of Height						
		5th	10th	25th	50th	75th	90th	95th	5th	10th	25th	50th	75th	90th	95th
6	50th	91	92	93	94	96	97	98	54	54	55	56	56	57	58
	90th	104	105	106	108	109	110	111	68	68	69	70	70	71	72
	95th	108	109	110	111	113	114	115	72	72	73	74	74	75	76
	99th	115	116	117	119	120	121	122	80	80	80	81	82	83	83
7	50th	93	93	95	96	97	99	99	55	56	56	57	58	58	59
	90th	106	107	108	109	111	112	113	69	70	70	71	72	72	73
	95th	110	111	112	113	115	116	116	73	74	74	75	76	76	77
	99th	117	118	119	120	122	123	124	81	81	82	82	83	84	84
8	50th	95	95	96	98	99	100	101	57	57	57	58	59	60	60
	90th	108	109	110	111	113	114	114	71	71	71	72	73	74	74
	95th	112	112	114	115	116	118	118	75	75	75	76	77	78	78
	99th	119	120	121	122	123	125	125	82	82	83	83	84	86	86
9	50th	96	97	98	100	101	102	103	58	58	58	59	60	61	61
	90th	110	110	112	113	114	116	116	72	72	72	73	74	75	75
	95th	114	114	115	117	118	119	120	76	76	76	77	78	79	79
	99th	121	121	123	124	125	127	127	83	83	84	84	85	87	87
10	50th	98	99	100	102	103	104	105	59	59	59	60	61	62	62
	90th	112	112	114	115	116	118	118	73	73	73	74	75	76	76
	95th	116	116	117	119	120	121	122	77	77	77	78	79	80	80
	99th	123	123	125	126	127	129	129	84	84	85	86	86	87	88

(continued)

Nephrology

27

Table 27.5 BP Levels for Boys and Girls by Age and Height Percentile *(continued)*

Girls

Age (yr)	BP Percentile	SBP (mm Hg) Percentile of Height							DBP (mm Hg) Percentile of Height						
		5th	10th	25th	50th	75th	90th	95th	5th	10th	25th	50th	75th	90th	95th
11	50th	100	101	102	103	105	106	107	60	60	60	61	62	63	63
	90th	114	114	116	117	118	119	120	74	74	74	75	76	77	77
	95th	118	118	119	121	122	123	124	78	78	78	79	80	81	81
	99th	125	125	126	128	129	130	131	85	85	86	87	87	88	89
12	50th	102	103	104	105	107	108	109	61	61	61	62	63	64	64
	90th	116	116	117	119	120	121	122	75	75	75	76	77	78	78
	95th	119	120	121	123	124	125	126	79	79	79	80	81	82	82
	99th	127	127	128	130	131	132	133	86	86	87	88	88	89	90
13	50th	104	105	106	107	109	110	110	62	62	62	63	64	65	65
	90th	117	118	119	121	122	123	124	76	76	76	77	78	79	79
	95th	121	122	123	124	126	127	128	80	80	80	81	82	83	83
	99th	128	129	130	132	133	134	135	87	87	88	89	89	90	91
14	50th	106	106	107	109	110	111	112	63	63	63	64	65	66	66
	90th	119	120	121	122	124	125	125	77	77	77	78	79	80	80
	95th	123	123	125	126	127	129	129	81	81	81	82	83	84	84
	99th	130	131	132	133	135	136	136	88	88	89	90	90	91	92
15	50th	107	108	109	110	111	113	113	64	64	64	65	66	67	67
	90th	120	121	122	123	125	126	127	78	78	78	79	80	81	81
	95th	124	125	126	127	129	130	131	82	82	82	83	84	85	85
	99th	131	132	133	134	136	137	138	89	89	90	91	91	92	93

(continued)

Table 27.5 BP Levels for Boys and Girls by Age and Height Percentile (continued)

Girls

Age (yr)	BP Percentile	SBP (mm Hg) Percentile of Height							DBP (mm Hg) Percentile of Height						
		5th	10th	25th	50th	75th	90th	95th	5th	10th	25th	50th	75th	90th	95th
16	50th	108	108	110	111	112	114	114	64	64	65	66	66	67	68
	90th	121	122	123	124	126	127	128	78	78	79	80	81	81	82
	95th	125	126	127	128	130	131	132	82	82	83	84	85	85	86
	99th	132	133	134	135	137	138	139	90	90	90	91	92	93	93
17	50th	108	109	110	111	113	114	115	64	65	65	66	66	67	68
	90th	122	122	123	125	126	127	128	78	79	79	80	81	81	82
	95th	125	126	127	129	130	131	132	82	83	83	84	85	85	86
	99th	133	133	134	136	137	138	139	90	90	91	91	92	93	93

From the National High Blood Pressure Education Program Working Group on High Blood Pressure in Children and Adolescents. The fourth report on the diagnosis, evaluation, and treatment of high blood pressure in children and adolescents. *Pediatrics.* 2004;114(Suppl):558–559, Tables 3 and 4.

Nephrology

27

ETIOLOGY

Primary

- Uncommon in children; diagnosis of exclusion
- Often associated with positive family history of HTN or cardiovascular disease
- Frequently clusters with other cardiovascular risk factors (obesity, low HDL and high triglyceride levels, abnormal glucose tolerance)

Secondary

- Intrinsic renal disease: GN, ATN, HUS, HSP, tumor
- Renal vascular: renal artery stenosis, renal artery thrombosis, renal vein thrombosis, fibromuscular dysplasia, vasculitis
- Cardiovascular: coarctation of aorta
- Endocrine: hyperthyroidism, hyperparathyroidism, congenital adrenal hyperplasia, Cushing syndrome, primary hyperaldosteronism, pheochromocytoma, neuroblastoma
- CNS: intracranial mass/hemorrhage, ↑ICP, Guillain-Barré syndrome
- Medications/toxins: corticosteroids, oral contraceptives, nasal decongestants, cocaine, sympathomimetic agents, vitamin D intoxication

INVESTIGATIONS

- Calculate BMI
- Four-limb BP measurements
- Urine: urinalysis, culture
- Serum: CBC, Cr, urea, electrolytes
- Renal Doppler US
- Further studies for underlying disorder as guided by history and physical examination:
  - ABPM
  - Plasma renin, plasma and urine steroid levels, plasma and urine catecholamines
  - Renovascular imaging
- Evaluation for comorbidities may include fasting lipid panel, fasting glucose, drug screen, polysomnography
- Evaluation for target-organ damage may include electrocardiogram (ECG), echocardiogram, retinal examination

MANAGEMENT

- See p. 28 for management of hypertensive crisis
- Primary HTN: weight reduction, exercise, dietary modification
- Secondary HTN: treat underlying cause

Pharmacologic Agents

- See Table 27.6
- Indications include secondary HTN and insufficient response to lifestyle changes in primary HTN
- Initiate therapy with single drug
- Use medication aimed at underlying mechanism of HTN

Table 27.6 Common Antihypertensive Agents for Outpatient Management (Oral)

Category	Drug Name	Dose	Action	Benefits	Adverse Effects
Calcium channel blockers	Amlodipine	0.1–0.3 mg/kg/dose od	Reduces vascular tone by inhibiting Ca^{2+} entry into arterial smooth muscle cells	Dosing (od), tasteless, odorless, suspension, 90% GI absorption	Facial flushing, tachycardia; may cause precipitous hypotension, edema
Diuretics	Hydrochlorothiazide	2–4 mg/kg/d ÷ q12h	Diuresis by inhibiting NaCl reabsorption in distal convoluted tubule	Effective in primary HTN	Not effective when GFR <50% normal; can cause $\downarrow K^+$, $\uparrow Ca^{2+}$, $\uparrow$ glucose, $\uparrow$ uric acid, hyperlipidemia
β-Blockers	Nadolol	1 mg/kg/d od or ÷ bid; $\uparrow$ to max of 4 mg/kg/d or 320 mg/d (whichever is less)	Nonselective β-blocker (blocks β_1 and β_2 receptors); $\downarrow$ peripheral vascular resistance	$\downarrow$HR, $\downarrow$ cardiac output, $\downarrow$ renin release	Contraindicated in asthma, diabetes, CHF, Raynaud disease; causes bronchospasm, bradycardia, vivid dreams
α_1-Blocker	Prazosin	0.05–0.1 mg/kg/d; max 0.5 mg/kg/d	Blocks α_1-mediated vasoconstriction of arterioles and venules	Effective in patients with renal failure, Raynaud disease, collagen vascular disease	Rarely used; causes nausea, palpitations, syncope, orthostatic hypotension with first dose
Vasodilators	Hydralazine	0.75–7 mg/kg/d ÷ q6h; max 7 mg/kg/d or 200 mg/d, whichever is less	Relaxes arteriolar smooth muscle	Rapid onset	Tachycardia, $\downarrow Na^+$, water retention; nausea; drug-induced SLE

(continued)

Table 27.6   Common Antihypertensive Agents for Outpatient Management *(continued)*

Category	Drug Name	Dose	Action	Benefits	Adverse Effects
ACE inhibitors	Captopril	Initial: 0.1–0.3 mg/kg/dose tid Maintenance: 0.3–4 mg/kg/d ÷ tid Max 6 mg/kg/d or 200 mg/d	Blocks conversion of angiotensin I to angiotensin II	↓ Proteinuria; preserves renal function; ↓ pulmonary vascular resistance and mean arterial pressure with little effect on HR	↑K⁺; transient hypotension; contraindicated in decreased renal perfusion; rarely associated with rash, cough, angioedema, marrow suppression
	Enalapril	Initial: 0.1 mg/kg/d od or ÷ bid Maintenance: 0.1–0.5 mg/kg/d od or ÷ bid Max 40 mg/d	As above		As above
Angiotensin II receptor antagonists	Losartan	0.7 mg/kg/d up to 50 mg/d od Max 1.0 mg/kg/d up to 100 mg/d	Blocks binding of angiotensin II to angiotensin I receptors	Avoids inhibition of ACE and degradation of bradykinin; not contraindicated in renal failure	Not well studied in children; dizziness most common side effect

All doses given as oral form only.

- Definition: >4 mg/m^2/h; nephrotic range >40 mg/m^2/h
- Pathologic if persistent or associated with hematuria, HTN, or renal dysfunction
- See Box 27.1

Box 27.1	Differential Diagnosis of Proteinuria

Benign
- Orthostatic
- Transient: fever, exercise, cold exposure, stress, epinephrine infusion

Pathologic

Glomerular
- Congenital: congenital nephrosis (Finnish), diffuse mesangial sclerosis, CMV, syphilis
- Acquired
  - Primary: minimal change, FSGS, membranous, MPGN
  - Secondary:
    - Infection: PSGN, shunt nephritis, SBE, hepatitis B or C virus, HIV, malaria, syphilis
    - Multisystem: SLE, HUS, HSP, sickle cell disease, Wegener granulomatosis, Goodpasture disease
    - Drugs: penicillamine, NSAIDs, captopril, gold, mercury, lithium
    - Neoplasia: leukemia, lymphoma, renal tumors
    - Renal/vascular: renal vein thrombosis, renal artery stenosis, HTN

Tubular
- Congenital/genetic: Fanconi syndrome, cystic/dysplastic renal disease
- Acquired: interstitial nephritis, pyelonephritis, ATN, transplant rejection, reflux nephropathy, drugs (aminoglycosides, analgesics, cyclosporine, cisplatin)

Nephrology

27

INVESTIGATIONS

- Urine microscopy and culture
- Asymptomatic patients: repeat first morning urinalysis 2–3× before extensive investigation
- Rule out orthostatic proteinuria with overnight (supine) urine sample collected separately from daytime (upright) sample
- Serum: CBC, electrolytes, urea, Cr, albumin, C3, C4
- Consider: antinuclear antibody, ASO titer, hepatitis serology, HIV, VDRL, abdominal US, renal biopsy (guided by history and physical examination of patient)

NEPHROTIC SYNDROME

- Definition: nephrotic-range proteinuria, hypoalbuminemia, edema, hyperlipidemia
- See Box 27.2

Primary

- Idiopathic (90% of pediatric patients)
  - Minimal change disease (85%)
  - FSGS (10%)
  - Mesangial proliferation (5%)
  - Finnish-type congenital nephrotic syndrome
  - Diffuse mesangial sclerosis

Secondary

- Infections (syphilis, HIV, hepatitis B or C, leprosy, malaria, schistosomiasis, toxoplasmosis)
- Malignancy (leukemia, lymphoma)
- Drugs (penicillamine, captopril, NSAIDs, mercury, gold, lithium, pamidronate, heroin)

PRIMARY IDIOPATHIC NEPHROTIC SYNDROME

Epidemiology

- Male:female ratio, 2:1
- Most commonly age 2–6 yr

Clinical Manifestations

- Periorbital and lower limb edema progressing to generalized edema, ascites, pleural effusions
- Anorexia, irritability, abdominal pain, diarrhea

Patient Subsets

- Steroid resistant: persistent proteinuria after 8 wk of steroid therapy
- Steroid dependent: relapses on alternate-day dosing with prednisone, or relapses within 14 d of prednisone discontinuation
- Frequent relapser: ≥ four relapses in 1 yr, or two relapses in 6 mo

Laboratory Features

- Nephrotic-range proteinuria (see tests for protein)
- Microscopic hematuria (20% of patients)
- Serum Cr usually normal; may be increased if intravascularly depleted
- Serum albumin <25 g/L
- ↑ Serum cholesterol and triglycerides

Treatment

- Low-salt diet
- Cautious use of diuretics, if necessary
- Consider use of 25% albumin infusion if symptomatic edema or if volume depleted

- Prednisone 60 mg/m^2/d × 4–6 wk, then taper to 40 mg/m^2/dose, given every other day × 4–6 wk
- Median time to remission is 10 d (urine shows negative or trace protein for 3 consecutive days)
- In steroid resistance, steroid dependence, or frequent relapser, cyclophosphamide, cyclosporine, tacrolimus, or mycophenolate mofetil are second-line options

Complications

- Intravascular depletion
- Pulmonary edema/respiratory distress
- Increased susceptibility to infections from encapsulated bacteria (decreased concentrations of IgG and factor B)
  - Rate of spontaneous bacterial peritonitis: 2–6%
- Increased risk of thromboembolic events (2–5% in children) due to decreased level of antithrombin III, increased platelet aggregation, volume depletion, and hyperviscosity
  - Use of diuretics, corticosteroids, and immobilization further increase risk

Prognosis

- Minimal-change disease has 95% response rate to steroid therapy; response rate 30% in FSGS
- Overall, relapse rate after steroid treatment 60–80%, although may be lowered to 30–40% with longer initial therapy course
- 5-yr risk of developing ESRD for patients with steroid-resistant nephrotic syndrome exceeds 40%

HEMATURIA

- See Figure 27.3

DEFINITION

- Hematuria: >5 RBCs/high-power field in spun urine
- Common causes of "dark urine," which could be mistaken for hematuria:
  - Drugs (rifampin, nitrofurantoin, methyldopa, levodopa, metronidazole)
  - Pigments (hemoglobin, myoglobin, bilirubin, beets, blackberries, urates)
- See Box 27.3 for differential diagnosis

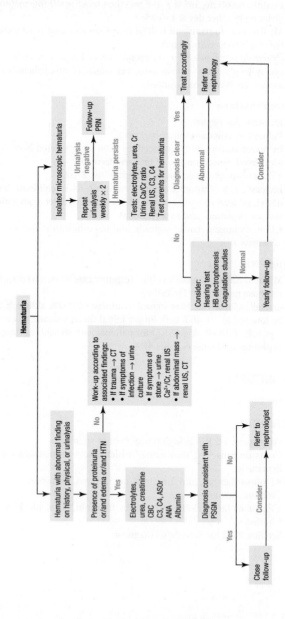

Figure 27.3 Approach to Hematuria

Hematuria

Hematuria with abnormal finding on history, physical, or urinalysis

Isolated microscopic hematuria

Repeat urinalysis weekly × 2

Urinalysis negative → Follow-up PRN

Hematuria persists

Tests: electrolytes, urea, Cr
Urine Ca/Cr ratio
Renal US, C3, C4
Test parents for hematuria

Diagnosis clear — Yes → Treat accordingly

No

Consider:
Hearing test
HB electrophoresis
Coagulation studies

Abnormal → Refer to nephrology

Normal

Yearly follow-up

Consider

Presence of proteinuria or/and edema or/and HTN

No → Work-up according to associated findings:
• If trauma → CT
• If symptoms of infection → urine culture
• If symptoms of stone → urine Ca²⁺/Cr, renal US
• If abdominal mass → renal US, CT

Yes

Electrolytes, urea, creatinine
CBC
C3, C4, ASOr
ANA
Albumin

Diagnosis consistent with PSGN

No → Refer to nephrologist

Yes

Consider

Close follow-up

Box 27.3   Differential Diagnosis of Hematuria

Upper Tract
Glomerular
- Thin basement membrane disease, PSGN, IgA nephropathy (Berger disease), systemic vasculitis, Alport syndrome, HUS, shunt nephritis, Goodpasture disease, MPGN, lupus nephritis

Tubulointerstitial
- Infection, tumors, nephrotoxins, cystic disease
- Nephrocalcinosis, hypercalciuria, nephrolithiasis

Lower Tract
- Infections
- Calculi
- Trauma
- Obstruction

Vascular
- Renal vein or artery thrombosis
- Coagulopathy, thrombocytopenia
- Sickle cell disease/trait

EPIDEMIOLOGY

- Prevalence of isolated microscopic hematuria in children and adolescents: about 1.5%
- Majority asymptomatic; do not develop significant renal disease
- Persistent microscopic hematuria (on three samples) should prompt further investigations
- Investigations to consider: CBC, electrolytes, Cr, urea, Ca^{2+}, C3, C4; urine: culture, Cr, protein, Ca^{2+}; renal US (see Figure 27.3)
  - If recent sore throat or skin infection, consider antihyaluronidase, anti-DNAse B, and ASO titers
  - If features of lupus, send ANA, anti-dsDNA; may require renal biopsy
  - If persistent, asymptomatic, isolated hematuria, screen other family members as workup of thin basement membrane disease

NEPHRITIC SYNDROME

- Definition: hematuria, proteinuria, and impaired renal function together with HTN, fluid overload, and edema
- See Box 27.4

| Box 27.4 | Differential Diagnosis of Low C3 Glomerulonephritis |

- Acute postinfectious GN
- Lupus nephritis
- Shunt nephritis
- Membranoproliferative GN
- SBE

COMMON RENAL PROBLEMS IN CHILDREN

ALPORT SYNDROME

- Definition: disorder of basement membrane due to an abnormality in type IV collagen
- Genetics: X-linked dominant (80% of patients) or AR

Features

- Renal: hematuria, proteinuria, HTN, renal insufficiency
- Ocular: anterior lenticonus, perimacular flecks
- Cochlear: high-frequency sensorineural hearing loss (50% patients)
- Leiomyomatosis
- Workup: renal US to rule out other pathology, renal biopsy
- Treatment: supportive, dialysis, renal transplant

IGA NEPHROPATHY (BERGER DISEASE)

- Results from deposition of IgA in glomerular mesangium
- Most common cause of GN in children
- M:F ratio, 2:1
- Presents at all ages but more commonly in the second and third decades of life
- Usually not associated with HTN or edema
- Workup: serum IgA may be ↑; clinical diagnosis confirmed by renal biopsy
- Therapy: immunosuppression and ACE inhibitors considered if significant proteinuria and/or HTN
- Prognosis: 25% progress to chronic renal insufficiency

POSTSTREPTOCOCCAL GN

- Presents 7–21 d after group A β-hemolytic streptococcal infection of throat or skin
- Occurs in all age groups; most cases found in ages 5–15 yr
- Features: tea-colored urine, edema, HTN, mild to moderate impairment of renal function
- If symptoms of nephritis are subclinical or missed, may present with isolated hematuria
- Antibiotic treatment will *not* prevent development of nephritis but should be prescribed for a patient with a positive throat culture
- ASO titer ↑ initially; serum C3↓ but returns to normal within 6–8 wk

- If C3 does not normalize by 6–8 wk, consider renal biopsy to establish diagnosis
- Microscopic hematuria generally resolves within 6–12 mo after onset of nephritis; may persist for up to 2 yr
- Treatment in acute phase: fluid and salt restriction, diuretics, antihypertensive medication, as indicated
- Excellent prognosis

HENOCH-SCHÖNLEIN PURPURA

- Small-vessel vasculitis
- Etiology unknown, but often follows a URTI
- Younger children most frequently affected; peak incidence between 4–5 yr of age
- Nonrenal features: maculopapular rash progressing to petechiae or palpable purpura, arthritis, edema, intermittent abdominal pain, intussusception
- Renal features may include hematuria, proteinuria, acute nephritic syndrome, nephrotic syndrome
- Renal manifestations can occur up to 12 wk after initial presentation
- Potential role for high-dose steroids or cytotoxic therapy (cyclophosphamide, azathioprine) in patients with crescentic GN or significant proteinuria
- Prognosis favorable; 2–5% progress to chronic renal failure

HEMOLYTIC UREMIC SYNDROME

- Leading cause of acute renal failure in North America in otherwise healthy children
- Most common in 9-mo–4-yr-old children
- Triad of microangiopathic hemolytic anemia, thrombocytopenia, renal insufficiency
- Subdivided into
  - Typical HUS, with Shiga-like toxin producing diarrhea (D+): 90%
  - Atypical HUS, without diarrhea (D–): 10%

TYPICAL HUS

- Usually caused by Shiga toxin–producing strains of *Escherichia coli*, most often O157:H7 subtype
- Presents with abdominal pain followed by bloody diarrhea; fever: low grade or absent
- Develops 2–14 d after diarrhea onset
- 40–50% with typical HUS will develop acute renal failure requiring dialysis
- CNS involvement occurs in 15–20% of patients
- Treatment is supportive

ATYPICAL HUS

- No diarrheal prodrome
- Etiology:
  - Infection: *Streptococcus pneumoniae*, HIV
  - Genetic: deficiencies in complement components, von Willebrand factor–cleaving protease; defects of vitamin B_{12} metabolism; idiopathic AR and AD disease
- Varied clinical presentation and course but tends to have high risk of disease recurrence, chronic renal disease, and death

ACUTE RENAL FAILURE

- Definition: clinical syndrome in which sudden deterioration of renal function results in the inability of the kidneys to maintain fluid and electrolyte homeostasis
- See Box 27.5

Box 27.5	Classification of Acute Renal Failure

Prerenal
- Volume depletion: diarrhea, vomiting, osmotic diuresis, burns, hemorrhage
- ↓Effective circulating volume: septic shock, anaphylactic shock, nephrotic syndrome
- Cardiac: ↓ function, ↓ systemic blood flow (anatomic malformation), arrhythmia, tamponade

Intrinsic Renal
- Glomerular: PSGN, lupus nephritis, HSP, IgA nephropathy, crescentic GN, SBE
- Vascular/hemodynamic: HUS, renal vein thrombosis, vasculitis, malignant HTN, NSAIDs, ACE-I
- Tubular (ATN): uncorrected prerenal or postrenal ARF, hypoxemia, obstruction by crystals, medications, toxins, tumor lysis syndrome
- Interstitial nephritis: allergic interstitial nephritis, malignant infiltrates, pyelonephritis, sarcoidosis

Postrenal
- UPJ obstruction, bilateral nephrolithiasis, neoplasm, bilateral megaureter, PUV, urolithiasis

---

INVESTIGATIONS

- Serum tests: Cr, urea, electrolytes, albumin, Ca^{2+}, phosphorus, uric acid, CBC, venous blood gas
- Urine tests: urinalysis, Na^+, Cr, osmolality
- Imaging: CXR (if signs of fluid overload), renal Doppler US

COMPLICATIONS

- Metabolic: ↑K^+, metabolic acidosis, ↑PO_4^-, ↓Ca^{2+}, uremia
- Systemic: fluid overload, HTN, anemia, altered mental status, platelet dysfunction, anorexia, nausea, vomiting

MANAGEMENT

- Treat metabolic acidosis
  - Oral sodium citrate or $NaHCO_3$
  - IV $NaHCO_3$; consider dialysis if persistent acidosis
- Treat $\uparrow K^+$ (see Chapter 16)
- Treat $\downarrow Ca^{2+}$
  - Resolves with correction of $\uparrow PO_4^-$ and dietary Ca^{2+}
  - If evidence of tetany, give IV Ca^{2+} gluconate or Ca^{2+} chloride
- Treat $\uparrow PO_4^-$ (see Chapter 16)
- Optimize nutrition
- Adjust medications for degree of renal failure
- Fluid management
  - Euvolemia: give insensible losses + urine output + other losses
  - Dehydration: give deficit + insensible losses + urine output + other losses
  - Fluid overload: give insensible losses + urine output, but subtract estimated volume of fluid to be deficited over given time period

CHRONIC KIDNEY DISEASE

- See Box 27.6

Box 27.6	Classification of Chronic Kidney Disease (National Kidney Foundation Guidelines, K-DOQI)

- Stage 1: kidney damage with normal or $\uparrow$GFR (GFR $\geq$90)
- Stage 2: kidney damage with mildly $\downarrow$GFR (GFR 60-89)
- Stage 3: moderate $\downarrow$GFR (GFR 30-59)
- Stage 4: severe $\downarrow$GFR (GFR 15-29)
- Stage 5: kidney failure (GFR $\leq$15, or patient on dialysis)

27

CLINICAL MANIFESTATIONS

- Presentation often insidious, highly variable
- May present antenatally with oligohydramnios or polyhydramnios
- FTT, fatigue, headache, anorexia, nausea, vomiting, pallor, rickets, edema, HTN
- Teenagers may present with delayed puberty, anemia, HTN
- Uncommonly pruritis, peripheral neuropathy

COMPLICATIONS

Renal Osteodystrophy

- Two types: osteitis fibrosa (high bone turnover) and adynamic bone disease (low bone turnover)
- Requires frequent monitoring of iCa, PO_4^-, alkaline phosphatase, PTH
- Management: low-phosphate diet, phosphate binders (Ca^{2+} carbonate, Ca^{2+} acetate, sevelamer), activated vitamin D

Growth Retardation

- Multifactorial etiology: inadequate intake of calories and protein, renal osteodystrophy, metabolic acidosis, anemia, and perturbations in the growth hormone–insulin-like-factor axis

Anemia

- Normochromic, normocytic anemia with ↓ reticulocyte count
- Due to ↓ production of erythropoietin, bone marrow inhibition, iron/B_{12}/folate deficiency, osteitis fibrosa
- Treatment with erythropoietin replacement highly effective

MANAGEMENT

- Monitor Hb, electrolytes, Cr, urea, Ca^{2+}, PO_4^-, albumin, total CO_2
- Measure PTH level to detect renal osteodystrophy
- Ensure all medications are adjusted for degree of renal impairment
- Echocardiogram
- Manage HTN, as indicated
- Optimize nutrition; may require G tube if unable to meet recommended caloric intake
- Growth hormone, erythropoietin, if applicable

RENAL REPLACEMENT THERAPY (DIALYSIS)

- See Box 27.7 and Table 27.7

Box 27.7	Indications for Dialysis

Short-Term Dialysis Indications
- Hyperkalemia with ECG abnormalities
- Severe uremic pericarditis
- HTN secondary to fluid overload
- Uremic encephalopathy
- Congestive heart failure due to fluid overload
- Toxins, poisons
- Inborn errors of metabolism

Long-Term Dialysis Indications
- GFR <15 mL/min/1.73 m^2
- Fluid overload, uremic symptoms (nausea, anorexia, lethargy), uncontrolled biochemical abnormalities, deceleration in growth rate

	Hemodialysis	**Peritoneal Dialysis**	**CRRT**
Table 27.7	**Modalities for Renal Replacement Therapy**		
Advantages	· Rapid ultrafiltration and solute clearance	· Easy access and technically simple · Continuous and gradual ultrafiltration and solute clearance · No need for systemic anticoagulation	· Continuous ultrafiltration and solute clearance · Usually tolerated even with cardiac instability
Technical aspects	· Double-lumen catheters can be used for short-term dialysis, inserted into internal jugular or femoral veins · Arteriovenous fistula is preferred access in children and teenagers receiving long-term dialysis · Need for anticoagulation	· CAPD (manual process of exchange) · APD (use of cycler)	· CVVH · CVVHD · CVVHDF · Need for anticoagulation
Complications	· Vascular access dysfunction · Hypotension · Infections · Clotting of extracorporeal circuit · Bleeding	· Exit site and tunnel infections · Peritonitis · Leakage · Hernia, lower back pain · Anorexia · Caregiver burnout	· Similar to hemodialysis

DEVELOPMENTAL ABNORMALITIES OF THE KIDNEYS

- Normal development requires presence and interaction of two embryologic structures: ureteric bud and metanephrogenic blastema

UNILATERAL RENAL AGENESIS

- Failure of formation of one kidney
- Usually isolated, sporadic anomaly
- Look for other anomalies, including cleft lip/palate, preauricular pits, cardiac and vertebral defects
- Consider VCUG to rule out VUR

HYPOPLASTIC

- Small kidney due to reduced number of otherwise normal nephrons
- Clinically significant if both kidneys affected; can progress to end-stage renal failure by late childhood

DYSPLASTIC

- Kidney lacks normally developed nephron structures
- Extent of renal dysfunction depends on degree of morphologic abnormalities

Multicystic Dysplastic

- Results from abnormal metanephric differentiation
- Second most common cause of flank mass in newborn
- Usually asymptomatic; not functional
- Contralateral kidney (20–30%) often has some limited dysplasia and/or VUR
- Follow-up US needed to monitor involution of multicystic dysplastic kidney and compensatory growth of contralateral kidney

ABNORMALITIES OF POSITION

- Includes ectopic, horseshoe, crossed fused ectopia
- Few long-term consequences unless associated with dysplasia, reflux, or obstruction

CYSTIC KIDNEY DISEASE

- See Table 27.8

SYNDROMES ASSOCIATED WITH RENAL CYSTS

- Tuberous sclerosis
- von Hippel-Lindau disease
- VACTERL association
- Smith-Lemli-Opitz
- Branchio-oto-renal

URINARY TRACT INFECTION

- Febrile UTI in infant or young child causes risk of renal scarring, secondary HTN, and ↓ renal function
- Febrile UTIs must therefore be detected and treated promptly

EPIDEMIOLOGY

- Occurs in 3–5% of girls and 1% of boys
- < 1 yr, M:F, 3–5:1; >1 yr, M:F, 1:10
- Risk factors include female gender, uncircumcised male, toilet training, dysfunctional voiding, neurogenic bladder, obstructive uropathy, VUR, constipation, labial adhesions, urethral instrumentation

	AR PKD	AD PKD
Table 27.8	**Polycystic Kidney Disease**	
Definition	Polycystic kidneys and congenital hepatic fibrosis; may have severe liver disease with dilation of bile ducts (Caroli disease)	Renal cysts throughout nephron
Presentation	Majority present in infancy; may present in childhood Often presents as large, palpable flank masses	Usually normal renal function throughout childhood Found on US screening in family known to have disease or presents in adulthood with HTN and renal failure
Features	HTN, pyuria, ↓Na⁺, renal insufficiency, respiratory insufficiency, hepatospleno-megaly, esophageal varices, hypersplenism, signs of liver failure	Renal features: HTN, UTI/pyuria, gross or microscopic hematuria, flank masses, urolithiasis, renal insufficiency Extrarenal features: mitral valve prolapse; GI diverticuli; cerebral aneurysms; hepatic, pancreatic, ovarian, and seminal vesicle cysts
Diagnosis	Based on clinical findings, imaging, and family history (absence of cysts in both parents but may have an affected sibling)	Based on clinical findings, imaging, and family history (gene mutation in one parent)
Management	Supportive treatment Blood pressure control Dialysis or transplant when patient progresses to ESRD	Supportive treatment Blood pressure control Dialysis or transplant when patient progresses to ESRD

PATHOGENESIS

- Pathogens: *E. coli* (75–90%), *Klebsiella*, *Enterococcus*, *Enterobacter*, *Proteus*, *Staphylococcus saprophyticus* (remember the acronym KEEPS)

CLINICAL PRESENTATION

- Cystitis: dysuria, urgency, frequency, suprapubic pain, incontinence, malodorous urine
- Pyelonephritis: fever, flank pain, malaise, nausea, vomiting

DIAGNOSIS

- Midstream urine sample considered positive if
  - $\geq 10^5$ CFU/mL and only one pathogen OR
  - $\geq 10^4$ CFU/mL, only one pathogen, and patient symptomatic
- Catheter specimen considered positive if $\geq 10^3$ CFU/mL and only one pathogen
- Suprapubic aspiration gold standard but rarely performed
- *Do not* use bag specimen (very high contamination rate); only valu-able if culture negative

MANAGEMENT

- Treatment of underlying cause of dysfunctional voiding, constipation, if applicable
- Symptomatic and positive urinalysis: empiric antibiotics; modify if appropriate once culture results available (see Chapter 24 for specific antibiotics)
- Treat acute cystitis for 7 d; treat pyelonephritis for 10–14 d

EVALUATION

Renal US

- Recommended in all patients with first UTI at the time of diagnosis
- Identifies anatomic abnormalities
- Useful to examine for hydronephrosis, renal or perirenal abscess; may show acute pyelonephritis as evidenced by enlarged kidney, but not sensitive or specific for VUR
- Only demonstrates 30% of renal scars

VCUG

- Consider evaluation for VUR in all children <5 yr of age with UTI, any child with a febrile UTI, school-aged girls with ≥2 UTIs, any male with UTI
- Can be performed early, as long as afebrile and not toxic

NEPHROCALCINOSIS

- Definition: increase in Ca^{2+} content of the cortex or medulla
- Most commonly associated with
  - Idiopathic hypercalciuria
  - Use of furosemide
  - Prematurity
  - Distal renal tubular acidosis

UROLITHIASIS

CLINICAL PRESENTATION

- UTI, dysuria
- Abdominal or flank pain
- Microscopic or macroscopic hematuria
- Incidental finding; asymptomatic

ETIOLOGY

- Underlying metabolic disease (40%)
- Stasis or obstruction (25%)
- Infection (10%)
- Idiopathic (25%)

DIFFERENTIAL DIAGNOSIS BY STONE COMPOSITION

Calcium

- 90% of urinary calculi in children
- Different types: Ca^{2+} phosphate (precipitates in alkaline urine); Ca^{2+} oxalate (precipitates in acid urine)
- Hypercalcemia may be due to hyperparathyroidism, hyperthyroidism, hypervitaminosis D
- Normocalcemic hypercalciuria may be familial, sporadic, or related to distal RTA or loop diuretics
- Hyperoxaluria may be due to intestinal malabsorption, pyridoxine deficiency, increased vitamin C intake, increased oxalate intake, or underlying metabolic disorder
- Treatment: thiazide diuretics can reduce urinary Ca^{2+} excretion by increasing tubular Ca^{2+} reabsorption; potassium citrate inhibits Ca^{2+} stone formation

Cystine

- Caused by cystinuria; causes 8–10% childhood stones
- Cystinuria characterized by AR inherited defect in renal tubular reabsorptive transport of cystine and dibasic amino acids (ornithine, arginine, and lysine)
- Treated by urine alkalinization and chelating agents

Magnesium Ammonium Phosphate (Struvite)

- 2–3% of pediatric kidney stones
- Precipitates in alkaline urine
- Associated with UTIs from urea-splitting organisms (commonly *Proteus*)

Uric Acid

- Uncommon in childhood
- Precipitates in acid urine
- Due to tumor lysis syndrome, lymphoproliferative or myeloproliferative disorders, gout, Lesch-Nyhan syndrome, G6PD, short gut
- Treatment: fluid intake, dietary purine restriction, urinary alkalinization, allopurinol trial

DIAGNOSIS

- Compositional analysis of passed stone or sediment from strained urine
- AXR: Ca^{2+} oxalate and Ca^{2+} phosphate stones densely opaque; struvite and cystine stones intermediate density; uric acid stones radiolucent
- US: assess urinary tract anatomy, obstruction, nephrocalcinosis
- Blood: electrolytes, Cr, urea, Ca^{2+}, Mg^{2+}, PO_4^-, albumin, uric acid, HCO_3^-, alkaline phosphatase
- Urine: urinalysis, pH, culture, Ca^{2+}, oxalate, citrate, PO_4^-, uric acid, cystine, Cr

TREATMENT

- High fluid intake (>2 L/1.73 m^2/d), preferably in the form of water
- Low salt intake (to reduce urinary calcium)
- Specific therapies based on underlying disorder and stone type, as already described
- Surgical correction for anatomic abnormalities predisposing to stones or infections
- Lithotripsy for large stones, refractory cases

FURTHER READING

Avner ED, Harmon WE, Niaudet P. *Pediatric Nephrology*. 5th ed. Philadelphia. Pa: Lippincott Williams & Wilkins; 2004.

Eddy AA, Symons JM. Nephrotic syndrome in childhood. *Lancet*. 2003;362: 629–639.

National High Blood Pressure Education Program Working Group in High Blood Pressure in Children and Adolescents. The fourth report on the diagnosis, evaluation, and treatment of high blood pressure in children and adolescents. *Pediatrics*. 2004;114:555–573.

Rees L, Webb N, Brogan P. *Paediatric Nephrology*. Oxford, England: Oxford University Press; 2007.

USEFUL WEB SITES

The National Kidney Foundation, Kidney Disease Outcomes Quality Initiative. Available at: **www.kidney.org/professionals/KDOQI**

Nephrology

27

Chapter 28 Neurology and Neurosurgery

Shruti Mehrotra

Teesta Soman

COMMON ABBREVIATIONS

ACTH	adrenocorticotropic hormone
ADEM	acute disseminated encephalomyelitis
AED	antiepileptic drug
CSF	cerebrospinal fluid
CTA	computed tomography angiogram
CTV	computed tomography venogram
DHE	dihydroergotamine
EEG	electroencephalography
EMG	electromyography
GCS	Glasgow Coma Scale
ICH	intracranial hemorrhage
ICP	intracranial pressure
IEM	inborn errors of metabolism
LOC	level of consciousness
LP	lumbar puncture
MR	mental retardation
MRA	magnetic resonance angiogram
MRI	magnetic resonance imaging
MRV	magnetic resonance venogram
NCS	nerve conduction studies
SEGA	subependymal giant cell astrocytoma
TIA	transient ischemic attack
TMJ	temporomandibular joint
VP	ventriculoperitoneal

NEUROLOGIC EXAMINATION

- See Table 28.1

DERMATOMES

- See Figures 28.1A and 28.1B

PRIMITIVE AND SECONDARY REFLEXES

- See Box 28.1

Table 28.1	Neurologic Examination
Components	**Description**
Higher cognitive function	Mini Mental Status Examination
Cranial nerves	I: Smell II: Visual acuity, visual fields, fundoscopy, pupillary light reflex III, IV, VI: Extraocular movements, pupillary light reflex V: Light touch (V_1, V_2, V_3), corneal reflex, pain/temperature, jaw movements VII: Taste (anterior ⅔ of tongue), facial expression, corneal reflex VIII: Nystagmus (vestibular), Rinne/Weber (auditory) IX, X: Swallowing, phonation, articulation, taste (post ⅓ tongue–IX) XI: Trapezius (shoulder shrug) and sternocleidomastoid muscles XII: Movements of tongue, atrophy, fasciculations
Motor system	Abnormal movements, posture, muscle bulk, tone, power, coordination, deep tendon reflexes
Sensory system	Light touch, pain/temperature, vibration and proprioception, two-point discrimination, graphesthesia, stereognosis
Stance and gait	Postural stability, Romberg sign, walk, tandem gait

Based on Hohol MJ. The Neurological Exam. University of Toronto, Faculty of Medicine. 2001. Retrieved at:
http://www.utoronto.ca/neuronotes/NeuroExam/main.htm.

Figure 28.1A   Anterior Aspect of the Body Showing the Distribution of Cutaneous Nerves on the Right and Dermatomes on the Left

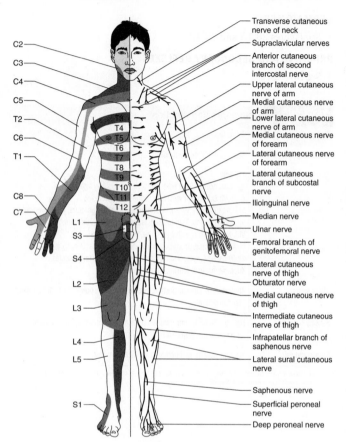

C2
C3
C4
C5
T2
C6
T1
C8
C7

T3
T4
T5
T6
T7
T8
T9
T10
T11
T12

L1
S3
S4
L2

L3

L4

L5

S1

Transverse cutaneous nerve of neck
Supraclavicular nerves
Anterior cutaneous branch of second intercostal nerve
Upper lateral cutaneous nerve of arm
Medial cutaneous nerve of arm
Lower lateral cutaneous nerve of arm
Medial cutaneous nerve of forearm
Lateral cutaneous nerve of forearm
Lateral cutaneous branch of subcostal nerve
Ilioinguinal nerve
Median nerve
Ulnar nerve
Femoral branch of genitofemoral nerve
Lateral cutaneous nerve of thigh
Obturator nerve
Medial cutaneous nerve of thigh
Intermediate cutaneous nerve of thigh
Infrapatellar branch of saphenous nerve
Lateral sural cutaneous nerve
Saphenous nerve
Superficial peroneal nerve
Deep peroneal nerve

Adapted from Snell R. *Clinical Neuroanatomy for Medical Students.* 5th ed. Baltimore, Md: Lippincott Williams and Wilkins; 2001. Reprinted by permission of Lippincott Williams and Wilkins.

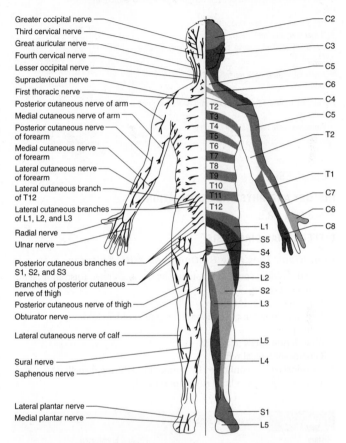

Figure 28.1B   Posterior Aspect of the Body Showing the Distribution of Cutaneous Nerves on the Left and Dermatomes on the Right

Greater occipital nerve
Third cervical nerve
Great auricular nerve
Fourth cervical nerve
Lesser occipital nerve
Supraclavicular nerve
First thoracic nerve
Posterior cutaneous nerve of arm
Medial cutaneous nerve of arm
Posterior cutaneous nerve of forearm
Medial cutaneous nerve of forearm
Lateral cutaneous nerve of forearm
Lateral cutaneous branch of T12
Lateral cutaneous branches of L1, L2, and L3
Radial nerve
Ulnar nerve
Posterior cutaneous branches of S1, S2, and S3
Branches of posterior cutaneous nerve of thigh
Posterior cutaneous nerve of thigh
Obturator nerve
Lateral cutaneous nerve of calf
Sural nerve
Saphenous nerve
Lateral plantar nerve
Medial plantar nerve

C2
C3
C5
C6
C4
C5
T2
T1
C7
C6
C8
L1
S5
S4
S3
L2
S2
L3
L5
L4
S1
L5

T2
T3
T4
T5
T6
T7
T8
T9
T10
T11
T12

Adapted from Snell R. *Clinical Neuroanatomy for Medical Students.* 5th ed. Baltimore, Md: Lippincott Williams and Wilkins; 2001. Reprinted by permission of Lippincott Williams and Wilkins.

Neurology and Neurosurgery

28

Box 28.1	Primitive and Secondary Reflexes*

Primitive Reflexes (present at birth; disappear between 3 and 5 mo)

Local
- Head: rooting, righting response
- Upper limbs: palmar grasp
- Lower limbs: plantar grasp, placing, stepping

General
- Asymmetric tonic neck reflex
- Moro reflex

Secondary Reflexes (appear between 4 and 10 mo and persist)
- Balancing
- Protective: parachute, lateral propping

*Abnormalities include absent or asymmetric reflexes and persistence of obligatory primitive reflexes.

SEIZURES

HISTORY AND PHYSICAL EXAMINATION
- See Table 28.2

DIFFERENTIAL DIAGNOSIS

Conditions That May Be Confused With Seizures
- Breath-holding spells: precipitated by trauma, anger, frustration, emotional stress
- Nightmares/night terrors
- Migraine: rule out confusional migraine in older children
- Syncope
- Shuddering spells in infancy
- Gastroesophageal reflux
- Pseudoseizures: confirmed by normal EEG during a spell
- Rage attacks (episodic loss/lack of control)

Table 28.2	Evaluation of Seizures	
History	**Physical Examination**
· Description of episode	· Vital signs; support airway
· Duration	· GCS, mental status
· Postictal assessment including mental status, focal neurologic signs*	· Note dysmorphism, fontanelle, head circumference, fundoscopic examination
· Events surrounding episode (fever, trauma, ingestion, underlying metabolic or CNS diseases)	· Meningeal signs
	· Trauma
· Review of systems: headache, vomiting, visual alterations, weight loss, change in behavior or LOC	· Thorough neurologic examination
· Developmental history	· Abdominal and dermatologic examinations
· Family history of epilepsy, CNS, metabolic pathologies	

*Absence of return to baseline suggests ongoing seizure activity, medication effect, or underlying disease.

TYPES

- Epilepsy may be diagnosed after having two or more unprovoked seizures in absence of concurrent illness/fever or acute brain injury
- See Chapter 26 for approach to neonatal seizures
- See Table 28.3 for classification of seizures
- See Table 28.4 for main seizure syndromes

Table 28.3	Classification of Seizures	
Seizure Type	**Clinical Features**	**Antiepileptic Drug of Choice**
Generalized		
Absence	Age of onset: 2–9 yr; abrupt cessation of activity; changes in facial expressions	(1) Ethosuximide (2) Valproate
Tonic–clonic	Most common; tonic phase: stiff limbs for 10–30 s; clonic phase: rapid jerks of limbs and trunk	(1) Phenobarbital* (2) Phenytoin (3) Valproate (4) Others—newer AEDs like topiramate, levetiracetam if not responsive to above
Clonic	Rhythmic and symmetric contractions of muscle groups	(1) Phenobarbital* (2) Phenytoin (3) Valproate (4) Others—newer AEDs like topiramate, levetiracetam if not responsive to above
Tonic	Increased tone in extension; high-pitched cry; <60 s	(1) Phenobarbital* (2) Phenytoin (3) Valproate (4) Others—newer AEDs like topiramate, levetiracetam if not responsive to above
Atonic	Sudden loss of muscle tone; rare	
Myoclonic	Brief involuntary muscle contractions; generalized or focal; single or repetitive; rhythmic or irregular	(1) Levetiracetam (2) Valproate (3) Lamotrigine (4) Topiramate
Partial		
Simple motor	Tongue, lips, hands commonly involved; may have spreading to involve other body parts (jacksonian march)	(1) Carbamazepine (2) Newer AEDs like topiramate, levetiracetam
Simple sensory	Numbness or dysesthesias in any body part; abnormal proprioception	(1) Carbamazepine (2) Valproate (3) Topiramate, levetiracetam useful for additive therapy

(continued)

Table 28.3	Classification of Seizures *(continued)*	
Seizure Type	**Clinical Features**	**Antiepileptic Drug of Choice**
Simple autonomic	Abdominal discomfort; sweating; dilated pupils	(1) Carbamazepine (2) Valproate (3) Lamotrigine (4) Gabapentin (5) Newer AEDs like topiramate, levetiracetam
Complex partial	Any partial seizure with loss of consciousness	(1) Carbamazepine (2) Valproate (3) Lamotrigine (4) Gabapentin (5) Newer AEDs like topiramate, levetiracetam

*First choice for children <2 yr.

FEBRILE SEIZURES

- 4% of children <5 yr; usually 6 mo–3 yr
- Typical features include generalized seizure <15 min, one seizure in 24 h, normal development, normal neurologic examination before and after the seizure

Investigations

- Geared toward cause of fever; imaging and EEG not indicated if typical febrile seizure
- Rule out meningitis if child <1 yr or recurrent prolonged seizures in past 24 h

Treatment

- Prophylactic anticonvulsants not indicated; rectal/sublingual lorazepam for prolonged recurrent seizures

FIRST UNPROVOKED AFEBRILE SEIZURE

- Stabilize child and determine whether a seizure has occurred, based on history and physical examination
- Determine cause of seizure:
  - Provoked: result of acute condition (hypoglycemia, electrolyte imbalance, toxin, intracranial infection, trauma, etc.)
  - Unprovoked: absence of such factors (unknown, remote pre-existing brain abnormality/insult, genetic)
- Children who have not returned to baseline and neonates require further investigation beyond that outlined here:
  - Laboratory tests (CBC, differential, glucose, urea, Cr, electrolytes, Ca^{2+}, Mg^{2+}, blood gas, toxicology screen): only on basis of suggestive history and examination
  - LP, only if possibility of meningitis or encephalitis

Table 28.4   Main Seizure Syndromes

Epilepsy Syndrome	Age at Onset	Type of Seizures	Investigations	Treatment
Infantile spasms	<1 yr	· Clusters of brief, symmetric myoclonic jerks (head and body tonic flexion followed by extension of head and adduction of arms) · Associated with developmental regression at onset of spasms · Usually evolves by 18 mo to different seizure disorder	· EEG shows hypsarrhythmia · Underlying cause found in 75% of patients based on history, physical, and imaging: perinatal asphyxia, congenital malformations, TS	· ACTH and/or vigabatrin (especially with TS) · Valproate may be effective Prognosis: · ⅓ relapse · Second trial of therapy effective in 75%
Benign familial neonatal seizures (fifth-day fits)	3–7 d	· Generalized tonic-clonic · Apnea	· EEG · MRI · Electrolytes · Metabolic workup	· Phenobarbital OR · Fosphenytoin · Treatment only needed in the acute phase of the illness
Benign familial infantile epilepsy	3 mo; no neonatal seizures	· Complex partial seizures ± generalization · Seizures stop spontaneously in 2–4 yr · Normal development past 5 yr	· Normal interictal EEG and neuroimaging	· Phenobarbital OR · Fosphenytoin
Benign myoclonus of infancy	Typically in early infancy, <6 mo of age	· Myoclonic jerks · Cluster at mealtimes · If only noted in sleep, known as benign sleep myoclonus	· Normal EEG	· Spontaneously stop usually after 3 mo of age; do not occur >2 yr

(continued)

Neurology and Neurosurgery

28

645

Table 28.4 Main Seizure Syndromes (continued)

Epilepsy Syndrome	Age at Onset	Type of Seizures	Investigations	Treatment
Lennox-Gastaut syndrome	Peak onset 3–5 yr	· Triad of seizures: atypical absence, atonic, myoclonic · 60% have identifiable cause: neurocutaneous syndromes, perinatal and postnatal brain injury · 20% history of infantile spasms · MR common by 5 yr	· EEG: 1.5–2-Hz spike-wave complex · Neuroimaging: normal or abnormal	· Corticosteroids · Antiepileptics
Juvenile myoclonic epilepsy	Onset 7–13 yr	· Generalized tonic–clonic, myoclonic, absence · Most myoclonic jerks in morning with intact consciousness	· Sleep-deprived and/or video EEG: generalized 4–6-Hz polyspike and wave complexes · Normal background · Photosensitivity · MRI: normal	· Valproic acid · Lamotrigine · Levetiracetam
Landau-Kleffner syndrome (also known as acquired epileptic aphasia)	3–8 yr	· Partial and generalized tonic–clonic (70–80%) seizures · Precede or accompany language deterioration	· Daytime and overnight EEG: temporal or parietal spikes or electrical status epilepticus in sleep · MRI: rule out structural lesions (typically normal) · Hearing tests normal	· Seizures: valproic acid, ethosuximide, clobazam · Language: corticosteroids or ACTH

TS, tuberous sclerosis.

- EEG for all patients with first seizure: for recurrence risk and to determine whether epilepsy syndrome (may be as outpatient after acute seizure)
- Neuroimaging: insufficient evidence for routine use, but if obtained, MRI preferred
- Treatment with AEDs: currently not indicated for epilepsy prevention; consider if benefits of reducing risk of second seizure outweigh risks of side effects of AEDs

MANAGEMENT

- See Chapter 3 for management of status epilepticus
- Treat underlying cause, if identified
- Parental education: first aid training, administration of sublingual lorazepam, support group

Anticonvulsants

- Goal to balance seizure control with drug toxicity
- Use monotherapy, if possible
- Monitor side effects and drug–drug interactions (Table 28.5)
- Wean gradually when seizure free for minimum of 2 yr and neurologically intact; higher risk of recurrence if neurologic deficit, focal seizures, and in first 6 mo after stopping medications

Ketogenic Diet

- For seizures refractory to anticonvulsants at nontoxic levels (especially myoclonic seizures, infantile spasms, atonic seizures, Lennox-Gastaut)
- Classic diet: 4:1 ratio fat to protein and carbohydrate (i.e., 90% calories from fat)
- MCT diet: 50% calories as MCT oil, 21% from other fats
- Adverse effects include abdominal pain, diarrhea, vomiting, renal stones, growth retardation
- Must be started in hospital under care of trained dietitian and neurologist

Surgery

- Intractable seizures with a definite seizure focus; never used as first-line therapy (see Table 28.5)

HEADACHES

HISTORY AND PHYSICAL EXAMINATION

- Onset, description, location, duration, frequency, associated symptoms (vomiting, visual disturbances, weakness), alleviating (drugs, sleep) and aggravating (coughing, bright light) factors, night awakening, precipitating factors (food, stress), and family history
- Growth variables, head circumference, skin, blood pressure, signs of ↑ICP (papilledema), neurologic deficits, cranial bruits, and evidence of sinusitis, otitis media, mastoiditis, or TMJ dysfunction

Table 28.5	Side Effects of Selected Antiepileptic Drugs		
AED*	**Side Effects**	**Monitor**	**Drug Interaction**
Carbamazepine	Leukopenia, diplopia, lethargy, ataxia, rashes, hepatic dysfunction	AED levels, CBC, LFTs	Erythromycin, cimetidine, fluoxetine, warfarin, cyclosporine, oral contraceptives, theophylline
Clonazepam	Tolerance, drowsiness, weight gain, excess salivation, cognitive impairment	–	–
Ethosuximide	Nausea, abdominal pain	AED levels	–
Gabapentin	Lethargy, dizziness, ataxia, rash	–	–
Lamotrigine	Rash, ataxia, diplopia, headache	–	Valproic acid (high risk of rash/SJS)
Levetiracetam	Behavioral changes	–	–
Oxcarbazepine	Drowsiness, hyponatremia	Serum Na$^+$	–
Phenobarbital	Hyperactivity, rash/SJS, drowsiness, impaired cognition	AED levels	Opiates, benzodiazepines, cough preparations, antihistamines, steroids, warfarin
Phenytoin	Hypersensitivity, gingival hypertrophy, hirsutism, ataxia, lymphadenopathy, rash/SJS, lupus-like illness, blood dyscrasias	AED levels	Cimetidine, isoniazid, estrogen, trimethoprim, steroids, cyclosporine, rifampin, warfarin
Topiramate	Lethargy, confusion, glaucoma, low appetite, renal stones	–	–
Valproate	Hepatotoxicity, fatal liver necrosis, weight gain, thrombocytopenia, pancreatitis, hyperammonemia (nausea)	AED levels, CBC, LFTs	ASA, lamotrigine
Vigabatrin	Short-term: GI upset, fatigue, confusion Long-term: visual field defects, behavior changes	Ophthalmologic examination Electroretinogram	–
Zonisamide	↓ Sweating, hyperthermia, drowsiness, anorexia	–	–

*See Section IV for dosages.
SJS, Stevens-Johnson syndrome.

DIFFERENTIAL DIAGNOSIS

- See Table 28.6 for common types
- Other causes include head injury, ↑ICP, seizure, headaches, CNS tumors, stroke, demyelination disorders, vasculitis, hypertension, drug-induced, eye strain, sinusitis, TMJ syndrome (arthritis of TMJ)

Table 28.6	Types of Headaches in Childhood	
Headache Type	Clinical Features	Management
Tension	· Chronic, low grade with long duration, bilateral, diffuse/band-like, dull/aching · Not aggravated by routine exercise · Associated with anxiety or depression · Normal neurologic examination	· Treat underlying stress · Rest · Ibuprofen or acetaminophen
Migraine	· 10% children 5–15 yr, family history often present *Without Aura (Common)* Diagnostic criteria: >4 attacks fulfilling criteria: 1) Attacks last 4–72 h 2) Two of following: unilateral, pulsating, moderate to severe pain, aggravated by routine physical activity 3) At least one of nausea, vomiting, photophobia OR phonophobia during headache *With Aura (Classic)* · Initial transient aura before headache: visual aberrations, dysesthesias, focal motor deficits, mental status changes · Triggers: stress, exercise, head trauma, menstrual cycle, food	· Avoid triggers · Take medication right away · Never use narcotics or other addictive drugs to treat · Rest *Acute attacks:* · Sleep · NSAIDs (e.g., ibuprofen) · Acetaminophen · Promethazine · Triptans (e.g., sumatriptan) *Prophylaxis:* · Amitriptyline · Propranolol · Valproate
Cluster	· Mainly boys, onset after 10 yr · Cluster of daily attacks lasting 2–12 wk · Few times per year, seasonal · Unilateral, sharp or burning, worse supine, associated with coryza, conjunctivitis, tearing, periorbital edema, or ptosis on ipsilateral side · Uncommon	· Prednisone (short-term) · Sumatriptan · Oxygen inhalation (100% 8–10 L/min) · Lithium (chronic)
Analgesic rebound	· Common in all ages · Cycle of headache–analgesic–headache · Diffuse, low intensity, dull, not aggravated by activity · Risk factors: migraine, daily analgesic use	· Stop all analgesics · Headache calendar · Avoid caffeine · Amitriptyline qhs for transition to analgesic-free state · Gabapentin

From Forsyth R, Farrell K. Headache in childhood. *Pediatr Rev.* 1999;20:39–45.

28

INVESTIGATIONS

- Children with no red flags and a normal neurologic examination do not require EEG or neuroimaging; should keep headache diary/calendar
- CT or MRI (with MRA/MRV) if red flags:
  - Signs: ↑ICP (see Raised ICP section)
  - Abnormal neurologic examination/focal neurologic signs
  - <2 yr of age
  - Headaches awaken child from sleep or occur in morning on awakening
  - Seizures or academic deterioration (EEG also indicated)
  - Complicated migraine (neurologic signs concurrent with the headache, not preceding it)
- LP if no signs of ↑ICP: measure opening pressure, CSF for cytology, culture, microscopy, virology; latex agglutination may be warranted if the child is already on antibiotics

MANAGEMENT OF STATUS MIGRAINOSUS

- Definition: daily or severe continuous headaches (intractable); generalized, throbbing, disabling; associated with vomiting or nausea; preceding history compatible with migraine
- Absence of prior headaches should raise concern about more serious cause: consider further investigation

Treatment

1. Chlorpromazine (Largactil) 0.1 mg/kg IV push over 20 min (keep child supine, check BP frequently, and hydrate with 20 mL/kg normal saline over 20–40 min), or prochlorperazine (Stemetil) 0.15 mg/kg IV given over 30 min; promethazine (Phenergan) is commonly used in the United Kingdom, Europe, and Asia; the antiemetic dosage is 0.25–1 mg/kg PO, PR, IM or IV, up to a maximum dose of 25 mg
OR
2. Metoclopramide 0.1 mg/kg IV over 20 min, followed by DHE 0.5 mg slow IV push or IM (repeat dosage if needed in 1 h) if over 16 yr
OR
3. Sumatriptan (Imitrex) nasal spray 5–10 mg, maximum 40 mg/d (off-label use in children <18 yr); it should not be used in basilar or hemiplegic migraine and in patients with uncontrolled hypertension, coronary artery disease, or in conjunction with other ergotamine preparations
- Chlorpromazine/prochlorperazine (phenothiazine group) and DHE cannot be used in sequence or together
- Refractory cases: consult neurologist and consider corticosteroids

RAISED ICP

- Infants: bulging fontanelle, failure to thrive, impaired upward gaze (setting sun sign), large head/macrocephaly, shrill cry
- Children: diplopia, headache (on bending, coughing, Valsalva maneuvers), mental changes, nausea and vomiting, papilledema

- Consult neurosurgeon if abnormal CT or MRI
- See p. 38 for management of ↑ICP

See p. 38 for management of ↑ICP

ACUTE HEMIPARESIS

HISTORY AND PHYSICAL EXAMINATION

- Sudden onset of focal weakness within hours
- Ask about location, hand preference in infants, developmental regression, if preceded by seizures (Todd paralysis), drug use, migraine, trauma, underlying medical conditions (systemic diseases, vascular and congenital malformations, coagulopathies, cardiac), preceding/concurrent infections, cognitive changes
- Vital signs, LOC, full neurologic examination: look for upper motor neuron signs, cardiac and dermatologic examinations

DIFFERENTIAL DIAGNOSIS

- Trauma: head injury, fractures (air, fat embolism)
- Infection: meningitis, focal encephalitis (e.g., herpes simplex)
- Cardiac disease: cyanotic CHD, arrhythmia, bacterial endocarditis
- Systemic disease: hemoglobinopathies (sickle cell disease), diabetes, MELAS, hypertension
- Cerebrovascular disease: occlusive (arteritis, moya moya, lupus), hemorrhagic (AVM, ICH)
- Epilepsy
- Tumor
- Demyelinating disease: MS, ADEM
- Hemiplegic migraine

STROKE

- Vascular lesion causing a focal neurologic deficit lasting >24 h
- TIA: focal deficit lasting <24 h; no new infarcts on CT or MRI

Clinical Presentation

- Hemiparesis (most common), visual field defects, hemisensory deficits, headache, seizures, and ↓LOC; neonates rarely present with focal signs—usually seizures only

Risk Factors

Ischemic Stroke

- Congenital/acquired heart disease (most common), sickle cell disease, dehydration, infections (meningitis, varicella), AIDS, coagulopathies, vasculopathy (vasculitis, dissection, migraine), hemolytic uremic syndrome, homocystinuria, Down syndrome, Williams syndrome, trauma

Hemorrhagic Stroke

- ITP and coagulopathies

History

- Past history of stroke, migraine, or seizures; head or neck trauma; chickenpox in preceding 12 mo; underlying medical conditions; family history of coronary artery, cerebrovascular, or venous occlusive disease before 60 yr of age; medications affecting coagulation

Physical Examination

- Evidence of ↑ICP, focal neurologic deficits, cardiovascular examination including head or neck bruits, evidence of sepsis, and skin lesions including hemangiomas

Investigations and Initial Management

- Further management should be guided in consultation with pediatric neurology or stroke specialists
- See Figure 28.2

Figure 28.2 Scheme of Investigation and Initial Management in a Stroke Patient

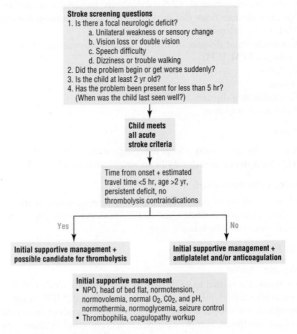

© The Hospital for Sick Children, Department of Neurology.

ACUTE GENERALIZED WEAKNESS

- See Figure 28.3

Figure 28.3 Differential Diagnosis of Generalized Weakness Based on Anatomic Lesion

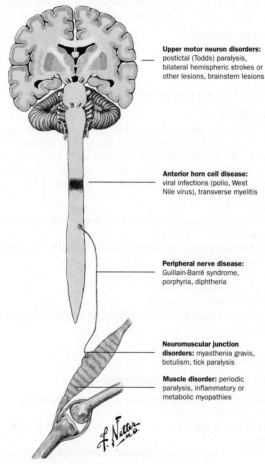

Upper motor neuron disorders: postictal (Todds) paralysis, bilateral hemispheric strokes or other lesions, brainstem lesions

Anterior horn cell disease: viral infections (polio, West Nile virus), transverse myelitis

Peripheral nerve disease: Guillain-Barré syndrome, porphyria, diphtheria

Neuromuscular junction disorders: myasthenia gravis, botulism, tick paralysis

Muscle disorder: periodic paralysis, inflammatory or metabolic myopathies

GUILLAIN-BARRÉ SYNDROME

- Rare disorder involving acute inflammation and demyelination of peripheral nerves
- Commonly preceded by infection, particularly in children <16 yr

Clinical Features

- Rapid onset of weakness (most common presentation) progressing from distal to proximal muscles, starting in legs, then arms; pain; sensory loss; ataxia; cranial nerve palsies in 30–40% of cases; respiratory symptoms (less common); autonomic disturbances
- Triphasic: symptoms reaching the maximum in 2–4 wk, plateau phase for several days to 4 wk, then recovery over weeks to months

Diagnostic Criteria

- Progressive motor weakness
- Areflexia
- ↑CSF protein
- Evidence of acute neuropathy on NCS

Investigations

- NCS, LP (may be omitted if primary infectious process not suspected), CBC, differential, LFTs, urea, Cr, CPK, quantitative immunoglobulins (if IVIG to be given), pulmonary function tests (2×/d × 48 h), CXR (if respiratory compromise), infectious disease workup (including stool culture for poliovirus), ECG (if autonomic dysfunction)

Management

- Monitor respiratory and cardiac function very closely as rapid deterioration can occur
- Watch for autonomic dysfunction (bowel and bladder or hypo/hypertension)
- Consider deep vein thrombosis prophylaxis
- IVIG: 2 g/kg divided over 2 d
- Appropriate pain management
- Physiotherapy: range of motion, monitoring muscle strength, and ambulation

THE FLOPPY INFANT

HISTORY AND PHYSICAL EXAMINATION

- Detailed obstetric history (maternal exposure to toxins or infections may suggest central lesion)
- Onset (floppy at birth if septic, whereas floppy 12–24 h after birth if IEM)
- Progression (static if central hypotonia but worsening in metabolic or degenerative diseases)
- Seizures (central lesion), delayed motor milestones (central or motor unit disease), and family history of neurologic disorders
- Dysmorphic features (CNS lesion/IEM), maternal myotonia (congenital myotonic dystrophy)
- For clues on physical examination, see Table 28.7
- UMN if floppy and strong; LMN if floppy and weak

Table 28.7					Neurologic Signs and Differential Diagnosis by Anatomic Localization in the Floppy Infant	
Localization	Power	Muscle Bulk	Deep Tendon Reflexes	Plantar Response	Differential Diagnosis	Investigations
Central	N or ↓	N or ↓	↑	Extensor	Perinatal asphyxia/HIE, ICH, IEM, genetic disorder, brain dysgenesis, benign congenital hypotonia, cervical spinal cord injury	MRI/CT, chromosomes, metabolic tests
Anterior horn cell	↓	Proximal atrophy	↓ to absent	Flexor to nonreactive	SMA, poliomyelitis	EMG, NCS, specific genetic tests
Peripheral nerve	↓	Distal atrophy	↓	Flexor to nonreactive	Congenital neuropathy, Charcot-Marie-Tooth, metabolic disorders, toxins, trauma	EMG, NCS, nerve and muscle biopsy, DNA analysis
Neuromuscular junction	Fluctuating weakness	N	N to ↓	Flexor	Myasthenia gravis, botulism	EMG, NCS, Tensilon test
Muscle	↓	↓	↓	Flexor	Congenital or metabolic myopathy; congenital muscular or myotonic dystrophy	EMG, NCS, muscle and nerve biopsy, DNA analysis, metabolic tests

N, normal; *Extensor*, upgoing toe; *Flexor*, downgoing toe; *HIE*, hypoxic ischemic encephalopathy; *SMA*, spinal muscular atrophy.
From Crawford TO. Clinical evaluation of the floppy infant. *Pediatr Ann.* 1992;21:348–354.

MOVEMENT DISORDERS

HISTORY AND PHYSICAL EXAMINATION

- Determine nature of movement: paroxysmal or intermittent; pattern or stereotyped, location and duration, presence during sleep, voluntary component, aggravating and alleviating factors
- Ask about underlying medical conditions; seizures, drugs, intoxications, trauma, other CNS pathology
- Ask parent to videotape movement
- See Table 28.8

NEUROLEPTIC MALIGNANT SYNDROME

- Neurologic emergency: most severe adverse reaction to neuroleptics
- Provoking agents: phenothiazines, butyrophenones, thioxanthenes
- Likely due to the blockade of dopaminergic receptors
- All ages, although young men predominate
- 20% mortality due to respiratory failure
- Clinical features: idiosyncratic response with muscle rigidity, akinesia, hyperthermia, altered LOC, autonomic dysfunction (pallor, tachycardia, diaphoresis, hypertension) lasting 1–3 d
- Differential diagnosis: malignant hyperthermia, acute serotonin syndrome
- Investigations: CBC (leukocytosis), differential, urea, Cr, CPK, LFTs, urine dip for myoglobin
- Management: withdraw neuroleptic agent; supportive care (control of hyperthermia, correction of metabolic abnormalities); dantrolene and bromocriptine

Table 28.8	Types of Involuntary Movements
Type of Movement	**Description**
Chorea	· Rapid movement of any body part ± voluntary component · Random, nonrhythmic
Athetosis	· Slow, writhing movement often seen with chorea
Ballismus	· High-amplitude, violent limb movement · Extreme form of chorea
Tardive dyskinesia	· Complex syndrome: buccolingual mastication movements (tongue protrusion, lip smacking, puckering, chewing) and/or extremities/trunk involvement (chorea, athetosis, dystonia, or tremor) · Commonly after exposure to dopamine antagonist (neuroleptics, antiemetics)
Dystonia	· Sustained contractions of agonist and antagonist muscles, resulting in abnormal postures, especially with movement
Tics	· Sudden, brief, complex, stereotyped movements (motor) or sounds (vocal) · Suppressible for short periods but uncomfortable to do so

ACUTE ATAXIA

DIFFERENTIAL DIAGNOSIS

- Idiopathic (acute cerebellar ataxia)
- Intoxication (e.g., drugs, alcohol, antiepileptics [phenobarbital])
- Cerebellar or brainstem tumors, neuroblastoma (opsoclonus–myoclonus–ataxia syndrome)
- Encephalitis
- Labyrinthitis
- Vascular disorders (e.g., lupus, cerebellar hemorrhage)
- Postinfectious/immune disorder (e.g., varicella, Guillain-Barré, multiple sclerosis)
- Trauma

ACUTE CEREBELLAR ATAXIA

Clinical Features

- Self-limiting process, commonly 1–4 yr of age; precedes or follows viral infection (varicella most common); associated with nystagmus, hypotonia, and tremors; recovery within 2 mo, but 30% have persistent neurologic deficit

History

- Previous infections, recent headaches, vomiting, presence of vertigo and neurologic findings, exposure to drugs or toxins, family history

Physical Examination

- Clumsy, wide-based, or staggering gait; difficulty sitting, dysarthria, dysmetria, dysdiadochokinesia, decreased tone, opsoclonus and nystagmus; no weakness or sensory loss

Investigations

- For most children with ataxia: CT or MRI, CSF analysis, viral titers
- Based on clinical presentation, consider metabolic workup, urine catecholamines to exclude neuroblastoma, toxicology screen, EEG

Management

- No specific treatment; ensure that child is safe from accidental self-injury

VENTRICULOPERITONEAL SHUNT FAILURE

- CSF VP shunting used to treat hydrocephalus
- Shunt failure can be due to obstruction (most common), infection, overdrainage, or loculated ventricles

HISTORY

- Signs of ↑ICP, abdominal pain, fever; prior similar history with proven shunt malfunction is best indication

INVESTIGATIONS

- CT or MRI to compare ventricular size with previous scans
- Shunt series (X-ray of skull, chest, and abdomen) to rule out shunt–tube disconnection
- CSF sample through subcutaneous reservoir for culture, if suspicion of infection

NEUROCUTANEOUS SYNDROMES

- See Table 28.9

SPINAL CORD LESIONS

ACUTE SPINAL CORD LESIONS

Clinical Features

- Back pain, deteriorating gait with weakness in lower extremities, alteration in bladder and bowel function, altered pinprick sensation in lower extremities (determine sensory level; see Figure 28.1), hypotonia and hyporeflexia, tenderness over the spine

Etiology

- Trauma (concussion, transection, or contusion of spinal cord), tumor (ependymoma, astrocytoma, neuroblastoma, lymphoma), infection (epidural abscess), transverse myelitis (infections, autoimmune disorders)

Investigations

- Careful neurologic and full physical examination indicated, CBC, CXR, urgent spinal MRI

Management

- Neurosurgical emergency: spinal cord decompression may be indicated

SPINAL DYSRAPHISM

- Neural tube defects resulting from failure of normal neuralation (spinal dysraphism refers to all forms of spina bifida)
- On spinal examination: look for dimpling, pigmentation or hair tufts in lower thoracic, lumbar, or sacral regions

Major Types

- Spina bifida occulta: midline defect of vertebral bodies; no protrusion of meninges or spinal cord; often asymptomatic
- Meningocele: protrusion of meninges through defect in posterior vertebral bodies
- Myelomeningocele: protrusion of meninges and spinal cord through defect in posterior vertebral bodies

Table 28.9 Findings in Neurocutaneous Syndromes

	Neurofibromatosis	Tuberous Sclerosis	Sturge-Weber Syndrome	Ataxia-Telangiectasia
Inheritance	AD (50%)	AD (30%)	Sporadic	AR
Skin findings	· Café au lait spots · Freckling (axilla and groin) · Neurofibromas	· Ash-leaf spots · Shagreen patch · Adenoma sebaceum (usually appears at puberty) · Café au lait spots · Periungual fibroma	· Facial angioma in V1 · Other cutaneous vascular malformations	· Telangiectases · Café au lait spots
Other findings	· Lisch nodules, seizures, developmental delay, bony lesions	· Infantile spasms, developmental delay, MR, calcified tubers in brain, retinal lesions	· Seizures, glaucoma, hemihypertrophy, intracranial AVM, MR	· Ataxia, immunodeficiency, abnormal ocular movement
Tumors	· Plexiform neuroma, optic glioma, acoustic neuroma (NF II), astrocytoma, meningioma, leukemia, pheochromocytoma, neuroblastoma, Wilms tumor	· Optic glioma, SEGA, cardiac rhabdomyoma, renal hamartoma, lung angiomyolipoma	· Intracranial calcifications	· Leukemia, lymphoma, solid tumors

NF, neurofibromatosis.

Management

- Assess for neurologic defects (distal motor paralysis, sphincter dysfunction), musculoskeletal deformity, evidence of hydrocephalus, other congenital anomalies
- Keep infant prone and apply sterile saline dressing to open defect
- Neurosurgical repair ± VP shunt
- Neurogenic bladder may require intermittent catheterization, prophylactic antibiotics, and urologic consultation
- Orthopedic referral
- Counseling: risk of recurrence; folic acid supplements for future pregnancies

TETHERED CORD

- Spinal cord becomes caught or tied down during vertebral column bone growth by scar tissue, fatty mass (lipoma), or a developmental abnormality resulting in stretching of cord
- May be associated with spinal dysraphisms
- Assess for cutaneous signs at base of cord and signs of acute spinal cord lesion
- Investigations: spinal US or MRI
- Surgical untethering of cord indicated if evidence of neurologic symptoms or deterioration

CHIARI MALFORMATIONS

- Chiari I malformation: herniation of cerebellar tonsils through foramen magnum into cervical spinal cord
  - May present as headache, neck pain, lower extremity spasticity, or urinary frequency
- Chiari II malformation: complex congenital malformation of brain, nearly always associated with myelomeningocele and progressive hydrocephalus
  - Downward displacement of the medulla, fourth ventricle, and cerebellum into the cervical spinal canal
  - Elongation of the pons and fourth ventricle, probably due to relatively small posterior fossa

FURTHER READING

Hirtz D, Berg A, Camfield C, et al. Practice parameter: treatment of the child with a first unprovoked seizure: report of the Quality Standards Subcommittee of the American Academy of Neurology and the Practice Committee of the Child Neurology Society. *Neurology*. 2003;60:166–175.

Hirtz D, Ashwal S, Berg A, et al. Practice parameter: Evaluating a first nonfebrile seizure in children: report of the Quality Standards Subcommittee of the American Academy of Neurology, the Child Neurology Society, and the American Epilepsy Society. *Neurology*. 2000;55:616–623.

Singer HS, Kossoff EH, Hartman AL, Crawford TO. *Treatment of Pediatric Neurological Disorders*. Boca Raton, Fl: Taylor & Francis; 2005.

USEFUL WEB SITES

The Neurologic Exam. Faculty of Medicine, University of Toronto. Available at: www.utoronto.ca/neuronotes/NeuroExam/credits_2.htm

American Academy of Neurology. Practice guidelines. Available at: http://www.aan.com/go/practice/guidelines

National Institute of Neurological Disorders and Stroke (NINDS). Available at: http://www.ninds.nih.gov/

Neurology Internet resources. Available at: www.toddtroost.com/mylinks2002.html

Neurology and Neurosurgery

28

Chapter 29 Oncology

Tony H. Truong
Kevin Weingarten
Oussama Abla

Chapter 29 Oncology

COMMON ABBREVIATIONS

ABV/E	adriamycin [doxorubicin], bleomycin, vincristine/etoposide
ALL	acute lymphoblastic leukemia
AML	acute myeloid leukemia
ANC	absolute neutrophil count
BMA	bone marrow aspirate
BMT	bone marrow transplant
COPP	cyclophosphamide, oncovin [vincristine], prednisone, procarbazine
CVL	central venous line
G-CSF	granulocyte colony-stimulating factor
HLA	human leukocyte antigen
HLH	hemophagocytic lymphohistiocytosis
HVA	homovanillic acid
ICP	intracranial pressure
IT	intrathecal
LCH	Langerhans cell histiocytosis
LP	lumbar puncture
MAS	macrophage activation syndrome
NHL	non-Hodgkin lymphoma
PET	positron emission tomography
PLT	platelet
PNET	primitive neuroectodermal tumor
pRBC	packed red blood cells
SVC	superior vena cava
TDM	therapeutic drug monitoring
TLS	tumor lysis syndrome
VMA	vanillylmandelic acid
VWD	von Willebrand disease

COMMON CLINICAL PRESENTATIONS OF MALIGNANCY

- See Table 29.1

APPROACH TO COMMON ONCOLOGY PRESENTATIONS

- See Table 29.2

DIFFERENTIAL DIAGNOSIS OF MEDIASTINAL MASS

- See Figure 29.1

Table 29.1	Common Clinical Presentations of Malignancy
Common Malignancies	**Signs/Symptoms**
Leukemia	Fever, bruising/bleeding, petechiae, fatigue, bone pain, hepato/splenomegaly, lymphadenopathy, skin lesions, chloromas (AML)
Lymphoma	Fever, night sweats, weight loss, fatigue, abdominal/chest/neck/head mass, pruritus, recurrent respiratory symptoms
Neuroblastoma	Mass anywhere (abdomen most common), emesis, hypertension, opsoclonus-myoclonus, periorbital ecchymoses, Horner syndrome, blue subcutaneous nodules ("blueberry muffin baby"), persistent respiratory symptoms
Wilms tumor	Abdominal mass or distension, hypertension, hematuria
Bone tumors	Limp, bone pain, joint pain
Brain tumors	Headache, vomiting, ataxia, seizures, focal deficits, vision changes, irritability, proptosis

DIAGNOSTIC TOOLS

- See Table 29.3

ONCOLOGIC EMERGENCIES

TUMOR LYSIS SYNDROME

- Breakdown of malignant cells and release of intracellular contents, leading to $\uparrow K^+$, $\uparrow$ urate (from release and metabolism of nucleic acids), $\uparrow PO_4^-$, with secondary $\downarrow Ca^{2+}$, and renal insufficiency
- Most common in Burkitt lymphoma, T-cell leukemia, T-cell lymphoma, and precursor B-cell ALL
- Uncommon in AML or other solid tumors (metastatic neuroblastoma, rhabdomyosarcoma may be exceptions)
- May occur spontaneously before therapy, and often after initiation of chemotherapy

Manifestations

- Renal failure: from urate and calcium phosphate crystallization in tubules, which may lead to
  - Cardiac arrhythmias from $\uparrow K^+$ or $\downarrow Ca^{2+}$
  - Seizures and tetany from $\downarrow Ca^{2+}$
  - Metabolic acidosis from massive cell lysis

Management

- See Figure 29.2
- Maintain good urine output, effectively lower urate levels, and monitor laboratory results so that other electrolyte disturbances may be corrected

Table 29.2 — Approach to Common Oncology Presentations

Presentation	History/Physical	Red Flags	Differential Diagnosis	Investigation/Management
Lymphadenopathy	· Duration of nodes, recent infections, fever, night sweats, weight loss, bone pain, travel history, ill contacts, pets (e.g., *Bartonella*), diet (e.g., brucellosis from raw milk) · Rashes, signs of Kawasaki disease, pharyngitis, hepato/splenomegaly, signs of systemic disease	· Noncervical (e.g., supraclavicular) · Asymptomatic, firm, fixed, ≥2.5 cm · Persistent/rapid enlargement · Systemic findings · Abnormal CXR, blood smear	· Infectious (e.g., viral URTI), rheumatologic, drug reaction, lymphoproliferative disorder, storage disease, granulomatous disease, malignancy	· Observe 2–3 wk if no red flags · Antibiotics if infectious · If enlarging, ≥2.5 cm, or not responding to antibiotics, consider CBC, cultures, PPD, viral serology · Biopsy if red flags present
Splenomegaly	· History of fever, bleeding, jaundice, bruising, hemolysis, neonatal illness (e.g., portal vein thrombus), travel, trauma, infection · Size of spleen, hepatomegaly, signs of liver disease, adenopathy, bruising, petechiae, signs of inflammatory or infectious diseases (e.g., SBE)	· Generally an abnormal finding needing further investigation	· Infectious (e.g., EBV, CMV, SBE, TB, malaria) · Hematologic (e.g., sickle cell sequestration, thalassemia, spherocytosis, myeloproliferative disorder) · Infiltration (e.g., storage disorder, malignancy) · Congestive (e.g., portal hypertension) · Rheumatologic (e.g., SLE, JIA)	· CBC, Coombs test, blood smear, LFTs, viral serology, ESR, C3, C4, ANA · US for organomegaly/lymphadenopathy, Doppler for portal vein thrombosis · Refer to pediatric center if persistent or accompanied by systemic symptoms, for BMA, or for bone marrow/lymph node biopsy
Abdominal mass	· Focus on GI/GU symptoms on history (e.g., stooling, pain, urinary symptoms) · Palpable painless mass often the presenting sign in malignant solid tumors	· Systemic symptoms · Hematuria · Enlarging mass	· 50% in neonates and infants are benign renal masses (hydronephrosis, poly/multicystic kidney) · Most common malignancies: Wilms, neuroblastoma · Others: leukemia, lymphoma, sarcoma, hepatoblastoma · Normal anatomy can be mistaken for masses (e.g., stool)	· CBC: polycythemia (Wilms); anemia; marrow involvement · Electrolytes, urea, creatinine · INR/PTT: acquired VWF deficiency (Wilms) · Urinalysis for hematuria · Urine VMA/HVA (neuroblastoma) · XR, US, CT

(continued)

Table 29.2 Approach to Common Oncology Presentations (continued)

Presentation	History/Physical	Red Flags	Differential Diagnosis	Investigation/Management
Mediastinal mass	· History of cough, wheezing, dyspnea without obvious source · Examine for SVC syndrome (see Table 29.4) · Often incidental finding on CXR	· Generally needs further investigation	· See Figure 29.1	· CXR, CT, MRI · Bone marrow studies (differentiate between infection/tumor) · May require emergency approach (see Table 29.4)
Bone lesion	· History of pain, systemic symptoms · Mass palpable in affected area · Often found after a pathologic fracture	· Pathologic fracture · Systemic symptoms	· Benign (more common than malignant); osteoid osteoma, osteochondroma, unicameral/aneurysmal bone cysts, LCH · Malignant: osteosarcoma, Ewing sarcoma, other malignant infiltration (e.g., leukemia)	· XR, CT, MRI, and bone scan · Differentiate between malignant and benign with a biopsy

ANA, Antinuclear antibody; *CMV,* cytomegalovirus; *EBV,* Ebstein-Barr virus; *LFTs,* liver function tests; *JIA,* juvenile idiopathic arthritis; *PPD,* purified protein derivative; *SBE,* subacute bacterial endocarditis; *SLE,* systemic lupus erythematosus; *URTI,* upper respiratory tract infection; *VWF,* von Willebrand factor.

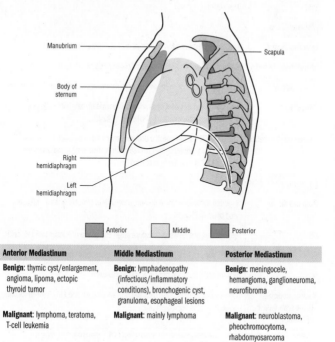

Figure 29.1 Differential Diagnosis of Mediastinal Mass on a Lateral Chest X-Ray

Manubrium

Scapula

Body of sternum

Right hemidiaphragm

Left hemidiaphragm

| Anterior | Middle | Posterior |

Anterior Mediastinum	Middle Mediastinum	Posterior Mediastinum
Benign: thymic cyst/enlargement, angioma, lipoma, ectopic thyroid tumor	**Benign**: lymphadenopathy (infectious/inflammatory conditions), bronchogenic cyst, granuloma, esophageal lesions	**Benign**: meningocele, hemangioma, ganglioneuroma, neurofibroma
Malignant: lymphoma, teratoma, T-cell leukemia	**Malignant**: mainly lymphoma	**Malignant**: neuroblastoma, pheochromocytoma, rhabdomyosarcoma

Management of Electrolyte Disturbances

- See Chapter 16 for details regarding management of ↑K^+
- Consider dialysis if $K^+ > 7$, creatinine >10× normal, urate >600 mmol/L and rising despite treatment, $PO_4^- > 3.2$ mmol/L, symptomatic ↓Ca^{2+}, volume overload, or oliguria
- Correct ↓K^+ or ↓PO_4^- with IV/PO supplementation with caution, considering specific clinical context and if symptomatic, with frequent monitoring of electrolytes

Steps for Management of ↓Ca^{2+}

- ECG/cardiac monitoring
- Observe for tetany and seizures
- Correct ↑PO_4^- by increasing hydration, aluminum hydroxide 30 mg/kg/dose PO tid–qid (50–150 mg/kg/d divided q4–6h) or sevelamer 400 mg PO bid (titrate dose to serum PO_4^-, up to 800–1600 mg/dose PO tid) (both to be given with meals)
- Do not give exogenous Ca^{2+} unless symptomatic from ↓Ca^{2+} or when $Ca^{2+} \times PO_4^-$ (in mmol) product is above 6 because treatment may promote metastatic calcification and renal failure

Oncology

29

Table 29.3	Diagnostic Tests in Cancer Evaluation
Test	**Description**
Laboratory Tests	
Light microscopy	Morphologic examination of marrow aspirate, biopsy, and tumor tissue
Immunohistochemistry	Antibodies to known antigens identify tumor's tissue of origin
Flow cytometry	Laser fluorescence of antibodies on cells determines clonal origin of malignancy
Cytogenetics	Cell culture and microscopy examines karyotype of malignant cells (e.g., Philadelphia translocation in leukemia: t(9;22))
Molecular cytogenetics	FISH and PCR identify specific DNA sequences that correspond to known chromosomal abnormalities (translocations, deletions) in malignancies (e.g., t(11;22) with Ewing sarcoma)
Diagnostic Imaging Tests	
Plain-film XR	For initial evaluation and follow-up, especially of thoracic disease, infection, and bone changes
US	For abdomen and pelvis to determine origin and nature of masses (solid vs. cystic)
CT	For CNS tumors, thoracic and abdominal masses, and adenopathy
MRI	Best modality for brain tumors and MSK tumors
Nuclear medicine (bone scan, gallium, PET, MIBG)	Bone scan to identify bone metastases; gallium scan and PET-CT for lymphoma; MIBG to assess neuroblastoma

FISH, fluorescent in situ hybridization; MIBG, meta-iodobenzylguanidine; PCR, polymerase chain reaction.

FEVER AND NEUTROPENIA

- See Figure 29.3 for fever and neutropenia management algorithm
- 10–20% will have bacteremia
- Algorithm also applies to patients within 6 mo of BMT regardless of ANC

Duration of Therapy

- Afebrile, ANC ≥500/µL, cultures negative at 48 h: discontinue antibiotics
- Afebrile, ANC <500/µL, evidence of hematologic recovery (↑ monocytes, neutrophils, or PLT), cultures negative at 48 h, IV antibiotics ≥48 h: consider discontinuing antibiotics (see Discharge Management section)
- Afebrile, ANC ≥500/µL, cultures positive: consider discontinuing broad-spectrum antibiotics; continue specific therapy
- Consider adding amphotericin after 5–7 d of persistent fever and initiate fungal/extended fever workup (e.g., sinus and chest CT, abdominal US/CT); caspofungin is acceptable first-line empiric agent if ≥2 yr old with AML, relapsed ALL, undergoing BMT, or abnormal renal function

Figure 29.2 **Tumor Lysis Syndrome Prevention Algorithm**

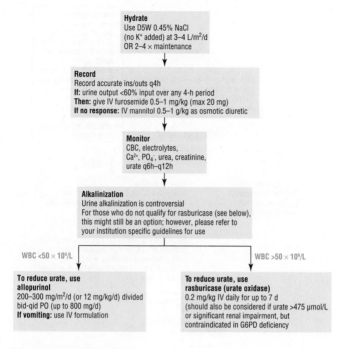

Hydrate
Use D5W 0.45% NaCl
(no K$^+$ added) at 3–4 L/m^2/d
OR 2–4 × maintenance

Record
Record accurate ins/outs q4h
If: urine output <60% input over any 4-h period
Then: give IV furosemide 0.5–1 mg/kg (max 20 mg)
If no response: IV mannitol 0.5–1 g/kg as osmotic diuretic

Monitor
CBC, electrolytes,
Ca^{2+}, PO$_4^-$, urea, creatinine,
urate q6h–q12h

Alkalinization
Urine alkalinization is controversial
For those who do not qualify for rasburicase (see below),
this might still be an option; however, please refer to
your institution specific guidelines for use

WBC <50 × 10^9/L   WBC >50 × 10^9/L

**To reduce urate, use
allopurinol**
200–300 mg/m^2/d (or 12 mg/kg/d) divided
bid-qid PO (up to 800 mg/d)
If vomiting: use IV formulation

**To reduce urate, use
rasburicase (urate oxidase)**
0.2 mg/kg IV daily for up to 7 d
(should also be considered if urate >475 µmol/L
or significant renal impairment, but
contraindicated in G6PD deficiency)

Oncology

29

Discharge Management

- No antibiotics recommended on discharge if
  - Negative blood cultures
  - Afebrile for minimum of 24 h
  - Fever no longer than 96 h
  - Clinically well
  - Evidence of marrow recovery: ↑ monocyte, neutrophil, or PLT counts
- May discharge patient with ANC <500/µL if 48 h IV antibiotics received and aforementioned criteria met
- Avoid routine use of oral antibiotics when discharging patients with the aforementioned criteria; other institutions may differ in approach
- If patient has localized infection and meets discharge criteria, consider discharging with appropriate therapy
- Hospitalize for IV therapy for localized infection if
  - Receiving induction therapy for malignancy known to significantly involve bone marrow
  - Known or suspected noncompliance
  - Clinical sepsis at presentation
- Recurrence of fever should be approached as new fever in neutropenic hosts; requires immediate re-evaluation

Figure 29.3 Fever and Neutropenia Management Algorithm

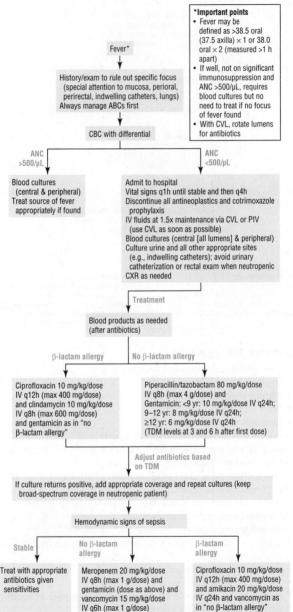

Fever*

History/exam to rule out specific focus
(special attention to mucosa, perioral,
perirectal, indwelling catheters, lungs)
Always manage ABCs first

*Important points
- Fever may be
  defined as >38.5 oral
  (37.5 axilla) × 1 or 38.0
  oral × 2 (measured >1
  h apart)
- If well, not on significant
  immunosuppression and
  ANC >500/µL, requires
  blood cultures but no
  need to treat if no focus
  of fever found
- With CVL, rotate lumens
  for antibiotics

CBC with differential

ANC >500/µL

Blood cultures
(central & peripheral)
Treat source of fever
appropriately if found

ANC <500/µL

Admit to hospital
Vital signs q1h until stable and then q4h
Discontinue all antineoplastics and cotrimoxazole
prophylaxis
IV fluids at 1.5x maintenance via CVL or PIV
(use CVL as soon as possible)
Blood cultures (central [all lumens] & peripheral)
Culture urine and all other appropriate sites
(e.g., indwelling catheters); avoid urinary
catheterization or rectal exam when neutropenic
CXR as needed

Treatment

Blood products as needed
(after antibiotics)

β-lactam allergy

Ciprofloxacin 10 mg/kg/dose
IV q12h (max 400 mg/dose)
and clindamycin 10 mg/kg/dose
IV q8h (max 600 mg/dose)
and gentamicin as in "no
β-lactam allergy"

No β-lactam allergy

Piperacillin/tazobactam 80 mg/kg/dose
IV q8h (max 4 g/dose) and
Gentamicin: <9 yr: 10 mg/kg/dose IV q24h;
9–12 yr: 8 mg/kg/dose IV q24h;
≥12 yr: 6 mg/kg/dose IV q24h
(TDM levels at 3 and 6 h after first dose)

Adjust antibiotics based
on TDM

If culture returns positive, add appropriate coverage and repeat cultures (keep
broad-spectrum coverage in neutropenic patient)

Hemodynamic signs of sepsis

Stable

Treat with appropriate
antibiotics given
sensitivities

**No β-lactam
allergy**

Meropenem 20 mg/kg/dose
IV q8h (max 1 g/dose) and
gentamicin (dose as above) and
vancomycin 15 mg/kg/dose
IV q6h (max 1 g/dose)

**β-lactam
allergy**

Ciprofloxacin 10 mg/kg/dose
IV q12h (max 400 mg/dose)
and amikacin 20 mg/kg/dose
IV q24h and vancomycin as
in "no β-lactam allergy"

SVC SYNDROME, SPINAL CORD COMPRESSION, AND HYPERLEUKOCYTOSIS

- See Table 29.4

SUPPORTIVE CARE

ANEMIA

- Common, usually due to chemotherapy-related myelosuppression, but consider malignant infiltration, secondary myelodysplasia, viral suppression, blood loss, hemolysis
- Recommended transfusion trigger: Hb 60–70 g/L and no signs of imminent marrow recovery, or symptomatic
- For procedures: ensure Hb >70–80 g/L for minimally invasive procedures (e.g., LP); >100 g/L for CVL insertion, other surgery (institutional practices vary)
- Give pRBCs 10–15 mL/kg: matched, leukocyte depleted, irradiated, and CMV negative (if applicable); in emergency, use whatever blood is available
- Leukocyte-depleted/-filtered blood decreases risk of alloimmunization to HLA antigens
- Irradiated blood reduces risk of graft-versus-host disease due to donor lymphocytes
- CMV-negative blood preferred for CMV-negative patients who have undergone or may undergo BMT; leukocyte-filtered/-depleted blood may reduce CMV risk if CMV-negative product unavailable

THROMBOCYTOPENIA

- Usually due to myelosuppression from chemotherapy or malignancy
- Risk of spontaneous hemorrhage increases when PLT <10,000/mm^3
- Transfusion recommended: active bleeding, or PLT <10,000/mm^3; many centers give transfusions to asymptomatic patients with PLT 10,000–20,000/mm^3 to avoid rare risk of intracranial hemorrhage
- For procedures: ensure PLT >50,000/mm^3 for minimally invasive procedures (e.g., LP) and 80,000–100,000/mm^3 for CVL insertion and other surgery
- When PLT transfusion necessary, give 1 unit/5 kg of random donor (pooled) PLT (max 5–6 units/transfusion)

NEUTROPENIA

- G-CSF: to reduce duration of neutropenia after chemotherapy; usual dose 5 mcg/kg SC once daily until neutrophil recovery, usually 10–14 d
- Adverse effects: bone pain (common); fever, nausea, rash (uncommon)

MANAGEMENT OF COMMON SYMPTOMS IN CHRONIC ILLNESS AND MALIGNANCIES

- See Table 29.5 for management of common symptoms in chronic illnesses, including malignancies

Table 29.4 Oncologic Emergencies: Superior Vena Cava Syndrome, Spinal Cord Compression, and Hyperleukocytosis

Emergency	Etiology	Signs/Symptoms	Investigations	Management
SVC/mediastinal syndrome: compression of SVC ± trachea	· Anterior mediastinal mass (NHL, Hodgkin lymphoma, germ cell tumor, ALL) · Thrombosis (e.g., CVL, CVS surgery/catheterization) · Granuloma · Infections	· Chest pain, cough, dyspnea, orthopnea, hoarseness, headache, stupor · Swelling of face, neck, upper extremities; engorged collateral veins; wheezing; pulsus paradoxus	· CXR for mediastinal mass · CBC, differential, blood smear for leukemia, lymphoma · α-Fetoprotein, β-hCG for germ cell tumor · Chest CT · ECG	· *Anesthetic risk* · Elevate head of bed >45°; do not lie patient supine; no sedation or stress, as may precipitate respiratory arrest · Do not intubate unless airway compromise · IV access · If critical airway compression, treat empirically with prednisone 40 mg/m²/d, urate oxidase, hydration, and defer biopsy, but not >48 h
Spinal cord compression	· Primary or metastatic tumor (e.g., neuroblastoma, sarcoma, lymphoma, leukemia, medulloblastoma)	· Back pain, localized tenderness, neurologic deficit; urinary/fecal retention or incontinence	· Spine XR (results may be normal) · Urgent MRI with contrast (gadolinium) or CT myelography if MRI unavailable	· Emergency (rapidly progressive neurologic dysfunction): dexamethasone 1–2 mg/kg IV bolus · Subacute emergency (possible cord compression): dexamethasone 0.25–0.5 mg/kg PO q6h · Urgent Neurosurgery consultation for decompression laminectomy · Other: urgent radiotherapy and chemotherapy
Hyperleukocytosis WBC >100 (× 1000/mm³)	· Presenting feature in ALL (10%), AML (20%) · Increased viscosity can cause widespread microvascular thrombi	· Delirium, lethargy, blurred vision, papilledema, focal deficits, seizures, tachypnea, dyspnea, oliguria, renal vein thrombosis, bleeding anywhere (CNS, GI, pulmonary)	· CBC, differential, blood smear, INR/PTT · Tumor lysis monitoring: include K⁺, Ca²⁺, PO₄⁻, urate, creatinine, urea · BMA and biopsy	· Tumor lysis prevention: hydration, urate oxidase · Chemotherapy as soon as safely possible · Transfuse PLT (1 U/kg) if manual count <50,000/mm³ and correct coagulopathy (FFP 10 mL/kg) to prevent CNS bleeding; avoid pRBC transfusion unless severe symptoms of anemia (if so, give 5 mL/kg) · Consider leukopheresis (temporary measure)

Table 29.5 Common Symptoms in Chronic Illness and Malignancies: Etiology and Management

Symptom	Possible Etiology	Treatment
Anorexia	Pain, nausea and vomiting, anxiety, thrush, drugs, depression, tumor burden	Address cause
Constipation	Inactivity, poor intake, ileus, drugs, fear (e.g., pain, rectal tears), social (e.g., uncomfortable not being at home for toileting)	*Prevention* a) Lubricant (e.g., mineral oil penetrates and softens) b) Surfactant (e.g., sodium docusate is like a detergent, ↑H$_2$0 content) c) Osmotic (e.g., glycerin tip, lactulose softens by osmosis and lubricates) d) Saline (e.g., sodium phosphate, milk of magnesia) releases bound H$_2$0 in stool, may cause peristalsis e) Peristalsis stimulator (e.g., anthracene [senna], polyphenolics [bisacodyl])
Cough	CHF, pulmonary disease, infection, lung metastases, neurodegenerative disorders, GERD, seizures, secretions	· Treat underlying cause; humidifier; positioning: PT; ipratropium/salbutamol; for secretions → suction, hyoscine patches, anticholinergic (glycopyrronium) · Treat with cough suppressors: mild (linctus or pholcodine); moderate (codeine linctus); severe (morphine or diamorphine linctus)
Dyspnea (subjective symptom, not based on measures like respiratory rate)	Anxiety, anemia, CHF, pulmonary disease, brain tumor, ascites, infection, mechanical, metabolic, ↑ICP, muscle dysfunction (neurodegenerative), etc.	*Treat cause* · O$_2$ supplementation by nasal prongs · Fan, cool breeze · Relaxation techniques and medications · Bronchodilators · Analgesia: morphine (PO) or diamorphine (SC) at ½ analgesia dose to ↓ anxiety and pain, settle respiratory center, ↓ pulmonary artery pressure

(continued)

Oncology

29

Table 29.5 Common Symptoms in Chronic Illness and Malignancies: Etiology and Management (continued)

Symptom	Possible Etiology	Treatment
Muscle spasm	Sequelae of neurodegenerative disorder, pain response, epileptic tonic spasms	May need to treat for QOL (e.g., so can sit/stand); PT assessment (positioning, handling, etc.) Diazepam (sedating); baclofen (may exacerbate epilepsy); dantrolene
Nausea and vomiting	a) Cerebellum → vestibular (movement, travel) b) Solitary tract nucleus → vagal/sympathetic/ glossopharyngeal (cough, cytotoxic drugs) c) Chemoreceptor trigger zone (drugs, uremia, ↑Ca²⁺) d) ↑ICP	a) Dimenhydrinate; prochlorperazine b) Domperidone; metoclopramide* (use with diphenhydramine to prevent extrapyramidal reactions) c) Ondansetron;* chlorpromazine; haloperidol d) Dexamethasone* Other options: granisetron, lorazepam,* nabilone
Urinary retention	Mechanical obstruction, neurologic, drugs (e.g. opioid, anticholinergic)	Bladder massage, switch opioid to fentanyl, catheterization, bethanechol, carbachol

*Commonly used in context of chemotherapy/radiotherapy.
CHF, congestive heart failure; GERD, gastroesophageal reflux disease; PT, physiotherapy; QOL, quality of life.
Excerpted from Jassal SS. Basic symptom control in paediatric palliative care. In: The Rainbows Children's Hospice Guidelines. 6th ed. 2006. Available at:
http://cnpcc.ca/documents/2006RainbowHospiceSymptomControlManual.pdf. Accessed September 12, 2007.
Table courtesy of Christine Newman, MD, and Maria Rugg, RN, MN, CHPCN(c). Palliative Care Service, The Hospital for Sick Children, Toronto, Ontario, Canada.

LEUKEMIA

- $>1/3$ of childhood cancer; peak age: 2–5 yr
- Acute: 95%; chronic: 5% (adult-type chronic myelogenous leukemia > juvenile myelomonocytic leukemia)
- See Table 29.6

LYMPHOMA

- See Table 29.7

NEUROBLASTOMA AND WILMS TUMOR

- See Table 29.8

HISTIOCYTIC DISORDERS

- Rare, diverse group of diseases characterized by infiltration and accumulation of antigen-processing and presenting cells (monocyte-macrophage-dendritic cells) in various tissues

LCH

- Accumulation of abnormally activated Langerhans cell histiocytes, lymphocytes, and macrophages; unpredictable course ranging from spontaneous remission to rapid progression and death
- Lesions common in bone, but also skin, bone marrow, lung, and liver

Clinical Features

- Localized (skin or bone) or multisystem (visceral organ involvement/dysfunction)
- Bone: painful lytic lesions in skull or long bones
- Skin: scaly lesions resembling seborrhea
- Lungs: tachypnea or dyspnea; may have nodules, cystic changes
- Liver: hepatomegaly and liver dysfunction
- CNS: diabetes insipidus most common

Treatment and Prognosis

- Observation for solitary bone lesions; chemotherapy for multisystem disease
- High rate of resolution with chemotherapy (68–90%)
- Higher mortality if poor response to initial therapy, multiorgan disease/dysfunction

Table 29.6 Comparison of Acute Lymphoblastic Leukemia vs. Acute Myeloid Leukemia

	ALL	AML
Epidemiology	• 80% childhood leukemia* • Majority B-cell lineage • Peak incidence: 2–6 yr • Males slightly more than females	• 15% childhood leukemia* • Subtypes generally uniform in incidence • Incidence stable from birth with increases in adolescence and during sixth decade of life • Morphology-based classification system (FAB) uses morphology and immunophenotype (M0–M7)
Risk stratification	Low risk: • Standard-risk patient with favorable cytogenetics Standard risk: • Age 1–9 yr • WBC <50 × 10⁹/L at presentation High risk: • Infants with MLL gene rearrangement • CNS disease • T cell Very high risk: • Certain cytogenetics • Induction failure	Low risk: • Favorable cytogenetics Standard risk: • Absence of either favorable or unfavorable cytogenetics and rapid response • Unfavorable cytogenetics in rapid responders High risk: • Induction failure • Secondary AML • Unfavorable cytogenetics
Signs/symptoms	• Bruising/bleeding, petechiae, hepato/splenomegaly, lymphadenopathy • Fever • Fatigue, pallor • Bone pain	Similar to ALL • DIC most common in M3 subtype • Neutropenia ± severe infections at presentation • Skin disease (i.e., chloroma: a malignant, green-colored tumor of myeloid cells)

(continued)

Table 29.6	Comparison of Acute Lymphoblastic Leukemia vs. Acute Myeloid Leukemia (continued)	
	ALL	**AML**
Investigations	· CBC with differential, PLT (manual), reticulocyte count, INR/PTT · Electrolytes, urea, creatinine, urate, Ca^{2+}, PO_4^-, LDH, LFTs, albumin · Immunoglobulins, serology for VZV, CMV, HSV, hepatitis · Urinalysis · CXR (to rule out mediastinal mass) · BMA and biopsy for morphology, flow cytometry, cytogenetics, and molecular genetics	
Treatment	· Prevent tumor lysis syndrome · Treat febrile neutropenia · Length: 2.5 yr (girls), 3 yr (boys) Induction (4 wk) includes prednisone/dexamethasone, PEG-asparaginase, vincristine, and IT methotrexate; daunorubicin added if high risk Consolidation includes PEG-asparaginase, IV and IT methotrexate, oral 6-MP Maintenance (2–2.5 yr) includes oral and IT methotrexate and oral 6-MP Issues during treatment: constipation, vincristine neuropathy (e.g., jaw pain), steroid side effects	· Common therapeutic agents: cytarabine, daunorubicin, etoposide Induction and consolidation (6 mo): remission in 75–90% BMT: · Poor responders, unfavorable cytogenetics, standard risk with matched sibling donor (60–70% have long-term remission) · Special cases: trisomy 21—majority cured with lower intensity
Prognosis	· Low risk: 85–95% cure · High risk: 70–80% cure · Minimal residual disease at end of induction is most important high-risk factor	· Low risk: 70% 5-yr event-free survival · High risk: 40% 5-yr event-free survival

*5% other (see text).

DIC, disseminated intravascular coagulation.

Table 29.7 Comparison of Hodgkin Lymphoma vs. Non-Hodgkin Lymphoma

	Hodgkin Lymphoma	Non-Hodgkin Lymphoma
Epidemiology	· 1/100,000/yr; common in older children · Peak at 15–34 yr and 50+ yr; rare <5 yr; male-to-female incidence: 3:1	· 1.5 /100,000/yr; common in younger children
Signs and symptoms	· Painless lymphadenopathy (90%): "rubbery" nodes; cervical and mediastinal most common · Pruritus, pain with alcohol ingestion, anorexia · B symptoms: weight loss >10% over 6 mo, unexplained recurrent fever, night sweats	· Cervical/axillary lymphadenopathy, mediastinal mass · Burkitt: intra-abdominal mass causing obstruction or intussusception, very fast growing; tumor lysis or renal failure are common complications
Classification	· Lymphocytic infiltrate with malignant multinucleated giant cells (Reed-Sternberg cells) and identification of one of four classic histologic subtypes	· Lymphoblastic (30%): rapidly progressive; usually T cell · Small noncleaved cell (Burkitt/non-Burkitt; 40–50%): B cell · Large cell (20%): B or T cell
Staging	· Each stage may be classified as A or B (if at least one B symptom) · Stage I: single lymph node region or single extralymphatic organ · Stage II: >2 nodes/extranodal regions on same side of diaphragm; may involve spleen · Stage III: tumor on both sides of diaphragm; may involve spleen · Stage IV: diffuse involvement of >1 organ, excluding spleen	· Stage I: single tumor/nodal region outside abdomen or mediastinum · Stage II: >1 nodal/extranodal site on one side of diaphragm · Stage III: tumors or nodes on both sides of diaphragm; all primary intrathoracic; extensive intra-abdominal disease; or any paraspinal or epidural tumors · Stage IV: bone marrow or CNS disease
Investigations	· CBC, liver and renal function, urate, ALP (bone, liver); ESR (active disease), ferritin, immunologic profile (T-, B-cell counts, T-cell function, immunoglobulins) · Staging: CXR; chest/abdomen/pelvis CT; gallium scan or PET; BMA + biopsy (bilateral) · Tissue diagnosis: biopsy	· CBC, liver and renal function, urate, PO_4^-, Ca^{2+}, LDH · Staging: CXR, chest/abdomen CT, bone scan, gallium scan or PET, BMA + biopsy (bilateral), CSF · Tissue diagnosis: biopsy
Treatment	· Combination chemotherapy ± radiotherapy · Chemotherapeutic combinations include COPP and ABV/E	· Manage SVC syndrome (see Table 29.4) and tumor lysis (see Figure 29.2) · Chemotherapy, CNS prophylaxis · Radiation not used in primary treatment
Prognosis	· Stages IA/B, IIA: >90% cure · Stages IIB, IIIA/B, IV: 80% cure · Significant incidence of second cancers	· Stages I, II cure rates: lymphoblastic lymphoma >85%, Burkitt >90%, large cell >90% · Stage III, IV cure rates: lymphoblastic lymphoma >75%, Burkitt 80%, large cell 75%

Table 29.8 Comparison of Neuroblastoma vs. Wilms Tumor

	Neuroblastoma	Wilms
Epidemiology/ etiology	· From neural crest cells; arise along sympathetic pathway · Most common tumor in infancy (8–10% of cancers)	· Also called nephroblastoma · Most common primary renal tumor (6% of all cancers) · Deletion of 11p13 in ~33% of patients · Peak age 3-4 yr
Signs/ symptoms	· Early stages often asymptomatic · In advanced disease, child systemically unwell Presentation varies: · Thoracic: dyspnea, Horner syndrome · Abdominal: palpable mass, vomiting, pain · Pelvic: constipation, urinary retention · Paraspinal: back pain, limp, leg weakness, hypotonia · Metastasis to bone marrow and skin: periorbital bruising (raccoon eyes) and skin nodules (blueberry muffin) · Paraneoplastic syndromes: opsoclonus-myoclonus, intractable watery diarrhea, hypertension, sweating	· Associated congenital anomalies (15%): hamartomas, hemihypertrophy, GU or MSK anomalies · Associated syndromes: Beckwith-Wiedemann, WAGR (Wilms, aniridia, GU anomalies, mental retardation), Denys-Drash (glomerulopathy, pseudohermaphroditism) · Generally asymptomatic · Abdominal mass ± hypertension and hematuria · Bleeding diathesis (acquired VWD) · Polycythemia
Investigations	· Urine VMA/HVA · Abdomen and chest CT · BMA and biopsy (bilateral) · Bone scan and MIBG scan, if available · Tissue biopsy	· If Beckwith-Wiedemann or hemihypertrophy: US q3mo until age 8 yr · CBC (polycythemia), INR/PTT, fibrinogen · Urinalysis (hematuria) · LFTs (metastases), creatinine, urea · Peripheral blood for chromosomal analysis · Abdomen US/CT (look at *both* kidneys) · Chest CT (metastases)

(continued)

Table 29.8 Comparison of Neuroblastoma vs. Wilms Tumor (continued)

	Neuroblastoma	Wilms
Staging	I: localized with complete excision IIA/B: localized with incomplete excision ± ipsilateral node determines A/B III: unresectable tumor crossing midline IV: any tumor with spreading to bone, bone marrow, distant nodes, liver, skin, or other organs (not IV-S) IV-S (limited to patients <1 yr old): localized primary tumor with spreading limited to skin, liver, bone marrow	I: limited to kidney, intact capsule, complete excision II: regional extension, complete excision III: residual tumor in abdomen IV: hematogenous metastases (lung, liver, bone, brain) V: bilateral involvement
Treatment	• Chemotherapy: cisplatin, vincristine, cyclophosphamide, doxorubicin, etoposide • If localized: surgery and short-course chemotherapy • If advanced: chemotherapy, radiation, surgery, and autologous BMT • Minimal treatment for stage IV-S (chemotherapy if organ dysfunction)	• Chemotherapy: dactinomycin, vincristine, ± doxorubicin • Surgery to attempt complete excision followed by chemotherapy, radiation added unless stage I/II with favorable histology • Length of treatment: 18 wk–6 mo (stage dependent)
Prognosis	• Good prognosis: age <1 yr, paraspinal site, opsoclonus, female, stage I, II, IV-S, low ferritin, VMA:HVA >1, aneuploid, favorable histology • Poor prognosis: N-MYC amplification, chromosome 11q and 1p deletions	• Good prognosis: low stage (I/II), favorable histology, no tumor rupture on excision

Adapted from Ater JL. Neuroblastoma. In: Behrman RE, Kliegman R, Jenson HB, eds. Nelson Textbook of Pediatrics. 17th ed. Philadelphia, Pa: WB Saunders; 2004;1709–1711; and from Jaffe N, Huff V. Neoplasms of the kidney. In: Behrman RE, Kliegman R, Jenson HB, eds. Nelson Textbook of Pediatrics. 17th ed. Philadelphia, Pa: WB Saunders; 2004;1711–1714.

HLH

- Life-threatening disorder characterized by unregulated T-cell activation, hemophagocytosis, and cytokine "storm"; often triggered by antecedent infections
- Features include fever, hepatosplenomegaly, skin rash, irritability, seizures
- See Box 29.1 for diagnostic criteria
- MAS may be considered a form of secondary HLH; may be initial presentation or complication of rheumatologic disease (e.g., systemic juvenile idiopathic arthritis); may differ from other forms of HLH (e.g., relative, not absolute cytopenia; increased AST)

Box 29.1 | **Revised Diagnostic Guidelines for Hemophagocytic Lymphohistiocytosis**

Diagnosis of HLH if either 1 or 2 is fulfilled:
1. A molecular diagnosis consistent with HLH
2. Diagnostic criteria for HLH fulfilled (5/8 criteria from A or B below)

A. Initial Diagnostic Criteria
1. Fever
2. Splenomegaly
3. Cytopenias (affecting ≥2 of 3 lineages in the peripheral blood):
   Hb <90 g/L (in infants <4 wk: Hb <100 g/L)
   PLT <100 × 10^9/L
   Neutrophils <1.0 × 10^9/L
4. Hypertriglyceridemia and/or hypofibrinogenemia:
   Fasting triglycerides ≥3.0 mmol/L (≥265 mg/dL)
   Fibrinogen ≤1.5 g/L
5. Hemophagocytosis in bone marrow or spleen or lymph nodes and no evidence of malignancy

B. New Diagnostic Criteria
6. Low or absent NK-cell activity (per local laboratory reference)
7. Ferritin ≥500 mcg/L
8. Soluble CD25 (soluble IL-2 receptor) ≥2400 units/mL

Adapted from Henter JI, Horne A, Aricó M, et al, for the Histiocyte Society. HLH-2004: diagnostic and therapeutic guidelines for hemophagocytic lymphohistiocytosis. *Pediatr Blood Cancer.* 2007;48:124–131.

BONE TUMORS

- See Table 29.9

BRAIN TUMORS

- Second most common group of malignancies in children (20%)
- >50% of children with brain tumors survive >5 yr

Table 29.9 Comparison of Osteosarcoma vs. Ewing Sarcoma

	Osteosarcoma	Ewing Sarcoma
Presentation	· Local pain and swelling, history of injury	· Local pain and swelling, fever
Predisposition	· Familial cancer syndromes, radiation	· None known
Age	· Second decade, peak during growth spurt	· Second decade, peak during growth spurt
Sex (M:F)	· 1.5:1	· 1.5:1
Site	· Metaphysis of long bones (femur 50%, tibia 26%)	· Diaphysis of long bones, flat bones
Investigations	· CBC, liver enzymes, LDH, ALP, urea, creatinine · CT/MRI of primary tumor; chest CT, bone scan to rule out metastases · Biopsy of lesion	· Studies as with osteosarcoma · Diagnostic molecular marker: t(11;22) · BMA and biopsy
Radiographic signs	· Sclerotic destruction or radiating calcification (classic sunburst pattern) in metaphyseal region; soft tissue extension	· Primarily lytic, multilaminar periosteal reaction ("onion skinning") · Bone destruction and soft tissue extension
Metastasis	· Lungs (10–20% at diagnosis), bones	· Lungs (30–40% at diagnosis), bones, bone marrow
Treatment	· Chemotherapy: methotrexate, doxorubicin, cyclophosphamide, ifosfamide, cisplatin · Limb-sparing surgery of primary tumor or amputation	· Chemotherapy: vincristine, doxorubicin, cyclophosphamide with ifosfamide and etoposide · Surgery for primary tumor, if resectable · Radiation for residual or unresectable disease
Outcome	· No metastases: 70% cured · Metastases at diagnosis: 20–40% survival · Poor prognosis: metastases, poor histologic response to chemotherapy	· No metastases: 60–70% cured · Metastases at diagnosis: 30–40% survival · Poor prognosis: proximal/axial skeleton tumor, large tumor, metastases, fever, anemia, aberrant molecular markers

Adapted from Arndt CAS. Neoplasms of bone. In: Behrman RE, Kliegman R, Jenson HB, eds. *Nelson Textbook of Pediatrics.* 17th ed. Philadelphia, Pa: WB Saunders; 2004:1717–1720.

CLASSIFICATION

- 50% supratentorial and 50% infratentorial
- Glial (75%), neuronal, primitive neuroectodermal, or pineal in origin

SIGNS AND SYMPTOMS

Increased ICP

- Vomiting, headache, lethargy
- Irritability, personality change, anorexia
- Cranial enlargement, papilledema, cranial nerve VI palsy (inability to abduct)
- Setting sun sign: impaired upward gaze in infants

Infratentorial Tumors

- Poor balance, truncal ataxia, incoordination
- Impaired conjugate/lateral gaze, facial nerve palsy

Supratentorial Tumors

- Seizures
- Upper motor neuron signs: hemiparesis, hyperreflexia, loss of sensation
- Behavioral problems
- Optic pathway: visual field deficits, nystagmus, head tilt
- Diencephalic syndrome: hypothalamic tumors; 6 mo–3 yr; child is emaciated, anorexic but hyperalert and euphoric
- Parinaud syndrome (pineal tumor): failure of upward gaze and pupillary light reaction

Dissemination to Spinal Cord

- Back/radicular pain, bowel and bladder symptoms, and paraparesis/paraplegia may occur with medulloblastoma and germ cell tumors

DIAGNOSIS AND TREATMENT

- CT for emergent imaging but MRI ± gadolinium best for posterior fossa, cystic/solid tumors, and to assess breakdown of blood–brain barrier
- Surgery: resect when possible for tissue diagnosis, relief of increased ICP
- CSF to assess for tumor cells
- Biopsy of brainstem gliomas often not done because of high morbidity and dismal prognosis
- Radiotherapy has major role as total resection often not possible, recurrence likely
- See Table 29.10 for comparison of brain tumors

Oncology

29

Table 29.10 Comparison of Astrocytoma, Medulloblastoma, Brainstem Glioma, and Craniopharyngioma

Tumor	Astrocytoma	Medulloblastoma	Brainstem Glioma	Craniopharyngioma
Epidemiology	· Usually in first decade	· 80% in <15 yr old · Peak in 3–4 yr old · Most common childhood malignant brain tumor	· Peak age 5–9 yr	· Peak age 5–10 yr
Description	· Glial origin · Low or high grade · Includes optic pathway tumors, as seen in NF-1	· Cerebellar embryonal neuroepithelial tumor · Also a PNET	· Arising from midbrain, pons, and medulla	· Mainly suprasellar, involves pituitary and hypothalamus
Presentation	· Can present as cerebellar, cerebral, optic tumor · See text for details	· CNS spread beyond primary tumor common at diagnosis · Most common brain tumor to metastasize extraneurally (bone/marrow)	· Diagnosis usually made radiographically · See text for details	· Short stature, delayed puberty, hydrocephalus, visual field defects · See text for details
Management	· Surgery for low grade but may use chemotherapy (vincristine, carboplatin)	· Needs MRI and CSF · Radiosensitive but avoid if <3 yr old · Very sensitive to chemotherapy (vincristine, lomustine, cisplatin)	· May surgically remove focal gliomas but surgery often not possible (high morbidity) · Radiotherapy may give initial response but most progress in 8–12 mo · Chemotherapy has a palliative role	· Can excise 75% of slow-growing sella lesions but often results in panhypopituitarism · Radiotherapy reduces recurrence with subtotal resection

(continued)

Tumor	Astrocytoma	Medulloblastoma	Brainstem Glioma	Craniopharyngioma
Outcome	Cerebellar tumor: · Usually not aggressive · Complete excision in 75–90%, >90% survival · Incomplete resection 70–90% survival with radiotherapy Cerebral tumor: · High or low grade · Prognosis related to resectability Optic pathway tumors: · Usually low grade · Common with NF-1	· Standard risk: age > 3 yr, no metastasis, complete/near complete resection · 5-yr survival >80% for standard risk, ~65% for high risk	· Resected focal glioma 80% 5-yr survival · Majority diffusely infiltrative with 90% dying within 18 mo of diagnosis · NF-1 patients are exceptions as tumors may be quiescent	· After total resection: 80% 10-yr survival · 50% 5-yr recurrence if subtotal resection

NF-1, neurofibromatosis type 1.

Adapted from Strother DR, Pollack IF, Fisher PG, et al. Tumors of the central nervous system. In: Pizzo PA, Poplack DG, eds. *Principles and Practice of Pediatric Oncology*. 5th ed. Philadelphia, Pa: Lippincott, Williams & Wilkins; 2006:778–785, 787–791, 795–798, 801–803.

Oncology

29

LATE EFFECTS IN CHILDHOOD CANCER SURVIVORS

- Up to 80% of children diagnosed with cancer survive to adulthood
- Treatment-related effects common: 62% have at least one chronic disease and 27% have a severe/life-threatening condition
- Neurocognitive late effects seen in brain tumor patients and patients with ALL after cranial irradiation and/or IT chemotherapy
- Endocrine late effects (short stature, delayed puberty, hypothyroidism, infertility) seen in patients after head/body irradiation and alkylating agents (cyclophosphamide, ifosfamide)
- Cardiac late effects due to anthracyclines (daunorubicin and doxorubicin) and chest irradiation
- Other therapy-related late effects include hearing loss, lung fibrosis, scoliosis
- Risk of relapse and secondary malignancies persists into adulthood

FURTHER READING

Lanzkowsky P. *Manual of Pediatric Hematology and Oncology.* 4th ed. Burlington, Ma: Elsevier Academic Press; 2005.

Nathan DG, Orkin S, eds. *Nathan and Oski's Hematology of Infancy and Childhood.* 6th ed. Philadelphia, Pa: WB Saunders; 2003.

Pizzo PA, Poplack DG, eds. *Principles and Practice of Pediatric Oncology.* 5th ed. Philadelphia, Pa: Lippincott Williams & Wilkins; 2006.

USEFUL WEB SITES

Abramson Cancer Center of the University of Pennsylvania. Available at: www.oncolink.com

American Cancer Society. Available at: www.cancer.org

British Columbia Cancer Agency. Available at: www.bccancer.bc.ca

National Cancer Institute. Available at: www.cancer.gov

Chapter 30 Ophthalmology

Radha Kohly

Nasrin Najm Tehrani

Chapter 30 Ophthalmology

COMMON ABBREVIATIONS

CN	cranial nerve
EOM	extraocular movement
FB	foreign body
ICP	intracranial pressure
OD	right eye
OS	left eye
OU	both eyes
ROP	retinopathy of prematurity
STI	sexually transmitted infection

COMMON OCULAR COMPLAINTS

- See Box 30.1

PHYSICAL EXAMINATION OF THE EYE

VISUAL ACUITY

- Always measure visual acuity before manipulating eye
- Test best corrected vision (wearing glasses, or through pinhole)
- Test at 6 m (20 ft) with Snellen chart (OD, OS, OU); record results as ratio (e.g., "20/50 $^{-2}$" indicates patient read line of letters at 20 feet that a normal eye could read at 50 feet; minus 2 indicates two mistakes made)
- In urgent cases, do crude test such as counting fingers, hand motion, or light perception

Assessment Options in Young Children

- Cover-uncover test: ensure central (corneal light reflection centered in cornea), steady (no nystagmus), and maintained (fixation maintained upon uncovering eye)
- Test fixation and following
- Cover testing to see whether objection to either eye being covered

PUPILS

- Assess if equal in size and reaction to light and accommodation
- Check for afferent pupillary defect using swinging flashlight test: check direct light reflex (pupil reacts to light), consensual light reflex (both pupils react when light is shone into one eye), then move light back and forth; see relative dilatation when light is brought back to affected eye

Box 30.1 | Differential Diagnosis of Common Ocular Complaints

Red Eye

Conjunctivitis, subconjunctival hemorrhage, trichiasis (lashes growing in toward the cornea), blepharitis, lagophthalmos (incomplete eyelid closure), acne rosacea, iritis, episcleritis, scleritis, dacryocystitis, contact lens related, traumatic (conjunctival, corneal abrasion), FB

Tearing

Nasolacrimal duct obstruction (most common), FB, congenital glaucoma

Discharge

Conjunctivitis, blepharitis, corneal ulcer, endophthalmitis

Photophobia

Conjunctivitis, corneal abnormality (abrasion/FB/ulcer/contact lens related), iritis, albinism, aniridia, congenital glaucoma, drugs (dilating drops), migraine, meningitis, optic neuritis

Blurry Vision

Refractive error, amblyopia, conjunctivitis, corneal abnormality (abrasion/FB/ulcer/contact lens related), iritis, vitritis, retinal pathology (e.g., detachment, vasculitis), optic nerve pathology (papillitis, optic neuritis, papilledema), drugs

Eyelid Swelling

Traumatic, stye/chalazion, contact dermatitis, herpes simplex, lid/lacrimal gland mass, dacryocystitis, preseptal or orbital cellulitis

Proptosis

Orbital cellulitis, orbital mass, retrobulbar hemorrhage, thyroid eye disease, cavernous sinus thrombosis, carotid cavernous fistula, idiopathic orbital inflammation (pseudotumor), pseudoproptosis (e.g., contralateral enophthalmos, high myopia, congenital glaucoma)

Transient Vision Loss

Seconds: papilledema
Minutes to hours: ocular migraine, transient ischemic attack, vertebrobasilar artery insufficiency, impending central retinal artery occlusion

Monocular Diplopia

Visual axis abnormalities, media opacities, corneal/pupil/lens-related problem (cataract, subluxed lens [e.g., in Marfan syndrome, homocysteinuria]), or retinal pathology

Binocular Diplopia

Decompensated phoria, posttrauma/surgery, orbital inflammatory disease (pseudotumor), myasthenia gravis, thyroid eye disease, internuclear ophthalmoplegia, CN III, IV, or VI palsy, carotid cavernous fistula

Flashing Lights

Retinal tear or detachment (flashes lasting seconds), ocular migraine (flashes lasting minutes), seizure (rare), oculodigital stimulation

Floaters

Posterior vitreous detachment, migraine, vitritis

SLIT LAMP EXAMINATION OR EXTERNAL EXAMINATION

Lids/Lashes/Lacrimal Gland

- Lacrimal gland: check for masses, tenderness
- Lids and lashes: look for redness, crusting, masses that may be associated with blepharitis (stye or chalazion), and trichiasis

Sclera/Conjunctiva
- Check for injected vessels (ciliary flushing around limbus: important finding in iritis)
- Check for nodules, cysts, nevi, tumors

Cornea
- Most common: punctate keratitis, abrasions, ulcers (chalky white spots on cornea through which iris detail cannot be seen), and FB

Anterior Chamber
- Assess depth; shallow or deep (use slit lamp or penlight); check for cells (WBCs, RBCs)

Iris
- Check for pigmentation, nodules, cysts, abnormal vessels, iridodialysis (traumatic separation of iris from ciliary body), tumors

Lens
- Check for cataracts and lens subluxation

COLOR VISION
- Use Ishihara color plates
- Check red saturation: ask patient to rate color red in each eye between 0% and 100%, 100% being full red saturation and 0% being none; eye with decreased red saturation is abnormal

CONFRONTATION TESTING FOR VISUAL FIELDS
- Test all four quadrants in each eye while occluding other eye (while facing the patient with patient fixing open eye on yours, test patient's ability to see target/finger you bring in from periphery to center with your own)

EXTRAOCULAR MOVEMENTS AND OCULAR ALIGNMENT
- Check range of movement in both eyes in following gaze positions: right, left, up, down, up right, up left, down right, and down left
- Check saccadic and smooth pursuit movements
- Check eye alignment with Hirschberg (light reflex) test (Figure 30.1): shine penlight at the eye; light reflection should be centered in pupil or just nasal to center; if one eye is not aligned with the other, light reflection is displaced in opposite direction of misalignment relative to pupil center

FUNDUS EXAMINATION
- Vitreous: if view of fundus is blurred, may have vitritis or vitreous hemorrhage
- Macula: area between temporal retinal vascular arcades; lesion here can decrease vision

Figure 30.1 Hirschberg Test. Light Reflection on Cornea Is Observed by Examiner

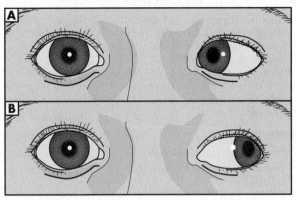

A, Left esotropia; in-turning of left eye; light reflection appears to be lateral to center of pupil. B, Left exotropia; out-turning of left eye; light reflection appears medial to center of pupil.

- Disc: assess for clear vs. blurry borders, pink vs. pale disc, disc hemorrhage
- Vessels: look for increased dilatation or tortuosity, hemorrhage, vascular sheathing

ROUTINE SCREENING

- See Table 30.1

Table 30.1	Routine Eye Screening	
Age	Screening Test	Referral to Ophthalmology Required
Premature neonates		See Chapter 26
Newborns	Red reflex at every well-child visit	Absent (black/white) or asymmetric red reflex
	Corneal light reflex test at every well-child visit	Ocular misalignment (strabismus)
	External examination at every well-child visit	Structural defect
Infants and toddlers	As above for newborns plus fixation and following, objection to cover test	As above for newborns plus abnormal eye movements, objection to covering of one eye as compared with the other
Yearly until age 10 yr, then every 2–3 yr	As above for infants/toddlers plus visual acuity test	As above for newborns plus, on repeated testing, ≥ 2-line difference between eyes, worse than 20/30 either eye before age 5 yr, or worse than 20/20 either eye after age 5 yr

HORDEOLUM (STYE) AND CHALAZION

- Obstruction of ducts of eyelid glands; on eyelid margins (stye, hordeolum) or within lid (chalazion); usually not infected despite swelling/discharge; chalazion may be chronic noninflamed painless lump
- Treatment: daily baby shampoo eyelash scrubs with cloth; warm compresses to lids od to bid; may add erythromycin or bacitracin/polymyxin B sulfate (Polysporin) ointment until symptoms subside; refer if symptoms affect vision or condition persists despite lid scrubs for 4–6 wk

BLEPHARITIS

- Inflammation, crusting, and scaling of lid margins; dry eye symptoms including burning and itching; may be associated with red eye
- May be associated with styes and/or chalazion
- Treatment: see Hordeolum (Stye) and Chalazion section

LID TRAUMA

- May result in ptosis secondary to ecchymosis, edema, or a laceration
- Complete dilated eye examination to rule out intraocular FB, globe perforation, or blunt injury; upper lid puncture wounds usually require imaging to rule out globe perforation
- Ophthalmologic consultation if full thickness lid laceration, lid margin involvement, loss of tissue (avulsion), or ptosis that persists after swelling resolved

PTOSIS

- Drooping of eyelid (usually upper eyelid); unilateral or bilateral; congenital or acquired; isolated or associated with other ocular disorders (e.g., lid tumors, congenital fibrosis syndrome, CN III palsy, Horner syndrome) or systemic disorders (e.g., myasthenia gravis, muscular dystrophy)
- Pseudoptosis: differential includes enophthalmos (after blow-out fracture), small eye (microphthalmia), eyelid lesion (e.g., chalazion/stye, tumor), eyelid swelling
- See Table 30.2

ORBIT

- See Table 30.3 for preseptal vs. orbital cellulitis

Table 30.2	Horner Syndrome vs. Cranial Nerve III Palsy	
	Horner Syndrome	**CN III Palsy**
Upper lid	Mild ptosis	More severe ptosis
Lower lid	Lower lid may be higher than other side (upside-down ptosis)	Unaffected
Pupil	Miosis	Mydriasis
Other features	Anhydrosis	Restricted adduction and elevation (eye "down and out")
Imaging	Head/neck/chest/abdomen CT to rule out neuroblastoma	Neuroimaging to rule out intracranial lesion
Surgical indications	To eliminate abnormal head posture, maintain binocular vision, improve visual field, or prevent amblyopia	

Table 30.3	Preseptal vs. Orbital Cellulitis	
	Preseptal Cellulitis	**Orbital Cellulitis**
Anatomy	Infection anterior to orbital septum	Serious infection posterior to orbital septum May spread posteriorly to cavernous sinus and brain (causing cavernous sinus thrombosis or meningitis)
Possible precipitants	Infection on eyelids or face (stye/chalazion, skin trauma), dental abscess	Paranasal sinusitis; less often from preseptal cellulitis, intraocular infection or tumor
Symptoms	Pain, redness, systemically well	Pain, redness, systemically unwell
Signs		
Fever	Afebrile	Febrile
Eyelids	Red, swollen	Red, swollen
Vision	Normal	Decreased acuity; decreased visual field (if optic nerve involved)
Proptosis	None	Present
EOMs	Normal, full	Decreased, painful EOMs
Pupils	Normal, reactive	Abnormal reaction (if optic nerve involved)
Common organisms	Nontraumatic: *Streptococcus pneumoniae*, group A streptococci, *Staphylococcus aureus*, *Haemophilus influenzae* Traumatic: *S. aureus*	
Workup	No imaging required	CT to look for sinusitis, orbital/subperiosteal abscess or cavernous sinus thrombosis (dilated superior orbital vein)
Treatment	Outpatient PO antibiotics (cloxacillin or cefazolin) unless infection severe, worsening on antibiotics, systemically unwell, immunocompromised, or <3 mo old	Prompt ophthalmology and ENT consults Inpatient IV antibiotics with aerobic and anaerobic coverage (cefotaxime or ceftriaxone with metronidazole); nasal decongestant if sinusitis Ophthalmology examination daily; consider surgical drainage if not improving or abscess present

NASOLACRIMAL DUCT OBSTRUCTION

- Seen in infants < 12 mo old; failure of canalization of nasolacrimal duct as enters nose
- Recurrent mild discharge that worsens on waking, typically with no conjunctival injection, ± tearing that worsens outdoors and during upper respiratory infection
- Often crusted lid margins and chronic lower lid skin changes
- Rarely develops acute infection of nasolacrimal sac (dacryocystitis; see next section)
- Treatment: massage several times per day (place index finger in sulcus between eye and side of nasal bridge and apply pressure downward; discharge may be expressed onto eye surface); clean crusted lids with moist cloth; if conjunctivitis, add topical antibiotics (e.g., trimethoprim sulfate/polymyxin B sulfate [Polytrim] or bacitracin/polymyxin B sulfate [Polysporin]) for 1 wk
- Majority resolve spontaneously by 1 yr of age; if persistent, refer to ophthalmologist

DACRYOCYSTITIS

- Rare acute infection of nasolacrimal sac with inflammation of surrounding tissues between eye and nose; may be associated with or preceded by lacrimal sac mucocele
- More common in infants < 1 mo old
- Treatment: consider IV antibiotics (e.g., cefazolin), then nasolacrimal probing

CONJUNCTIVA

OPHTHALMIA NEONATORUM

- Form of conjunctivitis in infants < 1 mo old; all newborns should be given prophylactic erythromycin ointment (or 1% silver nitrate drops, if others unavailable) for prevention of chlamydial and gonococcal conjunctivitis
- Must evaluate newborn for other STIs (HIV, syphilis, hepatitis B); arrange for testing and treatment of mother and partner(s)
- Note: conjunctivitis in newborn can also be caused by various other bacteria and viruses

Neisseria gonorrhoeae Conjunctivitis

- Marked purulent discharge and lid edema; vision-threatening emergency
- Stat Gram stain shows intracellular gram-negative diplococci
- Treat with IM cephalosporin ± topical erythromycin (after cultures and *Chlamydia* testing); frequent ocular lavage with normal saline to reduce bacterial load

- If gram negative but clinically purulent, admit for treatment until culture negative; must consult ophthalmologist as gonorrhea keratitis can rapidly result in corneal perforation

Chlamydia Conjunctivitis

- Milder conjunctivitis, less discharge and lid edema compared with gonococcus
- Eye swab for rapid immunologic tests, Giemsa stain, and culture
- Treat with erythromycin 40–50 mg/kg/d PO divided qid for 14–21 d to prevent subsequent pneumonitis, in addition to topical erythromycin

CONJUNCTIVITIS BEYOND NEONATAL PERIOD

- See Table 30.4 for differential diagnosis of conjunctivitis

Subconjunctival Hemorrhage

- Causes: blunt trauma (most common), Valsalva maneuver, forceful coughing (e.g., pertussis), vomiting, bleeding diathesis, severe hypertension, suffocation
- If extensive (180–360°) and history of trauma, suspect ruptured globe
- Treat with artificial tears for comfort; blood resorbs over few weeks

FB

- May be hidden in recesses of fornices; have patient look in all directions; may need upper lid eversion; fluorescein stain (rule out laceration, corneal abrasion); remove with forceps after placing anesthetic drop into eye

CORNEA

ABRASION

- Symptoms may include pain, tearing, photophobia, decreased vision; pain improves with topical anesthetic (diagnostic and temporarily therapeutic); may have minimal symptoms
- Fluorescein stain shows area of absent corneal epithelium; if vertical linear abrasion(s), suspect conjunctival FB under upper lid and perform lid eversion
- Look for chalky white lesion (i.e., ulcer) on slit lamp examination; urgent referral if present
- If no ulcer, treat with polymyxin B or erythromycin ointment plus cycloplegic agent (cyclopentolate 1% or homatropine 2%); refer to ophthalmologist if symptomatic after 24–48 h, large central abrasion, or poor healing
- Topical anesthetics should not be prescribed as they delay healing and may cause an ulcer
- No need to patch eye (does not improve healing or pain); may patch if patient prefers
- Note: patch should *never be used* for contact lens wearers, *even after* contact lens removed (increased risk of infection) or in those who have abrasion secondary to vegetable matter in eye (e.g., tree branch)

Table 30.4 Differential Diagnosis of Conjunctivitis

Feature	Bacterial (Nonchlamydial)	Viral (Nonherpetic)	Herpetic	Chlamydial	Allergic	Chemical
Discharge	Purulent	Clear or mildly purulent	Clear	Clear or mildly purulent	Clear	Rare acutely
Lid swelling	Moderate to severe	Mild to severe	Mild	Mild	Mild to severe	Mild to severe
Onset	Subacute	Subacute	Acute	Subacute or chronic	Hyperacute (exposure) or chronic (seasonal)	Acute
Injection	Severe	Moderate to severe	Moderate	Moderate	Mild to severe	Mild to severe; white eye more worrisome (tissue necrosis)
Cornea fluorescein stain	Nonspecific	Nonspecific	Superficial punctate keratitis, dendritic ulcer	Nonspecific	None	Nonspecific
Unilateral/bilateral	Uni/bilateral	Usually bilateral (second eye affected days later)	Unilateral (bilateral may be seen if history of atopy)	Usually bilateral	Usually bilateral	Uni/bilateral
Contact history	Common	Common	No	Common (STI)	Rare	Common
Preauricular node	Common	Common	Occasional	Occasional	None	None
Other associations	Otitis media	Otitis media, pharyngitis	History of eyelid or oral lesions	Genitourinary infection	Chemosis*	Chemosis*, limbal ischemia. Alkali injury worse than acid

(continued)

Table 30.4 — Differential Diagnosis of Conjunctivitis (continued)

Feature	Bacterial (Nonchlamydial)	Viral (Nonherpetic)	Herpetic	Chlamydial	Allergic	Chemical
Treatment	Erythromycin, polymyxin B, or polymyxin/trimethoprim Avoid sulfa agents, aminoglycoside, quinolones[†]	Symptomatic relief: cool compresses, artificial tear drops, as needed; hand hygiene important to prevent spread	Trifluridine[†] (Viroptic): 1 drop, 5–9×/d × 14 d Consult Ophthalmology NEVER prescribe steroids	Systemic and adjunctive topical antibiotics Consult Ophthalmology	Avoid allergens; consider artificial tears, mast cell stabilizers (e.g., cromolyn drops), systemic antihistamines	Irrigate eye with water × 20 min ASAP after instillation of anesthetic drops In ER: copious lavage with saline; use 2 L or until pH equal to nonaffected eye (average pH 7) After lavage, treat as corneal abrasion and consult Ophthalmology

*Chemosis: conjunctival swelling.
[†]See Table 30.7 for antimicrobial eye medications.

Ophthalmology

30

CLOUDY CORNEA

- May indicate glaucoma or systemic disease (e.g., mucopolysaccharidosis)
- Congenital glaucoma may also present with enlarged eyeball (buphthalmos), watery eyes, photophobia, blepharospasm
- Urgent Ophthalmology consultation in all cases to treat/prevent amblyopia

ANTERIOR CHAMBER

HYPHEMA

- Blood in anterior chamber (behind cornea in front of iris)
- Almost always sign of severe ocular trauma; urgent Ophthalmology consultation
- Treatment: bed rest, eye shield, topical steroids, cycloplegics, and antiglaucoma drops, if necessary
- Recurrent hemorrhage and secondary glaucoma may occur, especially in first 3–5 d; daily ophthalmic follow-up during this period

IRITIS (UVEITIS)

- Inflammation of uvea (iris, ciliary body, and choroid); consider traumatic, inflammatory, infectious, and malignant causes
- Diagnosis: ciliary flush (conjunctival injection at corneal–scleral junction), endothelial precipitates, iris nodules, cells and flare in the anterior chamber, vitritis, and chorioretinitis
- Treatment: refer to ophthalmologist for topical cycloplegics and steroids; oral and/or IV steroids and other immune-modulating drugs in severe cases

HYPOPYON

- Collection of white cells (pus) or tumor cells in anterior chamber
- Causes include internal ocular infection (endophthalmitis), retinoblastoma, leukemia, severe iritis; refer promptly to ophthalmologist

PUPIL AND IRIS

AFFERENT PUPIL DEFECT (MARCUS GUNN PUPIL)

- Unilateral or asymmetric defects of anterior prechiasmal optic pathway (e.g., optic neuritis) or extensive retinal dysfunction (e.g., total retinal detachment); pupils should still be of equal size due to intact pupil–light reflex
- Diagnosed using bright light in swinging flashlight test

ANISOCORIA

- Pupils of unequal size; must ascertain which pupil abnormal by examining under different illuminations: if anisocoria worse in dim light, smaller pupil is abnormal (does not dilate properly [e.g., Horner syndrome]); if anisocoria worse in bright light, larger pupil is abnormal (does not constrict normally [e.g., CN III palsy, traumatic or pharmacologic mydriasis])
- May be physiologic (approximately 20% of population); relative difference (usually 1 mm) in pupil size is same in bright or dim illumination

COLOBOMA

- Inferior nasal defect in iris ("keyhole" pupil)
- May be associated with microphthalmia (small eye) or cataract and chorioretinal coloboma; refer to ophthalmologist

LEUKOCORIA

- White pupil
- Ocular emergency; retinoblastoma until proven otherwise
- Other causes include cataract, infection (*Toxoplasma*, *Toxocara*), retinal detachment

ABSENT RED REFLEX

- Absent (black) reflex
- Light unable to pass because of obstruction (e.g., corneal opacity, hyphema, cataract, vitreous hemorrhage)
- Requires consultation with ophthalmologist
- Most common cause is small pupils; no referral needed if normal red reflex after pharmacologic dilation of pupils

RETINA

RETINAL HEMORRHAGES

- On retinal surface (preretinal), within layers of retina (intraretinal), under retina (subretinal)
- Common in newborns, after routine vaginal delivery; resolves within weeks
- Most common cause after birth in <4 yr is shaken baby syndrome; must consider and evaluate for child maltreatment (see Chapter 10)
- Other rare causes include leukemia, vasculitis, meningitis, cyanotic congenital heart disease, endocarditis, sepsis, blood dyscrasia, severe life-threatening accidental head trauma (<3%); in these entities, hemorrhages tend to be few and confined to posterior retina (around optic nerve and macula)
- Note: sickle cell disease, diabetes, and seizures *do not* cause retinal hemorrhages in first few years of life

CLINICAL FEATURES OF OPTIC NERVE DISEASE

- Reduced vision
- Impaired color vision (may be preserved)
- Afferent pupil defect
- Visual field loss
- ± Pain with EOMs

PAPILLEDEMA

- Usually from increased ICP; also consider optic nerve infiltration by malignancy, TB, sarcoidosis
- Earliest signs: blurred disc margins with diminished view of vessels on disc surface; splinter hemorrhages, disc elevation, loss of optic nerve central cup, dilation and tortuosity of retinal veins, retinal exudates
- Vision usually unaffected but may get transient bilateral visual blurring or loss (transient visual obscurations); in chronic papilledema, fibrosis/atrophy may cause visual loss with visual field constriction
- Other manifestations include tinnitus, diplopia (CN VI palsy)
- Papillitis (unilateral or bilateral) looks similar on examination, but vision decreased early and often severely affected
- Treatment depends on underlying cause

OPTIC ATROPHY

- Characterized by disc pallor (white disc): may be congenital or acquired
- Requires thorough ophthalmic and neurologic investigations

OPTIC NERVE HYPOPLASIA

- Congenital anomaly; may maintain good vision in mild cases; severe forms can cause legal blindness (<20/200 vision) and nystagmus
- Diagnosis is clinical: smaller optic nerve than normal; may have surrounding halo of retinal pigmentation (double-ring sign)
- Mostly unilateral; if bilateral, require neurologic assessment for CNS abnormalities (e.g., septo-optic dysplasia or pituitary insufficiency); MRI of brain and visual pathways recommended

STRABISMUS AND AMBLYOPIA

- Strabismus: any abnormal eye alignment
- Assess with Hirschberg test (see Figure 30.1); normal in pseudo-esotropia/pseudoexotropia
- Refer child with strabismus after 3–4 mo of age because eyes should be straight and move in tandem by this age—sooner if eyes extremely misaligned or not moving normally
- Children with neurologic problems (e.g., cerebral palsy or after head trauma) can display various abnormalities of eye alignment

30

- Strabismus is only emergent when eye(s) cannot move fully in all directions; may indicate paretic muscle (e.g., CN palsy) or restriction (see Blow-Out Fracture in Table 30.5)

AMBLYOPIA

- Subnormal vision in absence of structural defect along visual pathway; may result from strabismus, refractive error, ptosis, cataract
- Strabismus may cause amblyopia in the misaligned eye, but in many cases, both eyes retain equal vision despite strabismus because of alternate fixation (no amblyopia if each eye used for equal amounts of time)
- Amblyopia can be unilateral or, less commonly, bilateral; most common pediatric cause of vision loss (up to 4% of population)

TRAUMATIC EYE INJURIES

- See Table 30.5

COMMON OPHTHALMIC MEDICATIONS

- See Table 30.6 for common ophthalmic agents
- See Table 30.7 for common ophthalmic antimicrobials

Table 30.5	Traumatic Eye Injuries		
	Corneal Lacerations or Ruptured Globe	**Blow-Out Fracture**	**Retrobulbar Hemorrhage**
Preceding trauma	Blunt or penetrating	Blunt	Blunt
Eye symptoms and signs	Abnormally shaped pupil, hyphema, prolapsed iris, tissue protruding from sclera, 360° subconjunctival hemorrhage, chemosis	Restricted EOMs; initially proptotic and later enophthalmic; hypoesthesia over inferior orbital skin (inferior floor fracture)	Decreased vision, proptosis
Diagnostic aids	Nonpressure techniques to gently examine: stop examination once confirmed	CT scan (axial + coronal)	Afferent pupil defect, raised intraocular pressure
Management	Eye shield; no pressure on eye; no eyedrops/patch	Surgery for severe enophthalmos, diplopia in primary position, >50% fracture, orbital roof fracture, failed medical management	Prompt canthotomy/cantholysis to release pressure
Referral to Ophthalmology	Immediate	Early	Immediate

Table 30.6 Common Ophthalmic Agents

	Description	Method of Use	Onset	Duration	Use
Anesthetic	Proparacaine HCl 0.5% Tetracaine 0.5%	Not for home use: toxic to corneal epithelium, delays healing May cause corneal ulcer	15–20 s	20 min	Renders corneal epithelium insensitive to pain from cornea/conjunctiva
Anti-inflammatory	Topical steroids	Must use only under care of ophthalmologist	–	–	Inflammatory eye conditions (e.g., uveitis) NB: worsens glaucoma, herpetic, bacterial, or fungal ulcers
Fluorescein dye	Water-soluble orange dye; becomes green when viewed under cobalt/fluorescent blue light	Moisten dry fluorescein strip with sterile water or saline, then apply to inferior bulbar conjunctiva	Spreads across cornea in a few blinks	Transiently turns tears orange	Diagnoses abrasions (corneal/conjunctival), corneal herpetic dendrites, FB
Mydriatic					
Parasympatholytic (paralyses iris sphincter)	Tropicamide	0.5% in preterm, otherwise 1%	30 min	4–5 h	Dilates pupils
Cycloplegic (paralyses accommodation)	Cyclopentolate HCl		30 min	Up to 12 h	
	Homatropine 2%	Use only in >1 yr old	60 min	24–48 h (cycloplegia)	
Adrenergic (dilates pupillary muscle)	Phenylephrine HCl 2.5%		15–30 min	2–6 h	Adjunct in corneal abrasion

HCl, hydrochloride.

Table 30.7 Common Ophthalmic Antimicrobials*

	Examples	Sample Prescription	Special Use	Precautions
Antibiotics				
Macrolides	Erythromycin (O)	bid-qid	Chlamydial conjunctivitis	
Fluoroquinolones	Ciprofloxacin (D)	1-2 drops q2-4h while awake		Reserve for severe cases (resistance)
	Ciprofloxacin (O)	bid-tid		
	Ofloxacin (D)	1-2 drops q2-4h × 2 d, then qid × 5 d	In >1 yr old	
	Gatifloxacin (D)	1 drop 5-8×/d × 2 d, then qid × 5 d	In >1 yr old	
Aminoglycosides	Tobramycin (D)	1-2 drops q4h		Risk of corneal toxicity
	Tobramycin (O)	bid-tid		
	Gentamicin (D)	1-2 drops q2-4h		
	Gentamicin (O)	q8-12h		
Sulfonamides	Sulfisoxazole (D)	1-2 drops q1-4h		Risk of Stevens-Johnson syndrome
	Sulfacetamide (D)	1-2 drops q2-3h		
	Sulfacetamide (O)	qid and qhs (5×/d)		
Other	Bacitracin (O) ± polymyxin B (O) (Polysporin)	q3-12h (max 6×/d)	Choice for common bacterial conjunctivitis	
	Trimethoprim + polymyxin B (O) (Polytrim)			
Antifungal	Natamycin	Consult ophthalmologist		
	Amphotericin B			
Antiviral	Trifluridine (D)	1 drop 5-9×/d	Herpetic conjunctivitis	
	Acyclovir (O)	5×/d		

*Typical duration of ophthalmic medication use: 7–10 d for bacterial conjunctivitis; varies depending on clinical context.
(D), drops; (O), ointment (apply 0.5-inch ribbon to fornix to affected eye).

30

Ophthalmology

703

FURTHER READING

Fleisher GR, Ludwig S, eds. *Textbook of Pediatric Emergency Medicine.* 4th ed. Philadelphia, Pa: Williams & Wilkins; 2005.

Sit M, Levin AV. Direct ophthalmoscopy in pediatric emergency care. *Pediatr Emerg Care.* 2001;17:199–204.

Young T, Levin AV. The afferent pupillary defect. *Pediatr Emerg Care.* 1997;13:61–65.

USEFUL WEB SITES

www.aapos.org

Ophthalmology

30

Chapter 31 Orthopedics

Fabio Ferri-de-Barros

Andrew W. Howard

COMMON ABBREVIATIONS

AP	anteroposterior
AVN	avascular necrosis
CRP	C-reactive protein
JIA	juvenile idiopathic arthritis
NSAIDs	nonsteroidal anti-inflammatory drugs
ROM	range of motion
SCFE	slipped capital femoral epiphysis
SLE	systemic lupus erythematosus
XR	X-ray

APPROACH TO THE LIMPING CHILD

- Comprehensive history and physical examination; always consider child maltreatment (see Chapter 10)
- With constitutional symptoms (e.g., fever, weight loss, fatigue, malaise), consider infection or neoplasm

DIFFERENTIAL DIAGNOSIS

- See Table 31.1

HIP

DEVELOPMENTAL DYSPLASIA

Before Walking Age

- Identify risk factors: family history, female, frank breech

Table 31.1	Differential Diagnosis for the Limping Child
Congenital/developmental	Developmental dysplasia of the hip, Legg-Calvé-Perthes disease, leg length discrepancy, Osgood-Schlatter disease, osteochondritis dissecans
Infectious	Cellulitis, septic arthritis, osteomyelitis, diskitis
Neoplastic	Leukemia, primary bone tumor, neuroblastoma
Musculoskeletal trauma	Stress fracture, SCFE
Vascular/hematologic	Hemarthrosis/hemophilia, sickle cell disease
Neuromuscular	Cerebral palsy, muscular dystrophy
Autoimmune	JIA, seronegative spondyloarthropathies, SLE, Henoch-Schönlein purpura
Other	Transient synovitis, maltreatment, hypermobility, psychogenic

Physical Findings

- Can be subtle
- Ortolani sign: dislocated hip reduces with flexion–abduction and ventral push over the greater trochanter; usually present up to 3 mo of age
- Barlow test: unstable hip dislocates with mild extension–adduction and posterior push
- Galeazzi sign: unilateral dislocated and irreducible hip; with hips and knees flexed, femur looks shorter on dislocated side from end of examination table

Investigations

- US: if physical findings suggestive, especially if identified risk factors
- Pelvis XR (AP and frog-leg) useful after ossification of the proximal femoral epiphysis (average age, 6 mo in girls and 7 mo in boys)

Treatment

- Positive physical findings confirmed with US: refer to pediatric orthopedist
- Goal is to obtain and maintain stable reduction; method is age dependent
- Pavlik harness widely accepted as first-line treatment
- Under 3 mo of age: 95% success with nonoperative treatment

Walking Age

- History: waddling gait, consistent limp or toe-walking
- Physical: apparent short femur (Galeazzi sign), decreased or asymmetric hip abduction, Trendelenburg gait
- Treatment: usually surgical; no clinical alternative

LEGG-CALVÉ-PERTHES DISEASE

- Idiopathic AVN of the femoral head
- Typically young (age 3–10 yr); male-to-female, 6:1
- Usually insidious onset, mild hip pain, and limp
- Physical: Trendelenburg gait, decreased internal rotation, decreased abduction, thigh and buttock atrophy
- Diagnosis confirmed with pelvic XR (AP + frog-leg positions): morphologic changes of the proximal femoral epiphysis

Principles of Treatment

- Maintain ROM with exercises: enables molding of femoral head to acetabulum
- Containment: keeps femoral head within acetabulum to evenly distribute weight-bearing forces; primarily achieved by ROM exercises ± operation
- Analgesia: to help establish ROM and containment
- Good prognosis: early onset (<6 yr), no deformity of femoral head at maturity

TRANSIENT/TOXIC SYNOVITIS

- May be difficult to differentiate from early septic arthritis of hip
- Typical features: afebrile or low-grade fever; child looks well; presents with reluctance to bear weight; painful passive hip ROM; <6 yr
- WBC, ESR, CRP help to distinguish from septic hip or osteomyelitis (Box 31.1)
- XR to assess joint and look for osteomyelitis
- Consult orthopedist if suspect septic hip

Box 31.1	Predictors of Septic Hip vs. Transient Synovitis
Fever >38.5° C	Retrospective data based on four predictors suggests:
Refusal to bear weight	0 predictors: 0.2% probability of septic hip
WBC >12.0 × 10^9/L	1 predictor: 3% probability of septic hip
ESR >40 mm/h	2 predictors: 40% probability of septic hip
CRP >20.0 mg/L	3 predictors: 93.1% probability of septic hip
	4 predictors: 99.6% probability of septic hip

Adapted from Caird MS, Flynn JM, Leung YL, Millman JE, D'Italia JG, Dormans JP. Factors distinguishing septic arthritis from transient synovitis of the hip in children. *J Bone Joint Surg.* 2006;88A:1253.

Treatment

- Activity restriction for comfort ± gentle ROM; gradual resumption of activity
- NSAIDs (e.g., naproxen)
- Careful observation, early re-examination to rule out early septic arthritis

SCFE

- Mechanical separation of femoral head through physis
- Typically 10–16 yr; more common in males, obese, or African descent
- Bilateral in 30%; 90% chronic; frequently delayed diagnosis
- Can present with prodrome of pain in groin, anterior thigh, or referred to the knee, and/or acute episode of sharp pain in same distribution (preslip)
- Consider endocrinopathy (e.g., hypothyroidism, hypogonadism, renal osteodystrophy) if outside typical weight range
- Younger skeletal age at greater risk of contralateral slip
- Physical findings: unable to bear weight if unstable, Trendelenburg gait, externally rotated leg during gait and when supine, flexion and limited internal rotation of involved hip

Investigations

- XR findings may be subtle; 2 views (AP pelvis and frog-leg lateral) of both hips essential (to rule out asymptomatic contralateral side)
- Findings: on lateral: femoral head is posterior, line along anterior metaphysis misses head, growth plate wide; on AP: femoral head

height loss, growth plate wide, head slipped medially, white blush in metaphysis
- Consult orthopedist if previous history of SCFE in contralateral hip, even in absence of XR abnormalities

Treatment
- Patient not to bear weight
- Urgent surgical pinning of hip
- Goal is to prevent further slip, AVN, and arthritis
- AVN is a devastating complication with no cure; prevention possible with early diagnosis and treatment
- AVN rare in stable slips (<5%); may progress to unstable (up to 50% AVN) if not treated

KNEE

- Knee pain may be referred from hip (e.g., SCFE); always examine the hip
- Meniscal injury rare in children: intra-articular fractures of inter-condylar eminence or dislocated patella more common
- Discoid lateral meniscus pain associated with locking and "clunking"

OSGOOD-SCHLATTER DISEASE
- Tendonitis of the tibial tubercle
- Typically older children and teenagers (10–15 yr); usually unilateral
- XR necessary to rule out other conditions

- Treatment: education, quadriceps and hamstring stretching, reassurance (lasts ≥18 mo); rest for symptom relief; physical activities as symptoms allow; patellar tendon brace

RECURRENT SUBLUXATION OF PATELLA
- Traumatic/developmental hypermobile patella (shifts laterally beyond midline)
- Triad "at risk": increased femoral anteversion, external tibial torsion, valgus knees
- Skyline knee XR (flexed 40°) may demonstrate hypoplastic lateral femoral condyle (developmental) or avulsed fragment (traumatic dislocation)
- Treatment: quadriceps (vastus medialis) strengthening, hamstrings stretching exercises

DIFFUSE NONSPECIFIC ANTERIOR KNEE PAIN
- Classically in teenage females with hypermobile joints
- Pain reproduced by compressing patella against femur
- XR normal; rule out bony lesions (tumors, infection)
- Also referred to as patellar chondromalacia
- Treatment: quadriceps strengthening, hamstrings stretching exercises

OSTEOCHONDRITIS DISSECANS

- Aching knee pain and "giving way"
- Typically in active adolescent males; >20% bilateral
- Deep tenderness over condyles when knee is flexed; restricted knee ROM
- Knee XR (tunnel view): notched lateral aspect of medial femoral condyle
- Restrict sports and refer to orthopedist

LOWER LIMB ALIGNMENT

PHYSIOLOGIC ALIGNMENT OF THE KNEES (VARUS/VALGUS)

- Varus at birth around 12°
- Gradually decreases to neutral alignment at age 18 mo
- Maximum valgus 12° around age 3 yr
- Final alignment 5–7° valgus at age 6 yr

NONPHYSIOLOGIC VARUS KNEE (BOWLEGS)

Causes

- Rickets or other forms of metabolic bone disease
- Infantile tibia vara (Blount disease)
- Skeletal dysplasias
- Physeal disturbance

Treatment

- Treatment depends on etiology
- Rule out or treat rickets before referring to orthopedist

FOOT SHAPE ABNORMALITIES

- Important to perform comprehensive neurologic examination
- Examine lower extremities and spine carefully
- See Table 31.2

Congenital Talipes Equinovarus

- Also known as *club foot*
- Four components to deformity: equinus, varus, cavus ("high arch"), adductus
- May be idiopathic, neurogenic, or syndromic; 50% bilateral
- Examine lower extremities and spine
- Treatment: weekly serial casting as soon as diagnosed, followed by Achilles tenotomy and orthotic management; occasionally surgical intervention

Table 31.2	Differential Diagnosis and Management of Foot Shape Abnormalities		
	Age of Presentation	Main Feature	Treatment
Clubfoot	Birth	Equinus, cavus, varus	Serial casts at birth, Achilles tenotomy, occasionally surgical correction
Calcaneovalgus	Birth	Opposite of equinus	Observation/casts
Metatarsus varus	Birth–3 mo	Forefoot adduction	Observation/casts/brace
Vertical talus	Birth–3 mo	Rocker-bottom sole	Usually requires surgical correction
Flexible flat foot	2+ yr	Arch appears on tiptoeing	Reassurance; special shoes or inserts not required
Pes cavus	10+ yr	Fixed high arch	Rule out neuromuscular conditions
Toe walking	3+ yr	Short calf muscle	Rule out neuromuscular conditions

SPINE

TORTICOLLIS

- Diagnosed during neonatal period due to muscular, articular, or bony abnormalities

Muscular Abnormalities

- Contracture (i.e., congenital torticollis) of sternocleidomastoid muscle
- Can be associated with hip dislocations and foot deformities
- Treatment with stretching; surgery for late diagnosis

Rotatory Displacement of C1–C2

- History, physical examination, and neck XR ± C1–C2 CT scan
- Typically associated with previous upper respiratory infection/abscess or surgery

Treatment

- Early presenting (1–2 wk): soft collar and physiotherapy for neck ROM exercises
- Late presenting (3–6 wk): may need orthopedic care for closed reduction or operative treatment depending on severity and symptoms

Bony Abnormalities

- Congenital fusion-associated syndromes (e.g., Klippel-Feil)
- Refer for specialist evaluation

BACK PAIN

- See Box 31.2

Orthopedics

31

Box 31.2 Differential Diagnosis of Back Pain

- Mechanical: spondylolysis, spondylolisthesis, Scheuermann kyphosis
- Infectious: osteomyelitis, diskitis
- Tumors and tumorlike conditions: eosinophilic granuloma, aneurysmal bone cyst, osteoblastoma, osteoid osteoma, leukemia
- Injury
- Idiopathic
- Psychogenic

Investigations

- Thorough history and physical examination
- AP and lateral XR, CBC, ESR, CRP for screening
- Bone scan (usually nonspecific)
- MRI/CT to confirm clinical suspicion of specific problems

SPONDYLOLISTHESIS

- *Spondylolysis* refers to pars interarticularis defect/fracture (collar of "Scotty dog")
- High suspicion in gymnasts and wrestlers (repetitive hyperextension exercises)
- *Spondylolisthesis* refers to vertebral body ventral subluxation
- L5–S1 segment most commonly involved
- Congenital (malformation of L5 pars) or acquired (traumatic)
- May present with cauda equina syndrome (see pp. 658–660): prompt specialized care required
- AP, lateral, oblique lumbosacral spine XR (lateral demonstrates grade of slippage)
- Grade of slippage refers to amount of subluxation of L5–S1 (25–100%)
- Greater potential for slip progression the younger the child

Treatment

- Low-grade (0–50%) asymptomatic slip: observe; no need to restrict activity
- Low-grade symptomatic slip: restrict sports, physiotherapy for abdominal- and back-strengthening exercises (avoid extension exercises)
- High-grade (75–100%) asymptomatic slip: treatment controversial (restrict contact sports and observe to skeletal maturity vs. fusion in situ)
- High-grade symptomatic slip: restrict activity and refer to orthopedist

SCOLIOSIS

- Coronal plane spinal deformity greater than 10%
- Etiology: idiopathic, congenital, neuromuscular, syndromic
- Idiopathic most common; infantile/juvenile/adolescent
- Adams forward bend test as part of routine physical examination (Figure 30.1)

Figure 31.1 Adams Forward Bend Test

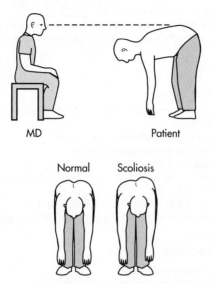

Seven percent of rotation using scoliometer is minimal value for requesting radiography of spine.

- Asymmetric rib prominence, waist line, or shoulder height suggests scoliosis
- History and physical: age at onset, pubertal stage, skin changes, and syndromic features (marfanoid body habitus, café au lait spots, midline skin defects), neurologic examination
- See Box 31.3 for red flags suggestive of an intraspinal canal problem

Prognosis

- Early presentation (up to age 6–7 yr) may compromise lung development
- Adolescent idiopathic scoliosis (late onset) affects body shape more than function, even if not treated

Box 31.3 Red Flags Suggestive of Intraspinal Canal Problems

- Left convex thoracic curve in adolescents and right convex thoracic curve in infants (the usual idiopathic pattern is the opposite)
- Cavus feet
- Asymmetric cutaneous abdominal reflex
- Rapidly progressive deformity
- Abnormal neurologic examination

Orthopedics

31

Treatment

- Clinical observation for curves < 25°
- Brace for progressive curves > 25° in skeletally immature patients; surgery considered for curves likely to progress after skeletal maturity

UPPER LIMB

PULLED ELBOW

- Common in children aged 2–5 yr; clinical diagnosis based on history and examination
- Caused by pull on pronated-extended forearm
- Child will not use arm (pseudoparalysis)
- Consider subtle fracture
- Gently supinate and flex forearm until hand's ulnar border touches shoulder; "click" is felt
- Pain resolved, ROM re-established (elbow unlocked)
- Occasionally requires second attempt by specialist/experienced physician

ELBOW DISLOCATION

- Swollen and deformed elbow
- Medial epicondyle may get entrapped in the joint
- If in doubt, do XR for contralateral elbow

SHOULDER DISLOCATION

- Rare in young children
- 90% anterior glenohumeral dislocations (palpable gap distal—anterior to the acromion)
- Perform full neurovascular examination before and after reduction; axillary nerve most commonly affected ("shoulder badge" area sensation, deltoid contraction)
- XRs confirm diagnosis
- Closed reduction can be achieved by different gentle traction maneuvers; may be assisted by conscious sedation; consult experienced physician

FRACTURES

- Fractures in infants < 18 mo: consider child maltreatment (see Chapter 10)
- Salter-Harris classification of growth plate injuries (Figure 31.2) uses the acronym SALTR (Box 31.4)
- Higher grades, usually from high-energy injuries, are likelier to lead to premature or asymmetric growth arrest (angular deformity, or limb length discrepancy in lower extremities)

Figure 31.2 **Classification of Growth Plate Injuries**

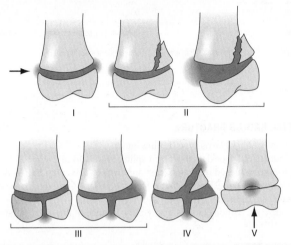

Adapted from Salter RB, Harris WR. Injuries involving the epiphyseal plate. *J Bone Joint Surg.* 1963;45A:599, 604, 606, 608, 609. Reprinted with permission from The Journal of Bone and Joint Surgery, Inc.

GENERAL MANAGEMENT

- Check neurovascular status of limb (Table 31.3)
- Look for any evidence of open fracture
- Examine joints above and below to rule out associated injuries
- NPO in case of potential reduction or surgery
- Intra-articular fractures (see Figure 31.2, types III and IV) may require open reduction
- Open fractures: ensure tetanus status up to date, cover wounds with sterile dressings, splint, prompt IV antibiotics, XR, urgent orthopedist consultation for specialized treatment
- See Chapter 6 for cast application
- See Table 31.4 for examples of common fractures

Box 31.4	Salter-Harris Classification of Growth Plate Injuries (SALTR)

- **S**table (type I): transverse through growth plate
- **A**bove (type II, most common): through metaphysis and along growth plate
- **L**ow (type III, intra-articular): through epiphysis and along growth plate
- **T**hrough (type IV, intra-articular): through epiphysis, metaphysis, and growth plate
- **R**am (type V): crush injury of growth plate

Table 31.3   Quick Neurologic Examination of the Hand

Nerve	Motor	Sensory
Radial	Thumb extension	Dorsal webbing between thumb and index finger
Median	Thumb and index DIP flexion	Lateral side of index finger DIP
Ulnar	Finger abduction	Medial side of pinky finger DIP

DIP, distal interphalangeal joint.

DISTAL RADIUS FRACTURE

- Usually Salter-Harris type II; ulna intact
- Undisplaced (buckle): short arm splint, follow up in 1 wk
- Displaced: closed reduction, cast application, follow up in 3–4 d with orthopedist; beware Salter-Harris type IV (subtle diagnosis; different prognosis)
- Long-term complication is growth disturbance of the distal radius

Table 31.4   Common Fractures

Type of Fracture	Obligatory Orthopedics Consultation	Cast/Splint
Clavicular	Tenting of skin, medial or lateral third of clavicle involved Sternoclavicular joint involved (may be subtle)	Triangular arm sling
Proximal humeral	Tenting of skin, ≥12 yr with fracture displaced >45° on XR or neurovascular compromise	Shoulder sugar tong (splint from the axilla extending caudally, around the elbow, and back cranially up to the acromioclavicular joint, involving the whole arm medially and laterally), and collar and cuff
Supracondylar humeral	Any displacement	Above-elbow posterior slab
Ulnar/radial	Forearm clinically deformed (soft tissue contour on XR)	Above-elbow posterior slab
Scaphoid	Visible displacement	Thumb spica splint
Boxer	Any finger rotation, >40–50° angulation of fifth metacarpal	Ulnar gutter cast
Tibial or fibular	Displaced/angulated fractures Proximal metaphysis involved	Above-knee cast
Metatarsal	Significant angulation	Posterior short-leg slab

MIDSHAFT RADIUS AND ULNA DIAPHYSEAL FRACTURES

- Greater potential for remodeling the younger the child
- Clinically deformed limb requires closed reduction and cast application
- Check neurovascular status and skin integrity (open vs. closed fracture)
- Follow up with orthopedist 3–4 d after reduction

RADIAL NECK FRACTURE

- Look for posterior fat pad sign (anterior fat pad present in 10% of normal elbows)
- If undisplaced, long-arm cast and follow-up in 1 wk
- If markedly displaced or angulated, consult orthopedist

LATERAL CONDYLE HUMERAL FRACTURE

- Tender lateral condyle with posterior fat pad sign on lateral elbow XR
- Fracture may not be obvious on AP and lateral XR: order oblique views
- Refer all lateral condyle humeral fractures to orthopedist immediately
- Long-term complications: nonunion, cubitus valgus, late-presenting ulnar nerve palsy

SUPRACONDYLAR HUMERUS FRACTURE

- Extension type is more common than flexion
- Look for break in the "hourglass" on lateral elbow XR
- Careful neurovascular examination, especially brachial and radial pulses
- Undisplaced with posterior cortex intact treated with standard long-arm cast
- Displaced fractures: do not attempt reduction; require splinting in ER; NPO with prompt referral to orthopedist for reduction or possible pinning
- Acute complication: neurovascular injury/compartment syndrome (see p. 718)
- Long-term complications: cubitus varus (gun stock deformity), stiffness

MONTEGGIA FRACTURE

- Fracture of proximal ulna and dislocated radial head
- Diagnosis often not obvious
- Axis of proximal radius must point to capitellum on all normal XRs
- Ulna may be bent (plastically deformed), not fractured
- Refer all proximal ulnar fractures to orthopedist immediately

PROXIMAL FEMUR FRACTURE

- If suspected: NPO, IV analgesia, splint using skin traction, then pelvic and femoral XRs
- Careful neurovascular examination before and after splint
- Refer to orthopedist immediately
- Main complication: AVN of the proximal femoral epiphysis

31

FEMORAL SHAFT FRACTURE

- Infants and toddlers: consider child maltreatment (see Chapter 10)
- Careful neurovascular examination for pulses and sciatic/femoral nerve function
- NPO, IV analgesia, splint in position of comfort
- Refer to orthopedist immediately

TIBIAL SHAFT FRACTURE

- High-energy (transverse or oblique) or low-energy (spiral) injury
- Requires careful neurovascular examination
- If undisplaced and spiral configuration: long-leg splint, follow up with orthopedist in 1 wk
- If angulated and/or displaced, refer to orthopedist immediately
- Infant and toddlers: consider child maltreatment (see Chapter 10)

ANKLE FRACTURE

- Evaluate position of talus within mortise on three views (AP, lateral, mortise XRs)
- Most common: Salter-Harris type I undisplaced fibular fracture
- Short-leg splint, non–weight bearing, follow up with orthopedist in 1 wk
- Salter-Harris types II and III distal tibial fractures require evaluation by orthopedist

FOOT FRACTURES

- Extra-articular phalangeal fractures treated with "buddy taping"
- Commonly undisplaced or minimally displaced metatarsal low-energy injuries treated with short-leg splints, non–weight bearing, and followed up in 1 wk
- Refer immediately to orthopedist: high-energy Lisfranc tarsometatarsal fracture/dislocation, intra-articular fractures, displaced fractures of the first metatarsal, and talus/calcaneus fracture (uncommon; suspect in setting of high-energy axial trauma)

COMPARTMENT SYNDROME

- Risk of muscle ischemia and neurovascular compromise (Volkmann contracture)
- Common predisposing conditions: supracondylar humerus fractures, displaced forearm fractures, proximal tibial metaphyseal fractures
- Early signs and symptoms: pain exacerbated by passive extension of fingers/toes, swollen extremity tense to palpation, constant/increasing pain unrelieved by analgesics
- Definitive treatment essential within 4–6 h to avoid permanent neuromuscular damage
- Emergent surgical decompression of involved compartments necessary

INFECTION

OSTEOMYELITIS

- May be acute, subacute, or chronic (gradual onset of pain, XR changes may resemble osteosarcoma/Ewing sarcoma)
- Osteomyelitis associated with point tenderness, often in metaphysis of long bone
- Recurrent, multifocal osteomyelitis: rare, bone pain in several sites; XR shows wide growth plates
- Osteomyelitis often spreads to joints with intra-articular metaphysis (e.g., proximal humerus, radius, femur, tibia–fibula), with risk of septic joint

Investigations

- CBC + differential, ESR, CRP, blood cultures (positive in 70%)
- IV antibiotics ± surgical drainage followed by oral antibiotics
- See Table 31.5 for diagnostic imaging considerations

Treatment

- Analgesia, immobilization
- Empiric antibiotics (see Chapter 24) until specific organism and sensitivities identified
- Antibiotics should be given IV initially; once signs of acute inflammation have resolved, switch to equivalent oral antibiotics if patient can tolerate oral medications, strict compliance is ensured, and follow-up can be maintained (weekly clinical evaluation, CRP, and ESR)

Duration of Antibiotic Treatment

- Controversial
- Acute osteomyelitis: minimum 21 d, until all clinical signs resolved and ESR normal
- *Pseudomonas* osteomyelitis secondary to foot puncture wound: 1–2 wk after debridement

Table 31.5	Diagnostic Imaging for Osteomyelitis	
Context	**Initial Diagnostic Imaging**	**Follow-Up Imaging***
Neonate	Plain films of localized area	May need whole body survey and specialized imaging as below
Older infants and children	Plain films of localized area (bone changes only evident after 7–10 d)	If generalized undefined area: bone scan If localized isolated area: MRI
Patient with sickle cell disease	Plain films of localized area (may be nondiagnostic)	As above; MRI may be useful to better define changes of sickle cell–related infarction or infection; may be needed to guide surgical drainage

*Done if initial diagnostic imaging negative and clinical suspicion persists.

Indications for Surgical Drainage/Debridement
- Poor response within 72 h and abscess or joint sepsis
- Vertebral osteomyelitis with neurologic signs
- Consider for foot puncture wound

SEPTIC ARTHRITIS
- Refer a suspected septic joint to orthopedist immediately
- History: fever; refusal to move affected joint/bear weight if lower extremity affected; may have sudden progressive swelling, erythema, tenderness of affected joint area (may be harder to identify in deeper joints, such as the hip)
- Physical: antalgic positioning of affected limb; child prefers position maximizing intracapsular volume (e.g., FABER: *F*lexed/*AB*ducted/*E*xternally *R*otated hip position); pain on passive motion with restricted ROM of affected joint
- May involve multiple sites in neonates or in patients with disseminated gonococcal infection
- Rule out nonmusculoskeletal causes (such as appendicitis for septic hip)

Investigations
- XR to exclude fracture/neoplasm
- US may confirm hip effusion/periosteal abscess
- MRI may be useful in atypical presentations
- Bone radionuclide scan (technetium, gallium) may be useful if generalized pain or unclear diagnosis (e.g., suspect pelvic neoplasm)
- CBC, ESR, CRP, blood cultures (approximately 70% positive)
- Joint aspiration under sterile conditions if high clinical suspicion of septic joint
- Thick pus may not come out through needle: beware false-negative result
- Test aspirate for WBC + differential, glucose, culture, Gram stain, latex agglutination

Treatment
- Prompt joint drainage (consult orthopedist), IV antibiotics, analgesia
- Empiric antibiotics (see Chapter 24) until specific organism and sensitivities identified
- Antibiotics should be given IV initially; switch to equivalent oral antibiotics as with osteomyelitis
- If aspiration for diagnosis is imminent, do not start antibiotics until afterward to increase diagnostic yield

Duration of Antibiotic Treatment

- Depends on clinical context and response
- Minimum 2 wk
- Shorter courses (1 wk) can be given for gonococcal arthritis
- Longer courses (3–4 wk) advised for *Staphylococcus aureus* arthritis of hip joint, neonates, immunocompromised patients, gram-negative arthritis, or underlying osteomyelitis (4–6 wk)

FURTHER READING

Beaty JH, Kasser JR. *Rockwood and Wilkins' Fractures in Children*. 5th ed. Philadelphia, Pa: Lippincott Williams & Wilkins; 2001.

Green NE, Swiontkowski MF. *Skeletal Trauma in Children*. 3rd ed. Philadelphia, Pa: WB Saunders; 2003.

Herring JA. *Tachdjian's Pediatric Orthopaedics*. 3rd ed. Philadelphia, Pa: WB Saunders; 2002.

Morrissy RT. *Lovell and Winter's Pediatric Orthopaedics*. 6th ed. Philadelphia, Pa: Lippincott Williams & Wilkins; 2005.

Wenger DR, Rang M. *The Art and Practice of Children's Orthopaedics*. New York, NY: Raven Press; 1993.

USEFUL WEB SITES

Wheeless' Textbook of Orthopaedics. Available at: **www.wheelessonline.com**

Orthopedics

31

Chapter 32 Otolaryngology

Gordon S. Soon
Paolo Campisi

Chapter 32 Otolaryngology

COMMON ABBREVIATIONS

ABR	auditory brainstem response
AOM	acute otitis media
DDAVP	desmopressin acetate
ENT	ear, nose, and throat
FB	foreign body
GABHS	group A β-hemolytic streptococcus
I&D	incision and drainage
ITP	idiopathic thrombocytopenic purpura
IVIG	intravenous immunoglobulin
OAE	otoacoustic emissions
OE	otitis externa
OM	otitis media
OME	otitis media with effusion
OSA	obstructive sleep apnea
PSGN	poststreptococcal glomerulonephritis
RCOF	ristocetin cofactor
RST	rapid strep test
TEF	tracheoesophageal fistula
TM	tympanic membrane
URTI	upper respiratory tract infection
vWD	von Willebrand disease

EAR

CERUMEN REMOVAL

- Often necessary to soften wax (cerumenolysis) before its removal
  - Cerumenolytic agents include 10% sodium bicarbonate (baking soda) solution; organic liquids (olive oil, mineral oil, baby oil); docusate; carbamide peroxide (e.g., Murine)
  - Use 2–3 times daily for 3–5 d before cerumen removal
- Syringing (irrigation): usually with warm water, normal saline, or sodium bicarbonate solution; adjust pressure and speed; gentle irrigation over long period less painful, safer
- Curette method: dislodge and remove cerumen

- Congenital: most nonsyndromic cases are autosomal recessive; syndromic cases include Waardenburg, Pendred, Treacher Collins, Alport syndromes
- Acquired: in utero infection (e.g., TORCH, see Chapter 24), prematurity, perinatal asphyxia, ototoxic medication (e.g., gentamicin), hyperbilirubinemia, meningitis, temporal bone injury
- May be conductive or sensorineural; unilateral or bilateral
- Early accurate diagnosis and referral to ENT (<6 mo of age) for effective rehabilitation, genetic consultation, and counseling
- Investigations may include OAE, ABR, sound field audiometry, CT of head and temporal bones (inner ear dysplasia) (Table 32.1)

Table 32.1	Newborn Hearing Screening
OAE	· Performed in well-infant nursery or within 1 mo of discharge · Result is either "pass," "refer," or "incomplete" · If "refer" or "incomplete" result, arrange ABR
ABR	· Performed in special care nursery, if risk factors* or if referred from OAE (see above) · If "refer" or "incomplete" result, arrange detailed audiologic evaluation by otolaryngologist
Sound field audiometry	· To assess behavioral responses; more accurate than OAE or ABR
Head/temporal bone CT	· To rule out structural anomalies of inner ear and assess suitability for cochlear implant

*Family history of permanent childhood hearing loss; in utero infections (e.g., TORCH); postnatal infections associated with sensorineural hearing loss such as bacterial meningitis; hyperbilirubinemia requiring exchange transfusion; persistent pulmonary hypertension associated with mechanical ventilation; stigmata associated with a syndrome known to include sensorineural or conductive hearing loss.

MASTOIDITIS

- Rare but potentially serious complication of OM
- Clinical presentation: protruding ear, postauricular swelling and tenderness
- Wide myringotomy, IV antibiotics usually necessary
- Chronic mastoiditis with chronic otorrhea: mastoid air cell loss/ coalescence on CT scan
- If subperiosteal abscess formation, surgical drainage may be required; if erythema behind ears and no radiologic evidence of coalescence, give parenteral antibiotics (e.g., cefuroxime)
- Need to rule out cholesteatoma with chronically draining ear

OE

- Localized infection: often *Staphylococcus aureus*; often furuncle in outer third of ear canal
- Diffuse infection: often *Pseudomonas aeruginosa* or *Candida*; predisposing factors include trauma, swimming, aggressive cleaning of canal
- Keep ear dry
- Debriding ear canal is an important part of therapy: if lack appropriate equipment or experience, refer to ENT surgeon to remove purulent discharge and epithelial debris from ear canal (by wet swabbing, gentle irrigation, and suctioning) if not responding to therapy
- Provide oral analgesia and ototopical agent
- See Table 32.2
- If periauricular swelling, regional adenopathy, signs of systemic infection present, systemic antibiotics required; antibiotic choice should be effective against *Pseudomonas*
- If difficulty differentiating furuncle of ear canal from mastoiditis with subperiosteal abscess, refer to ENT surgeon

Table 32.2	Topical Management of Otitis Externa		
Agent*	Dosing†	Advantages	Disadvantages
Neomycin/polymyxin B/hydrocortisone	4 drops q6h	Commonly used	Increasing resistance patterns Potential ototoxicity
Ofloxacin	5 drops q12h	Only twice daily No risk of ototoxicity	Potential for resistance
Ciprofloxacin/ dexamethasone	4 drops q12h	Only twice daily No risk of ototoxicity	Potential for resistance

*Gentamicin-based drops not listed because of higher risk of ototoxicity and development of newer agents; however, occasionally used if no alternative when faced with fluoroquinolone-resistant infections.
†In general, treat for 3 d beyond cessation of symptoms (usually 5–7 d total); in more severe cases, may need to treat for 10–14 d.

OM

- Classified as AOM or OME
- Diagnosis of AOM based on
  1. Rapid onset
  2. Signs of middle ear effusion (bulging TM, limited mobility of TM, air–fluid level behind TM, or otorrhea)
  3. Middle ear inflammation (erythema of TM or distinct otalgia) (Figure 32.1)
- Persistent OME (i.e., effusion without signs or symptoms of infection) is normal for 2–3 mo after therapy; does not require retreatment

Figure 32.1 Tympanic Membrane: Landmarks and Pathology

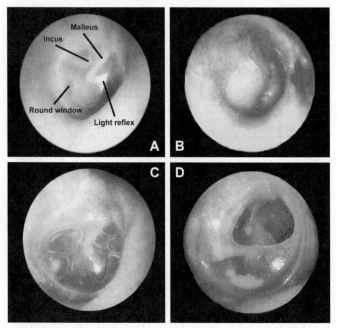

A, Landmarks of normal TM. B, AOM: bulging, hyperemic TM with indistinct landmarks. C, OME: air bubbles and serous fluid behind retracted TM. D, Perforated TM.

A, B, C from Scott EG, Powell KR. Acute otitis media. *Infect Med.* 2003;20:224–229. Available at: http://www.medscape.com/viewarticle/455529_3. Accessed November 20, 2007; D adapted from Isaacson JE, Vora NM. Differential diagnosis and treatment of hearing loss. *Am Fam Physician.* 2003;68:1125–1132. Available at http://www.aafp.org/afp/20030915/1125.html. Accessed November 20, 2007. A,B,C: Copyright 2003, *Infections in Medicine,* CMPMedica. All rights reserved. D: Copyright 2003, American Academy of Family Physicians. All rights reserved.

AOM

- Most common organisms: *Streptococcus pneumoniae, Haemophilus influenzae, Moraxella catarrhalis, Streptococcus pyogenes*
- Viruses including RSV, *Rhinovirus, Coronavirus,* parainfluenza, adenovirus, *Enterovirus*
- Always assess and treat pain: mild–moderate (acetaminophen, ibuprofen); moderate–severe (consider benzocaine otic [Auralgan] 2–3 drops q4–6h prn)
- Observation option: defer antibiotics for 48–72 h if reliable follow-up and (1) age 6 mo–2 yr with nonsevere presentation (mild otalgia and fever <39°C) AND uncertain diagnosis or (2) age ≥2 yr with nonsevere presentation OR with uncertain diagnosis (Table 32.3)
- Treat initially for 5–7 d in children ≥2 yr with nonsevere presentation and 10 d for children <2 yr or with severe presentation (fever ≥39°C and/or severe otalgia) or with underlying medical conditions

- For perforation with discharge (in absence of fever), treat with antibiotic drops (ciprofloxacin/dexamethasone bid × 7–10 d); if fever, add systemic antibiotics
- Myringotomy indicated for the following:
  - Recurrent AOM
  - Intractable pain
  - Bulging TM and severe pain after 48–72 h of therapy
  - AOM with complications (e.g., meningitis, mastoiditis, facial nerve palsy)
  - Persistent OME causing hearing loss >3–4 mo after AOM
  - Immunosuppressed patient (e.g., on chemotherapy)
  - Tympanocentesis in infants <6 wk

Recurrent AOM
- Defined as ≥3 documented episodes per 6 mo or ≥4 episodes per 12 mo
- Antibiotic prophylaxis generally discouraged
- Consider myringotomy and tympanostomy tube insertion

OME
- OME lasting >3 mo may require therapy
- Prolonged OME most common cause of conductive hearing loss
- If undiagnosed or left untreated, may result in delayed onset of speech, learning problems in susceptible children (e.g., Down syndrome, cleft palate)
- Asymptomatic: follow until OME resolves (tympanometry useful)

Table 32.3	Systemic Antibiotic Treatment of Otitis Media	
	Fever ≥39°C and/or Severe Otalgia	
Clinical Assessment	**No**	**Yes**
Requires initial treatment with antibiotic*	Amoxicillin† 80–90 mg/kg/d	Amoxicillin‡ 90 mg/kg/d with clavulanate 6.4 mg/kg/d
Failure at 48–72 h of observation option	Amoxicillin† 80–90 mg/kg/d	Amoxicillin‡ 90 mg/kg/d with clavulanate 6.4 mg/kg/d
Failure at 48–72 h despite initial antibiotic treatment	Amoxicillin‡ 90 mg/kg/d with clavulanate 6.4 mg/kg/d	Ceftriaxone 50 mg/kg/dose IM daily × 3 d
Failure at 10–28 d despite antibiotic treatment	Amoxicillin-clavulanate, cefuroxime, or ceftriaxone; consider tympanocentesis and culture§	Amoxicillin-clavulanate, cefuroxime, or ceftriaxone; consider tympanocentesis and culture§

*When observation option is not appropriate.
†If allergic, consider cefuroxime, azithromycin, clarithromycin, or erythromycin-sulfisoxazole.
†If allergic, consider ceftriaxone or clindamycin (note: clindamycin not effective against *H. influenzae* and *M. catarrhalis*; allow culture to guide treatment).
§Culture-guided treatment may be considered in management of treatment failures.
Adapted from American Academy of Pediatrics, Subcommittee on Management of Acute Otitis Media. Diagnosis and management of acute otitis media. *Pediatrics.* 2004;113:1451–1465.

- Medical management: antihistamines and decongestants ineffective, not recommended; antibiotics and corticosteroids no long-term efficacy, not recommended for routine management
- Surgical candidates (myringotomy and tympanostomy tube insertion):
  - OME >4 mo with persistent hearing loss or other signs and symptoms
  - Persistent OME in at-risk children
  - OME and structural damage to TM or middle ear
  - If patient requires second set of tubes, consider adenoidectomy

TRAUMATIC PERFORATION OF THE TYMPANIC MEMBRANE

- See Fig. 32.1D
- Consult ENT surgeon immediately; emergency exploration and repair *may* be required
- Audiometric assessment and follow-up in 3–4 wk with ENT surgeon
- Must keep water out of ear until perforation closes; avoid swimming; ear plugs during bathing

NOSE

EPISTAXIS

- Bleeding usually from Little's area (anterior septum)
- Bleeding more common during acute URTIs and in allergic rhinitis

MANAGEMENT

- Mild: firm persistent pressure between fingers for 10 min
- More persistent, see Box 32.1
- Prevention: keep fingernails short to avoid digital trauma; apply petroleum jelly (Vaseline) to affected nostril daily; use humidification in dry season

FRACTURED NOSE

- Examine nose for septal hematoma or dislocation (causes nasal obstruction and/or pain; may result in late nasal deformity); septal hematoma requires urgent surgical drainage
- Nasal XR not necessary; even if negative, may still be serious pathology
- If no swelling, contact ENT surgeon to reduce deformity early (within 2–3 h of injury)
- If swelling, may observe 3–4 d; should refer all cases to ENT clinic for 3–7 d follow-up to check for late septal hematoma, abscess formation, or deformity (noted after swelling subsides)

Box 32.1 | Management of Epistaxis

Child Actively Bleeding ≥30 Min Despite Appropriate Local Pressure

Initial Approach
1. Assess severity of bleeding (vital signs, quantity, controlled with anterior pressure?)
2. Obtain relevant medical history (ITP, VWD, hemophilia, transplant, oncology, etc.)
3. Ensure IV access, CBC, crossmatch, fluids, PRBCs, epistaxis tray at bedside
4. Consult ENT surgeon

Local Management at Bedside
1. Visualize (head mirror or light); may be facilitated by sedation
2. Control bleeding with pressure and cotton pledgets moistened with cocaine 4–5% (max 3 mg/kg) or 0.25% phenylephrine/3% lidocaine solution
3. Consider nasal decongestion (e.g., xylometazoline [Otrivin])
4. Intranasal examination:
   - If defined bleeding: cauterize with AgNO$_3$ stick behind bleeding point of vessel followed by dry cotton pack for 5 min; do *not* cauterize both sides of septum; apply topical ointment (petroleum jelly [Vaseline] or bacitracin/polymyxin B [Polysporin]) for 7–10 d to prevent dryness
   - If no source seen: initial packing (gelatin sponge [Gelfoam]); secondary packing (petroleum jelly [Vaseline] gauze); tertiary packing (posterior pack)
5. If bleeding persistent, take to OR for endoscopic examination, electrocautery, and repacking

Management of Hematologic Disease
1. **ITP:** IVIG 1 g/kg IV; platelets 1 unit/5 kg only if hemodynamically unstable
2. **vWD:** DDAVP 0.3 mcg/kg/dose IV/SC (max 20 mcg/dose); if DDAVP nonresponder, consider RCOF 40 IU/kg Humate-P IV
3. **Hemophilia A:** 30 units/kg FVIII IV
4. **Hemophilia B:** 50 units/kg FIX IV
5. **Anticoagulation:** may need to reverse with FFP (10–20 mL/kg); vitamin K 1 mg IV; protamine sulfate

© The Hospital for Sick Children, 2006. Adapted from Price V, Campisi P, Blanchette V. *Guidelines for the Investigation and Management of Epistaxis in Children* [internal document]. Toronto, Ontario, Canada: Hospital for Sick Children; 2005, 2006.

32

SINUSITIS

- Ethmoid and maxillary sinuses present at birth; sphenoid sinuses by age 5 yr; frontal sinuses appear ages 7–8 yr
- Sinusitis: obstruction of sinus drainage, retention of secretions in paranasal sinuses
- Etiology: *S. pneumoniae, H. influenzae, M. catarrhalis, S. aureus,* anaerobes
- Patients at risk for prolonged infection and/or atypical organisms: cystic fibrosis, immotile cilia syndrome, metabolic disorders, immunocompromised states, smokers

DIAGNOSIS

- Acute bacterial sinusitis is a clinical diagnosis with infection lasting <30 d (Box 32.2)
- Gold standard: recovery of bacteria in high density (>10 CFU/mL) from paranasal sinus; not commonly done
- Imaging not necessary ≤6 yr (history as predictive as imaging); in children >6 yr, imaging controversial; XRs are difficult to interpret: poor specificity (high false-positive rate), especially with preceding URTI
- Imaging (XR, CT, MRI) can only support clinical history; reserved for patients who do not recover or who worsen despite antimicrobial therapy
- Three views: Waters occipitomental projection for maxillary sinuses; Caldwell occipitofrontal projection for ethmoid and frontal sinuses; lateral projection for sphenoid sinuses
- CT scans of paranasal sinuses only if surgery being considered or if complications of acute sinusitis

COMPLICATIONS

- Orbital: periorbital cellulitis/edema, subperiosteal abscess, orbital cellulitis/abscess
- Intracranial: cavernous sinus thrombosis, meningitis, subdural empyema, epidural or brain abscess
- Osteomyelitis: frontal (Pott puffy tumor), maxillary bone

MANAGEMENT

- Antibiotics for acute bacterial sinusitis; same as for AOM (see AOM section, p. 726)
- In nonresponders, moderate or severe, or those attending day care: high-dose amoxicillin-clavulanate, cefuroxime, ceftriaxone
- Duration of therapy: until symptom free plus additional 7 d
- Adjuvant therapy: limited evidence; consider nasal irrigation, antihistamines, decongestants, mucolytic agents, topical intranasal steroid
- If persistent: refer to ENT surgeon for sinus lavage and drainage

Box 32.2	Diagnostic Criteria for Acute Bacterial Sinusitis	
2 major criteria OR 1 major and 2 minor criteria		
Major Criteria*		**Minor Criteria***
Facial pain/pressure		Headache
Facial congestion/fullness		Dental pain
Purulent nasal discharge		Ear pain/pressure
Nasal obstruction		Fatigue
Postnasal drip		Halitosis
Hyposmia/anosmia		Cough
Fever		

*Listed in order of relative frequency.

THROAT

ABSCESSES

- See Table 32.4

Table 32.4	Peritonsillar and Retropharyngeal Abscesses	
	Peritonsillar Abscess	**Retropharyngeal Abscess**
General	· Most common complication of untreated or partially treated acute tonsillitis	· More correctly, *infection of the retropharyngeal and parapharyngeal spaces*; difficulty differentiating abscess from cellulitis/phlegmon
Differential diagnosis	· Retropharyngeal abscess, parapharyngeal infection, cervical adenitis, dental abscess, submandibular/sublingual abscess (Ludwig angina)	· Peritonsillar abscess, parapharyngeal infection, cervical adenitis, dental abscess, submandibular/sublingual abscess (Ludwig angina)
Typical bacteria	· Typically mixed organisms: GABHS, anaerobes (*Prevotella, Peptostreptococcus*, etc.), *S. aureus, H. influenzae, S. pneumoniae*	· GABHS, *S. aureus*, anaerobes (*Bacteroides, Prevotella*, etc.), *H. influenzae*
Clinical presentation	· Commonly >10 yr · Sore throat or neck pain, increasing unilateral odynophagia or dysphagia, uvular deviation, muffled "hot potato" voice, trismus, neck adenopathy, fever >38°C	· Commonly <6 yr (due to paramedian chains of lymph nodes) · Sore throat or neck pain, fever >38°C, torticollis, dysphagia, neck mass, preceding URTI · Toxic appearance ± stridor as infection progresses
Investigations and diagnosis	· CBC, throat culture · Lateral soft tissue neck XR may help rule out retropharyngeal abscess (see Chapter 14) · US: high specificity; cost-effective; fast; however, few technicians are trained, US probe often painful · CT: consider in children <7 yr; failed I&D; failed antibiotic therapy (consider extension to the parapharyngeal spaces)	· CBC · Lateral soft tissue neck XR (in extension and during inspiration); abnormal if prevertebral space >7 mm anterior to C2 (half the vertebral body) or >14 mm anterior to C6 (width of vertebral body) (see Chapter 14) · CT: high clinical suspicion of retropharyngeal abscess or equivocal lateral neck XR; can help differentiate between cellulitis and abscess
Management	· Small abscess, nontoxic patient: consider PO or IV antibiotics (clindamycin; second-generation cephalosporin; or amoxicillin-clavulanate) · Fluctuant mass: IV antibiotics and consider needle aspiration or I&D; if prior history of tonsillar disease, consider tonsillectomy	· If no immediate risk of airway compromise: surgical drainage *recommended*; start IV antibiotics (clindamycin; first- or second-generation cephalosporin and metronidazole) · If risk of airway compromise or failed response to antibiotics within 24–48 h, *immediate* surgical drainage; start IV antibiotics

- Pharyngeal tonsils (adenoids), palatine tonsils (tonsils), lingual tonsils form ring of lymphatic tissue (Waldeyer ring) within oral cavity and nasopharynx
- Multiple organisms can infect tonsils; superficial swab cultures may not yield causative organism:
  - Bacterial: GABHS, *H. influenzae*, *S. aureus*, *S. pneumoniae*, *M. catarrhalis*
  - Viral: adenovirus, influenza A, herpes simplex, EBV, coxsackievirus A
  - Fungal: *Candida*

COMMON COMPLICATIONS

Adenotonsillar Hypertrophy

- May cause snoring, mouth breathing, nasal congestion, rhinorrhea, dysphagia
- If severe, may lead to OSA and cardiopulmonary abnormalities (e.g., pulmonary hypertension, cor pulmonale)

Tonsillitis

- Acute (<3 wk), subacute (3 wk–3 mo), or chronic (>3 mo)
- Chronic or recurrent tonsillitis: ≥7 well-documented, clinically important, adequately treated episodes in one year; ≥5 in each of two successive years; or ≥3 in each of three successive years
- Suppurative complications: peritonsillar abscess; infection of retropharyngeal and parapharyngeal spaces; OM; sinusitis
- Nonsuppurative complications of GABHS infections: rheumatic fever; glomerulonephritis

MEDICAL MANAGEMENT

- Antibiotic coverage for GABHS and β-lactamase–producing bacteria (e.g., *S. aureus*, *H. influenzae*)
- Prophylactic antibiotics not recommended for recurrent or chronic infections because of increasing resistance patterns
- Corticosteroids may provide short-term benefit for OSA from adenotonsillar hypertrophy; does not prevent adenotonsillectomy in long term

ADENOTONSILLECTOMY

- See Table 32.5

Management of Acute Hemorrhage

- Resuscitate if clinically appropriate (see Chapter 1)
- Establish IV access
- CBC; INR/PTT; crossmatch

Table 32.5

Table 32.5	Indications, Contraindications, and Complications of Adenotonsillectomy	
	Tonsillectomy	**Adenoidectomy**
Absolute indications	· OSA due to hypertrophy · Suspected malignancy · Recurrent hemorrhage · Severe dysphagia	· OSA due to hypertrophy · Suspected malignancy · Severe dysphagia
Relative indications	· Recurrent tonsillitis · Recurrent peritonsillar abscesses	· Chronic and recurrent adenoiditis or OME · Speech distortions · Dental/facial maldevelopment · Chronic sinusitis
Relative contraindications	· Medical contraindications (e.g., bleeding disorders) · Risk for velopharyngeal insufficiency: greater risk in cleft palate, bifid uvula, orofacial anomalies (e.g., Treacher Collins; Pierre Robin), neuromuscular disorders (e.g., Arnold-Chiari malformations; myotonic dystrophy; Down syndrome)	
Complications	· Hemorrhage: primary (<24 h after surgery); secondary (5–8 d after surgery), usually secondary to infection · Avoid NSAIDs pre- and postoperatively due to antiplatelet effect	

NSAIDs, nonsteroidal anti-inflammatory drugs.

- Start IV antibiotics (e.g., clindamycin)
- Admit for minimum 24 h of observation
- If severe or patient uncooperative, return to OR for bleeding localization and control

Otolaryngology

32

CORROSIVE BURNS OF UPPER GASTROINTESTINAL TRACT

- Common sources of acids: toilet bowl or drain cleaners, automotive tire or metal cleaners, rust removers, tile cleaners, battery fluid
- Common sources of alkali: toilet bowl or drain cleaners, oven cleaners, household bleach, pool chlorination system tablets, dishwashing or clothing detergents, button batteries
- Acids cause coagulation necrosis, which limits extension of injury (except hydrofluoric acid, which behaves similar to alkalis); alkalis cause liquefaction necrosis, which continues to penetrate deeply into tissue, much more dangerous
- Degree of visible burns in mouth and pharynx may not reflect extent of esophageal involvement
- Presence of >2 symptoms and signs (e.g., oral discomfort, swelling, burning, numbness, dysphagia, refusal to swallow, shortness of breath, chest pain) correlates with esophageal burns

MANAGEMENT

- Emergent ENT consultation
- Determine nature (acid/alkali/other) and form (solid/liquid) of ingested material
- Do NOT give emetic; do NOT attempt gastric lavage
- Do NOT give anything by mouth (e.g., milk or water for acid, alkali, or bleach)
- Observe for respiratory distress secondary to laryngeal involvement (hoarseness, stridor, dyspnea); consider IV steroids to temporize laryngeal edema
- Monitor vital signs closely
- Severe chest pain and abdominal pain may be indicative of visceral perforation
- Esophagoscopy usually performed after oral burns improve (3–5 d) to assess extent of esophageal stricture, which develops in approximately 15% of caustic ingestions
- NG tube placement should be done at time of esophagoscopy to maintain lumen

FOREIGN BODY

- Must have proper equipment and ability to visualize
- Blind attempts at removal should be avoided
- Neutral objects (e.g., bead, piece of plastic) are generally not urgent
- See Table 32.6

Table 32.6	Approach to Foreign Body in the Ear, Nose, and Aerodigestive Tract
Anatomic Site	**Approach**
Ear	· Visualize FB with head mirror or headlamp and attempt removal; if deep in ear canal, consult ENT surgeon before attempting removal · Soft material: use loop · Hard smooth object: use hook or loop · If insect: kill it before removal by instilling rubbing alcohol; syringing with warm water is helpful · If vegetable matter, foam, or paper, manual debridement recommended because object may swell with irrigation · If TM perforated, consult ENT surgeon for emergency exploration and possible repair; arrange audiometric assessment and follow-up in 3–4 wk with ENT
Nose	· FB is most common cause of unilateral (usually foul-smelling) nasal discharge · Visualize FB with head mirror or light · Anesthetize and shrink nasal mucosa by inserting cotton packs soaked with cocaine 4–5% (max dose 3 mg/kg) or 0.25% phenylephrine/3% lidocaine solution · Suction discharge surrounding FB · Soft material (e.g., paper, cotton): use forceps · Solid object: use hook

(continued)

Table 32.6	Approach to Foreign Body in the Ear, Nose, and Aerodigestive Tract *(continued)*
Anatomic Site	**Approach**
Esophagus	· History of ingestion, dysphagia, regurgitation, vomiting, drooling; may be several months' duration · Examination may be normal; stridor may be present if trachea compressed · AP *and* lateral XR; FB (e.g., coin) may be seen head-on in AP view · Remove FB endoscopically under general anesthesia · Disk battery in esophagus is an *acute emergency* that requires immediate consultation and removal; may see "double-halo sign" on XR
Larynx and tracheobronchial tree	· Consider FB in any child with difficult-to-diagnose chronic cough, wheezing, chest disease, dysphagia · Usually history of choking or cyanotic episode, but sometimes no acute presentation · Aphonia + airway distress indicates laryngeal FB · Stridor, wheezing, unequal expansion of chest, decreased air entry unilaterally; however, examination may be normal · Investigations: 　· Inspiratory and expiratory XRs; two views essential (bilateral decubitus if uncooperative) 　· Collapse suggests complete obstruction; hyperinflation suggests ball-valve obstruction · Management: 　· Positive history, despite normal examination ± normal XR, necessitates endoscopy 　· FB in larynx may cause complete obstruction and require immediate removal; if bronchoscopist not available, direct laryngoscopy and removal with Magill forceps followed by endotracheal intubation may be life saving 　· Cricothyroidotomy is last resort; use only for laryngeal/pharyngeal obstruction

PHARYNGITIS

- Infectious (~90% viral; ~10% bacterial; rarely fungal)
- No sign or symptom clearly distinguishes GABHS infection from viral causes
- Primary concern is that untreated GABHS may cause rheumatic fever

BACTERIAL PHARYNGITIS

- GABHS most common; rarely, other pathogens can include *Corynebacterium diphtheriae*, *S. aureus*, *H. influenzae*, groups C and G hemolytic streptococci, anaerobes, *Chlamydia trachomatis*, *Mycoplasma pneumoniae*, *Neisseria gonorrhoeae* (gonococcal pharyngitis: occurs in sexually active patients; characteristic greenish exudate)

GABHS Pharyngitis (Strep Throat)

- Peak prevalence 5–10 yr; rare under 2 yr
- Children with acute onset of sore throat (<12 h), pharyngeal exudate, odynophagia, fever >38.5°C, and enlarged tender anterior cervical lymph nodes warrant testing for GABHS
- Children with manifestations suggestive of viral infection (e.g., coryza, conjunctivitis, hoarseness, cough, anterior stomatitis, discrete ulcerative lesions, diarrhea) generally should not be tested for GABHS

Testing

- RST: result in 10–20 min; sensitivity 80–90%; specificity 95%; if +ve start treatment; if –ve, plate throat culture
- Throat culture (gold standard): result available in 1–2 d
- Culture only appropriate patients (10% are carriers; have GABHS but lack clinical symptoms, are generally not contagious, and not at risk for rheumatic fever)

Treatment

- Penicillin V is drug of choice
  - In patients <27 kg: penicillin V 250 mg tid for 10 d
  - In patients ≥27 kg: penicillin V 500 mg tid for 10 d
- Penicillin allergy: first-generation cephalosporin (10 d); erythromycin (10 d); clarithromycin (10 d); azithromycin (5 d)
- To prevent rheumatic fever, start therapy within 9 d of illness and complete course
- Complications can be suppurative (cervical adenitis; submandibular/sublingual/peritonsillar/retropharyngeal abscess); nonsuppurative (scarlet fever; rheumatic fever, PSGN)

VIRAL PHARYNGITIS

- Usually associated with sneezing, rhinorrhea, cough
- Adenovirus, *Rhinovirus*, EBV, HSV 1, HSV 2, influenza, parainfluenza, *Coronavirus*, *Enterovirus* (including coxsackievirus and echovirus), RSV, CMV, HIV
- EBV pharyngitis: see Chapter 24
- Herpetic pharyngitis: see Chapter 24

TRACHEOSTOMY

INDICATIONS

- Most common: bilateral vocal fold paralysis, subglottic stenosis

TUBES

- Metal, polymeric silicone (Silastic), polytef (Teflon), polyethylene, and rubber
- Cuffed or uncuffed; may have single lumen or removable inner cannula
- In pediatrics, most common to use uncuffed single-lumen tube

COMMON PROBLEMS

Obstructed Tracheostomy Tube

- If presents with respiratory distress, assume obstruction: usually inspissated mucus
- Give high-flow oxygen and suction; if unsuccessful, inject 5–10 mL normal saline and resuction
- If unsuccessful, remove and replace tube

- Patient may breathe better through stoma or may require oral or nasal intubation
- Consider other causes (e.g., low tracheal stenosis, pneumonia, aspiration)

Displaced Tube and Stomal Closure

- Do not try to force tube: may cause hemorrhage
- Replace with smaller-sized tube; stoma may be gradually enlarged on daily basis

False Passage

- May occur when replacing tube with excessive force
- Can be recognized by failure of positive-pressure ventilation to inflate lungs and rapid development of subcutaneous emphysema
- Use catheter as guide before removal and insertion of new tube

Hemorrhage

- Life-threatening emergency in immediate postoperative period
- Tracheoinnominate artery fistula (between trachea and brachio-cephalic artery) may occur 1–3 wk postoperatively
- May present as coughing of >10 mL of blood from tube or notice-able pulsating tube movement
- Requires immediate bronchoscopy and tube removal
- If minor (<10 mL) superficial bleeding site is found, it may be packed or cauterized
- If significant hemorrhaging continues, must apply direct pressure until emergency sternotomy

Infection

- Infection is rare, but colonization (especially with *Pseudomonas*) is common
- If peristomal cellulitis occurs, treat with oral antibiotics to cover *S. aureus* (e.g., clindamycin)
- Paratracheal abscess requires prompt drainage and IV antibiotics to prevent mediastinitis

UPPER AIRWAY OBSTRUCTION

STRIDOR

- Results from turbulent airflow through narrowed passageway
- *Inspiratory stridor*: usually extrathoracic obstruction, most commonly at vocal folds and above
- *Inspiratory and expiratory stridor*: associated with fixed lesions, most commonly at vocal folds or subglottis
- *Expiratory stridor*: wheezing; usually intrathoracic obstruction, most commonly tracheobronchial lesions
- See Figure 32.2

Figure 32.2 **Upper Airway Obstruction: Stridor**

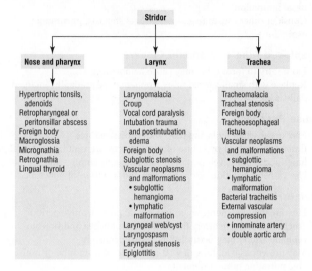

Nose and pharynx	Larynx	Trachea
Hypertrophic tonsils, adenoids Retropharyngeal or peritonsillar abscess Foreign body Macroglossia Micrognathia Retrognathia Lingual thyroid	Laryngomalacia Croup Vocal cord paralysis Intubation trauma and postintubation edema Foreign body Subglottic stenosis Vascular neoplasms and malformations • subglottic hemangioma • lymphatic malformation Laryngeal web/cyst Laryngospasm Laryngeal stenosis Epiglottitis	Tracheomalacia Tracheal stenosis Foreign body Tracheoesophageal fistula Vascular neoplasms and malformations • subglottic hemangioma • lymphatic malformation Bacterial tracheitis External vascular compression • innominate artery • double aortic arch

FB

- See Table 32.6

Congenital Causes

Nasal

- Newborns are obligate nose breathers
- Bilateral choanal atresia: common in CHARGE (see p. 374); unilateral choanal atresia does not cause respiratory distress unless contralateral side becomes obstructed
- Nasal mass: encephalocele, glioma, dermoid cyst
- Symptoms: cyanosis in newborn, relieved by crying
- Diagnosis: inability to pass rubber catheter through nares bilaterally, flexible nasal endoscopy, CT
- Treatment: oral airway and surgical repair of choanal obstruction

Pharyngeal

- Causes: retrognathia, lingual thyroid, enlarged tongue, tonsillar hypertrophy
- Symptoms: nighttime apnea, cyanosis
- Diagnosis: physical examination
- Treatment: nasopharyngeal airway, surgical intervention

Laryngeal
- Laryngomalacia: most common cause of stridor in children < 2 yr; due to intrinsic defect or delayed maturation of supporting structures of larynx; worse when supine, crying, during URTI; most resolve spontaneously by 2 yr
- Other causes: laryngeal cysts/webs, subglottic hemangioma, subglottic stenosis (congenital vs. acquired secondary to intubation), vocal fold paralysis
- Symptoms: inspiratory stridor, hoarseness, weak cry
- Diagnosis: endoscopy (flexible or rigid)
- Treatment: observation; consider laser excision; rarely tracheotomy

Tracheal
- Tracheomalacia: due to abnormal flaccidity of trachea, abnormal collapse during expiration; may occur with laryngomalacia but often occurs independently
- Other causes: tracheal stenosis, TEF, lymphangioma/hemangioma (external compression), vascular ring (aortic arch or pulmonary artery anomalies)
- Symptoms: expiratory stridor, "dying spells" (apneic or cyanotic spells)
- Diagnosis: airway fluoroscopy and barium swallow to assess dynamic airway and evidence of vascular compression; may require MRI and echocardiography
- Treatment: observation; surgical correction of underlying cause as needed (e.g., repair TEF, aortopexy, possible stenting)

Neoplastic Causes

Benign
- Squamous papillomas: 50% of mothers have history of genital condylomas at delivery
- Symptoms: stridor and hoarseness
- Diagnosis: laryngeal endoscopy
- Treatment: multiple laser or mechanical resections

Malignant
- Lymphoma, neuroblastoma, teratoma, rhabdomyosarcoma

Infectious Causes
- Laryngotracheitis (croup)
- Peritonsillar abscess
- Infection of retropharyngeal and parapharyngeal spaces
- Submandibular/sublingual abscess (Ludwig angina)
- Bacterial tracheitis
- Supraglottitis (epiglottitis)

FURTHER READING

American Academy of Pediatrics. Clinical practice guideline: management of sinusitis. *Pediatrics*. 2001;108:798–808.

American Academy of Pediatrics, Subcommittee on Management of Acute Otitis Media. Diagnosis and management of acute otitis media. *Pediatrics*. 2004;113:1451–1465.

American Academy of Pediatrics, Joint Committee on Infant Hearing. Year 2007 position statement: principles and guidelines for early hearing detection and intervention programs. *Pediatrics*. 2007;120:898–921.

Paradise JL, Bluestone CD, Colborn DK, Bernard BS, Rockette HE, Kurs-Lasky M. Tonsillectomy and adenotonsillectomy for recurrent throat infection in moderately affected children. *Pediatrics*. 2002;110:7–15.

Pickering LK, Baker CJ, Long SS, McMillan JA, eds. *Red Book: 2006 Report of the Committee on Infectious Diseases*. 27th ed. Elk Grove Village, Ill: American Academy of Pediatrics; 2006.

Price V, Campisi P, Blanchette V. *Guidelines for the Investigation and Management of Epistaxis in Children* [internal document]. Toronto, Ontario, Canada: Hospital for Sick Children; 2005.

USEFUL WEB SITES

eMedicine. Available at: **www.emedicine.com/ent/**
ENTLinx.com. Available at: **www.entlinx.com/index.cfm**

Chapter 33 Plastic Surgery

Ksenia Slywynska

Christopher R. Forrest

Chapter 33 Plastic Surgery

COMMON ABBREVIATIONS

DIP	distal interphalangeal
ICP	intracranial pressure
IPJ	interphalangeal joint
MCP	metacarpophalangeal
PIP	proximal interphalangeal
Td	tetanus and diphtheria toxoid
Tdap	tetanus toxoid, diphtheria toxoid, and acellular pertussis

WOUND MANAGEMENT

ABRASIONS

- Anesthetize as necessary to ensure adequate cleansing
- Scrub area to remove embedded dirt; use scrub brush, if necessary
- Use dilute antiseptic (e.g., povidone-iodine [Betadine]) to avoid irritation

CONTUSIONS

- An injury that does not break the skin but results in discoloration; a bruise
- Ice/saline-soaked cold compresses in early stages to minimize swelling (24–48 h)
- Consider consultation with plastic surgeon if hematoma suspected
- Watch for signs of tissue compromise due to expanding hematoma

AVULSION

- Flap of tissue that is torn/lacerated
- If partial and tissue is viable, retain all tissue and secure it back into position with simple sutures
- If complete, consult plastic surgeon: may be able to thin tissue and secure as a graft

PUNCTURE

- If contaminated (particularly bites), should leave open; treat larger cleaner punctures in anatomically prominent areas (face) with copious cleansing with iodine and reapproximation
- Explore for foreign body (e.g., glass), as may have more severe injury than expected from outward appearance

- Watch for cat claw puncture wounds, which have a tendency for infection
- XR to help rule out radio-opaque foreign body (e.g., metal); some wood is radio-opaque in case of penetrating wounds
- Tetanus status and rabies prophylaxis (see Chapter 23) should be considered in all animal bites; antibiotic management (Tables 33.1 and 24.3)

High-Risk Wounds

- Primary closure should *not* be considered; prophylactic antibiotics recommended
- Key to preventing infection is adequate irrigation and satisfactory debridement of devitalized tissue; antibiotic use is of secondary importance; remember, infections usually have a cause (hematoma, closed space, dead tissue)

Examples

- Crush injuries
- Puncture wounds
- Bites involving the hands
- Dog bite wounds with delayed presentation; >6–12 h (arm/leg) or >12–24 h (face)
- Cat or human bites, except those to the face
- Bite wounds in immunosuppressed hosts

Table 33.1	Common Bites, Organisms, and Antibiotic Therapy		
Type of Bite	**Common Organisms**	**Management**	**Comments**
Dog	*Staphylococcus* spp., *Streptococcus* spp., anaerobes (e.g., *Pasteurella canis*, *Bacteroides*)	· Role of prophylactic antibiotics uncertain · Rx: penicillin or amoxicillin/clavulanate	· Often crush injury
Cat*	*Pasteurella multocida*, anaerobes (e.g., *Bacteroides*)	· Prophylaxis recommended · Rx: amoxicillin/clavulanate or penicillin or clindamycin + TMP/SMX	· Puncture wound · May be associated with lymphadenopathy · Frequently presents infected
Human	*Streptococcus* (α- and β-hemolytic), *Staphylococcus aureus*, *Eikenella corrodens*, anaerobes	· Rx: amoxicillin/clavulanate or penicillin + dicloxacillin or cefazolin or erythromycin	· Prone to developing infection · Must consider child maltreatment

*Bites of other animals (rodents, squirrels, rabbits, guinea pigs) should be treated as cat bites.
TMP/SMX, trimethoprim-sulfamethoxazole.

33

EXTRAVASATION INJURIES

- Stop infusion as soon as detected
- Elevate extremity
- Watch for signs of compartment syndrome
- Most are managed expectantly
- Delayed debridement and wound closure when tissue loss declared

LACERATIONS

Management

Immunization

- Clean wounds do not require Td unless patient not fully immunized or has been >10 yr since booster
- All dirty wounds require Td unless fully immunized and <5 yr since booster
- If incomplete immunization status or uncertain status, need Td + tetanus immune globulin
- Tdap may be more appropriate than Td for adolescents aged 14–16 yr (see Chapter 23)

Anesthesia

- Infiltrate area with 1% lidocaine with 1:200,000 epinephrine (no epinephrine for appendages [e.g., fingers, toes, ears, nose])
- Dose limits: 7 mg/kg with epinephrine, 5 mg/kg without epinephrine
- May need to consider sedation, depending on child and extent of wound

Cleansing

- Use dilute antiseptic
- Be aggressive in wound cleansing and debridement of devitalized tissue
- Wounds with heavy bacterial inoculum at time of injury and clean wounds open for >6 h should be considered contaminated
- Closing these wounds requires copious irrigation, attention to balance of infection risk vs. cosmesis, and early follow-up

Suturing

- Always consider two-layer closure unless mucosa, palm, sole, or skin too thin
- For skin closure, use monofilament 5-0 or 6-0 (absorbable, for young children <5 yr, or nonabsorbable, nylon or polypropylene [Prolene]); do not use silk for skin closure
- For layered closure, use 4-0 or 5-0 polyglactin 910 (Vicryl) or polyglecaprone 25 (Monocryl) to reapproximate dermis
- Remove sutures after 7–14 d (e.g., 7 d for face, 2 wk for lower extremity)
- 2-Octylcyanoacrylate (Dermabond) should only be used for shallow lacerations with clean edges (never for animal bites or dirty wounds) in areas that are not stressed by movement (e.g., not across joints)

Facial Lacerations

- May be closed outside of 6 h window because of healthy blood supply and cosmetic concerns
- Consult plastic surgeon for eyelid lacerations, lacerations crossing vermilion border, concern of injury to facial nerve or parotid duct, ear lacerations involving cartilage, or with suspected hematoma or complex/stellate lacerations

SCAR MANAGEMENT

- Scars take up to 2 yr to mature; be patient
- Scar management consists of massage (4–5 × daily), direct pressure, silicone gel patches, and use of sunscreen (>30 SPF for cosmetically sensitive areas for 12 mo)
- Vitamin E convenient lubricant but not proven to be of special benefit
- Hypertrophic scar: growth limited to scar; conservative treatment (intralesional/topical corticosteroids)
- Keloid: growth beyond boundaries of scar; treatment includes combination of pressure, topical/intradermal steroids, intralesional excision

FACIAL FRACTURES

EVALUATION

- First stabilize patient and evaluate cervical spine
- Check skin/scalp for lacerations and abrasions, evidence of basal skull fracture (Battle sign, "raccoon eyes," hemotympanum, CSF otorrhea or rhinorrhea)
- Palpate for pain, crepitations, asymmetry, "step" deformity
- Check midface stability (palpate craniofacial skeleton for crepitations and irregularities, look for facial asymmetry of bony structures) and malocclusion
- Check sensation at forehead, cheek/upper lip, and chin (branches of trigeminal nerve)
- Test for visual acuity and extraocular movements
- Examine for intraoral lacerations and loose dentition

RADIOGRAPHIC ASSESSMENT

- CT with thin cuts and coronal reconstruction if suspect facial fracture
- Panoramic radiography (Panorex) if mandibular fracture suspected
- Plain facial XR of no practical value in diagnosis of facial fractures
- Refer to plastic surgeon if suspect fracture

CLEFT LIP AND PALATE

- Immediate impact on feeding, airway (in association with micrognathia), and parental well-being
- Long-term impact on speech, hearing, dentition, facial growth, cosmesis
- Refer to regional cleft palate team promptly
- Unilateral cleft lip most common, followed by cleft lip and palate, followed by isolated cleft palate
- Examine child carefully to rule out other malformations (especially cardiac)
- Additional structural abnormalities occur in up to 50% of newborns with isolated cleft palate and 20% with cleft lip and palate; typically involve CNS and cardiovascular systems
- Associated syndromes, in presence of other anomalies, include DiGeorge, Treacher Collins, orofaciodigital syndrome
- Lip repair at 3 mo; palate repair at approximately 1 yr
- If parent has cleft, increased risk that child will have cleft; if first child affected, increased risk of second child having cleft lip and/or palate (see p. 385)

CRANIOSYNOSTOSIS

- Premature fusion of one or more sutures (coronal, sagittal, metopic, lambdoid) in cranial vault or base, resulting in abnormal growth of the skull
- Classified as primary vs. secondary, single vs. multiple sutures, syndromic vs. nonsyndromic; majority (95%) single suture, nonsyndromic
- Secondary causes (e.g., rickets, bone metabolic disorders, achondroplasia, prematurity, shunt/biomechanical)
- Incidence: most common sagittal—1 in 2000; infrequent lambdoid— 1 in 150,000
- Functional problems: increased ICP (14% of single suture, 40% of multiple suture), aesthetic
- See Figure 33.1

DEFORMATIONAL PLAGIOCEPHALY

- Positional; "flattened" occiput, nonsynostotic
- Parallelogram-shaped skull
- Ipsilateral ear anteriorly positioned compared with opposite side
- Extremely common due to amount of time babies spend supine
- Incidence increased when baby has untreated congenital torticollis

Management

- Awake time in an alternate position (supervised tummy time)
- Place toys and mirrors or both sides of the crib/car seat
- Physiotherapy for torticollis
- Severe cases: molding helmets worn throughout most of the day; most effective if started between 4–6 mo; less effective after 12 mo

Figure 33.1 Craniosynostosis

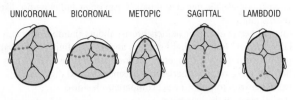

HAND INJURY

EXAMINATION

Vascular

- Pulses, capillary refill, color, tissue turgor

Allen Test

- Used to test for integrity of ulnar and radial arteries
- Hand is squeezed in a fist for 30 s; radial and ulnar arteries are occluded and hand should appear blanched (see nail beds); ulnar artery pressure is released, and color should return to hand in <5 s (if ulnar artery intact); reverse order to assess radial artery

Sensory

- See Figure 33.2
- Assess light touch, two-point discrimination, vibration, proprioception
  - Median nerve: radial side index finger
  - Ulnar nerve: ulnar side little finger
  - Radial nerve: snuffbox at base of thumb on dorsum
  - Digital nerves: radial and ulnar

Figure 33.2 Nerves of the Hand

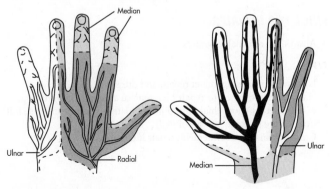

Median

Ulnar

Radial

Ulnar

Median

Plastic Surgery

33

Motor

- Movement of specific muscles; if patient can open and close fist, likely motor is intact
  - Median nerve: abductor pollicis brevis; abduct thumb from palm
  - Ulnar nerve: abductor digiti minimi; abduct little finger or do paper test between digits for finger adduction (patient tries to maintain hold on piece of paper between adjacent extended digits while examiner tries to pull it away; compare both sides)
  - Radial nerve: wrist extension

Tendons

- Five flexor and nine extensor zones to describe location of injury
- Flexor
  - Flexor digitorum profundus: assess by asking patient to flex DIP while stabilizing PIP
  - Flexor digitorum superficialis: assess by asking patient to flex PIP
  - Mass action of all finger flexor tendons may be assessed by squeezing forearm and watching for gross finger flexion; useful in infants and young children
  - Flexor pollicis longus: ask patient to flex IPJ of thumb
- Assess extensor tendons by asking patient to make a fist and open hand
- Remember, intrinsic muscles flex MCP and extend IP
- Any deep injury to the flexor surface should be explored
- All flexor tendon repairs should be done in the OR
- Extensor tendons may be repaired in the ER
- Watch for partial laceration of extensor tendons over dorsum of finger with late boutonnière deformity

MANAGEMENT

- "Safe" position for splinting: wrist at 45° extension, MCP joints at 90°, IP joints extended, and thumb abducted in opposed position

FINGERTIP INJURIES

- Always use resorbable sutures

TYPES

- Laceration: cleansing, direct repair, and dressing
- Nail bed: remove nail to repair bed, replace as stent if laceration extends across eponychial fold to prevent late synechiae (may use foil from suture package instead of nail)
- Crush: cleansing, debridement, repair if possible, dressing

Amputation

- Controversy regarding benefits of replacement (biologic dressing) vs. secondary healing (better neurosensory recovery)
- Young children have better chance of piece taking as composite graft
- Distal to DIP: vessels too small to repair
- Proximal to DIP: place part in sterile gauze in plastic bag on ice and consult plastic surgery
  - Partial: replace and repair, dress
  - Complete:
    - Bone exposed: trim bone back and replace/dress
    - No bone exposed: replace vs. dress
- Dressings to fingertips best left intact for 7–10 d to allow healing
- Polysporin/Band-Aids with soap and water washes good for high-risk cases
- XR hand for evidence of tuft fracture; useful for prognostic information only; if fracture present, may benefit from splint for comfort

OBSTETRIC BRACHIAL PLEXUS INJURY

- Risk factors: large birth weight, breech presentation, shoulder dystocia
- Look for lack of limb movement
- Usually right sided; Erb palsy (C5, C6) most common: limb seen in adduction, prone, and internally rotated positions; 5% have associated phrenic nerve paresis
- Total palsy (C5–T1): loss of grasp and lack of wrist movement; may have associated Horner syndrome
- Treat with physiotherapy; some have spontaneous partial to good recovery; better prognosis if some improvement in first 2 wk of life; many require surgical repair
- Early referral (2–3 months) to plastic surgeon essential; surgery generally done around 6 mo of age

BURNS

- Majority of pediatric burns are scalds or contact burns
- Prevent severe immersion burns by keeping water temperature at home at recommended setting of 49°C (120°F)
- Cold water immersion of burned area may be helpful immediately after burn or within first hour (do not use ice)
- Careful history (including social) and physical examination noting degree, location, and extent of burn; be wary of nonaccidental injury (see Chapter 10)

MANAGEMENT

- See Chapter 3 for resuscitation and acute management

Outpatient

- Diagram burn area, noting degree (Table 33.2 and p. 50)
- Cool part; eliminate inciting agent (copious irrigation with water if chemical burn)
- Cleanse with 0.9% NaCl (use sterile gloves); leave intact blisters alone
- Debride broken blisters and loose debris; apply antibiotic ointment (e.g., Polysporin) and then framycetin sulfate (Sofra-Tulle)
- Dress with wet 0.9% NaCl gauze, dry gauze, and secure with conforming gauze (Kling) bandage; frequency of changes are dependent on state of burn, usually once or twice daily
- Review tetanus immunization status (see Chapter 23); oral analgesics prn for pain, and re-evaluate in 2–5 d
- Discuss signs of infection (erythema, edema, green/violaceous discoloration, fever, malaise) with caregivers

Inpatient

- See Box 3.2 (p. 5) for criteria for hospitalization of patients with burns

Burn Care

- Evaluate and document burn size, location, and depth
- Cleanse in burn bath (lukewarm salt water at 38°C [100°F]) and debride loose tissue and broken blisters; leave intact blisters alone
- Apply silver sulfadiazine cream to burn areas on body and Polysporin ointment to burns on face

Fluid Management

- Insert urinary catheter for bladder decompression and monitoring of urine output if burn >15% BSA
- Record accurate hourly input and output
- Parkland formula (see p. 49) is only a guide for initial fluid management and must be reassessed and adjusted:
  - If urine output <1 mL/kg/h, consider 0.9% NaCl bolus
  - If urine output 1–3 mL/kg/h, continue with Parkland formula
  - If urine output >3 mL/kg/h, decrease fluids to ⅔ Parkland formula
  - In addition to Parkland formula, for children <2 yr of age, give maintenance fluid requirements
  - Note: no K^+ to be given in IV fluids over first 48 h due to K^+ release secondary to cell death

Table 33.2	Severity of Burn	
Degree	Level of Burn	Characteristics
First	Epidermis	Erythema, pain
Second · Superficial · Deep	Superficial dermis Deep dermis	Blisters, pain Eschar, ± pain
Third	Subcutaneous tissue	Leathery eschar, insensate

Supportive Care

- NPO with NG tube in severe burns, H_2 blocker
- Begin enteral feeding within the first 8 h after injury; maximize feedings (e.g., PO or NG) on second postburn day; remember, these children are hypermetabolic
- Pain management critical with IV opioids as needed (see Chapter 5)
- Take swabs for culture and sensitivity from nose, throat, and burn wound
- Review tetanus immunization status; tetanus prophylaxis, if not up to date
- May require high environmental temperature (i.e., 28–30°C [82–86°F]) to prevent heat loss
- Transfuse with albumin, plasma, or blood as needed
- Observe carefully for sepsis

CIRCUMFERENTIAL BURNS

- Loss of capillary integrity leads to massive swelling with resuscitation
- Circumferential eschar constriction may compromise distal circulation
- Consider immediate escharotomy

FURTHER READING

Milerad J, Larson O, Hagberg C, Ideberg M. Associated malformations in infants with cleft lip and palate: a prospective, population-based study. *Pediatrics*. 1997;100:180–186.

Thorne CH, Beaseley RW, Bartlett SW. *Grabb and Smith's Plastic Surgery*. 6th ed. Philadelphia, Pa: Lippincott Williams & Wilkins; 2006.

Plastic Surgery

33

Chapter 34 Respirology

Tania Samanta

Joanna Swinburne

Hartmut Grasemann

Chapter 34 Respirology

COMMON ABBREVIATIONS

ABPA	allergic bronchopulmonary aspergillosis
BAL	bronchoalveolar lavage
BPD	bronchopulmonary dysplasia
CCAM	congenital cystic adenomatoid malformation
CCHS	congenital central hypoventilation syndrome
CF	cystic fibrosis
CFTR	cystic fibrosis transmembrane conductance regulator
CHD	congenital heart disease
CLD	chronic lung disease
DIOS	distal intestinal obstruction syndrome
DLCO	carbon monoxide diffusing capacity of the lung
FEV_1	forced expiratory volume in 1 s
hMPV	human metapneumovirus
IPH	idiopathic pulmonary hemosiderosis
IRT	immunoreactive trypsin
LVH	left ventricular hypertrophy
NO	nitric oxide
OSA	obstructive sleep apnea
PDA	patent ductus arteriosus
PEF	peak expiratory flow
PEG	polyethylene glycol
PEP	peak expiratory pressure
PFT	pulmonary function test
PHT	pulmonary hypertension
PJP	*Pneumocystis jiroveci* pneumonia
PPHN	persistent pulmonary hypertension
PSG	polysomnography
RSV	respiratory syncytial virus

Respirology

34

RESPIRATORY VARIABLES

PaO_2	arterial PO_2
PAO_2	alveolar PO_2
$PaCO_2$	arterial PCO_2
$PACO_2$	alveolar PCO_2 approximates $PaCO_2$
R	respiratory quotient (CO_2 produced/O_2 consumed) = approximately 0.8
PiO_2	partial pressure of inspired O_2 = approximately 150 mm Hg at sea level in room air
P_B	atmospheric pressure = 760 mm Hg at sea level
P_{H20}	pressure of water vapor = 47 mm Hg

NORMAL RANGES FOR RESPIRATORY RATES

- See Table 34.1

Table 34.1	Normal Ranges for Respiratory Rates
Age	**Respiratory Rate**
Neonate	30-60
Infant	20-50
1 yr	20-40
2 yr	20-35
3 yr	15-30
Adolescent	12-18

Adapted from Rusconi F, Castagneto M, Gagliardi L, et al. Reference values for respiratory rate in the first 3 years of life. *Pediatrics.* 1994;94:350–355; and from Hooker EA, Danzl DF, Brueggmeyer M, Harper E. Respiratory rates in pediatric emergency patients. *J Emerg Med.* 1992;10:407–410.

FORMULAS

ALVEOLAR GAS EQUATION

$$PAO_2 = PiO_2 - (PACO_2/R)$$
$$PiO_2 = FiO_2 \times (P_B - P_{H2O})$$

ALVEOLAR–ARTERIAL O$_2$ GRADIENT

$$A\text{-a gradient} = PAO_2 - PaO_2$$

- Obtain ABG measuring PaO_2 and $PaCO_2$ with patient on 100% O_2 for at least 10 min
- Calculate PAO_2 (see above) and A-a gradient:
  - Normal is <50 mm Hg in 100% O_2 or <20–30 mm Hg in room air
  - >450 mm Hg indicates severe respiratory failure

OXYGENATION INDEX

$$OI = (\text{mean airway pressure} \times FiO_2 \times 100)/PaO_2$$

- Normal, <5; severe respiratory failure in children, >20; severe respiratory failure in neonates, >40
- Consider ECMO if severe respiratory failure

PULMONARY FUNCTION TESTS

- Used to provide objective measurements of lung/airway function, volumes, gas diffusion, changes over time

- Spirometry plots airflow vs. lung volume; usually reliable in those aged >6 yr; may be completed before and after bronchodilators to assess reversibility of airway obstruction or after bronchial challenge (e.g., methacholine) to assess airway hyperreactivity (Table 34.2)
- See Figure 34.1 for lung volume subdivisions

Table 34.2	Interpretation of Pulmonary Function Testing		
Measurement		Restrictive	Obstructive
Volumes			
Total lung capacity (TLC)		↓	↑
Residual volume (RV)		↓↑	↑
Forced vital capacity (FVC)		↓	N or ↓
Forced expiratory volume in 1 s (FEV$_1$)		↓	↓
Flows			
Maximal mid expiratory flow (MMEF)		↓	↓
Forced expiratory flow from 25–75% of VC (FEF$_{25-75}$)			↓
FEV$_1$/FVC		N or ↑	↓

Adapted from Schmidlow DV, Smith DS. *A Practical Guide to Pediatric Respiratory Diseases*. Philadelphia, Pa: Hanley and Belfus; 1994.

Figure 34.1 **Lung Volume Subdivisions**

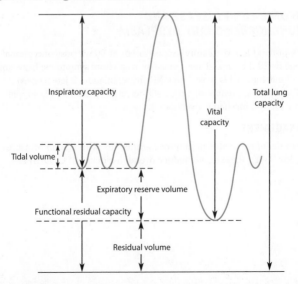

- See Table 34.3

Table 34.3	Oxygen Delivery Systems		
Mode of Oxygen Delivery	Fraction of Inspired O_2 (FIO_2) Effectively Delivered	Flow Rate (L/min)	Notes
Nasal prongs	0.22–0.40	0.25–4	Unpredictable O_2 delivery
Simple mask	0.35–0.55	6–10	Flow must be sufficient to flush out CO_2
Partial rebreathing mask	0.60–0.95	>6	Flow must be sufficient to maintain inflation of reservoir bag
Nonrebreathing mask	Up to 1.0	>6	Reservoir bag must remain inflated; one-way valve prevents mixing
Venturi mask	24–50%		Predictable O_2 delivery
O_2 hood/head box		Must be at least 10	May achieve high O_2 concentration

© The Hospital for Sick Children, 2009. New artwork created by The Hospital for Sick Children, for *The Hospital for Sick Children Handbook of Pediatrics*, 11th edition.

CONGENITAL MALFORMATIONS OF THE LUNG

- See Table 34.4

CHRONIC LUNG DISEASE AND BRONCHOPULMONARY DYSPLASIA

- Persistent O_2 ± ventilatory support needs at 36 wk postconceptional age or 28 d postnatal age; persistent respiratory symptoms; hazy small-volume lung fields typical on CXR (hyperinflation at later stages)
- Risk factors: prematurity, neonatal respiratory distress, O_2 supplementation, mechanical ventilation

MANAGEMENT

- No definitive treatment; improved outcomes with certain measures (Box 34.1); these do *not* reduce overall incidence of CLD/BPD

34

Table 34.4

Congenital Malformations of the Lung

Malformation	Etiology / Anatomy	Presentation	Diagnosis	Comments
Pulmonary sequestration	· Segment of nonfunctioning lung tissue, no communication with tracheobronchial tree, blood supply via systemic arterial collateral vessel · Intralobar: more common (90%), adjacent to normal lung · Extralobar: completely separated from normal lung by pleura; 10% below the diaphragm	· Intralobar often asymptomatic, may present early as neonatal heart failure or later as result of secondary infection · Extralobar may be associated with other congenital malformations, often detected in first year of life	· Prenatal US, CXR, or chest CT; MRI if diagnosis unclear	
CCAM	· Overgrowth of terminal bronchioles occurring early in fetal development, connected to tracheobronchial tree · May occur in any area of lung; blood supplied via pulmonary circulation	· Feeding difficulties, tachypnea, cyanosis, acute respiratory distress; symptoms may be due to pulmonary infection	· Prenatal US; CXR, chest CT	· Prenatal complications: polyhydramnios, hydrops (rare), lung hypoplasia · Postnatal complications: recurrent lung infections, PHN, malignant transformation (rare) · No treatment if asymptomatic; may opt for surgical removal due to risk of malignancy or if infections occur
Bronchogenic cysts	· Thin-walled islands of bronchial tissue left behind during branching of airways early in fetal development	· May be asymptomatic or present with respiratory distress, depending on size and location	· CXR, confirmed on CT	
Congenital diaphragmatic hernia	· Abnormalities in development of diaphragm; usually left posterior lateral aspect · Abdominal contents herniated into thorax	· Can result in significant lung hypoplasia, respiratory insufficiency from birth; PHN	· Prenatal US; detection before 25 wk gestation associated with poor outcome	· Intubate immediately at delivery, without bag and mask ventilation; insert NG tube, set to continuous suction; may require high-frequency oscillatory ventilation or ECMO before corrective surgery
Congenital lobar emphysema	· Congenital overinflation of pulmonary lobe	· 50% present by 4 wk of age, some may remain asymptomatic	· CXR showing hyperinflation	· Upper > lower lobes, left > right, M > F · Associated with CHD in 10–20% of cases

Medications
- Prenatal steroids
- Exogenous surfactant
- Diuretics
- Inhaled bronchodilators

Ventilation
- Decreased use of high supplemental O_2
- Regulation of ventilated airway pressure/volume
- Patient-triggered ventilation
- Permissive hypercapnia

Other
- Closure of symptomatic PDA
- Improved nutrition

© The Hospital for Sick Children, 2009. New artwork created by The Hospital for Sick Children, for *The Hospital for Sick Children Handbook of Pediatrics*, 11th edition.

OUTCOMES

- Improvement of lung function with time (lung growth/remodeling); few patients remain on O_2 past 2 yr of age
- ↑ Risk of wheezing, asthma, pulmonary infections
- Complications: PHT ± cor pulmonale, LVH, systemic HTN, delays in cognitive/motor function
- Routine monitoring of growth, development, and systemic BP recommended
- Currently no guidelines for screening for PHT in premature infants or BPD, but recommendations include echocardiography for extremely premature infants (GA <25 wk or birth weight <600 g), infants requiring prolonged mechanical ventilation, O_2 requirement out of proportion with lung disease or poor growth; ECG for patients with lower risk of PHT
- Poor prognosis associated with prolonged ventilation, IVH, PHT, cor pulmonale, O_2 dependence >1 yr of life

UPPER RESPIRATORY TRACT INFECTIONS

- See Table 34.5

BRONCHIOLITIS

- Infection of lower respiratory tract characterized by wheezing; distinct features as follow

Table 34.5	Comparison of Upper Respiratory Tract Infections		
Factor	**Epiglottitis**	**Croup**	**Bacterial Tracheitis**
Age	Usually older (2–6 yr)	Usually younger (6 mo–4 yr)	Any age
Gender incidence	M = F	M > F	M = F
Agents	Bacterial: GAS, H. influenzae type B	Viral: parainfluenza 1, 2, 3; RSV; influenza, Rhinovirus	Bacterial: S. aureus, pneumococcus, H. influenzae
Seasons	Winter, spring	Late fall, early winter	Any time
Clinical features	Toxic, severe airway obstruction, drooling, tripod sit, stridor, sternal recession	Nontoxic, may be restless, cyanotic, not drooling, stridor common, sternal recession common, barking cough, hoarseness, coryza	Toxic; crouplike cough, stridor
Progression	Rapid	Usually slow	Moderately rapid
Recurrence	Rare	Fairly common	Rare

CLINICAL FEATURES

- Infants and children <2 yr (80% <1 yr)
- Typically preceded by upper respiratory tract infection
- Signs/symptoms: fever, poor feeding, irritability, dyspnea, tachypnea, intercostal indrawing, wheezing, crackles; bilateral otitis media in 16–50%
- Increasing severity indicated by apnea, hypoxemia, hypercapnia, tachycardia or bradycardia, increasing tachypnea, cyanosis; risk factors: age <6 wk, prematurity, CLD, CHD, neurologic disease, immunodeficiency

ETIOLOGY

- Common causes:
  - Viral: RSV (70%), hMPV (3–12%), influenza virus, parainfluenza virus, adenovirus, Rhinovirus
  - Bacterial: pertussis

INVESTIGATIONS

- CXR: not recommended routinely; nonspecific findings (hyperinflation, peribronchial thickening, ↑ linear markings, atelectasis)
- Consider nasopharyngeal swab for respiratory viruses, pertussis

MANAGEMENT

- Supportive measures: O_2 saturation monitoring, humidified O_2, hydration (oral/IV), antipyretics
- Trial of inhaled salbutamol or nebulized epinephrine; should be discontinued if no response
- Ribavirin controversial, not routinely recommended; in immunodeficient children, consider using with advice from specialist in infectious diseases
- Systemic steroids, anticholinergics (ipratropium bromide) not routinely recommended
- Antibiotics only if pertussis or bacterial superinfection suspected
- See Chapter 23 for prophylaxis recommendations

OUTCOMES

- Generally self-resolving
- Complications: apnea, dehydration, electrolyte disturbances (usually hyponatremia), bacterial superinfection, myocardial dysfunction, myocarditis; rarely respiratory failure requiring intubation
- Subsequent recurrent wheezing/asthma in up to 30% after RSV bronchiolitis

PNEUMONIA

ETIOLOGY

- Viral (most common): RSV, parainfluenza, influenza A and B, adenovirus, hMPV, *Rhinovirus*
- Bacterial: pneumococcus, *Mycoplasma*; consider *Staphylococcus* if pneumatocele or empyema; consider oral anaerobes if aspiration suspected
- Hospitalized patients: oral anaerobes, *S. aureus*, enteric bacilli; consider fungal in immunocompromised patients
- See Chapter 24 for etiology and empiric treatment by age group

INVESTIGATIONS

- CBC with differential, blood culture, CXR
- Consider: ABG (if respiratory distress), throat swab for *Mycoplasma*, sputum culture, NP swab, tuberculin skin test, diagnostic thoracentesis (if significant pleural fluid)
- Flexible bronchoscopy with BAL may be indicated in immunocompromised patients (especially if PJP is suspected) or if deterioration with optimized therapy

MANAGEMENT

- Supportive care including PO/IV fluids, humidified O_2
- See Chapter 24 for antibiotic coverage
- Associated empyema and/or pleural effusion may require chest tube drainage

PLEURAL EFFUSION

CLINICAL FEATURES

- Pleuritic chest pain, dullness to percussion; may be associated with significant pneumonia or pneumonia unresponsive to therapy

INVESTIGATIONS

- Pleural fluid for cell count (WBC, differential, RBC), cytologic examination, biochemistry (protein, glucose, pH, LDH, triglycerides if chylous), microbiology (Gram stain, culture, acid-fast staining, virology); immunologic investigations when appropriate (complement studies)
  - *Transudates* associated with CHF, nephrotic syndrome, acute glomerulonephritis, cirrhosis, myxedema
  - *Exudates* associated with infection, collagen vascular diseases, malignancy, pancreatitis, subdiaphragmatic abscess
- See Table 34.6

Table 34.6	Constituents of Pleural Effusions	
Test	**Transudate**	**Exudate**
Protein	<3 g/dL	>3 g/dL
Pleural-to-serum ratio, protein	<0.5	>0.5
Pleural-to-serum ratio, LDH	<0.6	>0.6
WBC	<1000/mm³; usually >50% lymphocyte or mononuclear cells	1000/mm³; >50% PMN (acute inflammation); >50% lymphocytes (TB, neoplasm)
pH	>7.3	<7.3 (inflammatory)
Glucose	= serum	< serum

MANAGEMENT

- Treat underlying cause
- Observation and supportive care if clinically stable
- Drainage: tap or chest tube placement for diagnostic and/or therapeutic indications (e.g., prolonged fever, respiratory distress) (see Chapter 6)

PNEUMOTHORAX

- Causes: trauma, iatrogenic (e.g., postintervention), CF, asthma, other lung diseases, infection, idiopathic/spontaneous
- Primary spontaneous pneumothorax may be more common in tall, young men > women, genetic disorders (e.g., Marfan, Ehlers-Danlos)
- Symptoms: sudden-onset dyspnea, pleuritic chest pain, shoulder/back pain, respiratory distress
- Signs: chest wall movement decreased on affected side, ipsilateral hyperresonance to percussion, ↓ breath sounds on auscultation, subcutaneous emphysema; with tension pneumothorax, contralateral tracheal shift, displaced heart sounds (mediastinal shift), jugular venous distension, tachycardia, hypotension, cyanosis

INVESTIGATIONS

- CXR; may need CT to differentiate pneumothorax from blebs or other cystic formations or to identify underlying lung pathology
- Tension pneumothorax—*clinical* diagnosis

MANAGEMENT

- Tension pneumothorax—*medical emergency!*
  - ABCs (see Chapter 1)
  - If unstable, requires *emergent needle aspiration* (see Chapter 6)
- Small pneumothoraces (<15% of hemithorax transverse diameter): observation only; resorption may occur more quickly with 100% O_2
- Large pneumothoraces: serial CXR to evaluate progress; chest tube drainage to underwater seal if clinically unwell
- Recurrent/persistent pneumothoraces: chemical pleurodesis, open thoracotomy, pleural bleb excision

PULMONARY HEMORRHAGE

CLINICAL FEATURES

- Acute: cough ± hemoptysis, respiratory distress, hypoxia; may have ↓ breath sounds, crackles, wheezing, cyanosis, hemodynamic instability
- Chronic: Fe deficiency anemia (fatigue, pallor); may have digital clubbing

DIFFERENTIAL DIAGNOSIS

- See Box 34.2

INVESTIGATIONS

- O_2 saturation, ABG
- Laboratory tests: CBC with MCV (low Hb, leukocytosis), reticulocyte count
- PFTs: ↑DLCO with acute bleeding; may have restrictive pattern if chronic due to fibrosis

Box 34.2 Differential Diagnosis of Pulmonary Hemorrhage

- Upper airway bleeding (nose, adenoids/tonsils, mouth/gums)
- Hematemesis
- Infection (e.g., TB, anaerobes)
- Foreign body
- Bronchiectasis (e.g., CF, PCD) with erosion into bronchial arteries
- CHD
- Trauma
- Infarction
- Other (rare): pulmonary renal syndromes (SLE, Wegener, Goodpasture, microscopic polyangitis, HSP), arteriovenous malformation (e.g., hereditary hemorrhagic telangiectasia), airway hemangioma, lung tumor, coagulopathy, IPH (often diagnosis of exclusion)

© The Hospital for Sick Children, 2009. New artwork created by The Hospital for Sick Children, for *The Hospital for Sick Children Handbook of Pediatrics*, 11th edition.

- Imaging: CXR (may not show changes if acute event); CT if massive or recurrent; radionuclide scan (technetium-99–labeled RBCs) for active bleeding
- Bronchoscopy to identify site(s) of bleeding, airway lesions; BAL 3–14 d after suspected bleeding for hemosiderin-laden macrophages
- Specific investigations for underlying etiology as appropriate (e.g., INR/PTT, autoantibodies, echocardiography, sweat chloride, urinalysis/microscopy)

MANAGEMENT

- ABCs (see Chapter 1) including ventilatory support or transfusion if necessary
- Focal bleeding: observation, possible embolization; selective bronchial intubation or lung resection if massive
- Diffuse hemorrhage: systemic steroids, immunosuppression, Fe therapy
- Identify and treat underlying cause if possible

ASTHMA

CLINICAL FEATURES

- Episodic or persistent symptoms of dyspnea, chest tightness, wheezing, sputum production, cough
- Reversible airflow limitation, variable degree of airway hyperresponsiveness to triggers (respiratory tract infections, allergens, cold air, exercise, chemical irritants, tobacco smoke, stress)
- Risk factors for developing asthma: personal history of eczema, allergic rhinitis, family history (parent/sibling) of asthma or eczema, eosinophilia
- Differential diagnosis of wheezing: FB aspiration, congenital airway anomalies (e.g., vascular ring), CF, BPD, gastroesophageal reflux, CHF, infection (pneumonia, bronchiolitis, pertussis, tuberculosis)

Respirology

34

INVESTIGATIONS

- Rule out other causes of wheezing/airflow limitation
- Objective measurements (PFTs) to confirm diagnosis and monitor lung function whenever possible (>6 yr of age)
- Airway obstruction indicated by ↓FEV_1 (<80% predicted), ≥12% ↑ in FEV_1 from baseline after inhaled bronchodilator administration, and/or airway hyperresponsiveness to challenge (e.g., methacholine)
- When spirometry not available, diagnosis based on history, physical examination, response to treatment
- Peak flows can be used at home as rough monitor of airway function and guide changes in therapy

GENERAL MANAGEMENT

Step 1: Determine Degree of Asthma Control

- See Table 34.7

Step 2: Identify and Modify Environmental Triggers

- Eliminate exposure to triggers (e.g., cigarette smoke, environmental allergens)
- History and skin prick testing helpful in establishing atopy

Step 3: Initiate Maintenance Therapy With Both Reliever and Controller Medications

- Relievers (short-acting β_2-agonists) used to relieve acute symptoms; only on demand; goal is minimum dose and frequency
- Controllers (anti-inflammatory medications) taken regularly to control symptoms; inhaled corticosteroids (most effective), leukotriene receptor antagonists (e.g., montelukast)
- See Table 34.8

Table 34.7	Criteria for Well-Controlled Asthma
Parameter	**Frequency or Value**
Daytime symptoms	<4 d/wk
Nighttime symptoms	<1 night/wk
Physical activity	Normal
Exacerbations	Mild, infrequent
Absent from school/work due to asthma	None
Need for β_2-agonist	<4 doses/wk (may use 1 dose/d to prevent exercise-induced symptoms)
FEV_1 or PEF	≥90% of personal best
PEF during diurnal variation*	<10–15%

*Calculated as [(highest PEF – lowest PEF) ÷ (highest PEF)] × 100]; calculated for morning and night, over 2-wk period.
From Becker A, Bérubé D, Chad Z, et al. Canadian Pediatric Asthma Consensus guidelines, 2003 (updated to December 2004). *CMAJ.* 2005;173(6 suppl):S13 [Table 2]. © 2005 Canadian Medical Association.

Table 34.8

Table 34.8 Mainstays of Asthma Therapy

Medication	Trade Name	Mechanism of Action	Indications	Usual Dose*
Salbutamol (albuterol)	Ventolin	β₂-agonist (bronchodilator)	Treats acute wheezing or cough; prevents exercise-induced symptoms	0.01–0.03 mL/kg/dose in 3 mL 0.9% NaCl via nebulizer q½–4h prn
Fluticasone	Flovent	Inhaled corticosteroid (reduces airway inflammation)	Controller medication, prevents exacerbations	100–500 mcg/d ÷ bid
Budesonide	Pulmicort	Inhaled corticosteroid (reduces airway inflammation)	Controller medication, prevents exacerbations	0.125–1.0 mg bid via nebulizer
Prednisolone	Pediapred	Systemic anti-inflammatory	May ↓ severity/shorten duration of exacerbation if given soon after onset of symptoms	1–2 mg/kg/d PO od for 5 d
Dexamethasone		Systemic anti-inflammatory	May ↓ severity/shorten duration of exacerbation if given soon after onset of symptoms	0.3–0.6 mg/kg/d IV/PO ÷ bid for 3 d
Montelukast	Singulair	Leukotriene receptor antagonist	Maintenance therapy; most beneficial in patients with atopic asthma	1–5 yr: 4 mg PO od 6–14 yr: 5 mg PO od >14 yr: 10 mg PO od
Salmeterol	Serevent	Long-acting β₂-agonist	Not used as monotherapy in children	

*See Section IV: Pediatric Drug Dosing Guidelines for details.

© The Hospital for Sick Children, 2009. New artwork created by The Hospital for Sick Children for *The Hospital for Sick Children Handbook of Pediatrics*, 11th edition.

Respirology

34

Step 4: Assess Effectiveness of Therapy After 4–6 Wk

- If inadequate control, may either ↑ dose of inhaled corticosteroid or consider adding leukotriene receptor antagonist or long-acting β_2-agonist
- Delivery devices: for optimal drug delivery, puffers should be used with aerochamber at all ages; powder inhaler devices such as Turbuhaler or Diskus require patient-generated flow (appropriate for patients >8 yr); techniques should be reviewed at each visit

Acute Medical Management

- See Chapter 3 for management of status asthmaticus
- Acute exacerbations (bronchodilator needed >q4h): treat with nebulized salbutamol (and ipratropium bromide), O_2 as needed, oral or IV prednisone (see Table 34.8)

CYSTIC FIBROSIS

CLINICAL FEATURES

- Multisystem disease secondary to defective electrolyte and water transport; pulmonary disease accounts for majority of morbidity/mortality
- Autosomal recessive; due to mutations in CFTR (chloride channel) gene
- Classic diagnostic triad (chronic pulmonary disease, pancreatic insufficiency, ↑ sweat chloride), but clinical features vary by age:
  - Neonate: meconium ileus ± peritonitis (pathognomonic)
  - Infancy: steatorrhea, rectal prolapse, FTT, heat prostration/hyponatremia, obstructive jaundice
  - Childhood: malabsorption, FTT, recurrent pneumonia/bronchitis, pansinusitis, nasal polyposis, intussusception, rectal prolapse, pancreatitis
  - Adolescence/adult: male infertility/azoospermia, reduced female fertility, chronic pulmonary disease, abnormal glucose tolerance, diabetes mellitus, CF liver disease (obstructive biliary cirrhosis), gallstones

INVESTIGATIONS

- Suspicion for CF based on clinical presentation (lung, sinus disease, pancreatic disease) ± family history
- Sweat chloride: quantitative analysis of NaCl content in sweat induced by pilocarpine iontophoresis
  - Minimum 100 mg of sweat needed; may be difficult to obtain in first weeks of life
  - Sweat chloride >60 mmol/L in 98% of CF patients; 40–60 mmol/L is borderline; <40 mmol/L is normal
  - False-positive tests with untreated Addison disease or hypothyroidism, ectodermal dysplasia, some glycogen storage diseases, nephrotic syndrome, nephrogenic diabetes insipidus, G6PD deficiency, evaporation
  - False-negative tests with edema, malnutrition, overdilution of sample

- Pancreatic insufficiency evaluated with 3–5-d fecal fat collection or stool elastase
- Genetic testing:
  - >1600 known sequence variants; screening is available for >30 common mutations (represents >85–90% of CF patients in the Caucasian population); negative genetic screen does not rule out CF
  - Whole gene sequencing available if strong clinical suspicion, known familial defect
  - Prenatal testing available
- Ontario newborn screening for CF done by IRT testing; infants with positive result confirmed by CFTR genetics undergo sweat test to confirm diagnosis

MANAGEMENT

Chronic Pulmonary Disease

- Progressive course punctuated by acute exacerbations
- Other pulmonary complications: bronchiectasis, hemoptysis, spontaneous pneumothorax
- Serial clinical evaluation with PFTs and sputum samples (deep throat swabs for younger children) for microbiology
- Typical CF lung organisms: *S. aureus, Haemophilus influenzae, Pseudomonas aeruginosa, Burkholderia cepacia*
- *B. cepacia* generally seen later in life, associated with more severe disease; risk of person-to-person transmission requires avoidance of contact between infected and noninfected patients

Therapy

- Physiotherapy (PEP mask, percussion and postural drainage) ± inhaled salbutamol
- DNAse, hypertonic saline to improve secretion clearance
- Long-term inhaled antibiotics for those chronically colonized with *Pseudomonas*

Acute Pulmonary Exacerbations

- Fever, ↑ coughing and sputum, shortness of breath, fatigue, hemoptysis, anorexia, weight loss; may have ↑ accessory muscle use, crackles, wheezing on examination
- ↓FEV_1 by >10% from baseline, changes in blood gas or on CXR; ↑WBC and ESR may be seen (especially with *B. cepacia*)
- Mild exacerbations treated with 2–3-wk trial of oral antibiotics based on most recent sputum cultures; close follow-up with repeated PFTs to assess response to therapy
- First growth of *Pseudomonas* on culture: attempt to eradicate with 1 yr of inhaled antibiotics (tobramycin 80 mg bid)
- Moderate to severe exacerbations require hospitalization, IV antibiotics (usually 14 d) appropriate for sputum culture results, inhalational therapy, physiotherapy, supplemental O_2, nutritional support

- If little clinical improvement, consider ABPA; diagnosis based on clinical presentation (wheezing) and
  - 2 of (1) immediate skin test reactivity to *Aspergillus* allergens, (2) precipitating antibodies to *Aspergillus* antigen, or (3) elevated serum IgE (>1000) *AND*
  - 2 of (1) peripheral eosinophilia >1, (2) pulmonary infiltrates, (3) *Aspergillus* growth in sputum, (4) elevated *Aspergillus*-specific IgG/IgE, or (5) response to steroids
- Mainstay of treatment is oral steroids (itraconazole may be added if poor response)

GI DISEASE

- DIOS managed with mineral oil, osmotic laxatives and/or PEG with electrolyte solution (e.g., GoLYTELY, MiraLax) PO/NG; meconium ileus managed with enemas and/or surgery
- Improved nutrition and stool quality reduces occurrence of rectal prolapse

Pancreatic Disease

Exocrine Dysfunction

- 85% of CF patients have pancreatic insufficiency and require pancreatic enzyme replacement, vitamin A, D, E, K supplementation, and a high-energy diet
- If adequate growth not achieved with optimal pancreatic enzyme therapy, assess compliance, possible CF-related diabetes or poor intake; consider adding inhibitors of gastric acid production to improve enzyme function

Endocrine Dysfunction

- CF-related diabetes in 4% of children, 25% of adults; due to scarring of pancreas; may require insulin therapy

OUTCOMES

- Current life expectancy >30 yr of age
- Predictors for poor outcome: young age of colonization with mucoid *Pseudomonas; B. cepacia, Mycobacterium abscessus*; CF-related diabetes
- Treatment for severe advanced lung disease is lung transplant; main criteria for transplantation are FEV_1 <30% predicted, rapid decline in PFTs, and poor quality of life
- Posttransplant 1-yr survival 70–80%; 5-yr survival 55–65% (in *B. cepacia*–negative patients)

PULMONARY HYPERTENSION

- Definition: mean pulmonary artery pressure ≥25 mm Hg at rest or ≥30 mm Hg during exercise

CURRENT WHO CLASSIFICATION (2003)

- See Box 34.3

Box 34.3   WHO Classification of Pulmonary Hypertension (2003)

1. **Pulmonary Arterial HTN**
   - Sporadic or familial
   - Related to collagen vascular disease, congenital systemic-to-pulmonary artery shunts, portal HTN, HIV infection, drugs, toxins, PPHN
2. **Pulmonary Venous HTN**
   - Left-sided atrial, ventricular, or valvular heart disease; compression of pulmonary veins; pulmonary veno-occlusive disease
3. **PHT Associated With Disorders of Respiratory System**
   - Chronic obstructive pulmonary disease, interstitial lung disease, sleep-disordered breathing, alveolar hypoventilation disorders, chronic exposure to high altitude, neonatal lung disease, alveolar-capillary dysplasia
4. **PHT Due to Chronic Thrombotic and/or Embolic Disease**
   - Thromboembolic obstruction of proximal or distal pulmonary arteries (pulmonary embolism, thrombus, tumor, sickle cell disease)
5. **PHT Due to Disorders Directly Affecting the Pulmonary Vasculature**
   - Inflammation (e.g., schistosomiasis, sarcoidosis), pulmonary capillary hemangiomatosis

---

CLINICAL FEATURES

- Often asymptomatic; symptoms and clinical presentation depend on underlying etiology
- Infants: signs of low cardiac output (FTT, poor feeding, lethargy, diaphoresis, tachypnea, tachycardia, irritability)
- Children: asthmalike symptoms, exertional cyanosis, dyspnea, syncope (usually exertional or postexertional), chest pain, hypoxic seizures (rare)
- Physical findings: may include tachypnea, tachycardia, loud second heart sound, systolic ejection murmur (tricuspid regurgitation)

INVESTIGATIONS

- If PHT suspected, refer to pediatric center with experience in PHT
- CXR, ECG, echocardiogram
- Rule out underlying conditions causing PHT
- PFTs, overnight oximetry, V/Q lung scan, cardiopulmonary exercise testing
- Blood work (CBC, liver enzymes, HIV test, antiphospholipid antibodies)
- Cardiac catheterization (gold standard for diagnosis, assessment of severity, treatment)
- Evaluation of pulmonary vasoreactivity to vasodilators (e.g., inhaled NO, IV epoprostenol, inhaled iloprost)

MANAGEMENT

- Optimize treatment of underlying condition
- Minimize hypoxemia with supplemental O_2
- Oral treatment with phosphodiesterase V inhibitor (e.g., sildenafil), endothelin receptor antagonists (e.g., bosentan)
- IV or SC prostacyclin (and derivates)
- Anticoagulation
- In acute situation, short-term therapy with inhaled NO may be useful
- Lung transplantation

OUTCOMES

- Fatal disease: death usually due to progressive right ventricular failure or sudden death (secondary to arrhythmias, acute pulmonary embolism, massive pulmonary hemorrhage, sudden right ventricular ischemia)
- Intercurrent illness (e.g., pneumonia) may be fatal due to alveolar hypoxia and further pulmonary vasoconstriction resulting in cardiogenic shock

SLEEP-DISORDERED BREATHING

DEFINITIONS

- Central apnea: absence of airflow secondary to absence of respiratory effort (20 s in length or >3 s with desaturation or arousal)
- Obstructive apnea: absence of airflow despite respiratory effort (paradoxic) ± desaturation, arousal
- Obstructive hypopnea: >50% reduction in airflow with paradoxic respiratory effort, associated with desaturation or arousal
- Periodic breathing: >3 central apneas with <20 s between events
- Sleep-disordered breathing includes OSA, central hypoventilation syndromes, and disorders of infancy (e.g., apnea of prematurity)

OSA

- Repeated events of partial or complete upper airway collapse on inspiration during sleep with disruption of normal gas exchange and sleep patterns
- Habitual snoring (sign of ↑ upper airway resistance) is found in up to 27% of children; ratio of habitual snoring to OSA is 5:1
- Peak prevalence in pre/early school age (2–8 yr)

Etiology

- Combination of structural and neuromuscular abnormalities
- Causes include adenotonsillar hypertrophy (common), obesity, allergic rhinitis, asthma, micrognathia, macroglossia, Down syndrome, craniofacial anomalies (e.g., Pierre Robin sequence), neuromuscular disorders (e.g., cerebral palsy, Duchenne muscular dystrophy)

Clinical Features

- Nighttime: snoring, difficulty breathing/snorting episodes, witnessed apnea, paradoxic chest/abdominal motion, cyanosis, sweating
- Daytime: mouth breathing, nasal obstruction, adenoid facies, hyperactivity, moodiness, poor school performance; daytime somnolence is a late symptom
- Complications: PHT ± cor pulmonale, systemic HTN, LVH, neurobehavioral deficits, FTT (less common)

Investigations

- History and physical examination are poor predictors for OSA
- Definitive study is overnight PSG; current American Academy of Pediatrics (AAP) guidelines recommend all children with snoring and features suggestive of OSA undergo PSG for diagnosis
- Components of PSG include sleep staging (EEG, chin EMG and EOG), detection of airflow, chest, abdominal/limb movements and gas exchange (SaO_2, PCO_2), ECG, video (for snoring, body position)

Management

- First line: tonsillectomy and adenoidectomy (shown to have a high cure rate in OSA); must be monitored closely postoperatively and should be re-evaluated after 8–10 wk with sleep study
- CPAP (or BiPAP)
- Treatment of underlying problems (e.g., weight loss for obesity, control of allergic rhinitis, reconstruction for craniofacial syndromes)
- Tracheostomy in severe cases

CENTRAL APNEA AND HYPOVENTILATION SYNDROMES

- Respiratory insufficiency in sleep with impaired ventilatory responses to hypercapnia and hypoxemia

Etiology

- Primary causes include CCHS and late-onset CHS
- Secondary causes include Arnold-Chiari type II malformation with myelomeningocele (most common), other causes of brainstem injury (e.g., trauma, encephalitis, tumor, CNS infarct, ↑ICP)

Diagnosis

- Persistent evidence of sleep hypoventilation on PSG with $PaCO_2$ >60 mm Hg and absence of cardiac, pulmonary, or neuromuscular causes
- Genetic testing may support diagnosis of CCHS

Management

- Management of cause (e.g., brainstem decompression), BiPAP, or tracheostomy with mechanical ventilation

34

FURTHER READING

American Academy of Pediatrics and the Canadian Paediatric Society. Joint statement. Postnatal corticosteroids to treat or prevent chronic lung disease in preterm infants. *Paediatr Child Health.* 2002;7:20–28.

Becker A, Bérubé D, Chad Z, et al. Canadian Pediatric Asthma Consensus guidelines, 2003 (updated to December 2004). *CMAJ.* 2005;173(6 suppl):S13.

Chernick V, Boat TF, Kendig EL. *Kendig's Disorders of the Respiratory Tract in Children.* 6th ed. Philadelphia, Pa: WB Saunders; 1998.

Infectious Diseases and Immunization Committee, Canadian Paediatric Society, and Fetus and Newborn Committee. Joint statement. Palivizumab and respiratory syncytial virus immune globulin intravenous for the prophylaxis of respiratory syncytial virus infection in high risk infants. *Paediatr Child Health.* 1999;4:474–480.

USEFUL WEB SITES

American Journal of Respiratory and Critical Care Medicine. Available at: ajrccm.atsjournals.org

American Thoracic Society. Available at: www.thoracic.org

Canadian Cystic Fibrosis Foundation. Available at: www.cysticfibrosis.com

Chest—the cardiopulmonary and critical care journal. Available at: www.chestjournal.org

Chapter 35 Rheumatology

Michelle Batthish
Shirley M.L. Tse

Rheumatology

COMMON ABBREVIATIONS

ANA	antinuclear antibody
c-ANCA	cytoplasmic antineutrophil cytoplasmic antibody
CREST	calcinosis, Raynaud's, esophageal dysmotility, sclerodactyly, telangiectasia
CRP	C-reactive protein
DIP	distal interphalangeal
IBD	inflammatory bowel disease
ILAR	International League of Associations for Rheumatology
JDM	juvenile dermatomyositis
JIA	juvenile idiopathic arthritis
KD	Kawasaki disease
MCP	metacarpophalangeal
MCTD	mixed connective tissue disease
MMF	mycophenolate mofetil
NLE	neonatal lupus erythematosus
NSAID	nonsteroidal anti-inflammatory drug
p-ANCA	perinuclear antineutrophil cytoplasmic antibody
PIP	proximal interphalangeal
RF	rheumatoid factor
ROM	range of motion
RNP	ribonucleoprotein
SLE	systemic lupus erythematosus

35

APPROACH TO THE CHILD
WITH RHEUMATOLOGIC DISEASE

HISTORY

- Swelling, pain quality, radiation, aggravating and alleviating factors, timing, overlying skin change/warmth
- Movement, gait, morning stiffness, weakness, enthesitis (heel pain)
- Fever, night pain, weight loss, fatigue, rash, photosensitivity, Raynaud phenomenon, hair loss, vision problems, ulcers, GI symptoms, dysuria
- Activity, school days lost, sleep, sexual activity (if applicable)
- Family history: psoriasis, IBD, joint/back problems, SLE, other autoimmune/connective tissue diseases
- Travel, specific exposure to TB or Lyme disease, trauma
- Treatment: medications (pharmacologic, nonpharmacologic, alternative), physiotherapy

PHYSICAL EXAMINATION

- Careful and thorough general examination
- Joints: heat, swelling, erythema, range of passive and active motion, tenderness, deformity
- Include localized bony tenderness, spine, sacroiliac, entheses (attachment of tendons to bone), leg length, growth disturbances
- Gait: normal walking, walking on heels, on toes
- Gowers test, muscle bulk, strength

INVESTIGATIONS TO CONSIDER

- CBC, differential, ESR, CRP
- Albumin, LFTs, CPK, LDH
- C3, C4
- Autoantibodies (Table 35.1)
- Coagulation, renal function, urinalysis, 24-h urine collection
- Radiologic imaging (XR, bone scan, MRI, US)
- Arthrocentesis (Table 35.2)
- Ophthalmologic examination

Table 35.1	Serologic Tests for Rheumatologic Diseases	
Test	**Disease Entity**	**Incidence/Comments**
ANA	Nonrheumatologic disease	<10% of normal children
	Risk factor for uveitis in oligo-JIA	60–80%
	SLE	Close to 100%, not very specific
	NLE	80–90%
	Dermatomyositis	50–75%
	Systemic sclerosis	~90%
	Localized scleroderma	50%
	MCTD	100% and very high titer
Anti-dsDNA	SLE	60–90%
Anti-Sm (Smith)	SLE	25–40%
Anti-RNP	SLE, MCTD	In very high titer, suggests MCTD
Anti-Ro/anti-La	SLE, NLE, Sjögren syndrome	Present in asymptomatic mothers of babies with NLE
Anti-Scl-70	Diffuse systemic sclerosis	Marker for severe disease
Anticentromere	Limited systemic sclerosis (CREST)	Very uncommon in childhood

(continued)

Table 35.1	Serologic Tests for Rheumatologic Diseases (continued)	
Test	**Disease Entity**	**Incidence/Comments**
c-ANCA	Wegener granulomatosis	Sensitive and specific
p-ANCA	Microscopic polyarteritis nodosa	Sensitive
RF	RF-positive poly-JIA	100%
Anticardiolipin	Antiphospholipid antibody syndrome SLE	IgG isotype most commonly associated with disease manifestations

Adapted from Laxer RM, Lee Ford-Jones E, Friedman J, Gerstle JT, eds. *The Hospital for Sick Children Atlas of Pediatrics.* Philadelphia, Pa: Current Medicine LLC; 2005:450.

Table 35.2	Synovial Fluid Analysis		
	Normal	**Inflammatory**	**Infectious**
Appearance	Transparent	Translucent	Cloudy
Viscosity	High	Low	Variable
WBC	$<2 \times 10^9$/L	$2\text{--}50 \times 10^9$/L	$>50 \times 10^9$/L
Neutrophils (%)	<10	Variable	>90
Glucose (mmol/L)	Equal to blood	<2.8	>2.8
Culture	Negative	Negative	Often positive

Adapted from Gerlag DM, Tak PP. Synovial fluid analyses, synovial biopsy, and synovial pathology. In: Harris ED, Budd RC, Genovese MC, Firestein GS, Sargent JF, Sledge CB, eds. *Kelley's Textbook of Rheumatology.* Vol 1. 7th ed. Philadelphia, Pa: WB Saunders; 2005:676-677.

DIFFERENTIAL DIAGNOSIS

- See Box 35.1

RED FLAGS

- See Box 35.2

JUVENILE IDIOPATHIC ARTHRITIS

- Onset <16 yr old
- At least 6 wk of arthritis
- Definition of arthritis: joint swelling (effusion) OR at least two of the following: joint pain/tenderness with palpation or motion, limited ROM, joint warmth
- See Table 35.3 for details of classification

Box 35.1   Differential Diagnosis of Limb Pain in Childhood

Inflammatory
- JIA (See Table 35.3)
- Transient synovitis
- Sarcoidosis
- Connective tissue diseases
- SLE
- JDM
- Scleroderma
- MCTD
- Sjögren syndrome
- Vasculitides (See Table 35.4)

Noninflammatory
- Fibromyalgia
- Reflex sympathetic dystrophy
- Hypermobility syndrome
- Growing pains
- Trauma

Infectious
- Primary
  - Bacterial: *Staphylococcus, Streptococcus, Haemophilus,* meningococcus, gonococcus, *Mycoplasma, Borrelia, Kingella kingae, Salmonella, Pseudomonas*
  - Viral: rubella, hepatitis, parvovirus, EBV
- Secondary
  - Rheumatic fever: poststreptococcal
  - Enteric: *Shigella, Salmonella, Yersinia, Campylobacter*
  - *Chlamydia*
  - Viral

Malignant
- Leukemia, neuroblastoma, lymphoma, primary bone/cartilage tumors

Hematologic
- Hemophilia
- Sickle cell disease

Orthopedic
- Legg-Calvé-Perthes disease
- Osgood-Schlatter disease
- Slipped capital femoral epiphysis

35

Box 35.2   Red Flags for Limb Pain in Childhood

- Night pain
- Fever
- Pain out of proportion to history/injury
- Weight loss
- Night sweats

Table 35.3 Classification of Juvenile Idiopathic Arthritis

ILAR JIA Subtype	Systemic	Oligoarthritis	Polyarthritis (RF−)	Polyarthritis (RF+)	Enthesitis-Related Arthritis	Psoriatic Arthritis	Undifferentiated
% of patients	10%	33–56%	11–28%	2–7%	3–11%	2–11%	11–21%
Gender differences	F = M	F > M	F > M	F > M	M > F	F > M	
Age at onset	Throughout childhood	Early childhood	2 peaks: 2–4 yr and 6–12 yr	Late childhood/ early adolescence	Late childhood/ adolescence	2 peaks: 2–4 yr and 9–11 yr	
Joints affected	Polyarticular or oligoarticular	4 or less joints during the first 6 mo Large joints Persistent: affects ≤ 4 joints throughout the disease course Extended: affects >4 joints after the first 6 mo	5 or more joints in the first 6 mo Symmetric C-spine and TMJ	5 or more joints in the first 6 mo Symmetric small and large joints Erosive joint disease	Weight-bearing joints, especially hip	Asymmetric or symmetric small and large joints	
Sacroiliitis	No	No	No	No	Yes	Rare	
Uveitis	Rare	Common, especially if ANA+, asymptomatic	Yes	Rare	Yes, symptomatic	Yes	

(continued)

Table 35.3	Classification of Juvenile Idiopathic Arthritis (continued)						
ILAR JIA Subtype	Systemic	Oligoarthritis	Polyarthritis (RF–)	Polyarthritis (RF+)	Enthesitis-Related Arthritis	Psoriatic Arthritis	Undifferentiated
Other features	Daily fever ≥2 wk + ≥1 of: rash, lymphadenopathy, hepatosplenomegaly, serositis	–	–	Rheumatoid nodules RF + twice ≥3 mo apart	Enthesitis, inflammatory spinal pain, family history HLA B27+, arthritis onset in boys >6 yr old	Nail pits, onycholysis, dactylitis, psoriasis, family history psoriasis	Unknown cause; ≥6 wk Does not fulfill criteria for any or fulfills criteria for >1 category
Ultimate morbidity	25–37% have severe destructive joint disease, especially hips, C-spine and TMJ 50% remit in 1 yr Risk MAS	Ocular damage 40% progress to extended course	10–15% severe arthritis	>50% severe arthritis	Risk of developing spondylitis in adulthood	Variable	–
RF	Negative	Negative	Negative	100% positive	Negative	Negative	–
ANA	Negative	60–80% positive	25% positive	75% positive	Negative	Positive	–
HLA-B27	Negative	Negative	Negative	Negative	75% positive	15% positive	–

TMJ, temporomandibular joint; MAS, macrophage activation syndrome.

Rheumatology

35

SLE

- Classification criteria: meets 4 of 11 criteria (Box 35.3)
- Female predominance, usually onset after puberty
- Often presents with generalized fever, fatigue, weight loss, and non-specific organ dysfunction

---

Box 35.3 | **Classification Criteria for Systemic Lupus Erythematosus**

Four of the following 11 criteria make it likely that a patient has SLE (95% specificity, 75% sensitivity):

1. Malar rash
2. Discoid rash
3. Photosensitivity
4. Oral and/or nasal ulcers
5. Nonerosive arthritis
6. Serositis (pericarditis, pleuritis)
7. Renal involvement (active sediment, proteinuria)
8. CNS involvement (seizures, psychosis)
9. Hematologic (hemolytic anemia, leukopenia, lymphopenia, thrombocytopenia)
10. Positive ANA
11. Positive immunoserology (positive anti-dsDNA, anti-Sm, anti-phospholipid antibody [anticardiolipin, lupus anticoagulant] false-positive VDRL)

Adapted from Tan EM, Cohen AS, Fries JF, et al. The 1982 revised criteria for the classification of systemic lupus erythematosus. *Arthritis Rheum.* 1982;25:1271–1277; and from Hochberg MC. Updating the American College of Rheumatology revised criteria for the classification of systemic lupus erythematosus. *Arthritis Rheum.* 1997;40:1725.

NLE SYNDROME

- Heart block, rash, thrombocytopenia, hepatitis
- Positive for ANA, anti-Ro, anti-La antibodies

JDM

- Heliotrope rash (violaceous discoloration of upper eyelids), Gottron papules (erythematous, atrophic scaly plaques over MCP, PIP, and DIP joints and extensor aspects of elbows and knees), proximal muscle weakness, ↑CPK and muscle enzymes, abnormal muscle biopsy, calcinosis, dysphonia (nasal voice), swallowing difficulties, capillary nailfold changes

SCLERODERMA

Localized

- Patchy (morphea) or linear fibrotic skin lesion

Systemic

- Diffuse: multiorgan sclerosis including upper GI, lung, cardiac, renal; skin involvement (proximal to wrists, ankles, and trunk), associated with anti-Scl 70 autoantibodies
- Limited: CREST, associated with anticentromere autoantibodies

MIXED CONNECTIVE TISSUE DISEASE

- Overlap of JIA, SLE, JDM, scleroderma
- High-titer ANA with speckled pattern and antibodies to U1-RNP

SJÖGREN SYNDROME

- Keratoconjuctivitis sicca (dry eyes and dry mouth)
- Antibodies (anti-Ro, anti-La)

VASCULITIS

APPROACH TO CHILDHOOD VASCULITIS

- See Table 35.4

Table 35.4	Classification of Primary Childhood Vasculitis	
Vasculitis	**Vessels Affected**	**Characteristics**
Predominantly Large-Vessel		
Takayasu arteritis	Muscular and elastic arteries; involvement of aortic arch and primary branches	Granulomatous inflammation, absent pulses, bruits, hypertension, stroke
Predominantly Medium-Vessel		
Kawasaki disease	Coronary and other muscular arteries	Fever, conjunctivitis, oral mucosal inflammation, cervical lymphadenopathy, rash, extremity changes, coronary artery lesions
Polyarteritis nodosa	Medium (often near bifurcations) and small muscular arteries and sometimes arterioles	Fever, arthritis, myalgia, abdominal pain, renal disease, hypertension, CNS disease, peripheral neuropathy, skin (nodules, purpura, livedo reticularis, ulcers); when disease limited to skin and joints only: cutaneous polyarteritis
Predominantly Small-Vessel Nongranulomatous		
Henoch-Schönlein purpura	Arterioles and venules, often small arteries and veins	Palpable purpura, subcutaneous edema, abdominal pain, intussusception, GI bleeding, arthritis, glomerulonephritis

(continued)

Table 35.4	Classification of Primary Childhood Vasculitis (continued)	
Vasculitis	**Vessels Affected**	**Characteristics**
Hypersensitivity vasculitis	Arterioles and venules	Fever, urticaria, purpura, arthritis, precipitated by medication or other agent
Microscopic polyarteritis nodosa	Necrotizing vasculitis affecting small vessels	Pulmonary infiltrates or hemorrhage, glomerulonephritis, skin lesions, p-ANCA
Granulomatous		
Wegener granulomatosis	Small arteries and veins, occasionally larger vessels	Sinusitis, pulmonary infiltrates, nodules or hemorrhage, glomerulonephritis, c-ANCA
Churg-Strauss syndrome	Small arteries and veins, often arterioles and venules	Asthma, sinusitis, pulmonary infiltrates, mononeuritis multiplex, eosinophilia
Other Vasculitides		
Behçet syndrome	Small vessels with immune complexes	Oral and genital ulcers, uveitis, skin involvement (erythema nodosum, pseudofolliculitis, papulopustular lesions), pathergy, GI involvement

Adapted from Cassidy JT, Petty RE, Lindsley CB, Laxer RM. *Textbook of Pediatric Rheumatology.* 5th ed. Philadelphia, Pa: Elsevier Saunders; 2006:494.

KAWASAKI DISEASE

- Involves small and medium vessels
- Peak: 3 yr old; incidence in Asian > Black > Caucasian

DIAGNOSTIC CRITERIA

- Fever >5 d and at least four of the following clinical signs:
  1. Bilateral nonpurulent (bulbar) conjunctivitis
  2. Mucosal changes (red fissured lips, strawberry tongue, pharyngeal erythema)
  3. Red edematous hands and feet with eventual desquamation
  4. Polymorphic nonvesicular rash, groin rash/peeling
  5. Cervical lymphadenopathy >1.5 cm (usually unilateral)
- If incomplete presentation (<4 criteria) but high index of suspicion with >5 d of fever or evidence of coronary or myocardial disease, consider treating for KD, especially with younger (<1 yr) or older (>8 yr) patients

CLINICAL COURSE

Acute Phase

- Up to 10 d (until resolution of fever)
- Myocarditis, endocarditis, pericarditis, arrhythmias

Subacute Phase

- 10–25 d (until resolution of disease)
- Associated with rise in platelets, ESR, CRP, and skin peeling of hands and feet; coronary aneurysm in 20% of untreated cases

Convalescent Phase

- >1 mo; child appears well but evolution of coronary dilatation; resolution of ↑ESR/CRP and thrombocytosis

Other Manifestations

- Aseptic meningitis with profound irritability, arthritis, gallbladder hydrops, hepatitis, sterile pyuria, gastroenteritis, pneumonitis, macrophage activation syndrome, uveitis

Laboratory Findings

- Leukocytosis with neutrophilia, mild anemia, thrombocytosis (after week 1), ↑ESR, ↑CRP, mild transaminitis, ↓ albumin, ↓Na^+

Differential Diagnosis

- Streptococcal/scarlet fever
- Staphylococcal scalded skin syndrome
- Viral: adenovirus, EBV, measles
- Stevens-Johnson syndrome
- Toxins

Management

- Acute phase: IVIG 2 g/kg (single infusion) and ASA 100 mg/kg/d (divided in 4 doses) until defervescence (>24–48 h); if persistent fever, consider additional doses of IVIG or corticosteroids; ECG, echocardiography before discharge; if no aneurysm, discharge on ASA 3–5 mg/kg/d until follow-up echocardiogram
- Subacute: ASA 3–5 mg/kg/d until platelets normalize or indefinitely if coronary disease
- Convalescent: follow-up with echocardiography at 2, 6, 12 mo

NONINFLAMMATORY/PAIN AMPLIFICATION SYNDROMES

- Definition: pain out of proportion with physical findings

FIBROMYALGIA

- Female predominance, tenderness in 11 of 18 symmetric "trigger" points
- Associated with fatigue, disturbed sleep, headaches, irritable bowel syndrome, anxiety, depression, school absence
- Treat with reassurance, simple analgesia, normalize sleep patterns, daily aerobic activity (30 min/d)
- Physiotherapy, as needed

REFLEX SYMPATHETIC DYSTROPHY

- Female predominance, often after trauma/surgery to distal extremity; associated with psychological factors
- Severe pain, discoloration, hypersensitivity, autonomic dysfunction (sweaty, shiny, cool)
- Treat with simple analgesics, physiotherapy, psychosocial counseling

HYPERMOBILITY/OVERUSE SYNDROMES

- Hypermobility: touch thumb to forearm, hyperextension of fingers parallel to forearm, hyperextension of elbows and knees >10°, touch palms to floor with knees straight
- Examples include recurrent dislocating patella, shin splints, tenosynovitis
- Competitive athletics at an early age may predispose to overuse syndromes

GROWING PAINS

- Affects children 4–12 yr old
- Poorly localized, often lower limbs, occurs at night but never persists until morning
- No physical or radiologic signs or disability
- Managed with supportive measures: massage, simple analgesia

RAYNAUD PHENOMENON

- Vasospastic ischemic blanching, secondary cyanosis, resolving hyperemic redness and pain
- Primary or associated with SLE, MCTD, scleroderma (especially if positive ANA and capillary nailfold changes)

MACROPHAGE ACTIVATION SYNDROME

- A form of secondary hemophagocytic lymphohistiocytosis (see p. 681)

PHARMACOLOGIC MANAGEMENT OF RHEUMATOLOGIC DISEASE

- Chronic arthritis: NSAIDs, intra-articular steroids; for uncontrolled disease activity, consider second-line agents and biologics used alone or in combination
- Connective tissue disorders: systemic steroids, second-line agents, cyclophosphamide; consider biologics in refractory cases
- See Table 35.5 for details

Table 35.5

Anti-inflammatory/Immunomodulatory Drugs Used in Rheumatology

Drug	Mode of Action
First-Line Agents	
NSAIDs	Cyclo-oxygenase 1 and 2 inhibition
Steroids	Suppress inflammatory cytokine production and T cells; inhibit mediators of leukocyte recruitment and inflammation
Second-Line Agents	
Methotrexate	Suppresses inflammatory cytokine production, inhibits dihydrofolate reductase; in high doses, inhibits lymphocyte proliferation
Cyclophosphamide	Depletes lymphocytes, B and T cells
Cyclosporine	Blocks transcription of T-cell genes
MMF	Inhibits B- and T-cell proliferation
Azathioprine	Inhibits T lymphocytes
Hydroxychloroquine	Inhibits phospholipid function and binds DNA
Sulfasalazine	Exact mechanism unclear, possesses anti-inflammatory (5-ASA) and antibacterial (sulfapyridine) properties
Leflunomide	Decrease activation and proliferation of immune cells, inhibits dihydroorotate dehydrogenase
Biologic Agents	
Anti-TNF *etanercept (Enbrel)* *infliximab (Remicade)* *adalimumab (Humira)*	Blocks action of TNF (inflammation, T- and B-cell signaling, and T-cell proliferation)
Anti-IL-1 *anakinra (Kineret), rilonacept*	Blocks the action of IL-1 as a receptor antagonist or antibody against IL-1
Anti-sIL-6R (soluble IL-6 receptor) *tocilizumab (Actemra)*	Humanized monoclonal antibody that blocks cell signaling by the complex of IL-6/IL-6R
Anti-CTLA4 *abatacept (Orencia)*	Blocks costimulation signal CTLA4 necessary for T-cell activation
Monoclonal antibodies to B cells *rituximab (Anti-CD20)*	Depletes premature and mature B-cell numbers

Adapted from Woo P, Laxer RM, Sherry DD. *Pediatric Rheumatology in Clinical Practice.* London, England: Springer-Verlag; 2007:17–18. With kind permission of Springer Science & Business Media.
TNF, tumor necrosis factor.

Rheumatology

35

FURTHER READING

Cassidy JT, Petty RE, Lindsley CB, Laxer RM. *Textbook of Pediatric Rheumatology*. 5th Ed. Philadelphia, Pa: Elsevier Saunders; 2006.

Fam AG. *Musculoskeletal Examination and Joint Injection Techniques*. Philadelphia, Pa: Mosby/Elsevier; 2006.

Szer I, Kimura Y, Malleson P, Southwood T. *Arthritis in Children & Adolescents*. New York: Oxford University Press; 2006.

Woo P, Laxer RM, Sherry DD. *Pediatric Rheumatology in Clinical Practice*. London, England: Springer; 2007.

USEFUL WEB SITES

The Arthritis Society. Available at: **www.arthritis.ca**

Juvenile Scleroderma Network. Available at: **www.jsdn.org**

Lupus Ontario. Available at: **www.lupusontario.org**

The Myositis Association. Available at: **www.myositis.org**

Pediatric Rheumatology International Trials Organization. Available at: **www.printo.it/pediatric-rheumatology/**

Chapter 36 Transplantation

Lindsay Teskey
Vicky Lee Ng

Chapter 36 Transplantation

COMMON ABBREVIATIONS

ACR	acute cellular rejection
AMR	antibody-mediated rejection
AZA	azathioprine
C_0	trough cyclosporine level
C_2	cyclosporine level taken 2 h after dose
CMV	cytomegalovirus
CNI	calcineurin inhibitor
EBV	Epstein-Barr virus
EMBx	endomyocardial biopsy
GFR	glomerular filtration rate
HTx	heart transplant
IS	immunosuppressive
PJP	*Pneumocystis jirovecii* pneumonia
PTLD	posttransplant lymphoproliferative disease
SOT	solid organ transplant
TDM	therapeutic drug monitoring
TMP/SMX	trimethoprim-sulfamethoxazole

OVERVIEW OF PEDIATRIC SOLID ORGAN TRANSPLANTATION

- See Table 36.1

IMMUNOSUPPRESSION/DRUG THERAPY

- See Table 36.2 for details of IS drugs

POSTTRANSPLANT COMPLICATIONS

REJECTION

- See Table 36.3

INFECTION

- See Table 36.4
- Most common nonrespiratory viruses affecting SOT recipients: CMV, EBV
- Splenectomized and/or functionally asplenic recipients should be immunized with pneumococcal vaccine and receive appropriate prophylaxis (see Chapter 23)
- Patients with indwelling central vascular access catheters and other drains are at risk of foreign body–related infections

Table 36.1 Indications and Survival for Solid Organ Transplantation

	Kidney[1]	Liver[2]	Heart[1]	Lung[1]	Intestine[3]
Most common indications	End-stage renal disease due to 1. Congenital structural abnormalities/obstruction 2. Glomerular disease 3. Reflux nephropathy	1. Biliary atresia 2. Metabolic disease 3. Fulminant hepatic failure	1. Congenital heart disease with no acceptable surgical option 2. Cardiomyopathy with end-stage heart failure despite optimal medical management 3. Malignant arrhythmias	End-stage lung disease due to 1. Cystic fibrosis 2. Primary pulmonary hypertension 3. Pulmonary fibrosis 4. Bronchiectasis 5. Chronic interstitial lung disease 6. Eisenmenger syndrome	Intestinal failure due to 1. Short-bowel syndrome (e.g., NEC) 2. Defective intestinal motility 3. Impaired enterocyte absorptive capacity (MVID)
Survival	Living donor: 95% at 1 yr 80% at 5 yr Deceased donor: 91% at 1 yr 69% at 5 yr	90% at 1 yr 85% at 5 yr	87% at 1 yr 72% at 5 yr	83% at 1 yr 50% at 5 yr	Isolated intestine[1] 72% at 1 yr 48% at 5 yr Liver + intestine[3] 63% at 1 yr 40% at 5 yr

MVID, microvillous inclusion disease; NEC, necrotizing enterocolitis.

[1] 2006 Annual Report of the U.S. Organ Procurement and Transplantation Network and the Scientific Registry of Transplant Recipients: Transplant Data 1996–2005. Health Resources and Services Administration, Health Care Systems Bureau, Division of Transplantation, Rockville, MD. Available at: http://www.optn.org/AR2006/default.htm. Accessed September 12, 2008.

[2] Studies of Pediatric Liver Transplantation (SPLIT) 2007 Annual Report registry reports.

[3] Grant D for the Intestinal Transplant Registry. 2003 Report of the Intestine Transplant Registry. *Ann Surg.* 2005;241(4):607–613.

Table 36.2 Immunosuppressive Drugs

Agent	Mechanisms of Action	Interactions	Side Effects	Comments
Corticosteroids	Inhibits IL-1 and -2 production, expression of histocompatibility antigens; anti-inflammatory effects by inhibiting arachidonic acid metabolism	Increased bioavailability with hypoalbuminemia and liver disease	Hypertension, hyperglycemia, weight gain, growth retardation, cushingoid habitus, gastric/peptic ulceration, psychosis, pancreatitis, osteoporosis, delayed wound healing, cataracts	—
Cyclosporine (CNI)	Binds cyclophilin; complex inhibits calcineurin phosphatase and T-cell activation	Trough levels: (1) decreased by phenytoin, phenobarbital, rifampin, carbamazepine; (2) increased by calcium channel blockers, erythromycin, metoclopramide, ketoconazole, grapefruit juice	Nephrotoxicity, hypertension, hirsutism, gingival hyperplasia, posttransplantation diabetes mellitus, hyperlipidemia, headache, HUS, seizures, tremors	TDM required (C_0 and/or C_2)
Tacrolimus (CNI)	Binds to FKBP-12; complex inhibits calcineurin phosphatase and T-cell activation	Trough levels: (1) decreased by carbamazepine, steroids, isoniazid, phenobarbital, phenytoin; (2) increased by cyclosporine, fluconazole, calcium channel blockers, erythromycin, doxycycline, grapefruit juice	Nephrotoxicity, hypertension, posttransplantation diabetes mellitus, hyperlipidemia, hypomagnesemia, seizures, tremors, HUS	TDM required
Azathioprine	Antimetabolite/interference with DNA synthesis	—	Bone marrow effects (leukopenia, macrocytosis), liver toxicity, pancreatitis	Consider blood count monitoring

(continued)

Table 36.2 Immunosuppressive Drugs (continued)

Agent	Mechanisms of Action	Interactions	Side Effects	Comments
Mycophenolate mofetil (MMF)	Selective inhibitor of purine biosynthesis; inhibition of T- and B-cell proliferation	–	GI symptoms (mainly diarrhea), neutropenia, mild anemia	TDM available, but utility varies by organ and institutional practice
Sirolimus	Inhibits IL-2-driven T-cell proliferation	–	Hyperlipidemia, thrombocytopenia, mouth ulcers, delayed wound healing, delayed graft function, pneumonitis, interstitial lung disease	· TDM, lipid monitoring required · Baseline PFTs recommended
Daclizumab; basiliximab	Humanized monoclonal anti-CD25 antibody/IL-2 receptor antagonist; chimeric monoclonal anti-CD25 antibody/IL-2 receptor antagonist	–	Hypersensitivity reactions, neutropenia	May have utility in renal impaired patients
Polyclonal antithymocyte globulin (Thymoglobulin)	Blocks T-cell membrane proteins causing altered function, lysis, and prolonged T-cell depletion	–	Cytokine-release syndrome (fever, chills, hypotension), pulmonary edema, serum sickness, cytopenias	–
Monoclonal anti-CD3/52/20 antibody	Binds to CD3/52/20 on surface of B and/or T cells causing lysis and prolonged depletion	–	Cytokine-release syndrome (fever, chills, hypotension), pulmonary edema, serum sickness, cytopenias	–

HUS, hemolytic uremic syndrome; *PFTs*, pulmonary function tests.

Transplantation

36

Table 36.3 Rejection in Solid Organ Transplantation

	Kidney	Liver	Heart	Lung
Clinical	· Usually asymptomatic · Low-grade fever, hypertension, graft tenderness	· Usually asymptomatic, may have unexplained fever in early postoperative period	· Usually asymptomatic · Irritability, low-grade fever, arrhythmia · Rejection with hemodynamic compromise rare	· May be asymptomatic · Low-grade fever, fatigue, shortness of breath, nonproductive cough
Laboratory testing	· No specific diagnostic laboratory investigations, but serum creatinine likely elevated	· Typically characterized by significant rise in serum enzymes (AST, ALT), ± rise in ALP, GGT, bilirubin	· No diagnostic laboratory investigations · Anti-HLA antibodies if suspicious of AMR	· No diagnostic laboratory investigations
Diagnostic testing	· Renal biopsy	· Liver biopsy: gold standard; ACR and chronic rejection graded according to Banff criteria	· ECG: voltage change, arrhythmia · Echo: effusion, wall thickening, decreased function · EMBx: gold standard; ACR and AMR graded according to ISHLT	· CXR: may have perihilar infiltrates, interstitial edema, pleural effusions · PFTs: decreased forced expiratory volume, forced vital capacity · Bronchoscopy with bronchoalveolar lavage and transbronchial biopsy
Surveillance	· Serial serum creatinine levels ± protocol biopsies	· Serial serum liver transaminases levels	· EMBx	· Protocol bronchoscopies with biopsy
Treatment	· Based on type (humoral vs. cellular) and severity · Steroids, augmented IS regimen, antibody therapies	· Most episodes responsive to pulse steroids · Refractory or recurrent rejection treated with antilymphocyte therapy (i.e., Thymoglobulin or OKT3)	· Based on type and severity, evidence of graft dysfunction, and time after transplant · Steroids, augmented IS regimen, antibody directed therapies for AMR	· Most episodes resolve with therapy · Based on type and severity: pulse steroids, augmented IS regimen

ISHLT, International Society for Heart and Lung Transplantation.

Table 36.4   Infectious Complications

Infection	Clinical	Prophylaxis	Treatment
EBV	· Spectrum from infectious mononucleosis to PTLD · PTLD very important in the pediatric population	· Dependent on donor and recipient mismatch as well as organ · Options: ganciclovir, valganciclovir and/or CMV hyperimmuneglobulin	· Depends on severity, organ type, and timing · Options: ganciclovir, valganciclovir and/or CMV hyperimmuneglobulin
CMV	· Spectrum from infectious mononucleosis-like syndrome to pneumonia, colitis, retinitis	· As above—see EBV prophylaxis	· As above
Candida species	· Oral candidiasis most common · Spectrum from mucocutaneous to disseminated disease	· PO nystatin · Kidney: 3 mo · Liver/heart: until maintenance steroids discontinued · Lung: indefinitely	· Oral: PO nystatin, fluconazole · Skin: topical nystatin, clotrimazole · More significant disease: amphotericin, fluconazole
PJP (previously *P. carinii* or PCP)	· Fever, nonproductive cough, tachypnea, dyspnea, oxygen desaturation, respiratory failure	· TMP/SMX · Kidney/heart: 6 mo · Liver: 1 yr · Lung: indefinitely	· TMP/SMX drug of choice · Can also use pentamidine, corticosteroids (moderate-severe disease)
Polyomavirus (BK and JC virus)	· Most frequently in renal and bone marrow transplant recipients · Kidney: occasionally present with hemorrhagic or nonhemorrhagic cystitis; usually renal dysfunction · Heart: can present with sudden deterioration in renal function	· No prophylaxis	· Reduce IS · Options for therapy include cidofovir, leflunomide, IVIG
RSV	· Bronchiolitis, pneumonia, exacerbation of underlying chronic lung condition	· Palivizumab or RSV IVIG · Recommended for new HTx recipients, <5 yr old transplanted during RSV season or within 3 mo before start of RSV season. · Also HTx recipients <5 yr of age with risk factors (premature birth, chronic lung disease) on an individual case basis	· Supportive measures · Decision to use ribavirin based on individual case

ISHLT, International Society for Heart and Lung Transplantation; *IVIG*, intravenous immunoglobulin.

Transplantation

36

Kidney Transplant Recipients

- Urinary tract and wound site are the most frequent sites of infection
- *Polyomavirus* (BK and JC virus) can cause nephropathy resulting in renal dysfunction; carries 50% risk of allograft loss

Liver Transplant Recipients

- Bacterial infections are commonly associated with cholangitis from biliary reconstruction and vascular anastomosis

Heart Transplant Recipients

- Higher incidence of invasive pneumococcal disease
- *Toxoplasma gondii* can be transmitted in allograft as a result of latency in cardiac muscle

Lung Transplant Recipients

- Pneumonia is major cause of morbidity and mortality, particularly within 90 d after transplant
- Pathogens include resistant bacteria, including *Pseudomonas aeruginosa/Burkholderia cepacia* (for patients with cystic fibrosis) and atypical mycobacteria, common viruses, ubiquitous molds (e.g., *Aspergillus*) (for all lung transplant patients)

PTLD AND OTHER MALIGNANCIES

- Because of chronic IS therapy and young age at transplant, recipients are at increased risk of developing PTLD and de novo malignancies
- PTLD is a heterogeneous spectrum of diseases involving lymphoid proliferation: reactive polyclonal lymphoid hyperplasia to monoclonal malignant lymphoma
- Most commonly associated with EBV infection
- Risk factors for PTLD include type of transplant, recipient's age, IS regimen, EBV-seropositive organ transplanted into seronegative recipient
- Therapy consists of withdrawal or reduction of IS therapy; depending on histopathology, antiviral drugs or chemotherapy may be warranted

Clinical Clues Suggestive of PTLD or Malignancy

1. History of fever, weight loss, diarrhea, GI bleeding, upper respiratory tract infection with lymphadenopathy unresolved after a course of antibiotics, sinusitis, persistent headaches, CNS symptoms
2. Physical findings suggestive of cancer: tonsillitis, lymphadenopathy (cervical, axilliary, inguinal), sinusitis, otitis media, moles
3. Laboratory investigations showing iron deficiency anemia, atypical lymphocytes, cytopenias, hypoalbuminemia

HYPERTENSION

- Posttransplant hypertension in all SOT recipients often caused by medications, especially steroids and CNIs (see Chapter 27 for normal BP ranges)
- 24-h ambulatory BP monitoring may be required
- See Chapter 27 for antihypertensive drugs

NEPHROTOXICITY

- Nephrotoxicity secondary to CNIs is a significant issue in all SOT recipients
- Can lead to chronic renal insufficiency
- Serial TDM required to maintain desired levels
- More vulnerable to acute renal insufficiency, particularly in setting of intravascular volume depletion
- Nephrotoxic medications should be used with caution or avoided, if possible
- A serum creatinine level in the "normal" range can be misleading
- Many SOT recipients have some degree of chronic kidney disease (GFR, <90 mL/min/1.73 m^2)
- Best method to determine renal function is by nuclear medicine GFR scan (measured GFR)
- Recommend periodic screening for proteinuria with urine dipstick
- If dipstick positive (>0.3 g/L), should quantify with spot urine protein:creatinine and urine albumin:creatinine ratios
- CNIs can also cause renal tubular acidosis

AVASCULAR NECROSIS OF BONE AND OSTEOPOROSIS

- Reported in 6–21% of SOT recipients
- Most commonly involved sites: femoral heads or condyles
- Risk factors: corticosteroid therapy and secondary hyperparathyroidism
- Presence of bone pain raises suspicion of avascular necrosis
- Consider screening SOT recipients for osteoporosis with bone mineral density scans
- Consider therapy with calcium, vitamin D supplements; encourage weight-bearing exercise

GROWTH RETARDATION

- Often seen pretransplant as consequence of chronic illness, frequent hospitalizations, various drug therapies
- Steroids are major contributors to growth retardation; however, after transplant, many recipients experience significant catch-up growth
- Human growth hormone has been used in kidney, liver, and heart transplant recipients to improve height with good outcome

FEVER

- Considered significant if single temperature reading >38.5°C or two readings 38.0–38.5°C 1 h apart
- History and full physical examination important
- In addition to typical pediatric infectious illnesses, consider
  - Presence of indwelling catheters (CVL, PICC, other drains)
  - Opportunistic infections
- Investigations as directed by clinical scenario:
  - CBC and differential
  - Blood and urine cultures
  - Viral PCRs (EBV, CMV, HSV 1 and 2)
  - Nasopharyngeal swab for respiratory viruses
  - Stool testing (culture, virology, ova, and parasites)
  - Scraping of lesions as appropriate for electron microscopy
- Decision to admit patient based on clinical status, suspected focus of infection, need for further evaluation and treatment (parenteral vs. oral therapy)
- See suggested antibiotic regimens on Chapter 24
- With liver/intestine transplantation, consider whether patient has been splenectomized; may need initial triple antibiotic coverage (including metronidazole) for intra-abdominal sepsis

VOMITING AND DIARRHEA

- May require medical attention if vomiting and diarrhea persists for >1 d, interferes with medication administration, or renders child unable to maintain adequate hydration
- Patient should have routine stool studies sent, including *Clostridium difficile* toxin assay if taking antibiotics; consider temporary change to IV medication, and give IV fluid for rehydration
- Diarrhea *increases* tacrolimus absorption and *decreases* cyclosporine absorption; suggest TDM
- Vomiting while taking AZA can cause elevation of serum liver enzyme levels; consider holding AZA until vomiting settles
- If intravascularly depleted and taking CNI, increased risk of acute renal failure exists; consider IV rehydration early and check renal function

MANAGEMENT OF INTERCURRENT ILLNESS

- See Table 36.5

CHICKENPOX EXPOSURE

- See Chapter 23

HERPES SIMPLEX INFECTION

- See Chapter 23

Table 36.5	Solid Organ Transplant–Specific Problems		
	Renal Transplant Recipient	**Liver Transplant Recipient**	**Any SOT Recipient**
Problem	· Increased serum creatinine	· Increased serum liver enzymes/bilirubin levels	· Increased serum creatinine
Differential diagnosis	· Rejection · CNI toxicity · UTI · Hypovolemia · Other drug toxicity · BK nephropathy · GU obstruction · Vascular complication · Recurrent disease	· Vascular complication · Biliary complication · ACR · Infection · Drug reaction · Autoimmune hepatitis · Recurrent disease	· Hypovolemia · CNI toxicity · Other drug toxicity · BK nephropathy
Workup and management	· Complete history/physical including medication review · Electrolytes, Ca^{2+}, Mg^{2+}, PO_4^-, urea, creatinine, TDM · Urinalysis and culture · Trial of IV fluid · Renal US (r/o obstruction and vascular complication) · Correct electrolyte abnormalities · ± Hold/decrease dose of medication causing toxicity · ± Antibiotics · Consider biopsy if no improvement with above	· Complete history/physical including medication review · US and Doppler study of liver · AST, ALT, ALP, GGT, bilirubin (conjugated and unconjugated), albumin, protein, CBC + differential, INR, PTT, IgG, autoantibodies, TDM · Consider liver biopsy	· Complete history/ physical including medication review · Electrolytes, Ca^{2+}, Mg^{2+}, PO_4^-, urea, creatinine, TDM · Urinalysis · Trial of IV fluid · Correct electrolyte abnormalities · ± Hold/decrease dose of medication causing toxicity

Transplantation

36

FURTHER READING

Avitzur Y, De Luca E, Cantos M, et al. Health status ten years after pediatric liver transplantation—looking beyond the graft. *Transplantation.* 2004;78:566–572.

Fishman JA. Infection in solid organ transplant recipients. *N Eng J Med.* 2007; 357: 2601–2614.

Halloran PF. Immunosuppressive drugs for kidney transplantation. *N Engl J Med.* 2004;351:2715–2729.

Horslen S, Barr ML, Christensen LL, Ettenger R, Magee JC. Pediatric transplantation in the United States, 1996-2005. *Am J Transplant.* 2007;7(s1):1339–1358.

USEFUL WEB SITES

Canadian Institute for Health Information (CIHI). Available at:
http://secure.cihi.ca/cihiweb/

Trillium Gift of Life Network Organ and Tissue Donation. Available at:
http://organdonationontario.org/

Web sites for specific organs:
Kidney and heart. Available at: http://www.childrenshospital.org/
Liver. Available at: http://digestive.niddk.nih.gov/ddiseases/pubs/livertransplant_ez/
Lung. Available at: http://www.chestnet.org/

Chapter 37 Urology

Briseida Mema
Darius J. Bagli

Chapter 37 Urology

COMMON ABBREVIATIONS

AUV	anterior urethral valves
CIC	clean intermittent catheterization
DMSA	dimercaptosuccinic acid
DTPA	diethylene triamine pentaacetic acid
EMLA	eutectic mixture of local anesthetic
GA	gestational age
IVC	inferior vena cava
NSAID	nonsteroidal anti-inflammatory drug
PUV	posterior urethral valve
RNC	radiopharmaceutical nuclear cystography
RPD	renal pelvic diameter
STI	sexually transmitted infection
TMP/SMX	trimethoprim-sulfamethoxazole
UPJ	ureteropelvic junction
UTI	urinary tract infection
VCUG	voiding cystourethrogram
VUR	vesicoureteral reflux

APPROACH TO THE PATIENT WITH ACUTE SCROTUM

HISTORY

- Age, past medical history, sexual history (if applicable)
- Known urogenital anomalies (corrected or not)
- Pain: onset (gradual, sudden, subtle), course, duration (hours, days, intermittent), precipitating trauma
- Associated symptoms: fever, nausea/vomiting, antecedent illness, abdominal and irritative urinary symptoms

PHYSICAL EXAMINATION

- Abdominal and general examination: important for referred and systemic causes of pain
- Erythema, swelling, skin integrity, discharge, position of testes (right testis may be normally somewhat smaller and/or positioned slightly higher in the scrotum)
- Changes in scrotal size with supine position or Valsalva
- Cremasteric reflex: stroking medial thigh should cause elevation of testicle on the same side; normally found in 40% of males from newborn to age 4 yr and 75% from age 4–16 yr; absence may suggest testicular torsion

- Always examine normal testis first
- Testicular location, lie, axis, tenderness, fluid collections, lymphadenopathy, epididymis, hydrocele, hernia, spermatic cord "knot"
- Transilluminate any masses (hydrocele and spermatocele will transilluminate; tumors and varicocele will not)

INVESTIGATIONS

- CBC (leukocytosis in torsion or epididymitis)
- Urinalysis and urine culture (pyuria in epididymitis)
- Evaluate for STIs if sexually active (Gram stain, culture, nucleic acid amplification testing of urethral discharge; see p. 433)
- Color Doppler US to evaluate perfusion of testis and rule out torsion
- Doppler perfusion *must be* intraparenchymal; perfusion to testis periphery only is *insufficient* and is consistent with torsion
- Doppler can fail to detect perfusion in normal infant testis

DIFFERENTIAL DIAGNOSIS

- Torsion of spermatic cord (testicular torsion) until proven otherwise
- If diagnosis unclear, color Doppler US recommended to *exclude* testicular torsion before discharging patient
- Differentiating causes of acute scrotal pain: see Table 37.1

Other Causes of Acute Scrotum (Best Investigated by US)

- Tumor
- Hydrocele
- Incarcerated inguinal hernia (see Chapter 18)
- Varicocele (up to 16% in adolescence; 10–15% will have fertility problems; size does not correlate well with infertility; rule out IVC obstruction in right-sided varicocele)
- Spermatocele (fluid collection not surrounding testis; usually at head of epididymis)
- Trauma

PHIMOSIS

- Narrowed opening of the prepuce results in nonretractile foreskin
- Normal foreskin may not fully retract until adolescence
- Should only retract as much as easily retractable without force; clean accessible areas when bathing
- Never forcefully retract foreskin as leads to tearing, scarring, and true acquired phimosis
- Foreskin may balloon during voiding; this is normal
- Pathologic phimosis: interferes with voiding, causes recurrent UTI, or interferes with sexual activity/erection; may treat with topical steroid cream or circumcision if severe (scarred foreskin, irreversible)

Table 37.1   Differentiating the Causes of Acute Scrotal Pain

	Testicular Torsion	Torsion of Appendage	Acute Epididymitis
History			
Peak incidence	Perinatal and pubertal	Prepubertal	Infant and postpubertal
Onset of pain	Abrupt "worst pain in entire life"	Abrupt to gradual, usually superior pole of testis	Gradual
Fever	Unusual	Unusual	Common; associated with urinary symptoms
Trauma	None to minor event	Unusual	Unusual
Dysuria	Rare	Rare	Common
Physical Examination			
Findings	Bell-clapper "high riding testis with transverse lie"; palpable knot in cord	Blue dot (uncommon)	Swollen epididymis (posterior to testes) ± erythema
Cremasteric reflex	Usually absent	Usually present	Usually present
Tenderness	Initially testicular	Initially appendage or upper testis	Initially epididymis
Investigations			
Pyuria	Unusual	Unusual	Common
Positive culture	No	No	Often
Leukocytosis	Common	Uncommon	Common
Color Doppler	Parenchymal perfusion decreased/absent vs. contralateral normal side (may be absent in normal infant testes)	Normal or ↑	Normal or ↑
Management			
	Immediate surgical exploration (6-hr window of opportunity) Manual detorsion if expect delay (rotate testis outward toward the thigh or whichever direction relieves the pain)	Pain control (NSAIDS, ice application for 10–15 min qh, rest) Surgery: persistent pain, difficulty, ruling out testicular torsion No long-term implication for fertility	Pain control Antibiotic coverage for UTI or STI after urine culture obtained If recurrent or associated with UTI (culture-proven), need to rule out underlying urogenital ductal anomalies (VCUG, US ± urodynamics)

Adapted from Burgher SW. Acute scrotal pain. *Emerg Med Clin North Am*, 1998;16:781; and Haynes BE, Bessen HA, Haynes VE. The daignosis of testicular torsion. *JAMA*, 1983;249:2522.

- "Trapping" of foreskin in retracted position causes ischemia, swelling, and pain of foreskin and glans; requires prompt reduction or surgical release
- Use of compressive elastic dressing for 20–30 min decreases edema and facilitates reduction or manual compression of glans penis between fingers
- Sedation and pre-emptive analgesia before maneuver (e.g., EMLA)

PENILE INFECTION/INFLAMMATION

- Balanitis: inflammation of glans skin
- Posthitis: inflammation of preputial skin
- Balanoposthitis: inflammation of both the glans and preputial skin
- True infection (i.e., cellulitis) is painful and requires antibiotics (e.g., cephalexin or cloxacillin)
- Smegma (whitish discharge from under foreskin): normal desquamated skin cells and mucus; usually misinterpreted as pus/infection; reassure only
- Reddened foreskin: barrier ointment if desired (e.g., petroleum jelly), dry after voiding

HYPOSPADIAS

- See Figure 37.1
- Congenital termination of urethra on ventral penile surface (glanular, subcoronal, distal and proximal penile, scrotal, or perineal)
- Often associated with chordee (ventral penile curvature) due to skin, fibrous tissue, or ventral corporeal disproportion
- Very proximal defects (penoscrotal, scrotal, perineal) more likely associated with upper tract anomalies (consider US, VCUG), but in general, imaging not required
- If severe or gonad(s) nonpalpable, consider disorder of sexual differentiation (see Chapter 15)
- Associated cryptorchidism (10–30%), inguinal hernia (10%)
- Surgical repair at 6–18 mo of age to normalize voiding pattern, sexual function, and appearance
- Very important not to circumcise newborn as preputial skin often used in repair (to reconstruct urethra or skin coverage); although complex, surgery usually outpatient

Figure 37.1 Hypospadias

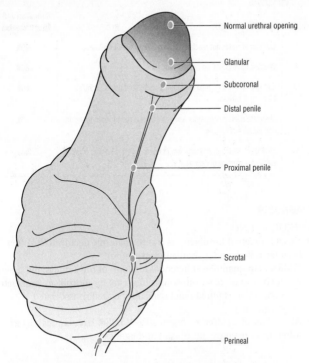

Normal urethral opening

Glanular

Subcoronal

Distal penile

Proximal penile

Scrotal

Perineal

VESICOURETERAL REFLUX

- Retrograde flow of urine from the bladder into the upper urinary tract
- Incidence 2% in children, 15% of those with antenatal hydronephrosis, 30–45% of those evaluated for UTI
- Primary VUR: reflux with no bladder dysfunction or obstruction
- Secondary VUR: high bladder pressures (functional or anatomic obstruction)
- Classified into five grades of severity on contrast VCUG (Table 37.2, Figure 37.2)

Urology

37

Table 37.2   Classification of Vesicoureteral Reflux

Grade	Appearance on VCUG	Resolution by 5 yr After Presentation
I	Contrast in ureter, not reaching renal pelvis, no ureteral dilatation	90%
II	Contrast up to pelvis, no ureteral dilatation	80%
III	Contrast up to pelvis, mild dilatation of ureter and pelvis, slight/no blunting of calyces	60%
IV	Moderate dilatation of ureter and pelvicalyceal system, mild tortuosity and blunting of calyces	30%
V	Significant dilatation and tortuosity of ureter, severe dilatation of pelvis, significant blunting of calyces	Rarely

DIAGNOSIS

- VCUG or RNC
- VCUG preferred for diagnosis (more anatomic detail); RNC often used for follow-up (less radiation exposure)
- DMSA scan quantifies differential function of the kidneys and assesses for cortical defects from congenital renal dysmorphism (associated with reflux) or acquired renal scarring (postreflux-associated pyelonephritis)
- About half of children with grade IV–V reflux have cortical defects (often from renal dysmorphism) at diagnosis

Figure 37.2   Grades of Vesicoureteral Reflux

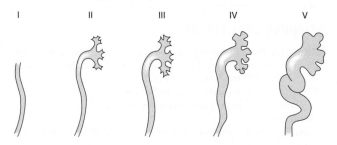

I   II   III   IV   V

MANAGEMENT

- Medical management principles include
  - Normalize voiding patterns (scheduled voiding q2–3h and double voiding)
  - Correct constipation
  - Prophylactic antibiotics (amoxicillin or trimethoprim in neonates; TMP/SMX or nitrofurantoin in children) and prompt full-dose treatment of infections
  - Follow-up yearly with US (kidney growth and hydronephrosis) and RNC (only for resolution, not grade)
- Surgical correction (ureteral reimplantation or gel injections) indications:
  - Documented, verified breakthrough febrile UTI, despite prophylactic antibiotics
  - Noncompliance with antibiotics (relative indication)
  - Reflux that persists into puberty
  - Evidence of new verified renal scarring, not confounded by existing renal dysmorphism
  - Surgical correction often discussed for grade V reflux, as spontaneous resolution unlikely, but correction not mandatory in the presence of structurally and functionally normal kidneys
- Management is evolving toward observation for those > age 4 yr with no resolution of reflux
- Can follow those with normal voiding patterns and no UTI without annual VCUG and UTI prophylaxis; decision must be discussed between patient's family and the pediatric urologist

ANTENATAL HYDRONEPHROSIS

- Dilated RPD on prenatal US: >7 mm at 18–23 wk GA and/or >10 mm at 30–34 wk GA
- See Figure 37.3 for management of antenatal hydronephrosis

OBSTRUCTIVE UROPATHY

APPROACH

- Obstruction may occur anywhere between urethral meatus to calyceal infundibula
- Classified as congenital, acquired, or functional (Table 37.3)

Figure 37.3 Management of Antenatal Hydronephrosis

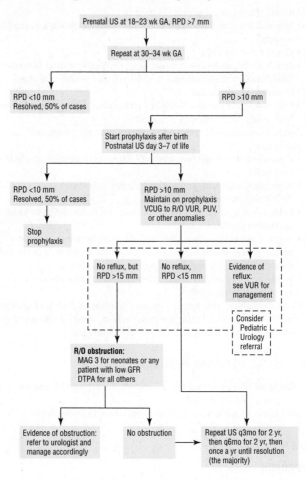

Prenatal US at 18–23 wk GA, RPD >7 mm

Repeat at 30–34 wk GA

RPD <10 mm
Resolved, 50% of cases

RPD >10 mm

Start prophylaxis after birth
Postnatal US day 3–7 of life

RPD <10 mm
Resolved, 50% of cases

Stop prophylaxis

RPD >10 mm
Maintain on prophylaxis
VCUG to R/O VUR, PUV,
or other anomalies

No reflux, but
RPD >15 mm

No reflux,
RPD <15 mm

Evidence of
reflux:
see VUR for
management

Consider
Pediatric
Urology
referral

R/O obstruction:
MAG 3 for neonates or any
patient with low GFR
DTPA for all others

Evidence of obstruction:
refer to urologist and
manage accordingly

No obstruction

Repeat US q3mo for 2 yr,
then q6mo for 2 yr, then
once a yr until resolution
(the majority)

UPJ OBSTRUCTION

- Most common site of urinary tract obstruction in children
- May be caused by segment of ureter that lacks peristalsis, muscular bands, or external compression from aberrant vessels
- 75% unilateral; mostly left; M:F, 2:1
- Complete UPJ obstruction associated with severe renal dysplasia

Table 37.3	Causes of Obstructive Uropathy	
Congenital	**Acquired**	**Functional**

Congenital infundibulopelvic stenosis
UPJ obstruction
Congenital obstructive megaureter
Ureteral ectopia
Ureterocele
Ureteral valves (PUV, AUV)
Urethral atresia (prune-belly syndrome)
	Obstruction anywhere in urinary tract from
	• Calculi
	• Trauma
	• Inflammatory (Crohn)
	• Infectious (TB)
	• Postsurgical
	• Neoplastic
		Neurogenic bladder
		• Neurologic etiology
		  • Neurospinal dysraphism (myelomeningocele)
		  • Degenerative diseases
		  • Guillain-Barré
		  • Postmyelitis
		• Anatomic
		• Myopathic
		• Psychological
		• Endocrine
		• Toxic

- Lesser degrees of obstruction result in hydronephrosis, increased risk of UTI
- Treatment: surgical removal of obstructed segment and reanastomosis of ureter to renal pelvis (pyeloplasty)

PRUNE-BELLY SYNDROME

- Triad: absent abdominal wall musculature, urinary tract anomalies, bilateral intra-abdominal cryptorchidism
- Urologic anomalies range from mild (urinary tract dilatation) to severe (renal failure)

PUV

- Urethral valve in prostatic urethra causes obstruction of urine outflow from bladder
- Spectrum; severe can cause dysplasia of both kidneys in utero; may present as oligohydramnios
- Milder presentations: straining to urinate, weak urinary stream, frequent UTIs
- Diagnose by VCUG or urethroscopy; suspect in newborn male with significant bilateral hydronephrosis
- 60% have secondary VUR
- Immediate treatment is adequate urine drainage via bladder catheter
- Definitive treatment is surgical ablation of the valves
- Long-term pediatric urologic follow-up of bladder and renal function required

NEUROGENIC BLADDER

- Cause of functional obstructive uropathy (see Table 37.3)

Management

- Control concomitant constipation
- Manage low sphincter tone with α-adrenergic medication (pseudoephedrine 0.4 mg/kg bid to 0.9 mg/kg tid PO) or surgery to increase outlet resistance (sling or artificial urinary sphincter)
- Manage unstable detrusor muscle function with oxybutynin (anticholinergic; 0.2 mg/kg bid–qid PO, up to 5 mg/dose) ± CIC, ± surgical augmentation cystoplasty if refractory to medical/CIC therapy
- Approximately half of those requiring CIC develop latex allergy (acquired IgE-mediated, secondary to repeated exposure); all myelomeningocele patients should follow latex precautions

Follow-Up

- Annual follow-up to detect change in pattern:
  - Urologic (continence, UTI) history, physical examination
  - US: renal growth and hydronephrosis, bladder stones
  - VCUG: bladder capacity, new trabeculation, diverticulum, VUR
  - Urodynamic studies: capacity, compliance (filling at low pressure to protect upper tract), detrusor stability (uninhibited contractions), adequate emptying

FURTHER READING

Ashfield JE, Nickel KR, Siemens DR, MacNeily AE, Nickel JC. Treatment of phimosis with topical steroids in 194 children. *J Urol.* 2003;169:1106–1108.

Current world literature. Pediatric urology. *Curr Opin Urol.* 2001;11:637–646.

Decter RM. Vesicoureteral reflux. *Pediatr Rev.* 2001;22:205–210.

Elder JS. Guidelines for consideration for surgical repair of vesicoureteral reflux. *Curr Opin Urol.* 2000;10:579–585.

Kaplan GW. Scrotal swelling in children. *Pediatr Rev.* 2000;21:311–314.

USEFUL WEB SITES

How the Body Works. Available at: **www.aboutkidshealth.ca/HowTheBodyWorks**

Section III Laboratory Reference Values

Section III Laboratory Reference Values

Fatoumah M.Y.M. Alabdulrazzaq
Khosrow Adeli
Wendy Lau

Clinical Biochemistry
Hematology
Toxicology
Therapeutic Drug Monitoring
Cerebrospinal Fluid
Stool
Urine
Microbial Serology
Blood Products
Useful Web Sites

CLINICAL BIOCHEMISTRY

Table III.1 Clinical Biochemistry

Test Name	Specimen Type	Age/Sex	Reference Interval/Units	Comments
α1-Acid glycoprotein (orosomucoid), plasma or serum	Blood		0.40–1.30 g/L	Acute phase reactant
Acid phosphatase, prostatic (PACP), serum	Blood		<2.3 mcg/L	
Acylcarnitines, plasma	Blood		Acetyl C2 4.65–35.39 μmol/L Propionyl C3 <1.08 μmol/L Butyryl/isobutyryl C4 <0.68 μmol/L Tiglyl C5:1 <0.09 μmol/L Isovaleryl/2-methylbutyryl C5 <0.47 μmol/L Hexanoyl C6 <0.32 μmol/L OHisoval/methylOHbutyryl-C5OH <0.14 μmol/L Octenoyl C8:1 <0.68 μmol/L Octanoyl C8 <0.30 μmol/L Malonyl C3DC <0.13 μmol/L Decenoyl C10:1 <0.29 μmol/L Decanoyl C10 <0.38 μmol/L Methylmalonyl/succinyl C4DC <0.13 μmol/L	

(continued)

Table III.1   Clinical Biochemistry (continued)

Test Name	Specimen Type	Age/Sex	Reference Interval/Units	Comments
			Glutaryl/3OHdecanoyl C5DC	<0.14 µmol/L	
			Dodecenoyl C12:1	<0.19 µmol/L	
			Dodecanoyl C12	<0.19 µmol/L	
			3OHdodecanoyl C12OH	<0.05 µmol/L	
			Tetradecadienoyl C14:2	<0.09 µmol/L	
			Tetradecenoyl C14:1	<0.21 µmol/L	
			Tetradecanoyl C14	<0.11 µmol/L	
			3OHtetradecenoyl C14:1OH	<0.05 µmol/L	
			3OHtetradecanoyl C14OH	<0.04 µmol/L	
			Palmitoleoyl C16:1	<0.09 µmol/L	
			Palmitoyl C16	<0.31 µmol/L	
			3OHpalmitoleoyl C16:1OH	<0.13 µmol/L	
			3OHpalmitoyl C16OH	<0.05 µmol/L	
			Linoleoyl C18:2	<0.14 µmol/L	
			Oleoyl C18:1	<0.28 µmol/L	
			Stearoyl C18	<0.10 µmol/L	
			3OHlinoleoyl C18:2OH	<0.03 µmol/L	
			3OHoleoyl C18:1OH	<0.04 µmol/L	
Adenosine diphosphate (ADP)	Blood		46–94%	
ADH, plasma	Blood			See antidiuretic hormone, plasma

Adrenal antibodies, serum	Blood		Not detected	
Adrenocorticotropic hormone (ACTH), plasma	Blood		<17 pmol/L Morning ACTH peak falls by half through the day	Take blood at 9 A.M. to use these values; for adequate interpretation, cortisol should be measured in same sample
ACTH stimulation test	Blood		A normal cortisol response is indicated by a doubling of the basal value and an absolute value of >500-550 nmol/L	Measures cortisol
Alanine aminotrans-ferase (ALT), plasma or serum	Blood	<1 yr ≥1 yr	≤ 60 units/L ≤ 40 units/L	
Albumin, plasma or serum	Blood	<1 mo 1-12 mo >1 yr	26-41 g/L 28-48 g/L 32-56 g/L	
Aldosterone, plasma or serum	Blood		Upright: 111-860 pmol/L Recumbent: 28-444 pmol/L	Request Na$^+$ and K$^+$ on same sample 24-h urine collection for Na$^+$ excretion rarely indicated; less useful than urine aldosterone, varies widely over short periods (depending on time of day, posture, Na$^+$ and K$^+$ intake); to demonstrate hyperaldosteronism in hypokalemic hypertension, give K$^+$ supplements until K$^+$ is in normal range before aldosterone is measured; diuretics (e.g., furosemide, spironolactone) and several other drugs (especially purgatives and liquorice derivatives [e.g., carbenoxolone]) should be discontinued (if possible) for 3 wk before assessment; indicate any drugs patient may still be taking

(continued)

Table III.1   Clinical Biochemistry (continued)

Test Name	Specimen Type	Age/Sex	Reference Interval/Units	Comments
Alkaline phosphatase, plasma or serum	Blood	Female: <1 yr 1-2 yr 3-8 yr 9-13 yr 14-15 yr 16-17 yr >18 yr Male: <1 yr 1-8 yr 9-11 yr 12-15 yr 16-17 yr 18 yr	185-555 units/L 185-520 units/L 185-425 units/L 160-500 units/L 90-400 units/L 45-140 units/L 25-100 units/L 175-600 units/L 175-400 units/L 180-475 units/L 200-630 units/L 100-455 units/L 80-210 units/L	Source: bone, liver, kidney, intestinal mucosa; isoenzymes exist for bone, liver, and intestine
Alkaline phosphatase isoenzymes, plasma or serum	Blood		ALP (fast liver): 8-61 units/L ALP (bone): 10-64 units/L	Include clinical indications for fractionation
Alpha fetoprotein (AFP), serum	Blood	<14 d 14-29 d 1 mo	8000-130,000 mcg/L 300-70,000 mcg/L 90-10,000 mcg/L	Tumor marker, especially gonadal germ cell or primary hepatic tumor; also raised during rapid liver regeneration (e.g., acute hepatitis)

	2 mo	40–1000 mcg/L	
	3 mo	20–300 mcg/L	
	4 mo	<300 mcg/L	
	5 mo	<100 mcg/L	
	6–7 mo	<40 mcg/L	
	8 mo	<20 mcg/L	
	9 mo–adult	<10 mcg/L	

Test	Sample	Values	Notes
ALT, plasma or serum	Blood		See alanine aminotransferase, plasma or serum
Aluminum, serum	Blood	Standard: <371 nmol/L On aluminum antacid medication: <1100 nmol/L	Aluminum toxicity signs may appear in dialysis patients when aluminum >2000 nmol/L
Amino acid screen, plasma	Blood	Qualitative assessment	Screening done by chromatography to detect genetic-metabolic disease; if screen abnormal, quantitative values should be obtained; reference values are age dependent, should be interpreted by specialist in metabolic disease
Amino acids quantitative, plasma or serum	Blood	(see table below)	Reference values are age dependent and should be interpreted by specialist in metabolic disease Units–μmol/L

Test	<7 d	7 d–7 mo	7 mo–3 yr
Alanine	325–425	239–345	99–313
Alloisoleucine	Not detected	Not detected	Not detected
Arginine	30–70	53–71	11–65
Argininosuccinic acid	Not detected	Not detected	Not detected
Aspartate	1–20	17–21	<9
Citrulline	1–26	1–47	<30

(continued)

Table III.1   Clinical Biochemistry (continued)

Test Name	Specimen Type	Age/Sex	Reference Interval/Units				Comments
			Test	**<7 d**	**7 d–7 mo**	**7 mo–3 yr**	
			Cystine	57–75	33–51	23–68	
			Glutamate	30–100	30–100	30–100	
			Glutamine	1–1043	1–746	1–746	
			Glycine	185–785	178–248	56–308	
			Histidine	30–70	64–92	24–112	
			Isoleucine	20–60	31–47	26–94	
			Leucine	45–95	56–98	45–155	
			Lysine	130–250	117–163	45–144	
			Methionine	30–40	15–21	3–29	
			Ornithine	70–110	37–61	10–107	
			Phenylalanine	70–110	45–65	23–69	
			Proline	155–305	141–245	51–185	
			Serine	195–345	104–158	24–172	
			Threonine	155–275	141–213	33–128	
			Tyrosine	20–220	33–75	11–122	
			Valine	80–180	123–199	57–262	
Ammonia, plasma		<30 d	<50 µmol/L				
		≥30 d	<35 µmol/L				
Amylase, plasma or serum			20–110 units/L				Source: pancreas, salivary glands

Androstenedione, plasma or serum	Blood	Male:		Source: ovaries, adrenals; can be considered "adrenal-specific" androgen until puberty in females and from 5 mo to puberty in males; in females, values are higher during luteal phase of cycle than during follicular phase but should still be within range shown
		1-5 mo	0.2-1.6 nmol/L	
		6-11 mo	0.2-1.0 nmol/L	
		1-5 yr	0.2-1.6 nmol/L	
		6-9 yr	0.2-1.9 nmol/L	
		10-11 yr	0.3-1.0 nmol/L	
		12-14 yr	0.7-3.0 nmol/L	
		15-18 yr	1.2-3.5 nmol/L	
		Female:		
		1-5 mo	0.2-1.2 nmol/L	
		6-11 mo	0.2-0.9 nmol/L	
		1-5 yr	0.2-1.4 nmol/L	
		6-9 yr	0.2-1.6 nmol/L	
		10-11 yr	0.9-2.8 nmol/L	
		12-14 yr	0.5-6.1 nmol/L	
		15-18 yr	1.9-7.0 nmol/L	
Angiotensin-converting enzyme (ACE), plasma or serum	Blood	Adult ref. range	12-54 units/L	Values not age dependent in children
			No ref. range established for children	
Antidiuretic hormone (ADH) (arginine vasopressin), plasma	Blood		0-6.7 ng/L	Interpret in relation to plasma osmolality

(continued)

Table III.1   Clinical Biochemistry (continued)

Test Name	Specimen Type	Age/Sex	Reference Interval/Units	Comments
Antithyroglobulin antibodies	Blood		<115 IU/mL	Referred out test; range subject to change
Anti-TPO antibody, plasma or serum (antithyroid peroxidase antibodies)	Blood		<35 IU/mL	Same as antimicrosomal antibodies
α_1-Antitrypsin, serum	Blood		0.90–2.00 g/L	
α_1-Antitrypsin phenotyping (PI typing), serum	Blood		Acute phase reactant; Order only if α_1-antitrypsin is abnormal; do not order repeat protease inhibitor (PI) typing following initial confirmation PI typing: · MM, normal (89% of population) · MS, normal variant (8%) · MZ, heterozygous for deficiency (<2%) · ZZ, homozygous for deficiency For clearance: falsely low values where lesion(s) in esophagus, stomach, or upper small bowel because low-pH environment degrades α_1-antitrypsin; collection must be free of urine; serum α_1-antitrypsin required (clotted blood collected during stool collection period or within 24 h after collection period)	Phenotyping may only be done if α_1-antitrypsin total is low

Apolipoprotein A-1, plasma or serum	Blood		0.92-1.96 g/L	
Apolipoprotein B, plasma	Blood		0.59-1.46 g/L	
Arginine stimulation test	Blood		Peak growth hormone, after stimulation >8 mcg/L	Includes glucose, growth hormone
Arginine vasopressin (ADH), plasma	Blood			See antidiuretic hormone (ADH)
Ascorbic acid (vitamin C), serum	Blood		>25 µmol/L	Wrap vial in foil to protect from light
Aspartate aminotransferase (AST), plasma or serum	Blood	<1 yr 1-9 yr ≥10 yr	≤110 units/L ≤45 units/L ≤36 units/L	Source: cardiac and skeletal muscle, liver, kidney, erythrocytes
Bicarbonate (calculated); arterial, capillary, or venous	Blood			See blood gas, arterial, capillary or venous
β2-microglobulin, blood	Blood		≤200 nmol/L	
Bile acids, plasma or serum	Blood		<8.2 µmol/L	
Bilirubin, conjugated; plasma or serum	Blood	≤15 d ≥16 d	≤10 µmol/L ≤2 µmol/L	

(continued)

819

Table III.1 Clinical Biochemistry *(continued)*

Test Name	Specimen Type	Age/Sex	Reference Interval/Units	Comments
Bilirubin, delta; plasma or serum	Blood	≤13 d ≥14 d	≤3 μmol/L 0 μmol/L	Delta bilirubin is albumin conjugated (long half-life) and associated with long-standing cholestasis
Bilirubin, unconjugated; plasma or serum	Blood	≤2 d 3–5 d 6 d–29 d ≥1 mo	<130 μmol/L <200 μmol/L <180 μmol/L <17 μmol/L	Refer to bilirubin value according to hour of age (see Neonatology)
Biotinidase screening, whole blood or serum	Blood		369–432 nmol/mL/h	

Blood gas; arterial, capillary, or venous	Blood	**pH**
		Arterial, capillary:
		  <1 mo
		  ≥1 mo
		  Venous
		PCO₂
		Arterial, capillary:
		  <1 yr
		  ≥1 yr
		  Venous
		PO₂
		  Arterial
		  <2 d
			
			7.30–7.49
			7.35–7.50
			7.32–7.42
			
			30–45 mm Hg
			32–45 mm Hg
			40–50 mm Hg
			
			60–70 mm Hg
				Blood gases (pH, PCO_2, PO_2, actual bicarbonate, base excess, and O_2 saturation calculation); normal values for capillary gas levels range from venous to arterial, depending on arterialization of sample site

		2 d	70–80 mm Hg	
		≥3 d	80–100 mm Hg	
		Venous	25–47 mm Hg	
		Bicarbonate		
		Arterial only:		
		≤6 d	17–26 mmol/L	
		7–29 d	17–27 mmol/L	
		1–5 mo	17–29 mmol/L	
		6–11 mo	18–29 mmol/L	
		≥1 yr	20–31 mmol/L	
Blood urea nitrogen, plasma or serum	Blood			See urea
C3 complement, serum	Blood	≤5 d	0.39–1.56 g/L	
		≥6 d	0.77–1.43 g/L	
C4 complement, serum	Blood	≤5 d	0.05–0.33 g/L	
		≥6 d	0.07–0.40 g/L	
Calcitonin, serum	Blood	Female	<7 ng/L	Measured after pentagastrin stimulation
		Male	<11 ng/L	
Calcium, ionized, whole blood	Blood		1.22–1.37 mmol/L	

(continued)

Table III.1 — Clinical Biochemistry (continued)

Test Name	Specimen Type	Age/Sex	Reference Interval/Units	Comments
Calcium, total; plasma or serum	Blood	<1 mo	2.00–2.75 mmol/L	Prolonged venous stasis (e.g., prolonged tourniquet use) alters result; low serum calcium levels; may be normal if hypoalbuminemia present; adjusted calcium should be in normal range For SI units: Adjusted Ca^{2+} (mmol/L) = total calcium (mmol/L) + [40 − albumin (g/L)] × 0.025 For traditional units: Adjusted Ca^{2+} (mg/dL) = calcium (mg/dL) − albumin (g/dL) + 4
		1–11 mo	2.17–2.70 mmol/L	
		1–3 yr	2.17–2.65 mmol/L	
		≥4 yr	2.19–2.60 mmol/L	
Carbohydrate-deficient transferrin, serum	Blood		Descriptive report	Also known as transferrin isoelectric focusing
Carboxyhemoglobin, whole blood	Blood		0.020	Specimen must be anaerobic; send stat; expressed as fraction of total hemoglobin
Carcinoembryonic antigen (CEA), serum	Blood		≤4.0 mcg/L	
Cardiolipin antibodies, plasma or serum	Blood		<19 arbitrary units	
Carnitine (free), serum	Blood	<16 d	12–60 µmol/L	
		≥16 d	26–60 µmol/L	

Carnitine (total), serum	Blood	<16 d	23-84 μmol/L
		≥16 d	32-84 μmol/L
Carotene, plasma or serum	Blood		0.9-3.7 μmol/L
Catecholamines, plasma	Blood	Epinephrine	<0.8 nmol/L	Drugs such as methyldopa, hydralazine (Apresoline), quinidine, epinephrine, or norepinephrine-related drugs (e.g., L-dopa) and renal function test dyes may interfere with catecholamine excretion and affect results
		Norepinephrine	0.8-3.4 nmol/L	Referred out test; range subject to change
Ceruloplasmin, serum	Blood	Female:		
		<10 yr	264-473 mg/L	
		10-13 yr	253-473 mg/L	
		≥14 yr	220-495 mg/L	
		Male:		
		<10 yr	264-473 mg/L	
		10-13 yr	242-396 mg/L	
		≥14 yr	154-374 mg/L	
Chloride, plasma or serum	Blood	<1 yr	96-106 mmol/L	
		1-18 yr	99-111 mmol/L	
		≥19 yr	98-106 mmol/L	
Cholesterol, plasma or serum	Blood	<3 mo	3.20-4.53 mmol/L	Values based on fasting states (before feeding in babies; after 12-h fast in older children); fasting not essential if total cholesterol requested without any other lipid determinations
		3 mo-1 yr	3.20-4.91 mmol/L	
		2-17 yr	3.20-4.40 mmol/L	
		≥18 yr	3.20-4.60 mmol/L	

(continued)

Table III.1   Clinical Biochemistry (continued)

Test Name	Specimen Type	Age/Sex	Reference Interval/Units	Comments
Chloride, sweat	Sweat	≥7 d	<40 mmol/L: negative 30–60 mmol/L: borderline/indeterminate >60 mmol/L: consistent with diagnosis of CF	A sweat chloride test result of 30–60 mmol/L is borderline for CF; repeat test within 2–4 wk Repeat test if first result ≥60 mmol/L Test is only accurate after 7 d of age
Cholesterol, HDL; plasma or serum	Blood	Female: <2 yr 2–6 yr 7–11 yr 12–15 yr 16–18 yr Male: <2 yr 2–6 yr 7–11 yr 12–15 yr 16–18 yr	0.21–1.58 mmol/L 0.31–1.66 mmol/L 0.60–2.07 mmol/L 0.65–2.15 mmol/L 0.54–1.99 mmol/L 0.21–1.58 mmol/L 0.60–1.81 mmol/L 0.65–2.05 mmol/L 0.49–1.97 mmol/L 0.67–1.94 mmol/L	Take blood before feeding for neonates and infants and after 12-h fast for older children
Cholesterol, LDL; plasma or serum	Blood	Female: <2 yr 2–9 yr 10–14 yr 15–19 yr	0.82–3.02 mmol/L 0.98–3.62 mmol/L 1.76–3.52 mmol/L 1.53–3.55 mmol/L	Take sample before feeding for neonates and infants and after 12-h fast for older children

		Male:	
		<2 yr	0.82-3.02 mmol/L
		2-9 yr	0.98-3.62 mmol/L
		10-14 yr	1.66-3.44 mmol/L
		15-19 yr	1.61-3.37 mmol/L
Cholinesterase, serum (pseudocholinesterase)	Blood	Cholinesterase total 620-1370 IU/L Dibucaine 77-83 IU/L Fluoride 56-68 IU/L Chloride 4-15 IU/L Succinylcholine (scoline) 87-92 IU/L	Clinical biochemist consultation required; for stat analysis only; cholinesterase phenotype includes chloride, cholinesterase-total, dibucaine, fluoride, scoline, and Ro 02-0683; collect 24 h after surgery
Cholinesterase, total activity; serum	Blood	620-1370 IU/L	
Chorionic gonadotropin, β subunit (qualitative); serum	Blood	Positive or negative	Pregnancy screen
Chorionic gonadotropin (quantitative HCG), serum	Blood	<5 IU/L	Tumor marker
Clonidine stimulation test	Blood	Peak growth hormone, after stimulation >8 mcg/L	Includes glucose, growth hormone
Complement, serum	Blood		See C3 and C4 complement

(continued)

Laboratory Reference Values

III

825

Table III.1 Clinical Biochemistry (continued)

Test Name	Specimen Type	Age/Sex	Reference Interval/Units	Comments
Copper, serum	Blood	Age: <3 mo 3-5 mo 6-11 mo 1-12 yr >13 yr	1.4-7.2 µmol/L 3.9-17.3 µmol/L 7.9-20.1 µmol/L 12.6-19.0 µmol/L 9.0-22.0 µmol/L	Do not use gel separator or plastic collection tubes
Coproporphyrin, erythrocytes	Blood		≤ 45 nmol/L	
Coproporphyrin, plasma or serum	Blood		≤ 45 nmol/L	Referred out test; range subject to change
Cortisol, plasma or serum	Blood		8 A.M.: 190-740 nmol/L 8 P.M.: 30-300 nmol/L	Result at 8 P.M. is <50% of the 8 A.M. value in 88% of cases; diurnal variation of cortisol may not develop until about 1 yr of age; in Cushing disease or syndrome, cortisol levels may be normal, but diurnal variation may be absent; other steroids produced in congenital adrenal hyperplasia or tumors may cross-react with cortisol assay; only poor diurnal variation may be evident; stress or shock can elevate cortisol levels
C peptide, plasma or serum	Blood		298-2350 pmol/L	Collect after overnight fast Do not use gel barrier tubes to collect

C-reactive protein (CRP), serum	Blood	≤8.0 mg/L

Creatine kinase (CK), plasma or serum	Blood	11 d–11 mo	≤390 units/L	Source: skeletal and cardiac muscle, smooth muscle, brain; elevated CK levels occur after physical activity and intramuscular injections; black people have significantly higher levels of CK than white people; bed rest for several days may drop CK levels by 20–30%
		1–3 yr	60–305 units/L	
		4–6 yr	75–230 units/L	
		7–8 yr	60–365 units/L	
		Female:		
		9–10 yr	80–230 units/L	
		11–13 yr	50–295 units/L	
		14–15 yr	50–240 units/L	
		≥16 yr	45–230 units/L	
		Male:		
		9–10 yr	55–215 units/L	
		11–13 yr	60–330 units/L	
		14–15 yr	60–335 units/L	
		≥16 yr	55–370 units/L	

Creatine kinase (CK) MB mass, serum	Blood	CK-MB mass	0.0–6.5 mcg/L	Approval required if CPK is <100 units/L
		CK-MB mass index	<20 ng/unit	Sources: CK-BB, predominantly brain; CK-MB, cardiac muscle, type II skeletal muscle fibers; CK-MM, skeletal muscle, cardiac muscle
				Purpose is to help differentiate skeletal from cardiac muscle disease or trauma
				CK-MB not specific for myocardial damage in first week or month after birth; if CK-MB is borderline, consider troponin T or I

(continued)

Table III.1 Clinical Biochemistry (*continued*)

Test Name	Specimen Type	Age/Sex	Reference Interval/Units	Comments
Creatinine, plasma or serum	Blood	≤6 d	19–99 µmol/L	
		7–60 d	10–56 µmol/L	
		2 mo–5 yr	<36 µmol/L	
		6–9 yr	<53 µmol/L	
		10–13 yr	<79 µmol/L	
		≥14 yr	<98 µmol/L	
Cryoglobulin, serum	Blood			Normally absent
7-Dehydrocholesterol, plasma or serum	Blood		µmol/L	Clinical biochemist consultation required. Referred out test; range will be included with the report
Dehydroepiandrosterone sulfate (DHEA-S), plasma or serum	Blood	Female:		
		≤5 mo	≤3.9 µmol/L	
		6 mo–7 yr	≤0.9 µmol/L	
		8–9 yr	≤2.9 µmol/L	
		10–12 yr	≤7.9 µmol/L	
		≥13 yr	1.0–12.0 µmol/L	
		Male:		
		≤5 mo	≤3.9 µmol/L	
		6 mo–7 yr	≤0.4 µmol/L	
		8–9 yr	≤2.9 µmol/L	
		10–12 yr	≤5.9 µmol/L	
		≥13 yr	3.0–12.0 µmol/L	

Deoxycorticosteroids, serum	Blood	Premature infants Newborns 1-12 mo 2-10 yr ≥11 yr	20-105 ng/dL See comments 7-49 ng/dL 2-34 ng/dL 2-19 ng/dL	Newborns: levels are markedly elevated at birth but decrease rapidly during first week to the range found in older infants Referred out test; range subject to change
11-Deoxycortisol, serum	Blood	 After metyrapone stimulation	≤22 nmol/L >200 nmol/L	Referred out test; range subject to change
Dihydropteridine reductase, whole blood	Blood		7-22 units/g Hb	
Dihydrotestosterone, serum	Blood	Male/female: 9 mo–puberty Adult male Adult female	31-317 nmol/L 217-1650 nmol/L 28-616 nmol/L	Arrange with biochemistry laboratory before blood collected
Epinephrine, plasma	Blood			See catecholamines, plasma
Estradiol, plasma or serum	Blood	Female: ≤11 mo 1 yr to adrenarche Puberty Adult Follicular phase Luteal phase	370 pmol/L <92 pmol/L Rising to adult values <165 pmol/L 110-183 pmol/L 550-845 pmol/L	

(continued)

Table III.1   Clinical Biochemistry *(continued)*

Test Name	Specimen Type	Age/ Sex	Reference Interval/Units	Comments
		Treated with synthetic estrogens	<165 pmol/L	
		Preovulating peak	550–1650 pmol/L	
		Male:		
		≤11 mo	370 pmol/L	
		1 yr to adrenarche	<92 pmol/L	
		Puberty	Rising to adult values	
		Adult	<165 pmol/L	
Estriol (unconjugated), serum	Blood	Gestational wk:	nmol/L:	
		15	2.42	
		16	3.14	
		17	4.07	
		18	5.28	
		19	6.85	
		20	8.88	
Fatty acid (free), serum	Blood	<10 d	≤1.85 mmol/L	
		≥10 d	0.22–0.88 mmol/L	
Ferritin, plasma or serum	Blood	Female:		Acute phase reactant
		1–15 d	46.0–237.0 mcg/L	
		16 d–3 yr	5.5–73.0 mcg/L	
		4–10 yr	9.0–73.0 mcg/L	

		11-14 yr	11.0-64.0 mcg/L
		15-20 yr	6.6-58.0 mcg/L
		Male:	
		1-15 d	32.0-233.0 mcg/L
		16 d-3 yr	5.5-62.0 mcg/L
		4-10 yr	13.0-73.0 mcg/L
		11-14 yr	15.0-70.0 mcg/L
		15-20 yr	10.0-82.0 mcg/L
Follicle-stimulating hormone (FSH), serum	Blood	Female:	
		≤5 mo	≤38.0 IU/L
		6 mo-1 yr	≤8.0 IU/L
		2-9 yr	≤4.0 IU/L
		≥10 yr	≤9.0 IU/L
		Male:	
		≤3 mo	≤15.0 IU/L
		4 mo-1 yr	≤3.0 IU/L
		2-10 yr	≤4.0 IU/L
		≥11 yr	≤7.0 IU/L
Free erythrocyte porphyrin	Blood	0-10 yr	0-0.61 mmol/L
		11 yr	0-1.32 mmol/L
Galactosemia screen	Blood		Qualitative test of RBC galactose 1-phosphate uridyltransferase activity; blood transfusion within 3 mo before this test may invalidate results; results may be falsely negative if child is not ingesting galactose-containing foods when blood is taken

(continued)

Table III.1   Clinical Biochemistry (continued)

Test Name	Specimen Type	Age/Sex	Reference Interval/Units	Comments
Gases, arterial, capillary, venous blood	Blood			See blood gas, arterial, capillary, venous blood
Gastrin, serum or plasma	Blood		0–89 ng/L	
GGT	Blood			See γ-glutamyltransferase, plasma or serum
Glucagon, plasma	Blood		59–177 pg/mL	
Glucagon stimulation test	Blood		After stimulation, peak growth hormone should exceed 8 mcg/L	Includes glucose and growth hormone
Glucose, plasma or serum; fasting, random, 2 h pc	Blood	<1 yr 1–2 yr 3–11 yr ≥12 yr	2.5–5.5 mmol/L 2.5–5.0 mmol/L 2.8–6.1 mmol/L 3.3–6.1 mmol/L	CSF glucose should be roughly ⅔ of blood glucose
γ-Glutamyltransferase (GGT), plasma or serum	Blood	<1 mo 1 mo 2–3 mo 4–6 mo 7 mo–14 yr ≥15 yr (female) ≥15 yr (male)	≤385 units/L ≤225 units/L ≤135 units/L ≤75 units/L ≤45 units/L ≤55 units/L ≤75 units/L	Source: liver, pancreas
Gonadotropins	Blood			See follicle-stimulating hormone (FSH) and luteinizing hormone (LH)
Growth hormone (GH), serum	Blood			Random samples have little diagnostic value Fetus has high GH, relative to children and adults

Growth hormone-releasing hormone stimulation	Blood		After stimulation, peak growth hormone should exceed 8 mcg/L	Includes glucose and growth hormone
Haptoglobin, serum	Blood		0.32-1.98 g/L	
HDL cholesterol, plasma or serum	Blood			See cholesterol, HDL; plasma or serum
Hemoglobin, plasma	Blood		≤ 29 mg/L	
Homocysteine, plasma	Blood	≤5 yr 6-12 yr 13-59 yr	0.5-11.0 μmol/L 5.0-12.0 μmol/L 5.0-15.0 μmol/L	Send specimen to laboratory on ice
Human chorionic gonadotropin screen, blood (β-HCG screen)	Blood			See chorionic gonadotropin screen
HCG stimulation test			Normal response will have a 3-4-fold increase in testosterone when 72-h post HCG level is compared with basal level	Measures testosterone
17-Hydroxyprogesterone, plasma or serum	Blood	<3 mo ≥3 mo Very sick and stressed infants <3 mo Borderline for nonclassic CAH	<10.0 nmol/L <6.0 nmol/L <30 nmol/L 6-10 nmol/L	Cord blood or sample taken during the first 24-48 h of life is unsatisfactory Clinical biochemist consultation required for stat analysis

(continued)

833

Table III.1   Clinical Biochemistry (continued)

Test Name	Specimen Type	Age/Sex	Reference Interval/Units	Comments
IgE, serum	Blood	Female:		
		<1 yr	<8 IU/mL	
		1–3 yr	<28 IU/mL	
		4–10 yr	<137 IU/mL	
		11–18 yr	<398 IU/mL	
		Male:		
		<1 yr	<12 IU/mL	
		1–3 yr	<90 IU/mL	
		4–10 yr	<163 IU/mL	
		11–18 yr	<179 IU/mL	
IgF$_1$, serum	Blood	Female:		
		≤15 d	3–43 mcg/L	
		16 d–6 mo	6–306 mcg/L	
		7 mo–8 yr	48–350 mcg/L	
		9–10 yr	80–446 mcg/L	
		11–12 yr	120–691 mcg/L	
		13 yr	187–817 mcg/L	
		14–16 yr	219–930 mcg/L	
		17–18 yr	160–689 mcg/L	
		19–20 yr	121–447 mcg/L	
		Male:		
		≤15 d	3–43 mcg/L	
		16 d–6 mo	6–306 mcg/L	

		7 mo–8 yr	48–350 mcg/L
		9–10 yr	66–446 mcg/L
		11–12 yr	99–701 mcg/L
		13 yr	170–886 mcg/L
		14–16 yr	212–1077 mcg/L
		17–18 yr	167–807 mcg/L
		19–20 yr	131–534 mcg/L
IGF-BP3, serum (IGF-binding protein 3)	Blood	Female:	
		≤15 d	0.3–1.4 mg/L
		16 d–6 mo	0.7–2.9 mg/L
		7 mo–1 yr	0.7–3.7 mg/L
		2–3 yr	0.8–4.4 mg/L
		4–6 yr	1.0–5.7 mg/L
		7–8 yr	1.7–6.7 mg/L
		9–11 yr	2.1–8.2 mg/L
		12–13 yr	2.9–9.2 mg/L
		14–16 yr	3.4–9.7 mg/L
		17–18 yr	3.2–8.8 mg/L
		19–20 yr	2.9–7.4 mg/L
		Male:	
		≤15 d	0.3–1.4 mcg/L
		16 d–6 mo	0.7–2.9 mcg/L
		7 mo–1 yr	0.7–3.7 mcg/L
		2–3 yr	0.8–4.4 mcg/L
		4–6 yr	1.0–5.7 mcg/L
		7–8 yr	1.3–6.4 mcg/L

(continued)

835

Table III.1 Clinical Biochemistry (continued)

Test Name	Specimen Type	Age/Sex	Reference Interval/Units	Comments
		9–11 yr	1.7–8.3 mcg/L	
		12–13 yr	2.5–9.8 mcg/L	
		14–16 yr	3.2–10.4 mcg/L	
		17–18 yr	2.9–8.7 mcg/L	
		19–20 yr	2.8–7.3 mcg/L	
IgA	Blood	<1 yr	≤0.8 g/L	
		1–3 yr	0.2–1.0 g/L	
		4–6 yr	0.3–2.0 g/L	
		7–9 yr	0.3–3.1 g/L	
		10–13 yr	0.5–3.6 g/L	
		≥14 yr	0.5–3.5 g/L	
IgG	Blood	<1 yr	2.3–14.1 g/L	
		1–3 yr	4.5–14.3 g/L	
		4–6 yr	5.0–14.6 g/L	
		7–9 yr	5.7–14.7 g/L	
		10–13 yr	7.0–15.5 g/L	
		≥14 yr	7.2–15.8 g/L	
IgM	Blood	<1 yr	≤1.7 g/L	
		1–3 yr	0.2–1.8 g/L	
		4–6 yr	0.2–2.5 g/L	
		7–9 yr	0.4–2.5 g/L	

		10-13 yr	0.4-2.9 g/L	Reference values may be higher in obese patients; hemolysis and insulin antibodies may lower values
		≥14 yr	0.2-3.1 g/L	
Insulin, plasma	Blood	Fasting		
		<1 yr	<90 pmol/L	
		1-18 yr	<118 pmol/L	
		Stimulation		
		30 min	170-1550 pmol/L	
		1 h	117-1850 pmol/L	
		2 h	108-1120 pmol/L	
		3 h	13-161 pmol/L	
Insulin antibodies, plasma	Blood		<0.4 kU/L	Arrange with clinical biochemist or endocrinologist before blood is collected
Insulin tolerance test	Blood		After stimulation, peak growth hormone should exceed 8 mcg/L	Includes glucose and growth hormone
Intralipid, plasma or serum	Blood		≤0.90 g/L	
Iron, plasma or serum	Blood	<4 mo	20.0-48.0 μmol/L	Hemolysis elevates results
		4-11 mo	5.0-13.0 μmol/L	
		≥1 yr	9.0-27.0 μmol/L	
Islet cell antibodies, serum	Blood		Not detectable	
Ketones, plasma or serum	Blood		Negative	

(continued)

Table III.1   Clinical Biochemistry *(continued)*

Test Name	Specimen Type	Age/ Sex	Reference Interval/Units	Comments
Lactate, plasma	Blood		≤ 2.4 mmol/L	Used in detection of inherited causes of lactic acidemia, acidosis, or sepsis. Delayed separation of serum from RBC and hemolysis both elevate result; transport sample on ice
Lactate dehydrogenase (LDH), plasma or serum	Blood	Female:		Rarely indicated and nonspecific; highest concentrations in heart, liver, skeletal muscle, erythrocytes, kidney; elevated in hemolyzed samples
		<6 d	934–2150 units/L	
		6 d–3 yr	500–920 units/L	
		4–6 yr	470–900 units/L	
		7–9 yr	420–750 units/L	
		10–11 yr	380–770 units/L	
		12–13 yr	380–640 units/L	
		14–15 yr	390–580 units/L	
		16–19 yr	340–670 units/L	
		>19 yr	310–620 units/L	
		Male:		
		<6 d	934–2150 units/L	
		6 d–3 yr	500–920 units/L	
		4–6 yr	470–900 units/L	
		7–9 yr	420–750 units/L	
		10–11 yr	432–700 units/L	
		12–13 yr	470–750 units/L	
		14–15 yr	360–730 units/L	
		16–19 yr	340–670 units/L	
		>19 yr	310–620 units/L	

Lactate dehydrogenase isoenzymes (total), serum	Blood	100-220 units/L	
Lead, blood	Blood	<0.48 µmol/L	Concentration of lead in whole blood 75 × greater than in serum or plasma
Lipase, plasma or serum	Blood	≤60 units/L	Indication: monitoring for toxicity when exogenous IV lipids administered Lipoprotein electrophoresis indication: investigation and classification of hyperlipidemia
Luteinizing hormone (LH), serum	Blood	Female:	Ovulatory values may reach 100 IU/L; values rise through puberty to adult values; LH values >7 IU/L after stimulation suggest onset of puberty
		1-15 d <1.0 IU/L	
		16 d-11 mo 0.1-6.5 IU/L	
		1-10 yr 0.1-4.0 IU/L	
		11-14 yr 0.1-13.0 IU/L	
		15-20 yr 0.4-30.0 IU/L	
		Male:	
		1-15 d <1.0 IU/L	
		16 d-11 mo 0.1-4.8 IU/L	
		1-10 yr 0.1-3.0 IU/L	
		11-14 yr 0.1-8.0 IU/L	
		15-20 yr 0.5-11.0 IU/L	
Magnesium, plasma or serum	Blood	<1 mo 0.75-1.15 mmol/L	
		1 mo-18 yr 0.70-0.95 mmol/L	
		≥19 yr 0.65-1.00 mmol/L	
Magnesium, ionized, blood	Blood	0.54-0.67 mmol/L	

(continued)

Table III.1 Clinical Biochemistry (continued)

Test Name	Specimen Type	Age/Sex	Reference Interval/Units	Comments
Manganese, serum	Blood		0.017–0.053 μmol/L	
Mercury, blood	Blood		<18.1 nmol/L	
Methemoglobin, blood	Blood		≤0.029	
Mitochondrial antibodies, serum	Blood		Not detectable	
Norepinephrine, plasma	Blood		nmol/L	See catecholamines, plasma
Orosomucoid, serum	Blood			See α_1-acid glycoprotein, serum
Osmolality, plasma or serum	Blood	<2 d	275–300 mmol/kg H_2O	
		2–7 d	276–305 mmol/kg H_2O	
		8–28 d	274–305 mmol/kg H_2O	
		≥29 d	282–300 mmol/kg H_2O	
Osteocalcin, serum	Blood	<24 yr	15–35 mcg/L	
Ovarian antibodies, serum	Blood		Positive or negative	

Overnight growth hormone	Blood		After stimulation, peak growth hormone should exceed 8 mcg/L
Oxygen saturation (measured); arterial, mixed venous, venous	Blood		Specimen must be anaerobic
P5N screen, blood	Blood		See pyrimidine 5'-nucleotidase, blood
Parathyroid hormone (PTH), serum (intact PTH)	Blood		9-55 ng/L
Parietal cell antibodies, serum	Blood		Detectable or not detectable
Phenylalanine, blood	Dried blood spot	≤6 d	70-110 µmol/L
		7 d-6 mo	45-65 µmol/L
		7 mo-2 yr	23-69 µmol/L
		3-10 yr	26-61 µmol/L
		11-12 yr	38-116 µmol/L
		≥13 yr	37-115 µmol/L
			For follow-up on diagnosed PKU patients
Phosphate, plasma or serum	Blood	<1 mo	1.62-3.10 mmol/L
		1-3 mo	1.55-2.62 mmol/L
		4-11 mo	1.30-2.20 mmol/L
		1-3 yr	1.16-2.10 mmol/L
		4-8 yr	1.16-1.81 mmol/L
		9-14 yr	1.07-1.71 mmol/L
		≥15 yr	0.87-1.52 mmol/L

(continued)

Table III.1   Clinical Biochemistry (continued)

Test Name	Specimen Type	Age/Sex	Reference Interval/Units	Comments
Porphobilinogen deaminase	Blood		20–43 μmol/L/h	
Potassium, plasma or serum	Blood	<7 d	3.2–5.5 mmol/L	Varies widely, depending on intake; increased by hemolysis in sample
		7–29 d	3.4–6.0 mmol/L	
		1–5 mo	3.5–5.6 mmol/L	
		6–11 mo	3.5–6.0 mmol/L	
		1–15 yr	3.7–5.0 mmol/L	
		16–18 yr	3.7–4.8 mmol/L	
Prolactin, serum	Blood	Birth	Average 194.0 mcg/L	May be very high; falls to about 53.0 mcg/L at 4 wk
		1 yr–puberty	3.0–15.0 mcg/L	
		Adult males	2.5–11.5 mcg/L	
		Adult females	3.0–19.0 mcg/L	
Protein, plasma or serum	Blood	<6 mo	45–75 g/L	Excessively high protein concentrations (> 5 g/L) can occur if spinal canal is blocked
		6 mo–1 yr	54–75 g/L	
		≥2 yr	53–85 g/L	
Protoporphyrin, erythrocytes	Blood		≤550 nmol/L	
Protoporphyrin, plasma	Blood		≤55 nmol/L	

Protoporphyrin, free erythrocyte (FEP)	Blood	<11 yr ≥11 yr	≤0.61 µmol/L ≤1.32 µmol/L	Investigation of severe lead poisoning, congenital erythropoietic porphyria, erythrohepatic protoporphyria; increased FEP occurs in iron deficiency anemia and anemia of chronic disease
Pyruvate, blood	Blood		0.03–0.08 mmol/L	Used in detection of inherited causes of lactic acidemia Lactate must be done at same time; pyruvate only analyzed if lactate is elevated
Renin, plasma	Blood	≤3 mo 3–11 mo 1–3 yr 4–14 yr ≥15 yr	<14.0 mcg/L/s ≤4.20 mcg/L/s ≤2.80 mcg/L/s ≤1.70 mcg/L/s ≤0.56 mcg/L/s	Normal values vary with method of assay, sodium intake, time of day, erect or supine posture, age These ranges assume normal salt intake, 9 A.M., supine, after 1–12 h rest Premature infants will have higher ranges
Selenium, serum	Blood	>6 mo Preterm Full term	1.27–2.09 µmol/L 0.44–1.19 µmol/L 0.72–1.21 µmol/L	
Sodium, plasma or serum	Blood	<1 yr 1–18 yr ≥19 yr	133–142 mmol/L 135–143 mmol/L 135–145 mmol/L	Urinary sodium should be interpreted in relation to serum sodium
Testosterone, free; plasma or serum	Blood	Prepuberty: Female Male Puberty–19 yr: Female Male	1.0–2.0 pmol/L 1.0–2.0 pmol/L 2.0–11.0 pmol/L 36–90 pmol/L	

(continued)

Table III.1 Clinical Biochemistry (continued)

Test Name	Specimen Type	Age/Sex	Reference Interval/Units	Comments
Testosterone, serum	Blood	Female: 1 mo–10 yr 11–14 yr 15–20 yr Male: 1–2 mo 3–4 mo 5 mo–10 yr 11–14 yr 15–20 yr	<0.7 nmol/L <2.1 nmol/L <2.9 nmol/L <16.0 nmol/L <3.1 nmol/L <0.7 nmol/L <20.3 nmol/L <30 nmol/L	
Thyroglobulin, serum	Blood		<53 pmol/L	Following thyroid ablation: <5 pmol/L
Thyroid antibodies, serum	Blood		Positive or negative	See anti-TPO antibodies and antithyroglobulin antibodies
Thyroid-stimulating hormone (TSH)	Blood		0.5–5.0 MU/L	
Thyrotropin-releasing hormone stimulation test	Blood		Normal: rises by at least 5 mU/L to peak of 5–20 mU/L at 20 min; decreases to 2–10 mU/L by 60 min	Measures TSH
Thyroxine, free (free T₄), serum	Blood	≤2 d 3–29 d ≥1 mo	20.0–45.0 pmol/L 18.0–35.0 pmol/L 10.0–23.0 pmol/L	

Thyroxine-binding globulin capacity (TBG)	Blood	≤30 d	129–1158 nmol/L
		1–11 mo	257–978 nmol/L
		1–4 yr	373–695 nmol/L
		5–9 yr	321–643 nmol/L
		10–15 yr	270–592 nmol/L
		≥16 yr	150–360 nmol/L
Transferrin, serum	Blood	<1 yr	16.0–50.0 mmol/L	Acute phase reactant
		1–9 yr	23.0–41.0 mmol/L
		≥10 yr	24.0–48.0 mmol/L
Triglyceride, serum or plasma	Blood	<18 yr	0.40–1.30 mmol/L
Tri-iodothyronine, free (free T₃); serum	Blood		2.2–5.3 pmol/L	Referred out test. Range subject to change.
Tri-iodothyronine, reverse	Blood		0.12–0.54 nmol/L	Referred out test. Range subject to change.
Tri-iodothyronine (total T₃), serum	Blood	Female:	
		<1 yr	1.6–4.4 nmol/L
		1–10 yr	1.8–4.1 nmol/L
		11–14 yr	1.1–4.0 nmol/L
		15–20 yr	0.9–4.0 nmol/L
		Male:	
		<1 yr	2.1–4.2 nmol/L
		1–5 yr	1.7–4.0 nmol/L
		6–10 yr	1.1–4.0 nmol/L
		11–14 yr	1.5–3.7 nmol/L
		15–20 yr	0.8–3.6 nmol/L

(continued)

Table III.1 Clinical Biochemistry (continued)

Test Name	Specimen Type	Age/Sex	Reference Interval/Units	Comments
Urate (uric acid), plasma or serum	Blood	Female Male: <14 yr ≥14 yr	120-360 mmol/L 120-360 mmol/L 180-420 mmol/L	Diet dependent
Urea, plasma or serum	Blood	<1 yr 1 yr ≥2 yr	2.9-10.0 mmol/L 1.8-5.4 mmol/L 2.9-7.1 mmol/L	
Uroporphyrin, plasma	Blood		≤35 nmol/L	
Vitamin A, plasma or serum (retinol)	Blood		0.7-2.1 µmol/L	
Vitamin B₁₂, serum	Blood		Normal: 150-600 pmol/L	
Vitamin C, serum	Blood			See ascorbic acid, serum
Vitamin D, 1,25-hydroxy; plasma or serum	Blood		70-250 nmol/L	
Vitamin D, 25-hydroxy; plasma or serum	Blood		General guidelines: Toxic: > 250 nmol/L Optimal: > 70 nmol/L Adequate: 50-70 nmol/L	Ranges shown apply to summer months; reference range for winter months are slightly lower

			Suboptimal: 35–50 nmol/L Deficient: <35 nmol/L	
Vitamin E, plasma or serum (α-tocopherol)	Blood		12.0–46.0 µmol/L	
Xylose, plasma	Blood		2.2–3.7 mmol/L	For investigation of intestinal absorption of xylose
Zinc, serum	Blood	<30 d	9.9–21.4 µmol/L	
		1–11 mo	9.9–19.9 µmol/L	
		1–4 yr	10.3–18.1 µmol/L	
		5–8 yr	11.8–16.4 µmol/L	
		Female:		
		9–12 yr	12.1–18.0 µmol/L	
		≥13 yr	9.8–20.2 µmol/L	
		Male:		
		9–12 yr	11.6–15.4 µmol/L	
		≥13 yr	9.8–20.2 µmol/L	

Table III.2	Hematology			
Test Name	Specimen Type	Age/ Sex	Reference Interval/Units	Comments
Activated partial thromboplastin time (APTT), plasma	Blood	≤3 mo >3 mo	25–53 s 23–35 s	
Antiphospholipid antibody, plasma	Blood		PNP negative TTI negative RVV negative	Also known as lupus anticoagulant PNP, platelet neutralization procedure; TTI, tissue thromboplastin inhibition; RVV, Russell viper venom
Antithrombin activity (AT III), plasma	Blood	<3 mo ≥3 mo	0.40–1.10 IU/mL 0.85–1.25 IU/mL	
APC resistance, plasma	Blood		3.0–3.9	Interval is ratio of APTT with activated protein C to APTT without activated protein C
Band cell count, blood	Blood		×10⁹/L	See WBC differential
Bleeding time, whole blood	Blood	<1 d 1 d–18 yr >18 yr	0.5–1.5 min 2.0–9.0 min 2.0–8.0 min	
Complete blood cell count (CBC)	Blood	**Hemoglobin, blood** ≤6 d 7–30 d 1 mo 2 mo 3–11 mo 1–4 yr 5–13 yr Female: ≥14 yr Male: ≥14 yr **Hematocrit** ≤6 d 7–30 d 1 mo 2 mo 3–11 mo 1–4 yr 5–13 yr	150–220 g/L 140–200 g/L 115–180 g/L 90–135 g/L 100–140 g/L 110–140 g/L 120–160 g/L 120–153 g/L 140–175 g/L 0.460–0.700 0.400–0.650 0.350–0.540 0.270–0.400 0.300–0.420 0.350–0.420 0.360–0.480	Test includes WBC, RBC, Hb, Hct, MCV, MCH, MCH concentration (MCHC), platelet count (PLT), and mean platelet volume (MPV) See WBC differential, blood

(continued)

Table III.2	Hematology *(continued)*			
Test Name	**Specimen Type**	**Age/ Sex**	**Reference Interval/Units**	**Comments**
		Female:		
		≥14 yr	0.360–0.450	
		Male:		
		≥14 yr	0.420–0.500	
		Mean cell hemoglobin		
		<3 mo	24.0–34.0 pg	
		≥3 mo	24.0–31.0 pg	
		Mean cell hemoglobin concentration		
			320–360 g/L	
		Mean cell volume		
		≤6 d	110.0–130.0 fL	
		7–13 d	105.0–113.0 fL	
		14–30 d	97.0–113.0 fL	
		1 mo	87.0–113.0 fL	
		2 mo	80.0–96.0 fL	
		3–11 mo	73.0–85.0 fL	
		≥1 yr	80.0–94.0 fL	
		Mean platelet volume		
			4.0–14.0 fL	
		Platelet cell count		
			$150\text{--}400 \times 10^9/\text{L}$	
		Red blood cell count		
		≤30 d	$3.50\text{--}6.00 \times 10^{12}/\text{L}$	
		1–2 mo	$3.50\text{--}5.50 \times 10^{12}/\text{L}$	
		3–11 mo	$3.50\text{--}5.00 \times 10^{12}/\text{L}$	
		1–4 yr	$4.00\text{--}5.00 \times 10^{12}/\text{L}$	
		5–13 yr	$4.50\text{--}5.50 \times 10^{12}/\text{L}$	
		Female:		
		≥14 yr	$4.10\text{--}5.10 \times 10^{12}/\text{L}$	
		Male:		
		≥14 yr	$4.50\text{--}5.70 \times 10^{12}/\text{L}$	
		White blood cell (leukocyte) count		
		≤6 d	$9.0\text{--}30.0 \times 10^9/\text{L}$	See WBC differential
		7–13 d	$5.0\text{--}21.0 \times 10^9/\text{L}$	
		14 d–2 mo	$5.0\text{--}20.0 \times 10^9/\text{L}$	
		3–11 mo	$5.0\text{--}15.0 \times 10^9/\text{L}$	
		1–4 yr	$5.0\text{--}12.0 \times 10^9/\text{L}$	
		≥5 yr	$4.0\text{--}10.0 \times 10^9/\text{L}$	
D-Dimer, plasma	Blood		≤449 ng/mL	Replaces fibrin degradation products

(continued)

Table III.2	Hematology (continued)			
Test Name	**Specimen Type**	**Age/ Sex**	**Reference Interval/Units**	**Comments**
2,3-Diphospho-glycerate, erythrocytes	Blood		1.6–2.6 µmol/mL	
Erythrocyte sedimentation rate (ESR), whole blood	Blood		1–10 mm/h	
Euglobulin clot lysis	Blood		>120 min	
Factor II activity, plasma	Blood	≤3 mo ≥3 mo–18 yr	0.25–1.10 units/mL 0.50–1.50 units/mL	Hematology consultation is advised
Factor V activity, plasma	Blood	≤3 mo ≥3 mo	0.35–1.30 IU/mL 0.70–1.34 IU/mL	Hematology consultation is advised
Factor VII activity, plasma	Blood	≤3 mo ≥3 mo	0.25–1.30 IU/mL 0.79–1.66 IU/mL	Hematology consultation is advised
Factor VIII activity, plasma	Blood	>3 mo	0.79–1.99 IU/mL	Hematology consultation is advised
Factor IX activity, plasma	Blood	≤3 mo ≥3 mo	0.15–1.30 IU/mL 0.79–1.59 IU/mL	Hematology consultation is advised
Factor X activity, plasma	Blood	≤3 mo ≥3 mo–18 yr	0.10–1.10 IU/mL 0.50–1.50 IU/mL	Hematology consultation is advised
Factor XI activity, plasma	Blood	≤3 mo ≥3 mo–18 yr	0.10–1.00 IU/mL 0.50–1.50 IU/mL	Hematology consultation is advised
Factor XII activity, plasma	Blood	≤3 mo ≥3 mo–18 yr	0.10–1.10 IU/mL 0.50–1.50 IU/mL	Hematology consultation is advised
Factor XIII screen, plasma	Blood		Wild type/mutant type	Hematology consultation is advised
Factor XIII immunologic testing	Blood		Wild type/mutant type	Hematology consultation is advised
Factor inhibitor quantitation	Blood		<0.5 BU	Hematology consultation is advised
Factor inhibitor screen	Blood		Positive or negative	
Fibrinogen, plasma	Blood		1.60–4.00 g/L	This test may be done with INR and PTT on 3-mL sample

(continued)

Table III.2   Hematology *(continued)*

Test Name	Specimen Type	Age/ Sex	Reference Interval/Units	Comments
Folate, erythrocytes	Blood		421–1462 nmol/L	
Folate, serum	Blood		7.0–28.1 nmol/L	
Glucose-6-phosphate dehydrogenase (G6PD), erythrocytes	Blood	≤1 mo ≥2 mo	7.0–13.0 units/g 5.0–11.0 units/g	
Granulocyte antibodies	Blood			See white blood cell antibodies
Heinz body preparation, blood	Blood		Positive or negative	
Hematocrit (Hct), blood	Blood			See complete blood cell count (CBC)
Hemoglobin (Hb), blood	Blood			See complete blood cell count (CBC)
Hemoglobin A, blood	Blood	<1 d 1–27 d 28 d–1 mo 2–3 mo 4–5 mo 6–11 mo ≥1 yr	8.2–28.5% 3.7–45.4% 11.8–81.0% 35.6–98.3% 84.4–98.3% 94.4–98.3% 95.7–98.3%	See hemoglobin analysis, blood
Hemoglobin A$_{1c}$, blood	Blood		0.040–0.060	Mix well Abnormal or variant hemoglobins and hemoglobin F may give falsely elevated levels
Hemoglobin A$_2$, blood	Blood	<1 d 1–27 d 28 d–1 mo 2–3 mo 4–5 mo >6 mo	0% ≤0.7% ≤1.6% ≤2.6% 1.5–2.6% 1.5–3.5%	
Hemoglobin analysis, blood	Blood			Replaces Hb electrophoresis Tests for HbF, HbA$_2$, HbS, HbC, HbD, HbE, HbH, Hb Bart's CBC required See hemoglobin A$_2$, blood; hemoglobin A, blood; and hemoglobin F, blood

(continued)

Table III.2	Hematology *(continued)*			
Test Name	Specimen Type	Age/ Sex	Reference Interval/Units	Comments
Hemoglobin F, blood	Blood	<1 d 1–27 d 28 d–1 mo 2–3 mo 4–5 mo 6–11 mo 12–17 mo 18–23 mo 2 yr 3 yr 4–12 yr ≥13 yr	71.5–91.8% 54.6–96.3% 19.0–88.2% 0.1–64.4% 0.1–4.1% 0.1–4.1% 0.1–2.9% 0.1–2.6% 0.1–1.9% 0.1–1.8% 0.1–1.3% 0.1–1.1%	See hemoglobin analysis, blood
Hemoglobin S, screen, blood	Blood		Positive or negative	For >6 mo only; if <6 mo, order hemoglobin analysis See hemoglobin analysis, blood
Heparin, low molecular weight; plasma	Blood		0.05–1.00 IU/mL	
Heparin, standard; plasma	Blood		0.35–0.70 IU/mL	
Heparin-induced thrombocytopenia	Blood		Positive or negative	
Inhibitor screen, plasma	Blood		Positive or negative	
International normalized ratio (INR), plasma	Blood	<3 mo ≥3 mo–18 yr	0.90–1.60 0.90–1.10	
Isopropanol precipitation test	Blood		Positive or negative	For unstable hemoglobin
Kleihauer test	Blood		Positive or negative	To detect fetal cells or HbF-containing cells Maternal blood is needed if test is for the detection of fetomaternal bleeding
LE preparation	Blood		Positive or negative	For systemic lupus erythematosus; gently swirl specimen 5 min to defibrinate Use glass vial containing beads

(continued)

Table III.2   Hematology *(continued)*

Test Name	Specimen Type	Age/ Sex	Reference Interval/Units	Comments
Leukemia immuno-phenotyping, bone marrow	Bone marrow		Positive or negative	
Leukemia immuno-phenotyping, peripheral blood	Blood		Positive or negative	
Leukocyte count, blood	Blood			See complete white blood cell count (CBC), blood
Lymphocyte count	Blood			See white blood cell (WBC) differential, blood
Lymphocytes, atypical, count	Blood		$\times 10^9$/L	See white blood cell (WBC) differential, blood
Malarial smear, blood	Blood			Initial result (within 2 h) is for presence or absence of malaria from thin smear. Thick smear and speciation performed at Provincial Health laboratory or comparable authority within North America
Mean cell hemoglobin (MCH), blood	Blood	<3 mo ≥3 mo	24.0–34.0 pg 24.0–31.0 pg	See complete blood cell count (CBC), blood
Mean cell hemoglobin concentration (MCHC), blood	Blood		320–360 g/L	See complete blood cell count (CBC), blood
Mean cell volume (MCV), blood	Blood			See complete blood cell count (CBC), blood
Mean platelet volume (MPV), blood	Blood			See complete blood cell count (CBC), blood
Metamyelocyte cell count, monocyte cell count, myelocyte cell count, neutrophil cell count, blood	Blood		$\times 10^9$/L	See white blood cell (WBC) differential, blood
Neutrophil oxidative burst index (NOBI)	Blood		32–300 ratio	Screens for chronic granulomatous disease. WBC count and differential required

(continued)

Table III.2	Hematology (continued)			
Test Name	**Specimen Type**	**Age/ Sex**	**Reference Interval/Units**	**Comments**
Nucleated cell count	Blood		/100 WBC	See white blood cell (WBC) differential, blood (nucleated cells)
Partial thrombo- plastin time (PTT)	Blood			See activated partial thromboplastin time
Platelet aggregation	Blood		ADP: 46–94% COLL: 65–109% EPIN: 54–114% RIS-1.5: 69–113% RIS-0.5: <15% AA: >50%	Hematology consultation is advised ADP, adenosine diphosphate; COLL, collagen; EPIN, epi- nephrine; RIS, ristocetin; AA, arachidonic acid
Platelet antibodies	Blood			See white blood cell (WBC) antibodies
Platelet cell count, blood	Blood			See complete blood cell count (CBC), blood
Protein C activity, plasma	Blood	<3 mo ≥3 mo	0.17–0.80 IU/mL 0.55–1.30 IU/mL	
Protein S antigen, plasma	Blood	Female: <3 mo >3 mo Male: <3 mo >3 mo	0.10–1.20 IU/mL 0.50–1.30 IU/mL 0.10–1.20 IU/mL 0.69–1.49 IU/mL	
Prothrombin time (PT), plasma	Blood			See international normalized ratio
Pyruvate kinase (PK), erythrocytes	Blood	≤1 mo ≥1 mo	13.0–21.1 units/g 11.1–18.9 units/g	
Red blood cell count (RBC), blood	Blood			See complete blood cell count (CBC), blood
Reptilase time, plasma	Blood		16–22 s	
Reticulocyte cell count, blood	Blood	<2 d 2–6 d 7–29 d 1 mo 2 mo 3–5 mo ≥6 mo	$200–300 \times 10^9$/L $15.0–250.0 \times 10^9$/L $5.0–50.0 \times 10^9$/L $5.0–100.0 \times 10^9$/L $5.0–150.0 \times 10^9$/L $5.0–250.0 \times 10^9$/L $10.0–100.0 \times 10^9$/L	
Ristocetin cofactor, plasma	Blood	Blood group O Non–blood group O	0.42–1.50 IU/mL 0.51–1.50 IU/mL	

(continued)

| Table III.2 | Hematology *(continued)* |

Test Name	Specimen Type	Age/ Sex	Reference Interval/Units	Comments
Thrombin time, plasma	Blood		20–25 s	
von Willebrand factor antigen, plasma	Blood	Blood group O Non–blood group O	0.37–1.50 IU/mL 0.50–1.50 IU/L	
White blood cell (WBC) differential	Blood	**Neutrophil count**		Also reported when applicable:
		≤6 d	$6.0–26.0 \times 10^9$/L	· Blast cell count;
		7–13 d	$1.5–10.0 \times 10^9$/L	metamyelocyte cell count;
		14 d–2 mo	$1.0–9.5 \times 10^9$/L	promyelocyte cell count;
		3–11 mo	$1.5–8.5 \times 10^9$/L	atypical lymphocyte
		1–4 yr	$1.5–8.5 \times 10^9$/L	count
		5–9 yr	$1.5–8.0 \times 10^9$/L	($\times 10^9$/L)
		≥10 yr	$2.0–7.5 \times 10^9$/L	
		Band cell count		· Nucleated cell count
		≤6 d	$\leq 4.50 \times 10^9$/L	(/100 WBC)
		7–13 d	$\leq 0.80 \times 10^9$/L	
		≥14 d	$\leq 0.01 \times 10^9$/L	
		Lymphocyte count		
		<6 d	$2.00–11.00 \times 10^9$/L	
		7 d–2 mo	$2.00–17.00 \times 10^9$/L	
		3–11 mo	$4.00–10.50 \times 10^9$/L	
		1–4 yr	$2.00–8.00 \times 10^9$/L	
		5–13 yr	$1.50–7.00 \times 10^9$/L	
		≥14 yr	$1.50–4.00 \times 10^9$/L	
		Monocyte cell count		
		≤6 d	$0.40–3.10 \times 10^9$/L	
		7–14 d	$0.30–2.70 \times 10^9$/L	
		14 d–2 mo	$0.20–2.40 \times 10^9$/L	
		3–11 mo	$0.05–1.10 \times 10^9$/L	
		>1 yr	$0.05–0.80 \times 10^9$/L	
		Eosinophil count		
		≤6 d	$0.02–0.85 \times 10^9$/L	
		7–13 d	$0.07–1.00 \times 10^9$/L	
		14 d–2 mo	$0.07–1.00 \times 10^9$/L	
		3–11 mo	$0.05–0.70 \times 10^9$/L	
		>1 yr	$0.02–0.50 \times 10^9$/L	
		Basophil count		
		≤6 d	$\leq 0.60 \times 10^9$/L	
		>7 d	$\leq 0.20 \times 10^9$/L	
White blood cell (WBC) antibodies	Blood		Positive/negative	Includes granulocyte, platelet, and HLA antibodies

Test Name	Specimen Type	Reference Interval/Units	Comments
Table III.3		**Toxicology**	
Acetaminophen (Tylenol), plasma	Blood	Not detected	Refer to Rumak-Matthew nomogram for toxicity levels In overdose situation, draw sample anytime
Barbiturates/ sedative screen, serum	Blood	Not detected or µmol/L **Toxic ranges** Amobarbital >40 µmol/L Barbital >320 µmol/L Butabarbital >45 µmol/L Butalbital >45 µmol/L Glutethimide >45 µmol/L Meprobamate >450 µmol/L Methaqualone >20 µmol/L Methyprylon >160 µmol/L Pentobarbital >40 µmol/L Phenobarbital >170 µmol/L Secobarbital >30 µmol/L	Includes barbital, butabarbital (Butisol), butalbital (Fiorinal), amobarbital (Amytal), pentobarbital (Nembutal), secobarbital (Seconal), phenobarbital, methyprylon (Noludar), meprobamate (Miltown), glutethimide (Doriden), methaqualone (Quaalude)
Benzodiazepine screen, serum	Blood	Not detected or positive	Screening test only for benzodiazepine class of drugs
Benzodiazepine screen, urine	Urine	Not detected or positive	Random urine
Drug screen, serum	Blood		5 mL clotted blood Quantitative testing for 1. Volatiles (ethanol, methanol, isopropanol, acetone) 2. Ethylene glycol and propylene glycol 3. Barbiturates and some sedatives (barbital, butabarbital, butalbital, amobarbital, pentobarbital, secobarbital, phenobarbital, methyprylon, methaqualone, glutethimide, meprobamate)

(continued)

Table III.3 Toxicology *(continued)*

Test Name	Specimen Type	Reference Interval/Units	Comments
			Qualitative screening for 1. Benzodiazepines 2. Tricyclic antidepressants (nonspecific) Special tests for 1. Trichlorethanol (metabolite of chloral hydrate) 2. Lithium 3. Ibuprofen 4. Salicylate 5. Acetaminophen 6. Formic acid
Drug screen, urine	Random urine		Useful for detecting drugs in overdose situations, suicide intent, accidental poisoning, and for street drugs See Box III.1, p. 873
Ethylene glycol, plasma or serum	Blood	Not detected; mmol/L >4.8 mmol/L Toxic	
Formic acid	Blood	Toxic >3.3 mmol/L	Toxic metabolite of methanol
γ-Hydroxybutyrate (GHB), serum	Blood	Not detected or positive	Classified as one of the "date rape" drugs
Glutethimide	Blood	Not detected or μmol/L	See barbiturates/sedative screen, serum
Ibuprofen, serum	Blood	Not detected or mg/L	
Isopropanol, blood	Blood	Not detected or mmol/L >6.7 mmol/L Toxic	See volatile screen, plasma or serum
Meprobamate, plasma or serum	Blood	Not detected, or μmol/L	See barbiturates/sedative screen, serum
Methanol, blood	Blood	Not detected or mmol/L >6.2 mmol/L Toxic	
Pentobarbital, plasma or serum	Blood	Not detected or μmol/L	See barbiturates/sedative screen, serum
Phenobarbital, serum	Blood	Therapeutic: 65–70 μmol/L Alert: >170 μmol/L Critical: >225 μmol/L	Trough 0–60 min before next dose

(continued)

Table III.3 — Toxicology (continued)

Test Name	Specimen Type	Reference Interval/Units	Comments
Salicylate (ASA, aspirin), plasma or serum	Blood	Not detected or mmol/L	Draw sample 0–60 min before next dose: in overdose, draw sample anytime Done nomogram can be used to predict severity of intoxication (see Figure 4.1, p. 67)
Thiocyanate, serum	Blood	Not detected or mmol/L	
Trichloroethanol (TCE), plasma or serum	Blood	Therapeutic: 1.5–15.0 mg/L Toxic: >40 mg/L	
Tricyclic screen, plasma or serum	Blood	Not detected or positive	False positives may be caused by other drugs, (e.g., phenothiazines, carbamazepine, cyclobenzaprine) Urine is required to identify which tricyclic drug may be present
Volatile screen, serum	Blood	Not detected or mmol/L	Includes ethanol, methanol (wood alcohol, windshield washer fluid), isopropanol (rubbing alcohol), acetone

THERAPEUTIC DRUG MONITORING

Table III.4 — Therapeutic Drug Monitoring

Test Name	Specimen Type	Reference Interval/Units	Comments
Amikacin, serum or plasma	Blood	Trough: 2.5–10.0 mg/L Peak: 20.0–35.0 mg/L	
Busulfan, plasma	Blood	Protocol dependent, µmol/L	
Caffeine, serum	Blood	Trough: 30–100 µmol/L Critical: >120 µmol/L	
Carbamazepine, serum or plasma	Blood	Trough: 17–50 µmol/L Critical: >63 µmol/L	Tegretol
Carbamazepine epoxide, serum or plasma	Blood	Trough: 5.0–12.0 µmol/L	

(continued)

Table III.4   Therapeutic Drug Monitoring *(continued)*

Test Name	Specimen Type	Reference Interval/Units	Comments
Cyclosporine, whole blood	Blood	*Transplant:* Liver: 92-425 mcg/L Renal: 92-235 mcg/L Heart: 50-300 mcg/L BMT (related): 100-150 mcg/L BMT (unrelated): 150-200 mcg/L	Trough
Chloramphenicol, serum or plasma	Blood	Trough: 2.0-10.0 mg/L Peak: 15.0-25.0 mg/L	
Digoxin, serum or plasma	Blood	Trough: 1.0-2.5 nmol/L Critical: >3.5 nmol/L	
Digoxin, free; serum or plasma	Blood	Trough: 0.8-2.0 nmol/L	
Ethosuximide, serum or plasma	Blood	Trough: 280-710 µmol/L	Zarontin
Gentamicin, serum or plasma	Blood	Trough: 0.6-2.0 mg/L Peak: 5.0-10.0 mg/L	
Lamotrigine, serum or plasma	Blood	Trough: 4.0-39.0 µmol/L	
Methotrexate, serum or plasma	Blood	Protocol dependent, µmol/L	
Phenobarbital, serum or plasma	Blood	Trough: 65-170 µmol/L Critical: >225 µmol/L	
Phenytoin, serum or plasma	Blood	Trough: 40-80 µmol/L Critical: >85 µmol/L	
Phenytoin, free; serum or plasma	Blood	Trough: 4.0-8.0 µmol/L	
Primidone, serum or plasma	Blood	Trough: 23-55 µmol/L	Mysoline
Sirolimus, whole blood	Blood	Trough: 5.0-15.0 mcg/L	Rapamycin
Tacrolimus, whole blood	Blood	Trough: 5.0-15.0 mcg/L	FK506
Theophylline, serum or plasma	Blood	Trough: 55-110 µmol/L Critical: >110 µmol/L	
Thiopental, serum or plasma	Blood	Trough: 80-120 µmol/L	

(continued)

Table III.4 — Therapeutic Drug Monitoring (continued)

Test Name	Specimen Type	Reference Interval/Units	Comments
Thiopurine metabolites, whole blood	Blood	6-TG: 235–450 pmol/8 × 10^8 RBC 6-MMP: <5700 pmol/8 × 10^8 RBC	
Tobramycin, serum or plasma	Blood	Trough: 0.6–2.0 mg/L Peak: 5.0–10.0 mg/L	
Valproic acid, serum or plasma	Blood	Trough: 350–700 µmol/L Critical: >1400 µmol/L	Depakene
Vancomycin, serum or plasma	Blood	Trough: 5.0–12.0 mg/L Peak: 25.0–40.0 mg/L	

CEREBROSPINAL FLUID

Table III.5 — Cerebrospinal Fluid

Test Name	Age/Sex	Reference Interval/Units	Comments
Cell count, CSF	≤1 mo	Neutrophils: 0 Lymphocytes: ≤11 × 10^6/L	Includes WBC, RBC, and WBC differential if WBC >10 × 10^6/L Bacterial meningitis: neutrophils usually 100–10,000 × 10^6/L (but may be normal), lymphocytes usually <100 × 10^6/L
	≥1 mo	Neutrophils: 0 Lymphocytes: ≤5 × 10^6/L	Viral meningitis: neutrophils usually <100 × 10^6/L, lymphocytes 10–1000 × 10^6/L (but may be normal)
Glucose, CSF		2.1–3.6 mmol/L	Bacterial meningitis: usually <0.4 mmol/L Viral meningitis: usually normal
IgG/albumin ratio, CSF		IgG: 0.005–0.060 g/L Albumin: 0.134–0.237 g/L IgG/albumin ratio: <0.25	
Immunoglobulin G (IgG), CSF		<0.08 g/L	
Lactate, CSF		≤2.4 mmol/L	
Protein, CSF	<8 d 8–30 d ≥1 mo	0.40–1.20 g/L 0.20–0.70 g/L 0.15–0.40 g/L	Bacterial meningitis: usually >1.0 (but may be normal); viral meningitis: usually 0.4–1.0 (but may be normal)

Table III.6	Feces			
Test Name	Specimen Type	Age/ Sex	Reference Interval/Units	Comments
α_1-Antitrypsin clearance, feces and serum	Feces and blood		<22 mL/d	
APT test	Feces, gastric aspirate, vomit		Presence of fetal or maternal cells	Must be bright red blood if present (fetal or maternal RBCs)
Coproporphyrin, feces	Feces		<10 µmol/kg	Referred out test; range subject to change
Eosinophil, fecal smear	Feces			Random collection
Fat, feces	Feces	Premature infants Term infants >3 mo	(Fraction of intake) <0.20 <0.15 <0.10	3- or 5-d stool collection required; accurate account of dietary fat necessary during period of stool collection; regular fat study measures only amount of long chain fatty acids in stool
Hemoglobin, feces	Feces		Positive or negative	Qualitative study; detected when there are 4 mL whole blood per 100 g feces (i.e., 6 mg Hb/g feces)
Occult blood, feces	Feces			See hemoglobin, feces
Uroporphyrin, feces	Feces		≤1.2 µmol/kg	See porphyrins—in urine and blood only Referred out test; range subject to change

Laboratory Reference Values

III

URINE

Table III.7 Urine

Test Name	Age/ Sex	Reference Interval/Units		Comments
Albumin, urine				See microalbumin, urine
Aldosterone, urine		**Na⁺ intake (mmol/d)**	**Aldosterone**	Normal salt diet is <25 mmol/d Na⁺
		<25	47-122	Referred out test; range subject to change
		100-200	16-69	
		>200	0-16	
Amino acids, quantitative, urine				
Alanine	<3 d	9-45 mmol/mol creatinine		Random or timed collection; keep specimen cool; order
	3 d-1 yr	95-668 mmol/mol creatinine		qualitative urine amino acid screen unless diagnosis known
	1-13 yr	14-194 mmol/mol creatinine		
	≥13 yr	<28 mmol/mol creatinine		
Alloisoleucine		Not detected		
Arginine	<3 d	1-9 mmol/mol creatinine		
	3 d-1 yr	1-20 mmol/mol creatinine		
	1-13 yr	1-72 mmol/mol creatinine		
	≥13 yr	1-2 mmol/mol creatinine		
Aspartate	<3 d	1-11 mmol/mol creatinine		
	3 d-1 yr	1-11 mmol/mol creatinine		
	1-13 yr	5-26 mmol/mol creatinine		
	≥13 yr	1-6 mmol/mol creatinine		

Citrulline	<3 d	1-23 mmol/mol creatinine
	3 d-1 yr	1-23 mmol/mol creatinine
	1-13 yr	1-3 mmol/mol creatinine
	≥13 yr	1-3 mmol/mol creatinine
Cystine	<3 d	5-59 mmol/mol creatinine
	3 d-1 yr	1-80 mmol/mol creatinine
	1-13 yr	2-23 mmol/mol creatinine
	≥13 yr	1-14 mmol/mol creatinine
Glutamate	<3 d	1-16 mmol/mol creatinine
	3 d-1 yr	1-468 mmol/mol creatinine
	1-13 yr	1-468 mmol/mol creatinine
	≥13 yr	1-4 mmol/mol creatinine
Glutamine	<3 d	18-314 mmol/mol creatinine
Glycine	3 d-1 yr	254-2341 mmol/mol creatinine
	1-13 yr	46-761 mmol/mol creatinine
	≥13 yr	1-205 mmol/mol creatinine
Histidine	<3 d	1-47 mmol/mol creatinine
	3 d-1 yr	46-801 mmol/mol creatinine
	1-13 yr	53-413 mmol/mol creatinine
	≥13 yr	1-120 mmol/mol creatinine

(continued)

Table III.7   Urine *(continued)*

Test Name	Age/ Sex	Reference Interval/Units	Comments
Amino acids, quantitative, urine *(continued)*			
Homocystine		Not detected	
Isoleucine	<3 d	1-29 mmol/mol creatinine	
	3 d-1 yr	1-28 mmol/mol creatinine	
	1-13 yr	1-6 mmol/mol creatinine	
	≥13 yr	1-4 mmol/mol creatinine	
Leucine	<3 d	1-11 mmol/mol creatinine	
	3 d-1 yr	1-19 mmol/mol creatinine	
	1-13 yr	5-29 mmol/mol creatinine	
	≥13 yr	1-6 mmol/mol creatinine	
Lysine	<3 d	14-72 mmol/mol creatinine	
	3 d-1 yr	1-499 mmol/mol creatinine	
	1-13 yr	8-143 mmol/mol creatinine	
	≥13 yr	1-43 mmol/mol creatinine	
Methionine	<3 d	1-5 mmol/mol creatinine	
	3 d-1 yr	1-32 mmol/mol creatinine	
	1-13 yr	1-23 mmol/mol creatinine	
	>13 yr	1-6 mmol/mol creatinine	

Ornithine	<3 d	1-2 mmol/mol creatinine
	3 d-1 yr	1-54 mmol/mol creatinine
	1-13 yr	4-38 mmol/mol creatinine
	≥13 yr	1-2 mmol/mol creatinine
Phenylalanine	<3 d	1-7 mmol/mol creatinine
	3 d-1 yr	1-151 mmol/mol creatinine
	1-13 yr	4-59 mmol/mol creatinine
	≥13 yr	1-7 mmol/mol creatinine
Phosphoethanolamine	1-13 yr	4-34 mmol/mol creatinine
	≥13 yr	5-16 mmol/mol creatinine
Proline	<3 d	<25 mmol/mol creatinine
	3 d-1 yr	<466 mmol/mol creatinine
	1-13 yr	Not detected
	≥13 yr	Not detected
Serine	<3 d	1-99 mmol/mol creatinine
	3 d-1 yr	124-185 mmol/mol creatinine
	1-13 yr	20-219 mmol/mol creatinine
	≥13 yr	1-53 mmol/mol creatinine

(continued)

Table III.7 Urine (continued)

Test Name	Age/Sex	Reference Interval/Units	Comments
Amino acids, quantitative, urine (continued)			
Threonine	<3 d	11-38 mmol/mol creatinine	
	3 d-1 yr	1-279 mmol/mol creatinine	
	1-13 yr	6-110 mmol/mol creatinine	
	≥13 yr	1-31 mmol/mol creatinine	
Tyrosine	<3 d	1-7 mmol/mol creatinine	
	3 d-1 yr	1-200 mmol/mol creatinine	
	1-13 yr	9-65 mmol/mol creatinine	
	≥13 yr	1-15 mmol/mol creatinine	
Valine	<3 d	5-32 mmol/mol creatinine	
	3 d-1 yr	1-45 mmol/mol creatinine	
	1-13 yr	1-27 mmol/mol creatinine	
	≥13 yr	1-7 mmol/mol creatinine	
Barbiturates screen			See drug screen, urine
β₂-Microglobulin		<14 nmol/L	
Calcium		Random <0.1 mmol/L/kg/d	
Catecholamines, free		**Norepinephrine**	Values represent 95th percentile (100th centile in parentheses)
	<2 yr	280 (375) μmol/mol creatinine	Drugs such as methyldopa, hydralazine (Apresoline), quinidine, and
	2-4 yr	80 (150) μmol/mol creatinine	epinephrine, norepinephrine-related drugs (e.g., L-dopa), and renal

	5-9 yr	60 (90) μmol/mol creatinine	function test dyes may interfere with catecholamine excretion and affect results; sample not acceptable if urine pH >3.0
	10-19 yr	55 (60) μmol/mol creatinine	
	Adult	76 (90) μmol/mol creatinine	
	Epinephrine		
	<2 yr	45 (150) μmol/mol creatinine	
	2-4 yr	35 (60) μmol/mol creatinine	
	5-9 yr	20 (40) μmol/mol creatinine	
	10-19 yr	20 (70) μmol/mol creatinine	
	Adult	14 (50) μmol/mol creatinine	
	Dopamine		
	<2 yr	2220 (3480) μmol/mol creatinine	
	2-4 yr	1130 (2230) μmol/mol creatinine	
	5-9 yr	770 (990) μmol/mol creatinine	
	10-19 yr	400 (510) μmol/mol creatinine	
	Adult	400 (580) μmol/mol creatinine	
Coproporphyrin, quantitative, urine			See porphyrins, quantitative, urine
Cortisol, free, urine	4 mo-10 yr	≤380 nmol/d	
	11-20 yr	≤73 nmol/d	
	≥21 yr	≤151 nmol/d	
		50-220 nmol/d	
Creatinine, urine		Reference value not applicable	Random, timed, or 24-h collection
			Specify specimen collection period
Creatinine clearance, urine	≤7 d	0.25-1.20 mL/s/1.73 m²	See metabolic study, urine
	8-30 d	0.80-1.20 mL/s/1.73 m²	24 h collection required
	1-5 mo	1.00-1.80 mL/s/1.73 m²	
	≥6 mo	1.30-2.40 mL/s/1.73 m²	

(continued)

Table III.7 Urine (continued)

Test Name	Age/Sex	Reference Interval/Units	Comments
Dopamine			See catecholamines, urine
Drug screen		Not detected or positive	Broad-spectrum qualitative screening for many drugs: see Box III.1, p. 873 Immunoassays: · Used to screen for a specific class of drugs (i.e., not the individual drugs) · Used to identify drugs not identified on the broad-spectrum drug screen: 1. Barbiturates 2. Benzodiazepines 3. Opiates 4. Cocaine metabolite 5. Cannabinoid metabolite (tetrahydrocannabinol [THC]) Date rape drugs (sensitive benzodiazepine screen): 1. Screen for γ-hydroxybutyrate (GHB) 2. Screen for flunitrazepam (Rohypnol)
Eosinophil		Positive	Random collection
Hexanoylglycine		≤1.69 μmol/mol creatinine	
Homovanillic acid (HVA)	≤1 yr 2–4 yr 5–9 yr 10–19 yr	≤20.0 (48.0) mmol/mol creatinine ≤14.0 (37.0) mmol/mol creatinine ≤9.0 (21.0) mmol/mol creatinine ≤8.0 (27.0) mmol/mol creatinine	Values represent 95th percentile (100th centile in parentheses)
Human chorionic gonadotropin screen, urine (β-HCG screen)		Positive or negative	

17-Hydroxycorticosteroids	Male	10–30 µmol/d	Urinary steroid measurements superseded by more specific and sensitive serum steroid assays
	Female:	5–25 µmol/d	
	<1 yr	<5.5 µmol/d	
	1–2 yr	1.4–6.9 µmol/d	
	2–4 yr	2.8–11.9 µmol/d	
	4–6 yr	2.8–13.2 µmol/d	
	6–8 yr	2.8–15.5 µmol/d	
	8–10 yr	2.8–19.3 µmol/d	
	>10 yr	4.1–22.1 µmol/d	
5-Hydroxyindoleacetic acid		≤50 µmol/d	
Iron		<5.0 µmol/d	
Ketones		mmol/L	Normally negative
17-Ketosteroids	0–4 yr	<7 µmol/d	Referred out test; range subject to change
	5–9 yr	<21 µmol/d	
	Female >10 yr	17–52 µmol/d	
	Male >10 yr	42–70 µmol/d	
Mercury		<20.0 nmol/d	
		≤5 µmol/mol creatinine	
Metanephrines	1 yr	≤2.8 mmol/mol creatinine	
	2–8 yr	≤1.9 mmol/mol creatinine	
	9–14 yr	≤1.2 mmol/mol creatinine	
	≥15 yr	≤0.6 mmol/mol creatinine	

(continued)

Table III.7 Urine (continued)

Test Name	Age/Sex	Reference Interval/Units	Comments
Microalbumin		<20 mg/d ≤15.1 mcg/min	
Mucopolysaccharides screen		Normally not detectable	Normal result does not rule out all mucopolysaccharidoses
Myoglobin		Normally not detectable	Reacts like hemoglobin on dipstick; confirmatory tests available
Nickel		<85.1 nmol/d	
Oligosaccharides screen		Positive or negative	
Organic acids screen		Positive or negative	
Orotic acid	<15 d 15 d–11 mo 1–9 yr ≥10 yr	1.4–5.3 mmol/mol creatinine 1.0–3.2 mmol/mol creatinine 0.5–3.3 mmol/mol creatinine 0.4–1.2 mmol/mol creatinine	
Osmolality	24 h, average fluid intake Random urine depending on fluid intake	300–900 mmol/kg H_2O 50–1200 mmol/kg H_2O	

Oxalate	Children 0–16 yr	140–420 μmol/d	Timed collection
	Female >16 yr	40–320 μmol/d	Random collection: Nephrology patients only
	Male >16 yr	80–490 μmol/d	Referred out test; range subject to change
	Random	No reference ranges; μmol/L	
pH		5–9	
Phenylpropionylglycine		1.00–1.01 μmol/mol creatinine	
Porphobilinogen, quantitative		μmol/d	
Porphobilinogen screen		Negative	
Porphyrins, quantitative			Quantitation of coproporphyrin and protoporphyrin; screening tests are of value only during acute attack of porphyria; urine porphobilinogen may be increased between and during attacks of acute intermittent porphyria; porphyrinuria may also occur in lead poisoning, liver disease, and conditions of increased erythropoiesis
Potassium		Not applicable on random urine	Depends on intake
Sodium		Not applicable on random urine	Depends on intake
Specific gravity		1.003–1.035	
Urate (uric acid)		μmol/L	Depends on intake
Uroporphyrin		≤35 nmol/L	See porphyrins, quantitative, urine

(continued)

Table III.7 Urine (continued)

Test Name	Age/Sex	Reference Interval/Units	Comments
Vanillylmandelic acid (VMA), spot or random urine	≤1 yr 2–4 yr 5–9 yr 10–19 yr	≤11.0 (34.0) mmol/mol creatinine ≤6.5 (12.0) mmol/mol creatinine ≤5.0 (5.5) mmol/mol creatinine ≤5.0 (8.0) mmol/mol creatinine	Random collection less satisfactory than 24-h collection Use small urine vial with preservative; minimum 20 mL urine; preservative: 0.5 mL preservative (6 N HCl) For small babies, try pooling multiple and send as one random sample Values represent 95th percentile (100th centile in parentheses)
Vanillylmandelic acid (VMA), timed collection	≤1 yr 2–4 yr 5–9 yr 10–19 yr	≤12.0 (16.0) µmol/d ≤15.0 (20.0) µmol/d ≤18.0 (44.0) µmol/d ≤30.0 (39.0) µmol/d	Nonspecific elevations occur in fever, asthma, chronic anemia, or after surgery Values represent 95th percentile (100th centile in parentheses)

Box III.1   Drugs Detected by Broad-Spectrum Urine Drug Screen

- Currently more than 900 drugs in broad-spectrum drug library (parent and metabolites)
- Reported as *Not Detected* or *Positive* based on sufficient drug present in urine to allow for proper identification on chromatograph

Antidepressants/Antipsychotics

- Amitriptyline/nortriptyline
- Imipramine/desipramine
- Doxepin
- Fluoxetine (Prozac)
- Fluvoxamine
- Paroxetine (Paxil)
- Citalopram (Celexa)
- Bupropion (Wellbutrin)
- Olanzapine (Zyprexa)
- Sertraline (Zoloft)
- Venlafaxine (Effexor)
- Chlorpromazine
- Perphenazine
- Methotrimeprazine
- Risperidone
- Loxapine/amoxapine
- Quetiapine (Seroquel)
- Trazodone

Stimulants

- Amphetamine ("Speed")
- Methamphetamine
- MDMA/MDA ("Ecstasy")
- Cocaine/BEG (benzoylecgonine)
- PCP ("Angel Dust")
- Methylphenidate (Ritalin)
- Ephedrine/pseudoephedrine
- Phenylpropanolamine

Narcotics

- Codeine
- Morphine
- Oxycodone
- Hydrocodone
- Hydromorphone (Dilaudid)
- MAM (monoacetylmorphine—heroin metabolite)
- Methadone

Sedative/Hypnotic

- Clozapine

Gastrointestinal

- Ranitidine

Cardiac/Pulmonary

- Lidocaine
- Verapamil
- Diltiazem

Miscellaneous

- Diphenhydramine
- Meperidine
- Ketamine ("Special K")

- Testing guidelines, methodology, and interpretation change frequently and are updated regularly; see local Web sites for the most up-to-date information (contain user-friendly search functions)
- For testing in Canada:
  - National Microbiology Laboratory, Public Health Agency of Canada: http://www.nml-lnm.gc.ca/english/guide
- For testing in Ontario:
  - Ontario Ministry of Health and Long-Term Care: http://www.health.gov.on.ca/english/providers/pub/labs/specimen.html

BLOOD PRODUCTS

ABBREVIATIONS

CMV	cytomegalovirus
DDAVP	desamino-8-D-arginine vasopressin
F	factor
FP	frozen plasma
Hb	hemoglobin
Hct	hematocrit
HLA	human leukocyte antigen
IVIG	intravenous immune globulin
IU	international units
RcoF	ristocetin cofactor
RDP	random donor platelets
SDP	single donor platelets
VWF	von Willebrand factor

Table III.8   **Blood Components**

Blood Components	Indications	Dosage	Description	Preparation Time	Infusion Instruction	Special Precautions
Red cell concentrate (in additive solution) (filtered prestorage)	To correct inadequate tissue O_2 delivery	15 mL/kg (increase Hb by 20–30 g/L)	Volume approximately 250 mL/u Hct approximately 0.60	Uncrossmatched, 5 min (physician request only) Urgent, 45 min Routine, 4–6 h	Use blood filter* Transfuse within 4 h after issue	Crossmatch required Must be ABO compatible
Dedicated unit	For neonates birth weight <1000 g	15–20 mL/kg	Hct approximately 0.60			
FP (frozen plasma)	Urgent reversal of warfarin effect or vitamin K deficiency Severe liver disease and coagulopathy Treatment of DIC Massive and exchange transfusions	10 mL/kg	Contains all coagulation factors and complement Approximately 200 mL	Urgent, 30 min Routine, 1–2 h	Use blood filter* Transfuse within 4 h after issue	Should be ABO compatible
Cryoprecipitate	Hypofibrinogenemia (fibrinogen <1 g/L) Dysfibrinogenemia	1 u/10 kg	Approximate volume 10 mL Contains fibrinogen (average, 200 mg/u), F VIII, vWF, F XIII	Urgent, 30 min Routine, 1–2 h	Use blood filter* or IV push filter Transfuse within 4 h after issue	Monitor recipient response

(continued)

Table III.8 Blood Components (continued)

Blood Components	Indications	Dosage	Description	Preparation Time	Infusion Instruction	Special Precautions
Cryoprecipitate-free FP (cryosupernatant)	Plasma infusion or plasma exchange for thrombotic thrombocytopenic purpura	10–50 mL/kg	Plasma deficient in high molecular weight multimers of vWF Approximately 250 mL	Urgent, 30 min Routine, 1–2 h	Use blood filter* Transfuse within 4 h of issue	Should be ABO compatible
Platelet concentrates	Bleeding from thrombocytopenia or platelet function abnormality Prophylaxis for platelet count <10 × 10⁹/L Prophylaxis for invasive procedures when platelet count <50 × 10⁹/L	Neonates: 15 mL/kg Others: 5–10 mL/kg, up to 300 mL (adult dose)	Available as RDP (50–60 mL), Buffy Coat pool (300 mL), or SDP (300 mL) One SDP product is equivalent to 5 RDP or Buffy Coat pool of 4	Urgent, 30 min Routine, 1–2 h	Use blood filter* or IV push filter Transfuse within 4 h of issue	Should be ABO compatible Monitor recipient response; 5–10 mL/kg raises platelet count by 30–60 × 10⁹/L 10 min–1 h post-transfusion (less in chemotherapy patients)
HLA-matched SDP	Refractory to RDP or BC due to HLA antibodies			48-h notice usually required by issuing laboratory	Use blood filter* Transfuse within 4 h of issue	
Albumin (5%) Albumin (25%)	Volume expansion	0.5–1 g/kg; max 6 g/kg/d	12.5 g (250 mL) 12.5 g (50 mL); 25 g (100 mL)	Issued on demand	No filter required	Order in g and mL

*Use 170–260-micron blood filter; 40-, 80-, or 150-micron blood filters are appropriate alternatives.

Table III.9 Factor Concentrate

Factor Concentrate	Trade Name	Indications	Source of Factor	Method of Viral Inactivation	Special Instructions*
Fibrinogen	Haemocomplettan-P (CSL Behring)	Congenital or acquired fibrinogen deficiency	Human plasma	Pasteurized	1 g (50 mL) = 5 u of cryoprecipitate SAP†
FVII	FVII concentrate (Baxter)	FVII deficiency requiring replacement therapy	Human plasma	Steam treated	Dose (IU) = desired % increase × body wt (kg)/2, given at 12-h intervals SAP†
FVIIa	Recombinant FVIIa/NiaStase	FVIII deficiency with high titer inhibitors Hereditary FVII deficiency	Recombinant	DNA technology	Vial sizes: 1200 mcg, 2400mcg, 4800mcg Reconstituted with diluent (water); 1 mL = 600 mcg Dose: 35–90mcg/kg, given at 2–6 h intervals Dose: 15–30 mcg/kg, given at 4–6 h intervals
FVIII	Kogenate FS (Bayer) Advate (Baxter)	FVIII deficiency requiring replacement therapy	Recombinant	DNA technology	Dose (IU) = desired % increase × body wt (kg)/2, given at 8–24-h intervals Usual dose: 25–40 u/kg
Anti-inhibitor coagulant complex (FII, VII, IX, X)	FEIBA VH IMMUNO (Baxter)	FVIII deficiency with inhibitors	Human plasma	Vapor heated	Dose range: 50–100 u/kg, given at 6–12-h intervals Daily maximum: 200 u/kg
vWF	Humate-P (CSL Behring) Wilate (Octapharma)	von Willebrand disease, nonresponsive to DDAVP	Human plasma	Pasteurized Solvent detergent	Dose (IU vWF:RcoF = desired % increase of vWF:RcoF (IU/dL) × body wt (kg)/1.5, given at 8–12-h intervals

(continued)

877

Table III.9 Factor Concentrate (continued)

Factor Concentrate	Trade Name	Indications	Source of Factor	Method of Viral Inactivation	Special Instructions*
F IX	BeneFix (Wyeth Canada)	Factor IX deficiency requiring replacement therapy	Recombinant	DNA technology	Dose (IU) = desired % increase × body wt (kg) × 1.2 Usual dose: 50 u/kg
F XI	Factor XI (BPL)	Factor XI deficiency requiring replacement	Human plasma	Heat treated	Dose (IU) = desired % increase × body wt (kg)/2 SAP†
F XIII	Fibrogammin P (CSL Behring)	Congenital factor XIII deficiency requiring replacement therapy	Human plasma	Pasteurized	Dose (u) = 10 u/kg, 4-wk intervals SAP†
Partial prothrombin complex (FII, VII, IX, X)	Octaplex (Octapharma) Prothromplex (Baxter)	Acquired or hereditary deficiency of factors II, V, IX, X	Human plasma	Solvent detergent Steam treated	Vial size: 500 IU FIX Vial size: 500 IU, SAP†
AT III	Antithrombin III (Baxter)	Congenital or acquired AT III deficiency	Human plasma	Heat treated	Dose (IU) = desired % increase × body wt (kg) Usual dose: ~100 IU/kg
Protein C	Ceprotin (Baxter)	Congenital and acquired protein C deficiency	Human plasma	Vapor heated	Dose according to clinical response and protein C levels SAP†
C1 inhibitor	Berinert P (CSL Behring)	Hereditary angioneurotic edema	Human plasma	Vapor heated	Dose (IU) = desired % increase × body wt (kg)/2 SAP†
Fibrin sealant	Tisseel (Baxter) FloSeal (Baxter)	Achieve hemostasis, seal, or glue tissue, support wound healing	Human plasma	Vapor heated	Vial sizes: 1.0 mL, 2.0 mL, 5.0 mL*

*Order dose to nearest vial size.
†SAP, Special Access Program, Canada.

Table III.10 | Immune Globulins

Immune Globulins	Indications	Dosage	Description	Infusion Instruction	Special Precautions
Immune globulin (human) (e.g., GamaSTAN)	Prophylaxis for hepatitis A contact	0.02 mL/kg	2 mL/vial	IM injection	
	For travel of less than 3 mo	0.02 mL/kg			
	For travel of more than 3 mo	0.06 mL/kg			
	Prophylaxis for measles	0.25–0.5 mL/kg			
Varicella zoster immune globulin (e.g., VariZig)	Prophylaxis against varicella zoster infection	125 u /10 kg Max 625 u	125 u/vial	IM injection	
Hepatitis B immune globulin (e.g., HyperHEP B)	Prophylaxis: Infants of mothers positive for hepatitis B surface Ag	0.5 mL	0.5-mL, 1-mL, 5-mL vials	IM injection	
	Post hepatitis B exposure	0.06 mL/kg			
Tetanus immune globulin	Prophylaxis for tetanus	>7 yr: 250 u <7 yr: 4 u/kg	250 u/vial	IM injection	
Rho(D) immune globulin (WinRho SDF)	Treatment of idiopathic thrombocytopenic purpura	40–50 mcg/kg (IV)	120 mcg (600 IU) 300 mcg (1500 IU) 1000 mg (5000 IU)	IV infusion No filter needed	For IM dose, consult product insert 50-mL platelets contain 0.4 mL red cell concentrate
	Transfusion of Rh-positive blood	9 mcg/mL whole blood or 18 mcg/mL red cell concentrate (IV)			

(continued)

Table III.10 Immune Globulins (continued)

Immune Globulins	Indications	Dosage	Description	Infusion Instruction	Special Precautions
IVIG (supplied mainly as 10% solutions) (Gamunex 10%, Gammagard Liquid 10%)	HIV infection	400 mg/kg/mo	Vial sizes: 2.5 g (25 mL) 5 g (50 mL) 10 g (100 mL) 20 g (200 mL)	IV infusion Gamunex 10% and Gammagard Liquid 10% No filter needed Compatible with D5W, not 0.9% NaCl	Rate of infusion: 0.6 mL/kg/h × 15 min 1.2 mL/kg/h × 15 min 2.4 mL/kg/h × 15 min 3.6 mL/kg/h × 30 min, then slowly increase rate if tolerated Maximum rate for Kawasaki disease patients = 3.6 mL/kg/h Maximum rate for Gammagard Liquid 10% = 8 mL/kg/h Maximum rate for Gamunex 10% = 8.4 mL/kg/h until finished
	Hypo/agammaglobulinemia	600 mg/kg/mo			
	Guillain-Barré syndrome	1 g/kg × 2 d			
	Juvenile idiopathic arthritis	1.5 g/kg/mo, max 70 g			
	Idiopathic thrombocytopenic purpura	0.8–1 g/kg and reassess in 24–48 h			
	Bone marrow transplant	200–500 mg/kg/wk			
	Dermatomyositis	1 g/kg × 2 d each month, max 70 g			
	Kawasaki disease	2 g/kg × 1 dose, max 70g			
CMV immune globulin (Cytogam)	CMV prophylaxis CMV disease	150 mg/kg/dose	2.5 g in 50 mL	IV infusion Use 15-micron filter	Consult specialist in infectious diseases
	Epstein-Barr virus disease	100–200 mg/kg every 2 d for 3 wk, then weekly for 3 wk			

Table III.11 Nonblood Products

Nonblood Products	Indications	Dosage	Description	Infusion Instruction	Special Precautions
Pentastarch 10% (Pentaspan)	Volume expansion	28 mL/kg/d (max 2000 mL/d)	250-mL bag 500-mL bag	IV infusion No filter needed	Not a substitute for red blood cells or coagulation factors in plasma Contraindications: bleeding disorders, CHF with volume overload, renal disease not related to hypovolemia May elevate amylase Disturbance of blood coagulation can occur
Hydroxyethyl starch 6% (Voluven)	Volume expansion	33 mL/kg/d (max 50 mL/kg/d)	250-mL bag 500-mL bag	IV infusion No filter needed	Not a substitute for red blood cells or coagulation factors in plasma Contraindications: renal failure not related to hypovolemia, dialysis, intracranial bleeding, severe hypernatremia/hyperchloremia May elevate amylase Disturbance of blood coagulation can occur

USEFUL WEB SITES

Ontario Ministry of Health and Long-Term Care. Specimen collection guide: Testing guidelines. Available at: **www.health.gov.on.ca/english/providers/pub/ labs/specimen.html**

Laboratory Reference Values

III

Section IV Pediatric Drug Dosing Guidelines

Elaine Lau

Section IV Pediatric Drug Dosing Guidelines

BODY SURFACE AREA NOMOGRAMS

Figure IV.1 Body Surface Area Nomogram for Children and Adults

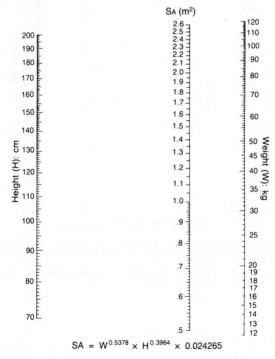

$$SA = W^{0.5378} \times H^{0.3964} \times 0.024265$$

To use the nomogram, a ruler is aligned with the height and weight on the two lateral axes. The point at which the center line is intersected gives the corresponding value for surface area. For the simplified formula to calculate BSA, see p. 285.

From Haycock GB, Schwartz GJ, Wisotsky DH. Geometric method for measuring body surface area: a height–weight formula validated in infants, children, and adults. *J Pediatr.* 1978;93:62–66.

Figure IV.2 Body Surface Area Nomogram for Infants

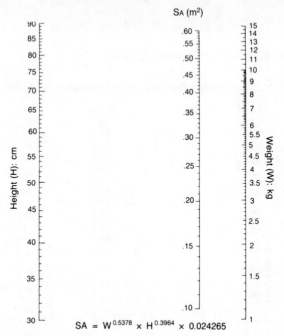

$$SA = W^{0.5378} \times H^{0.3964} \times 0.024265$$

To use the nomogram, a ruler is aligned with the height and weight on the two lateral axes. The point at which the center line is intersected gives the corresponding value for surface area. For the simplified formula to calculate BSA, see p. 285.

From Haycock GB, Schwartz GJ, Wisotsky DH. Geometric method for measuring body surface area: a height–weight formula validated in infants, children, and adults. *J Pediatr.* 1978;93:62–66.

IDEAL BODY MASS NOMOGRAM

Figure IV.3 **Nomogram for Estimating Ideal Body Mass**

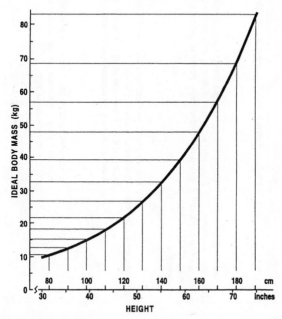

IBM (kg) = 2.396 $e^{0.01863}$ [height (cm)]

Effective body weight (kg) = IBM + 0.4 (total body weight − IBM)

Note: This nomogram is useful for estimation of ideal body mass (IBM) in children aged 1–17 yr; its accuracy is slightly diminished when used to estimate IBM for patients taller than 154 cm. IBM should be used for calculating dosage only if IBM is *less than* total body weight.

From Traub SL, Kichen L. Estimating ideal body mass in children. *Am J Hosp Pharm*. 1983;40:107–110. Copyright 1983. American Society of Health-System Pharmacists, Inc. All rights reserved. Reprinted with permission (R0317).

Table IV.1 — Drug Dosage Guidelines for Neonates* (Where Specified), Infants, and Older Children

Drug†‡§	Dose	Dose Limit	Comments
Abacavir Tab 300 mg Liquid 20 mg/mL	*3 mo–16 yr:* 16 mg/kg/d PO ÷ bid	600 mg/d	If hypersensitivity rash develops, rechallenge is contraindicated
Acetaminophen Tab 325, 500 mg Chew tab 80 mg Drops/susp 80 mg/mL Rectal suppos 120, 325, 650 mg	*Neonates:* 10–15 mg/kg/dose PO/PR q4–6h *Infants and older children:* 10–15 mg/kg/dose PO q4–6h prn 10–20 mg/kg/dose PR q4–6h prn	*Neonates:* 60 mg/kg *Infants and older children:* 75 mg/kg/d PO or 80 mg/kg/d PR or 4 g/d if >12 yr of age, whichever is less	For doses ≤80 mg, oral drops (not susp) may be administered rectally Single rectal loading doses of 30 mg/kg (in neonates) and 40 mg/kg (infants, older children) may be used for perioperative analgesia
Acetazolamide Tab 250 mg SR cap 500 mg Susp (HSC) 25 mg/mL	**Glaucoma** *Children:* 15–30 mg/kg/d PO/IV ÷ tid–qid *Adolescents:* 250–500-mg regular tabs PO tid–qid; 500-mg SR cap PO bid; 250–500 mg IV up to qid **Epilepsy** 4–15 mg/kg/d PO in divided doses	30 mg/kg/d or 1 g/d, whichever is less	Dose adjustment in renal impairment, moderate: q12h, severe: avoid TPD authorization is required for injection Use low end of dosing range when adding to antiepileptic drug therapy; extended-release caps not recommended for treatment of epilepsy
Acetylcysteine Injection 2 g/10 mL, 6 g/30 mL (20%) Liquid 200 mg/mL (20%) Liquid (HSC) 5%, 10%	**Prevention of contrast-induced nephropathy** 10 mg/kg PO bid × 4 doses (starting the day before the procedure)		For oral administration, the 20% IV solution can be diluted with water, juice, soft drinks, or chocolate milk to a final concentration of 5% and administered within the hour

Acetylsalicylic acid (ASA, aspirin) Chew tab 80 mg Tab 325 mg Enteric-coated tab 81, 325 mg Suppos 150, 650 mg	**JIA, pericarditis, rheumatic fever** 60–100 mg/kg/d PO + qid **Kawasaki disease** 100 mg/kg/d PO + q6h until defenvescence × 24 h, then 3–5 mg/kg/d PO qam **Antithrombotic therapy** 3–5 mg/kg/dose PO once daily	Max initial dose: 5.4 g/d 150 mg/kg/d 325 mg/d	Not recommended for antipyresis (risk of Reye syndrome); give with food; do not use enteric-coated tablets with milk, dairy products, antacids; use extreme caution in hepatic impairment Round dose to nearest ¼ tab Enteric-coated tabs cannot be split
Activated charcoal Susp 25 g/112.5 mL	If unknown quantity of toxin ingested, initial dose: 1 g/kg PO/NG If known quantity of toxin ingested, initial dose: 10 g activated charcoal per 1 g toxin ingested		Subsequent doses: only as advised by local Poison Control Center for particular indications
Acyclovir Susp 40 mg/mL Tab 200, 400, 800 mg Inj 6 mg/mL (HSC) Ophthalmic ointment 3% (Special Access drug)	*Neonates:* **Herpes simplex infections** >32 wk PCA and ≥1200 g: 60 mg/kg/d IV + q8h × 21 d *Infants and older children (dose on ideal body mass, see p. 887):* **Herpes simplex encephalitis** 1 m–12 yr: 60 mg/kg/d IV + q8h × 14–28 d >12 yr: 30 mg/kg/d IV + q8h × 14–28 d		Dosage should be calculated based on ideal body mass (see p. 887) Maintain optimal hydration (1½ × maintenance) and urine output of at least 1 mL/kg/h; measure baseline SCr; minimize use of concurrent nephrotoxins For neonates, dose interval adjustment in renal impairment: moderate (SCr, 70–109 μmol/L), q12h; severe (SCr, 110–130 μmol/L), q24h; failure (SCr >130 μmol/L or urine output <1 mL/kg/h), 10 mg/kg/dose q24h

*Guidelines apply to all neonates until a postconceptional age of >38 wk *and* a postnatal age of >4 wk have been achieved.

CR, controlled release; GA, gestational age (time from conception to birth); ODT, oral disintegrating tablet; PCA, postconceptional age (age since conception; GA + PNA); PE, phenytoin equivalents; PNA, postnatal age (chronologic age since birth); SCr, serum creatinine; SR, sustained-release; tPA, tissue plasminogen activator; VPA, valproic acid.

†Drug dosage forms listed may be used as a guide only and are not reflective of all dosage forms available.

Δsymbol represents Dissolve 'n' Dose system (available through PharmaSystems Inc.) indicated for use with some drugs when a liquid formulation is unavailable and the required dose cannot be obtained from the tablet form; can be used only for water-soluble drugs; not all drugs can be "dissolved and dosed."

§Liquids and suspensions noted with "HSC" (Hospital for Sick Children, Toronto, Ontario, Canada) are manufactured preparations; most formulations can be found at http://www.sickkids.ca/pharmacy/.

(continued)

Table IV.1 Drug Dosage Guidelines for Neonates* (Where Specified), Infants, and Older Children (continued)

Drug†‡§	Dose	Dose Limit	Comments
Acyclovir—cont'd	**Other herpes simplex, including gingival stomatitis** 15–30 mg/kg/d IV ÷ q8h **Genital herpes and other recurrent HSV infections** 200 mg PO qid		For infants, older children, dose adjustment in renal impairment: moderate, q12h; severe, q24h GFR <10 mL/min, 50% of dose q24h Oral therapy not recommended in neonates; for infants and older children, may be given PO with food; patients receiving >30 mg/kg/d should have CBC + diff weekly
	Prophylaxis in immunocompromised hosts (not HIV; for HIV-positive patients, see below) 50 mg/kg/d PO ÷ qid	1 g/d PO	
	Herpes simplex in HIV-positive patients Treatment: 40–80 mg/kg/d PO ÷ q8h × 7–14 d Maintenance viral suppression: 20 mg/kg/d PO ÷ bid	1200 mg/d PO 800 mg/d PO	
	Varicella or zoster in immunocompromised hosts <1 yr: 30 mg/kg/d IV q8h ≥1 yr: 1500 mg/m²/d IV ÷ q8h PO dosing (following IV therapy): 80 mg/kg/d PO ÷ qid		
	Varicella in immunocompetent host 80 mg/kg/d PO ÷ qid × 5 d	3.2 g/d PO	
	CMV prophylaxis in immunocompromised host 50–80 mg/kg/d PO ÷ tid-qid	3.2 g/d PO	

Adenosine Inj 3 mg/mL	**Supraventricular tachycardia** *Neonates:* 0.05 mg/kg/dose IV increasing in increments of 0.05 mg/kg to a max of 0.25 mg/kg/dose *Infants and older children:* 0.1 mg/kg/dose IV/IO; repeat q2min at 0.2 mg/kg/dose IV/IO	First dose: 6 mg Repeat dose: 12 mg	Administer by rapid IV/IO bolus over 1–2 s followed by 0.9% NaCl flush
Adrenaline	See epinephrine		
Albumin Inj 5%, 25%	0.5–1 g/kg/dose IV	6 g/kg/d	
Albuterol	See salbutamol		
Aldactazide Susp (HSC) Spironolactone 5 mg/mL and hydrochlorothiazide 5 mg/mL Tab spironolactone and hydrochlorothiazide, 25 mg each	*Neonates, infants, and older children:* 2–4 mg of each component/kg/d PO ÷ bid	Usual adult dose: 2–4 tabs/d	Give with food or milk; ineffective when GFR <30 mL/min
Allopurinol Susp (HSC) 20 mg/mL Tab 100 mg	200–300 mg/m²/d PO ÷ bid–qid 12 mg/kg/d PO ÷ bid–qid	800 mg/d	Maintain fluid intake; dose adjustment in renal impairment: moderate, 50%; severe, 25–30%

***¹§Refer to legend on p. 889.

(continued)

Pediatric Drug Dosing Guidelines

IV

Table IV.1 Drug Dosage Guidelines for Neonates* (Where Specified), Infants, and Older Children (continued)

Drug††§	Dose	Dose Limit	Comments
Alprostadil Inj 500 mcg/vial	*Neonates:* 0.01–0.1 mcg/kg/min IV via continuous infusion		May cause apnea; formula for dilution: 500 mcg in 80 mL at 1 mL/kg/h = 0.1 mcg/kg/min
Alteplase (tPA) Inj 2, 50 mg/vial Inj (HSC) 1 mg/mL	**See guidelines for blocked venous lines, p. 470** **Systemic thrombolytic therapy** 0.5 mg/kg/h IV × 6 h and re-evaluate; use unfractionated heparin (10 units/kg/h) during infusion		Systemic thrombolytic therapy indicated for arterial occlusions, massive pulmonary embolism, and pulmonary embolism not responding to heparin therapy; may also be indicated for acute extensive DVT and should be limited to situations in which risk of loss of life, organ, or limb due to thrombosis is present *Contraindications:* active bleeding, significant potential for local bleeding, general surgery within previous 10 d, neurosurgery within previous 3 wk, hypertension, AV malformations, recent severe trauma *Precautions:* no IM injections; minimal manipulation of the patient; avoid concurrent use of warfarin or antiplatelet agents; no urinary catheterization, rectal temperature, or arterial punctures; take blood samples from superficial vein or indwelling catheter; maintain platelets at >100 × 10^9/L Monitor INR, aPTT, fibrinogen; maintain fibrinogen at >1 g/L by infusions of cryoprecipitate
Aluminum hydroxide (aluminum and magnesium hydroxides) Aluminum hydroxide	**Antacid** *Infant:* 2.5–5 mL PO q1–2h *Child:* 5–15 mL PO pc and qhs *Adult:* 15–45 mL PO pc and qhs		

Susp 64 mg/mL Chew tab 600 mg Diovol Ex: magnesium hydroxide 60 mg/mL + aluminum hydroxide 99 mg/mL	**Hyperphosphatemia** *Child:* 50–150 mg/kg/d PO ÷ q4-6h; titrate to normal serum phosphate level *Adult:* 30–40 mL PO tid-qid	
Amantadine Liquid 10 mg/mL Cap 100 mg	**Influenza A prophylaxis and treatment** 5 mg/kg/d PO ÷ q12h	*<10 yr:* 150 mg/d *≥10 yr:* 200 mg/d	Continue prophylaxis for at least 10 d after exposure or throughout epidemic; active treatment should continue for 48 h after disappearance of symptoms; avoid alcohol; dose adjustment in renal impairment: mild, q24h; moderate, q2d; severe, q7d
Amikacin Inj 250 mg/mL Inj (HSC) 10, 250 mg/mL	*Neonates:* *<2 kg, 0–7 d:* 15 mg/kg/d IV/IM ÷ q12h *<2 kg, >7 d:* 20 mg/kg/d IV/IM ÷ q8h *≥2 kg, 0–7 d:* 20 mg/kg/d IV/IM ÷ q12h *≥2 kg, >7 d:* 30 mg/kg/d IV/IM ÷ q8h		
	Infants and older children: 15–30 mg/kg/d IV/IM ÷ q8h **Hematology/oncology and HPCT patients with fever and neutropenia** 20 mg/kg/dose IV q24h	500 mg/dose before TDM 1500 mg/d	Calculate dose according to effective body weight Monitoring of serum concentrations recommended; dose interval adjustment in renal impairment: moderate, q12h; severe, q24–48h
5-Aminosalicylic acid (5-ASA)	See mesalamine		

***§Refer to legend on p. 889.

(continued)

893

Table IV.1   Drug Dosage Guidelines for Neonates* (Where Specified), Infants, and Older Children *(continued)*

Drug††§	Dose	Dose Limit	Comments
Amiodarone Inj 50 mg/mL Tab 200 mg Cap (HSC) 5, 20 mg	Loading dose: 5 mg/kg IV over 1 h, followed by infusion of 5-15 mcg/kg/min 10 mg/kg/d PO as a single daily dose or ÷ bid × 7-10 d Maintenance: 5 mg/kg/d PO as a single daily dose	Usual adult loading dose: 800-1600 mg/d PO Usual adult maintenance dose: 200-400 mg/d PO	Dose may require reduction in patients with liver impairment; reduce digoxin dose by 50% during concurrent therapy Reduce warfarin dose by 33-50% during concurrent therapy Will increase phenytoin concentrations (monitor for toxicity) Monitor thyroid, liver, lung, eye function; nausea/vomiting occur frequently with loading dose
Amlodipine Tab 5 mg Oral susp (HSC) 1 mg/mL	Initial: 0.1-0.2 mg/kg/d PO once daily Maintenance: 0.1-0.3 mg/kg/d PO once daily	15 mg/d	Reduce initial dose in patients with liver impairment and titrate to effect; because of long half-life, dosage adjustments should not be made more frequently than q3-5d
Amoxicillin Susp 50 mg/mL Cap 250, 500 mg	50 mg/kg/d PO ÷ q8h High-dose therapy: 80-90 mg/kg/d PO ÷ q8h ***Helicobacter pylori*-associated ulcer** *Children:* 50 mg/kg/d ÷ bid *Adolescents, adults:* 1000 mg/dose PO bid × 1-2 wk with omeprazole and clarithromycin (2 wk preferred in children) **Prophylaxis for asplenic patients (alternative to penicillin)** *2-5 yr:* 20 mg/kg/d PO ÷ bid	4 g/d	Dose interval adjustment in renal impairment: moderate, q12h; severe, q24h; may be given with food
Amoxicillin/clavulanic acid (Clavulin) Susp 25 mg/mL Amoxicillin and 6.25 mg/mL	*<3 mo:* 30 mg amoxicillin/kg/d ÷ q12h given as 25 mg/mL susp *≥3 mo, ≤38 kg:* 25-45 mg amoxicillin/kg/d PO ÷ q8-12h given as 40 mg/mL susp	Usual adult dose: 750-1750 mg/d amoxicillin	Use with caution in patients with creatinine clearance <30 mL/min; adjust dose in renal failure: severe, 50-75% of standard dose or adjust interval; moderate, q12h; severe, q24h; tabs are not recommended in children <12 yr because of higher ratio of clavulanic acid

clavulanate; 40 mg/mL amoxicillin and 5.7 mg/mL clavulanate Tab 150 mg amoxicillin and 125 mg clavulanate	**Bites** ≥3 mo, ≤38 kg: 40 mg amoxicillin/kg/d ÷ q8–12h as 40 mg/mL susp >38 kg: 500 mg amoxicillin PO q8h as 500 mg tab *Otitis media* *Standard dose:* 40 mg amoxicillin/kg/d PO ÷ q8h as 40 mg/mL susp *High dose:* 80–90 mg amoxicillin/kg/d PO ÷ q8–12h given as 40 mg/mL susp	to amoxicillin; tabs are not equivalent to susp; various formulations of susp exist; are not all equivalent; administer with food to reduce GI upset; if possible, limit clavulanic acid to ~10 mg/kg/d in children to reduce GI symptoms; bid dosing may also reduce adverse GI effects such as diarrhea
Amphotericin B Inj (HSC) 0.1 mg/mL	*Neonates:* 1 mg/kg/d IV as a single daily dose *Infants, older children:* 1 mg/kg/d IV as a single daily dose	70 mg/d or 1.5 mg/kg/dose, whichever is less	Monitor serum potassium and renal function; consider premedication with meperidine, diphenhydramine Sodium load as tolerated
Amphotericin B lipid formulations	Amphotericin B lipid complex (Abelcet). **Documented/suspected fungal infection and empiric therapy** 5 mg/kg/d IV once daily Amphotericin B liposomal (AmBisome) **Empiric therapy in hematology/oncology and HPCT patients with febrile neutropenia** 3 mg/kg/d IV once daily **Documented/suspected fungal infection and empiric therapy** 5 mg/kg/d IV once daily		Consider in patients unable to receive conventional amphotericin because of toxicity (renal impairment, hypokalemia, infusion-related reactions) or treatment failure

(continued)

***Refer to legend on p. 889.

Table IV.1   Drug Dosage Guidelines for Neonates* (Where Specified), Infants, and Older Children (continued)

Drug^{††§}	Dose	Dose Limit	Comments
Ampicillin Inj 250, 500, 1000, 2000 mg/vial	*Neonates:* *<2 kg, 0–7 d* **Meningitis** 100 mg/kg/d IV ÷ q12h **Other** 50 mg/kg/d IV ÷ q12h *<2 kg, >7 d* **Meningitis** 150 mg/kg/d IV ÷ q8h **Other** 75 mg/kg/d IV ÷ q8h *≥2 kg, 0–7 d* **Meningitis** 150 mg/kg/d IV ÷ q8h **Other** 75 mg/kg/d IV ÷ q8h *≥2 kg, >7 d* **Meningitis** 200 mg/kg/d IV ÷ q6h **Other** 100 mg/kg/d IV ÷ q6h **Group B streptococcus meningitis** *PNA ≤ 7 d:* 200 mg/kg/d IV ÷ q8h *PNA > 7 d:* 300 mg/kg/d IV ÷ q6h **UTI prophylaxis** 50 mg/kg/d IV ÷ q12h		Reduce dose in renal impairment

	Infants and older children: **Meningitis** 200–300 mg/kg/d IV ÷ q6h **Other** 100–200 mg/kg/d IV ÷ q6h	12 g/d 4 g/d	Dose interval adjustment in renal failure: moderate, q6–12h; severe, q12h
Atenolol Tab 25, 50 mg	**Children ≥5 yr** 0.5–1.5 mg/kg/d as a single daily dose or ÷ bid	2 mg/d or 100 mg/d, whichever is less	Dose interval adjustment in renal failure: CrCl 15–35 mL/min: max 50 mg or 1 mg/kg/dose PO once daily CrCl <15 mL/min: max 50 mg or 1 mg/kg/dose PO q2d
Atorvastatin Tab 10, 20 mg	**Hyperlipidemia, heterozygous familial hypercholesterolemia** 10–17 yr: 10 mg PO once daily, may increase to 20 mg once daily	Children: 20 mg Adult: 80 mg	Monitor liver function tests (liver enzyme changes generally occur in first 3 mo); rhabdomyolysis has occurred rarely (risk increased with concurrent administration of certain drugs); in patients with impaired renal function, use lowest dose possible (max 10 mg)
Atropine Inj 0.6 mg/mL; preloaded inj 0.5 mg/5 mL	*Neonates:* **Resuscitation** 0.01–0.02 mg/kg/dose IV/IM/SC/ETT q20min prn *Infants and older children:* **Resuscitation** 0.02 mg/kg/dose IV/IO q5min prn 0.03 mg/kg ETT, repeat once prn min. dose: 0.1 mg max dose: 0.5 mg (children), 1 mg (adolescents)		ETT route to be used only if IV route not possible; dilute/follow dose by 1 mL 0.9% NaCl Incompatible with sodium bicarbonate

(continued)

***§Refer to legend on p. 889.

Table IV.1   Drug Dosage Guidelines for Neonates* (Where Specified), Infants, and Older Children *(continued)*

Drug[†‡§]	Dose	Dose Limit	Comments
Atropine—cont'd	**Preoperative** 0.01–0.02 mg/kg/dose IM/PO 30–60 min preop; min. dose: 0.1 mg	0.6 mg/dose	
	Cholinergic crisis 0.05 mg/kg IV q5min until secretions dry	2 mg/dose	
Azathioprine Susp (HSC) 50 mg/mL Tab 50 mg Inj (HSC) 10 mg/mL	**Transplantation** *Heart:* 2 mg/kg/d IV/PO as a single daily dose *Lung:* 1.5 mg/kg/d IV/PO as a single daily dose		Adjust dose in renal impairment: moderate, q36h or give 75% of standard dose; severe, q48h or give 50% of standard dose; give PO dose with food
Azithromycin Tab 250 mg	**Chlamydial urethritis, cervicitis, and pelvic inflammatory disease** ≥16 yr: 1 g PO stat		Clearance of other drugs, including tacrolimus, cyclosporine, and phenytoin, may be decreased
Baclofen Tab 10 mg Liquid (HSC) 5 mg/mL	≥2 yr: 10–15 mg/d PO ÷ q8h, titrate dose q3d by 5–15 mg/d	2–7 yr: 40 mg/d ≥8 yr: 60 mg/d Adult max: 80 mg/d	Avoid abrupt withdrawal of drug; use with caution in patients with seizure disorder, impaired renal function
Belladonna and opium Suppos 65 mg opium + 15 mg belladonna extract	**Ureteral spasm** 8–16 kg: ¼ suppos PR q4–6h prn 16–32 kg: ½ suppos PR q4–6h prn ≥32 kg: 1 suppos PR q4–6h prn		Min dose: ¼ suppos
Bisacodyl Tab 5 mg Suppos 5, 10 mg	0.3 mg/kg/dose PO 6–12 h before desired effect ≤6 yr: 5–10 mg PR 15–60 min before desired effect >6 yr: 10 mg PR 15–60 min before desired effect	15 mg PO	Do not divide or chew tabs; do not administer PO with dairy products or antacid

Budesonide Susp for inhalation 0.25 mg/2 mL, 0.5 mg/ 2 mL, 1 mg/2 mL	*Neonates:* 0.25–0.5 mg bid via nebulizer; acute distress, 0.5–1 mg bid via nebulizer **Severe acute asthma** *Children:* 0.5–1 mg bid via nebulizer *Adults:* 1–2 mg bid via nebulizer **Maintenance** *Children:* 0.25–0.5 mg bid via nebulizer *Adults:* 0.5–1 mg via nebulizer	Dilute to a total of 3 mL with 0.9% NaCl if required; may be mixed with salbutamol, ipratropium, or tobramycin solutions immediately before use
Caffeine citrate Inj 10 mg base/mL (Special Access drug)	*Neonates:* Loading: 10 mg base/kg IV/PO Maintenance: 3–5 mg base/kg/d IV/PO once daily, starting 24 h after loading dose	Injection may be given PO; dose expressed as caffeine base: 2 mg caffeine citrate = 1 mg caffeine base
1-α-calcidiol Drops 2 mcg/mL Cap 0.25 mcg	Initial dose 0.02–0.04 mcg/kg/d PO once daily	Adjust dose according to plasma calcium and phosphate concentration (also PTH for chronic kidney disease)
Calcitriol (1,25-dihydroxycholecalciferol) Cap 0.25, 0.5 mcg Inj 1 mcg/mL Liquid 1 mcg/mL	**Hypoparathyroidism, vitamin D–resistant rickets, dialysis** 0.015–0.025 mcg/kg/d PO ÷ bid; increase prn gradually to 0.5–1 mcg/d	Adjust dose according to plasma calcium concentration

***Refer to legend on p. 889.

(continued)

Table IV.1 Drug Dosage Guidelines for Neonates* (Where Specified), Infants, and Older Children (*continued*)

Drug††§	Dose	Dose Limit	Comments
Calcium Inj 100 mg/mL calcium gluconate (10%) = 9.3 mg elemental calcium/ mL = 0.23 mmol elemental calcium/mL Inj 100 mg/mL calcium chloride = 27 mg elemental calcium/mL = 0.68 mmol elemental calcium/mL Susp (HSC) 200 mg/mL calcium carbonate = 80 mg elemental calcium/mL = 2 mmol elemental calcium/mL Tab 625 mg calcium carbonate = 250 mg elemental calcium = 6.25 mmol elemental calcium	*Neonates:* **Resuscitation** 0.5–2 mL/kg/dose of 10% calcium gluconate solution (50–200 mg/kg/dose of calcium gluconate) IV q10–20min prn **Hypocalcemia** Initial: 0.12–0.46 mmol/kg/dose of elemental calcium (50–200 mg/kg/dose calcium gluconate) IV over 30 min Maintenance: 0.46–1.84 mmol/kg/d elemental calcium/kg/d (200–800 mg/kg/d calcium gluconate) IV 50–150 mg elemental calcium/kg/d PO ÷ qid		Avoid extravasation; central line preferred; oral calcium preparations are hyperosmolar; administer with feedings
	Infants and older children: **Resuscitation** 20 mg/kg/dose calcium chloride IV/IO q10–20min prn (0.2 mL/kg/dose of 10% calcium chloride)	1 g (10 mL)	

		Titrate dose according to serum PO_4^- or to corrected serum Ca^{2+}
	Calcium deficiency, initial dose for phosphate binding in chronic renal failure patients *Infants:* 125 mg elemental calcium/dose PO tid *Children:* 250 mg elemental calcium/dose PO tid	
Calcium polystyrene sulfonate (Resonium Calcium) Powder	**Hypocalcemia** 0.1–0.2 mmol calcium/kg/h IV; adjust IV rate q4h according to plasma calcium concentration	Avoid extravasation; central line preferred
	Initial: 1 g/kg/d PO/PR in divided doses **Maintenance:** 0.5 g/kg/d PO/PR in divided doses	Contains 8% w/w calcium (1.6–2.4 mmol/g); use in patients with hyperkalemia and restricted sodium intake
Captopril Tab 6.25, 12.5, 25, 50 mg Solution: Dissolve 'n' Dose system Δ	**Hypertension** **Initial:** 0.1–0.3 mg/kg/dose PO q8h **Maintenance:** 0.3–4 mg/kg/d PO ÷ q8h **CHF** **Initial:** 0.1 mg/kg/dose PO q8h **Maintenance:** 1.5–6 mg/kg/d PO ÷ q8-12h	6 mg/kg/d or 200 mg/d	Dose adjustment in renal impairment: moderate, 75%; severe, 50%
Carbamazepine Susp 20 mg/mL Tab 200 mg Tab CR 200, 400 mg Chew tab 100 mg	**Initial:** 10 mg/kg/d PO ÷ once or twice daily **Maintenance:** up to 20–30 mg/kg/d PO ÷ bid-qid; increase dose gradually over 2–4 wk		Chewable tabs must be thoroughly chewed and not swallowed whole; CR tabs may be split; give with food or milk; dose may require reduction in liver impairment; tabs, susp: dose tid-qid CR tabs: dose bid-tid

*†‡§Refer to legend on p. 889.

(continued)

Table IV.1   Drug Dosage Guidelines for Neonates* (Where Specified), Infants, and Older Children (continued)

Drug††§	Dose	Dose Limit	Comments
Carvedilol Tab 3.125 mg Susp (HSC) 1.67 mg/mL	**CHF** *< 4 yr:* 0.1 mg/kg/d PO ÷ q8–12h, increase to 0.8–1 mg/kg/d PO ÷ q8–12h *>4 yr:* 0.1–2 mg/kg/d PO ÷ q12h	50 mg PO bid	Reduce digoxin dose by 25% when carvedilol added to therapy
Caspofungin Inj 50 mg/vial Inj (HSC) 5 mg/mL	**Empiric therapy in hematology/oncology and HPCT patients** 50 mg/m²/d IV once daily	70 mg/dose	
	Documented or suspected invasive infection in any patient *Children 2–11 yr:* loading dose, 70 mg/m²/d IV on day 1, then 50 mg/m²/d IV *Children ≥12 yr:* loading dose, 70 mg IV on day 1, then 50 mg IV once daily	70 mg loading dose, 50 mg maintenance dose	
Cefazolin Inj 500 mg, 1 g, 10 g/vial	*Neonates:* *< 2 kg:* 40 mg/kg/d IV/IM ÷ q12h *≥ 2 kg, 0–7 d:* 40 mg/kg/d IV/IM ÷ q12h *≥ 2 kg, >7 d:* 60 mg/kg/d IV/IM ÷ q8h		Reduce dose in renal impairment
	Infants and older children: **Mild to moderate infections** 50–100 mg/kg/d IV/IM ÷ q8h	3 g/d	Dose interval adjustment in renal impairment: moderate, q12h; severe, q24h
	Severe infections 100–150 mg/kg/d IV/IM ÷ q8h	6 g/d	

Cefixime Susp 20 mg/mL Tab 400 mg	8 mg/kg/d PO once daily **Gonorrhea** 8 mg/kg PO × 1 dose	400 mg/dose	Dose adjustment in renal impairment: moderate, 75% standard dose; severe, 50% standard dose
Cefotaxime Inj 1 g/vial, 2 g/vial Inj (HSC) 250 mg/mL	*Neonates:* <*1200 g,* 100 mg/kg/d IV/IM ÷ q12h *1200–2000 g,* ≤*7 d:* 100 mg/kg/d IV/IM ÷ q12h *1200–2000 g,* >*7 d:* 150 mg/kg/d IV/IM ÷ q8h >*2000 g,* ≤*7 d:* 100–150 mg/kg/d IV/IM ÷ q8-12h >*2000 g,* >*7 d:* 150–200 mg/kg/d IV/IM ÷ q6-8h		Reduce dose in renal impairment
	Infants and older children:		Dose interval adjustment in renal impairment: moderate, q8-12h; severe, q12-24h
	Mild to moderate infections 100 mg/kg/d IV/IM ÷ q8h	6 g/d	
	Severe infections 150-200 mg/kg/d IV/IM ÷ q6-8h	8 g/d	
	Meningitis in infants 1-3 mo 200 mg/kg/d IV/IM ÷ q6h	10 g/d	
	Sickle cell disease (meningitis not suspected) 200 mg/kg/d IV ÷ q6-8h	10 g/d	

***†§Refer to legend on p. 889.

(continued)

Table IV.1 Drug Dosage Guidelines for Neonates* (Where Specified), Infants, and Older Children (continued)

Drug††§	Dose	Dose Limit	Comments
Cefoxitin Inj 1, 2 g/vial Inj (HSC) 200 mg/mL	**Mild to moderate infections** 80–100 mg/kg/d IV/IM ÷ q6–8h	4 g/d	Dose interval adjustment in renal impairment: moderate, q8–12h; severe, q24–48h
	Severe infections 100–160 mg/kg/d IV/IM ÷ q4–6h	12 g/d	
	Pelvic inflammatory disease 2 g/dose IV q6h		
Ceftazidime Inj 1, 2, 6 g/vial Inj (HSC) 250 mg/mL	*Neonates:* <2 kg, 0–7 d: 100 mg/kg/d IV/IM ÷ q12h <2 kg, >7 d: 150 mg/kg/d IV/IM ÷ q8h ≥2 kg, 0–7 d: 100 mg/kg/d IV/IM ÷ q8h ≥2 kg, >7 d: 150 mg/kg/d IV/IM ÷ q8h		Reduce dose in renal impairment
	Infants and older children: **Mild to moderate infections** 100 mg/kg/d IV/IM ÷ q8h	3 g/d	Dose interval adjustment in renal impairment: mild, q12 h; moderate, q24h; severe, q48h
	Severe infections 125–150 mg/kg/d IV/IM ÷ q8h	6 g/d	
	CF patients 200 mg/kg/d IV/IM ÷ q6h	6 g/d	
Ceftriaxone Inj 2 g/vial	**Meningitis in children >3 mo** 100 mg/kg/dose IV at 0, 12, and 24 h, then 100 mg/kg/dose IV q24h	2 g/dose	For meningitis, administration of dexamethasone before first dose of ceftriaxone may be considered; divide doses > 2 g/d (q12h); in neonates, may induce hyperbilirubinemia, *Candida* overgrowth; fatal

		cases of calcium-ceftriaxone precipitation have been reported in neonates (avoid concurrent administration with calcium-containing products)
Otitis media treatment failure 50 mg/kg/dose IM daily × 3 d	1 g/d	
Other infections 100 mg/kg/dose IV/IM q24h		
Uncomplicated gonorrhea <45 kg: 125 mg/dose IM × 1 dose ≥45 kg: 250 mg/dose IM × 1 dose	2 g/dose	Treat uncomplicated gonorrhea with combination of ceftriaxone and either doxycycline × 10 d or azithromycin × 1 dose
Cefuroxime Inj 750, 1500 mg/vial	75–100 mg/kg/d IV/IM ÷ q8h	6 g/d	Not to be used for the treatment of meningitis; dose interval adjustment in renal impairment: moderate, q12h; severe, q24h
Cefuroxime axetil Susp 25 mg/mL Tab 250, 500 mg	**Otitis media** 30 mg/kg/d PO ÷ bid as susp or (≥12 yr) 250 mg PO bid as tabs	1 g/d	Dose interval adjustment in severe renal impairment: q24h; dosages for liquid and tabs are not interchangeable; oral bioavailability is increased by food; bioavailability of tabs is 52% in adults when given with food; bioavailability of susp is 91% that of tabs, or ~47%; give with food, milk, or formula; susp may be mixed with small amount of orange/grape juice or chocolate milk immediately before administration; do not crush tabs (taste is very bitter)
	Pharyngitis 20 mg/kg/d PO ÷ bid as susp	500 mg/d	
	Other infections (≥12 yr) Mild to moderate: 125–250 mg PO bid as tabs Moderate to severe: 250–500 mg PO bid as tabs		
Cephalexin Susp 50 mg/mL Tab 250, 500 mg	25–50 mg/kg/d PO ÷ qid	4 g/d	May give with food Dose interval adjustment in renal impairment: moderate, q8–12h; severe, q12–24h
	Osteomyelitis (after IV therapy) 100–150 mg/kg/d PO ÷ q6h		
Charcoal, activated	See activated charcoal		

*†‡§¶Refer to legend on p. 889.

(continued)

Table IV.1 Drug Dosage Guidelines for Neonates* (Where Specified), Infants, and Older Children (*continued*)

Drug††§	Dose	Dose Limit	Comments
Chloral hydrate Syrup 100 mg/mL	*Neonates:* 10–50 mg/kg/dose PO/PR 3 or 4 times daily **Sedation preprocedure** 25–50 mg/kg/dose PO/PR *Infants and older children:* **Hypnotic** 50 mg/kg/dose PO/PR 20–45 min before examination; 25 mg/kg/dose PO/PR qhs prn **Sedation** 80–100 mg/kg PO/PR 20–45 min before procedure, may repeat with 40 mg/kg in 1 h	 1 g/dose 2 g/dose	Reduce dose in patients with CNS, renal or liver impairment. May cause gastric irritation; if possible, dilute dose or administer after feeding
Chloramphenicol sodium succinate Inj 1 g (base)/vial	**Meningitis** 75–100 mg/kg/d IV ÷ q6h **Other** 50–75 mg/kg/d IV ÷ q6h	4 g/d	Reduce dose in renal impairment; avoid in liver impairment; monitoring of serum drug concentration recommended
Chloroquine Tab 250 mg chloroquine phosphate = 150 mg base	**Malaria prophylaxis** 5 mg base/kg/dose PO given once weekly beginning 1–2 wk before entering malaria zone and continuing for 4 wk after leaving malarial area **Malaria treatment** 10 mg base/kg/dose PO × 1 dose, 5 mg base/kg/dose PO 6 h later, then 5 mg base/kg/d PO daily × 2 d	300 mg base/dose First dose: 600 mg base; subsequent doses: 300 mg base	Give PO with food or milk; drug extremely bitter; tabs may be crushed and mixed with cereal, jam, or chocolate syrup; widely available as syrup in malaria-endemic countries

Chlorpromazine Tab 25, 50, 100 mg Suppos 100 mg Inj 25 mg/mL	**Nausea/vomiting** 0.5–1 mg/kg/dose PO q4–6h 0.5–1 mg/kg/dose IV/IM q6–8h 1 mg/kg/dose PR q6–8h **Psychosis** 0.5–1 mg/kg/dose PO q4–6h 0.5–1 mg/kg/dose IV/IM q6–8h	*<5 yr:* 40 mg/d IM/IV *5–12 yr:* 75 mg/d IM/IV	May cause significant hypotension when given IV; use with caution and monitor BP; give PO with food or milk
Ciprofloxacin Inj 2 mg/mL Tab 250, 500, 750 mg Susp 100 mg/mL	**Cystic fibrosis** 40 mg/kg/d PO ÷ bid; 30 mg/kg/d IV ÷ q8h **Fever/neutropenia** 20 mg/kg/d IV ÷ q12h **Urinary tract infection** 20–30 mg/kg/d PO ÷ bid; 15–20 mg/kg/d IV ÷ bid **Other indications** 30 mg/kg/d PO ÷ bid; 20 mg/kg/d IV ÷ q12h **Selected cases** 30 mg/kg/d IV ÷ q8h	1500 mg/d PO, 1200 mg/d IV 800 mg/d IV 1000 mg/d PO, 800 mg/d IV 1500 mg/d PO, 800 mg/d IV 1200 mg/d IV	Dose interval adjustment in renal impairment: moderate to severe, q18–24h; avoid concurrent administration with antacids, iron; may decrease clearance of warfarin, tacrolimus, cyclosporine, and other drugs Use with caution in patients with seizure disorders; monitor for arthralgias, tendonitis; maintain adequate fluid intake to prevent crystalluria
Cisapride Tab 10 mg (Special Access drug)	0.2 mg/kg/dose PO tid–qid Usual adult dose: 5–10 mg/dose up to qid	0.8 mg/kg/d or 40 mg/d, whichever is less	Need to assess risk for QT interval prolongation before prescribing; reduce dose in renal or liver impairment; contraindicated in premature infants <36 wk GA, from 0–3 mo after delivery date Many potential drug interactions; may alter absorption of other drugs
Clarithromycin Tab 250, 500 mg Susp 25 mg/mL	15 mg/kg/d PO ÷ q12h ***Mycobacterium avium complex*** 15–30 mg/kg/d PO ÷ q12h	1 g/d	Dose reduction in renal impairment: severe, 50%, give 1–2 doses daily; may decrease clearance of tacrolimus, cyclosporine, other drugs

(continued)

***§Refer to legend on p. 889.

907

Table IV.1 Drug Dosage Guidelines for Neonates* (Where Specified), Infants, and Older Children (continued)

Drug†§	Dose	Dose Limit	Comments
Clarithromycin—cont'd	**Helicobacter pylori–associated ulcer** *Children:* 15 mg/kg/d PO ÷ bid *Adolescents:* 250–500 mg/dose PO bid × 1–2 wk with omeprazole and amoxicillin or metronidazole; 2 wk of therapy preferred in children		
Clavulin	See amoxicillin/clavulanic acid		
Clindamycin (palmitate) Oral solution 15 mg base/mL Phosphate oral liquid (HSC) 30 mg base/mL Cap 150 mg Inj 900 mg/vial	*Neonates:* *<2 kg, 0–7 d:* 10 mg/kg/d IV ÷ q12h *<2 kg, >7 d:* 15 mg/kg/d IV/PO ÷ q8h *≥2 kg, 0–7 d:* 15 mg/kg/d IV/PO ÷ q8h *≥2 kg, >7 d:* 20 mg/kg/d IV/PO ÷ q6h		Do not administer PO to neonates <7 d old; use clindamycin phosphate (not palmitate) in neonates ≥7 d old for oral doses
	Infants and older children: **Mild to moderate infections** 20–30 mg/kg/d PO/IV ÷ q6–8h	1.8 g/d PO 2.7 g/d IV	Give cap PO with food or full glass of water to avoid esophageal ulceration
	Severe infections 30–40 mg/kg/d IV ÷ q6–8h	3.6 g/d IV	
	Penicillin-allergic neutropenic patient with fever 30 mg/kg/d IV ÷ q8h	600 mg/dose IV	
	Chloroquine-resistant *Falciparum* malaria 20–40 mg/kg/d IV/PO ÷ tid	2.7 g/d PO	Use with quinine/quinidine for chloroquine-resistant malaria only if patient is unable to take doxycycline or tetracycline

Clobazam Tab 10 mg Cap (HSC) 1, 1.5 mg	Initial dose: 0.25 mg/kg/d PO once daily hs or ÷ bid; increase gradually to 0.5 mg/kg/d PO ÷ bid-tid	Initial dose: 10 mg Max dose: 1 mg/kg/d or 80 mg	
Clonazepam Susp (HSC) 0.1 mg/mL Tab 0.5, 2 mg	≤ 30 kg, initial dose: 0.05 mg/kg/d PO ÷ bid or tid; increase by 0.05 mg/kg/d q3d pm up to 0.2 mg/kg/d >30 kg, initial dose: 1.5 mg/d PO ÷ tid, increasing by 0.5–1 mg/d q3d up to 20 mg/d PO ÷ tid	20 mg/d	Reduce dose in liver impairment
Clonidine Tab 0.1 mg Susp (HSC) 0.1 mg/mL	**Growth hormone stimulation test** SA (surface area) ≤ 0.39 m^2: 0.05 mg/dose 0.4–0.7 m^2: 0.1 mg/dose 0.71–1.1 m^2: 0.15 mg/dose >1.1 m^2: 0.2 mg/dose **Preoperative dose** 4 mcg/kg/dose PO 90 min before operation (0.004 mg/kg/dose)	0.2 mg/dose	
Clopidogrel Tab 75 mg	**Cardiac patients with stents** *Initial*: 1 mg/kg/dose PO once daily **Stroke** 10–<30 kg: ¼ tab (18.75 mg) 30–<50 kg: ½ tab (37.5 mg) 50–<70 kg: ¾ tab (56.25 mg) ≥ 70 kg: 1 tab (75 mg)	75 mg/d	Use with caution in liver impairment

(continued)

***§Refer to legend on p. 889.

Pediatric Drug Dosing Guidelines

IV

Table IV.1 — Drug Dosage Guidelines for Neonates* (Where Specified), Infants, and Older Children (continued)

Drug†‡§	Dose	Dose Limit	Comments
Cloxacillin Susp 25 mg/mL Cap 250, 500 mg Inj 0.5, 2 g/vial	*Neonates:* *<2 kg, 0–7 d:* **Meningitis** 100 mg/kg/d IV ÷ q12h **Other** 50 mg/kg/d PO/IV ÷ q12h *<2 kg, >7 d:* **Meningitis** 150 mg/kg/d IV ÷ q8h **Other** 75 mg/kg/d IV/PO ÷ q8h *≥2 kg, 0–7 d:* **Meningitis** 150 mg/kg/d IV ÷ q8h **Other** 75 mg/kg/d IV/PO ÷ q8h *≥2 kg, >7 d:* **Meningitis** 200 mg/kg/d IV ÷ q6h **Other** 100 mg/kg/d IV/PO ÷ q6h		
	Infants and older children: **Mild to moderate infections** 50–100 mg/kg/d PO/IV/IM ÷ q6h	4 g/d PO/IV/IM	Give PO on empty stomach (1 h ac or 2 h pc)
	Severe infections 150–200 mg/kg/d IV/IM ÷ q6h	12 g/d IV/IM	

Codeine Syrup 5 mg/mL Tab 15, 30 mg Inj 30 mg/mL	**Analgesic** 3-6 mg/kg/d PO ÷ q4-6h prn	1.5 mg/kg/dose Usual adult analgesic dose: 30-60 mg/dose	Max dose should not be given for >24 h; IM route should not be used; not recommended for IV use because of potential adverse effects
	Antitussive 0.8-1.2 mg/kg/d PO ÷ q4-6h	Antitussive dose: 20 mg/dose	
Colistin Inj 150 mg sodium colistimethate/vial (75 mg colistin base/mL)	150 mg base/d inhaled ÷ bid		
Cotrimoxazole Susp trimethoprim 8 mg/mL + sulfamethoxazole 40 mg/mL Pediatric tab trimethoprim 20 mg + sulfamethoxazole 100 mg Adult tab trimethoprim 80 mg + sulfamethoxazole 400 mg Inj (HSC) trimethoprim 16 mg/mL + sulfamethoxazole 80 mg/mL	**Bacterial infection, treatment** 8-12 mg trimethoprim/kg/d PO/IV ÷ q12h (includes 40-60 mg/kg/d sulfamethoxazole) **Prophylaxis: urinary tract infection** 2-5 mg trimethoprim/kg/d PO once daily **Prophylaxis: asplenia and <6 mo of age** 5 mg trimethoprim/kg/d PO once daily **Pneumocystis jiroveci (carinii)** **Treatment** 20 mg trimethoprim/kg/d IV/PO ÷ q6h (includes 100 mg/kg/d sulfamethoxazole) **Prophylaxis, hematology/oncology** 150 mg trimethoprim/m²/d or 5 mg/kg/d PO given as single daily dose or ÷ bid on 3 d/wk (consecutive or alternate days)	320 mg TMP/d (160 mg TMP/dose)	Maintain fluid intake; may be given with food; dose interval adjustment in renal impairment: moderate, q18h; severe, q24h Use with caution in patients with G6PD deficiency Do not give to infants <1 mo old

***§Refer to legend on p. 889.

(continued)

Table IV.1 Drug Dosage Guidelines for Neonates* (Where Specified), Infants, and Older Children (continued)

Drug†‡§	Dose	Dose Limit	Comments
Cotrimoxazole—cont'd	**Prophylaxis, HIV-infected / exposed children** 5 mg trimethoprim/kg/d 3 or 7 d/wk PO ÷ bid **Prophylaxis, other immunocompromised children** 2.5–5 mg trimethoprim/kg/d PO 3 × weekly as a single daily dose		
Cromoglycate sodium Inhalation solution 20 mg/2 mL Nasal drops 2% Ophthalmic drops 2%	**Inhalation solution** 20 mg bid-qid via nebulizer **Nasal drops:** 1–2 drops into each nostril up to 6 times/d **Ophthalmic drops** 2 drops into each eye qid		
Cyclosporine Regular (Sandimmune) Inj 50 mg/mL Microemulsion (Neoral) liquid 100 mg/mL Cap 10, 25, 50, 100 mg	Initial dose before TDM: **Bone marrow transplantation** 3 mg/kg/d IV ÷ q12h **Lung/renal transplantation** 10 mg/kg/d PO ÷ q12h **Cardiac transplantation** 1 mg/kg/d IV as continuous infusion or 3 mg/kg/d IV ÷ q12h		Monitoring of serum drug concentration recommended; maintenance doses must be individualized, based on factors such as disease state or type of transplant/time since transplantation; reduce dose in liver impairment Oral to IV dose conversion as follows: Solid organ transplant: 3:1 BMT: 2.3:1 Microemulsion may be taken with or without food as long as this is done consistently; it should always be taken with the same beverage (not grapefruit juice); may interact with many other medications

Danaparoid Inj 750 units/0.6 mL	30 units/kg IV loading dose, then 1.2-2.0 units/kg/h continuous IV infusion; 18 units/kg/dose SC q12h (36 units/kg/d)		Monitor anti-factor Xa activity immediately after bolus dose, then q4h until steady state has been achieved, then daily to maintain therapeutic level of 0.4–0.8 units/mL; contraindicated in severe renal impairment; warfarin considered contraindicated by some experts
Dapsone Tab 100 mg Susp (HSC) 2 mg/mL	**Pneumocystis pneumonia prophylaxis (hematology/oncology, BMT)** 2 mg/kg/d PO once daily	100 mg/d	Caution in patients with G6PD deficiency, hypersensitivity to sulfonamides; may cause photosensitivity; do not administer with antacids
Darbepoetin Inj	**Anemia of chronic renal failure** Initial dose: 0.45 mcg/kg IV/SC weekly	100 mg/d	Titrate dose according to hemoglobin level; in some patients, the dose interval may be extended and the dose adjusted proportionally
Desmopressin Intranasal solution 0.25 mg/2.5 mL Intranasal spray 0.25 mg/2.5 mL (10 mcg/spray) Inj 4, 15 mcg/mL Tab 100, 200 mcg	**Diabetes insipidus** Nasal: 5–20 mcg/d intranasally once daily or ÷ bid Oral: 100–1200 mcg/d PO ÷ bid-tid		Consider PO route for patients with diabetes insipidus who are unable to tolerate intranasal administration; start with low dose and titrate to effect; for enuresis, maintain lowest effective dosage × 4 wk, then taper by decreasing dose by 10 mcg/night each month, if possible
	Coagulopathy 0.3 mcg/kg/dose IV/SC	Coagulopathy: 25 mcg/dose	
	Enuresis Initial: 20 mg (10 mg in each nostril) qhs × 7 d; may increase dose q7d in 10-mcg increments up to 30–40 mcg qhs	Enuresis: 40 mcg/d	

***§Refer to legend on p. 889.

(continued)

Table IV.1 Drug Dosage Guidelines for Neonates* (Where Specified), Infants, and Older Children (continued)

Drug†‡§	Dose	Dose Limit	Comments
Dexamethasone Susp (HSC) 1 mg/mL Tab 0.5, 4 mg Inj 4 mg/mL	*Neonates:* Short course: 0.3–0.6 mg/kg/d IV/PO ÷ bid × 3 d Intermediate course: 0.3–0.6 mg/kg/d IV/PO ÷ bid × 3 d, then 0.15–0.3 mg/kg/d IV/PO ÷ bid × 3 d, then 0.075–0.15 mg/kg/d IV/PO ÷ bid × 3 d Long course (18 d): 0.5 mg/kg/d IV/PO ÷ bid × 3 d, then 0.25 mg/kg/d IV/PO ÷ bid × 3 d, then 0.125 mg/kg/d IV/PO ÷ bid × 3 d, then 0.06 mg/kg/d IV/PO once daily × 3 d, then 0.06 mg/kg/dose IV/PO every other day × 7 d Long course (42 d): 0.5 mg/kg/d IV/PO ÷ bid × 3 d, then 0.25 mg/kg/d IV/PO ÷ bid × 3 d; reduce dose by 10% q3d until day 34, then 0.1 mg/kg/d IV/PO × 3 d, then 0.1 mg/kg/dose every other day × 7 d		Avoid in children with peptic ulcer disease; give PO with food or milk; to discontinue in patients receiving therapy for ≥10 d, reduce dose by 50% q48h until 0.3 ± 0.1 mg/m²/d achieved, then reduce dose by 50% q10–14d; in meningitis, administer first dose before antibiotics; dexamethasone may be contraindicated if the antineoplastic protocol prohibits its use as an antiemetic or in patients receiving treatment for brain tumors; this contraindication may be re-evaluated based on patient response
	Subglottic edema 1 mg/kg/dose PO/IV tid × 2 d, then reassess	20 mg/dose	
	Infants and older children: **Extubation (if previous difficulties)** 1–2 mg/kg/d PO/IV/IM ÷ q6h beginning before extubation and continuing 24–48 h afterward		
	Increased ICP 0.2–0.4 mg/kg IV, then 0.3 mg/kg/d IV/IM ÷ q6h; may be useful in cerebral tumors and malaria but not in head injuries	Initial dose: 10 mg	

		20 mg/dose (PO)	
	Croup 0.6 mg/kg IV × 1 1 mg/kg/dose PO, usually × 1 dose		
	Acute asthma: 0.3 mg/kg/d PO once daily **Meningitis:** 0.6 mg/kg/d IV ÷ q6h × 4 d		
	Antiemetic for antineoplastic regimens Very highly emetogenic regimen: 8 mg/m²/dose PO/IV prechemotherapy, then q12h thereafter	20 mg/dose	
	Highly emetogenic regimen: 4.5 mg/m²/dose PO/IV prechemotherapy, then once daily thereafter	8 mg/dose	
Dextromethorphan Liquid 3 mg/mL	1 mg/kg/d PO ÷ q6-8h	1 mg/kg/d (usual adult dose: 10-20 mg PO q4h prn)	
Dextrose Inj, preloaded 500 mg/mL (50%)	*Neonates:* Transient hypoglycemia: 5-7 mg/kg/min IV Acute hypoglycemia Loading dose: 0.1-0.2 g/kg IV Maintenance dose: 5-7 mg/kg/min IV		Dilute to 25% for neonates and young children; follow bolus dose by a continuous dextrose infusion; except in emergency, administer solutions >15% via central line
	Infants and older children: **Hypoglycemia** 0.5-1 g/kg/dose IV (1-2 mL/kg/dose)	Usual adult dose: 10-25 g	

(continued)

***§Refer to legend on p. 889.

Table IV.1 Drug Dosage Guidelines for Neonates* (Where Specified), Infants, and Older Children *(continued)*

Drug††§	Dose	Dose Limit	Comments
Diazepam Tab 2, 5 mg Inj 5 mg/mL Inj (Diazemuls) 5 mg/mL	*Neonates:* 0.1–0.2 mg/kg/dose IV *Infants and older children:* 0.1–0.8 mg/kg/d PO ÷ q6h **Status epilepticus** 0.3 mg/kg/dose IV q10min × 2 or 0.5 mg/kg/dose PR × 1 **Preoperative** 0.1–0.5 mg/kg/dose PO 30–90 min before surgery **Sedation** 0.1 mg/kg/dose IV; 0.2 mg/kg/dose PO given 45–60 min before procedure	2–10 mg/dose bid–qid PO Status epilepticus <5 yr: 5 mg/dose IV ≥5 yr: 10 mg/dose IV 20 mg/dose PO Usual adult dose for sedation: 5–10 mg/dose IV; 20 mg/dose PO	Neonates: administer at rate not to exceed 0.05 mg/kg/min May cause hypotension and apnea when given IV; Diazemuls is preferred product for IV sedation; for rectal doses, administer diazepam injection, undiluted; reduce dose in liver impairment
Didanosine Susp 10 mg/mL (Special Access drug) EC caps: 125, 200, 250, 400 mg	*<4 mo:* 100 mg/m²/d PO ÷ bid *4–8 mo:* 200 mg/m²/d PO ÷ bid *>8 mo:* usual dose 240 mg/m²/d PO ÷ bid (range: 180–300 mg/m²/d PO ÷ bid) EC caps: 240 mg/m²/d PO as single daily dose	Adult usual dose: ≥60 kg: 400 mg/d <60 kg: 250 mg/d	Reduce dose in renal impairment; use with caution in hepatic impairment; may cause pancreatitis, peripheral neuropathy, headache, diarrhea; give higher doses if risk of CNS disease, especially in developmental delay
Digoxin Elixir 50 mcg/mL Tab 62.5, 125, 250 mcg Inj (HSC) 10, 50 mcg/mL	*Neonates, infants, and older children:* **Digitalization (or loading) dose:** (3 doses: first stat, second in 6 h, third in another 6 h) *<37 wk PCA:*	Total digitalization dose: 1000 mcg	Do not administer IM; calculate dose according to ideal body weight; reduce dose in renal and hepatic impairment Digitalization (or loading) dose adjustment in renal impairment: severe, 50–65%; maintenance dose adjustment in renal impairment:

7 mcg/kg/dose PO; 5 mcg/kg/dose IV ≥37 wk PCA–2 yr: 17 mcg/kg/dose PO; 12 mcg/kg/dose IV >2 yr: 13 mcg/kg/dose PO; 10 mcg/kg/dose IV		moderate, 25–75%; severe, 10–25%; dose reduction for drug interactions: amiodarone, propafenone, quinidine–50%; carvedilol–25%; many other drugs may interact with digoxin; once-daily dosing may be satisfactory, especially in patients >2 yr Dose conversion: IV dose = oral dose × 0.7 Oral dose = IV dose × 1.4 Digoxin antibody (Digibind) is available to treat potentially life-threatening digoxin toxicity
Maintenance dose *<37 wk PCA:* 4 mcg/kg/d PO ÷ q12h 3 mcg/kg/d IV ÷ q12h *≥37 wk PCA–2 yr:* 10 mcg/kg/d PO ÷ q12h 7 mcg/kg/d IV÷ q12h *>2 yr:* 8 mcg/kg/d PO ÷ bid or as a single daily dose	Maintenance dose: 250 mcg/d	
Dimenhydrinate Liquid 3 mg/mL Tab 50 mg Suppos 25, 50 mg Inj 50 mg/mL	5 mg/kg/d PO/IV/IM/PR ÷ q6h	300 mg/d	

(continued)

Table IV.1 Drug Dosage Guidelines for Neonates* (Where Specified), Infants, and Older Children (continued)

Drug[††§]	Dose	Dose Limit	Comments
Dinoprostone (PGE₂) Solution: Dissolve 'n' Dose system Tab 500 mcg	*Neonates:* 40–50 mcg/kg/dose PO q2h; titrate dose and frequency to effect		Monitor for fever, diarrhea; tab may be administered by Dissolve 'n' Dose system: dissolve 1 tab in 10 mL water immediately before use to make 50 mcg/mL solution
Diphenhydramine Elixir 2.5 mg/mL Cap 50 mg Tab 25 mg Inj 50 mg/mL	**Antihistamine:** 5 mg/kg/d PO/IV/IM ÷ q6h **Anaphylaxis:** 1–2 mg/kg/dose IV	300 mg/d 50 mg/dose	
Dipyridamole Susp (HSC) 10 mg/mL Tab 25, 50 mg Inj 5 mg/mL	5 mg/kg/d PO ÷ tid	400 mg/d	Give on an empty stomach (1 h ac or 2 h pc)
Dobutamine Inj 250 mg/vial	*Neonates:* 5–25 mcg/kg/min IV *Infants and older children:* 2–30 mcg/kg/min IV	40 mcg/kg/min	Avoid extravasation; administer via central line, whenever possible
Docusate sodium Liquid 4 mg/mL Cap 100 mg	5 mg/kg/d PO ÷ q6–8h or as a single daily dose	Usual adult dose: 100–200 mg/d	Dilute liquid in milk or juice Onset of action, 24–72 h

Domperidone Tab 10 mg Susp (HSC) 5 mg/mL	1.2-2.4 mg/kg/d PO ÷ tid-qid; give 15-30 min ac + qhs	80 mg/d; usual adult dose: 10 mg tid-qid	Dose adjustment in renal impairment: extend interval to once or twice daily; consider dose reduction in more severe impairment; use with caution in patients with hepatic impairment
Dopamine Inj 200 mg/250mL (800 mcg/mL), 800 mg/ 250 mL (3200 mcg/mL)	*Neonates, infants, and older children:* 5-20 mcg/kg/min via continuous IV infusion	20 mcg/kg/min	Neonates may be less sensitive to dopamine than older infants and children; avoid dopamine >10 mcg/kg/min in neonates with PPHN; avoid extravasation; administer via central venous line whenever possible; do not dilute premixed bags
Dornase alfa Inj 1 mg/mL	2.5 mg via nebulizer once daily (twice-daily dosing may be used if forced vital capacity is >85%)		Administer undiluted; do not mix with other drugs in nebulizer
Doxazosin Tab 1, 2, 4 mg	*Initial:* 1 mg/d PO as single daily dose *Maintenance:* 1-4 mg PO daily	Adult max dose: 16 mg/d	Dose should be titrated q2wk until adequate blood pressure is achieved or dose-limiting side effects appear Monitor for syncope and postural hypotension with first dose
Doxycycline Susp (HSC) 5 mg/mL Cap 100 mg	2-4 mg/kg/d PO ÷ q12h	200 mg/d	May be given with food; not recommended for children <8 yr
	Chloroquine-resistant (*Falciparum*) malaria *Treatment:* 4 mg/kg/d PO ÷ bid × 7 d *Prophylaxis:* 2 mg/kg/d PO as single daily dose	200 mg/d 100 mg/d	
	Pelvic inflammatory disease ≥8 yr: 100 mg/dose PO bid		

continued

***§Refer to legend on p. 889.

Table IV.1 Drug Dosage Guidelines for Neonates* (Where Specified), Infants, and Older Children (continued)

Drug†‡§	Dose			Dose Limit	Comments
Edrophonium Inj 10 mg/mL	**Supraventricular tachycardia** 0.2 mg/kg/dose IV over 3 min			10 mg/dose	Have atropine ready
EMLA (lidocaine-prilocaine) Cream 5, 30 g Patch 1 g (25 mg/g lidocaine, 25 mg/g prilocaine)	**Age** >1–3 mo >3–12 mo and >5 kg 1–6 yr and >10 kg 7–12 yr and >20 kg	**Max skin area (cm²)** 10 20 100 200	**Dose** 1 g/h 2 g/4h 10 g/4 h 20 g/4 h		Methemoglobinemia risk; do not give to children 0–12 mo of age who are receiving other methemoglobin-inducing agents Contraindicated in G6PD deficiency
Enalapril Tab 2.5, 5 mg Susp (HSC) 1 mg/mL	**Hypertension, CHF** *Initial:* 0.1 mg/kg/d PO as single daily dose or ÷ bid				Dose adjustment in renal impairment: moderate, 75–100% of standard dose; severe, 50% of standard dose; use lower initial doses in patients with hyponatremia or hypovolemia or in patients receiving concurrent diuretics
	Maintenance: 0.1–0.5 mg/kg/d PO as a single daily dose or ÷ bid			40 mg/d	
Enalaprilat Inj 2.5 mg/2 mL	5–10 mcg/kg/dose IV q8–24h				Monitor blood pressure and renal function; IV (enalaprilat) and PO (enalapril) doses are *not* equivalent
Enoxaparin Inj 100 mg/mL	*Neonates and infants:* ≤2 mo: Initial treatment dose: 1.75 mg/kg/dose SC q12h Initial prophylactic dose: 0.75 mg/kg/dose SC q12h OR 1.5 mg/kg/dose SC once daily			Age ≤ 2 mo: 6 mg/kg/d	See protocol for low molecular weight heparin therapy, p. 468, for more information; hold for 2 doses before invasive procedures such as lumbar puncture and measure anti-factor Xa (low molecular weight heparin level)

Epinephrine Inj 0.1 mg/mL (1:10,000), 1 mg/mL (1:1000)	**>2 mo–18 yr:** Initial treatment dose: 1 mg/kg/dose SC q12h Initial prophylactic dose: 0.5 mg/kg/dose SC q12h OR 1 mg/kg/dose SC once daily	Age >2 mo: 4 mg/kg/d (treatment), 40 mg once daily (prophylaxis)	
	Neonates: **Resuscitation** 0.01 mg/kg/dose (0.1 mL/kg/dose of 1:10,000 solution) IV or 0.05 mg/kg/dose (0.5 mL/kg/dose of 1:10,000 solution) ETT q3–5min prn **Other** 0.05–1 mcg/kg/min IV		Verify concentration of solution before use; for ETT administration, follow or dilute with 0.5–1 mL 0.9% NaCl; incompatible with sodium bicarbonate; administer via central venous line, whenever possible
	Infants and older children: **Anaphylaxis** 0.01 mg/kg/dose (0.01 mL of 1:1000 solution/kg/dose) SC/IM q10–20min prn, min 0.1 mg/dose	0.5 mg/dose	
	Resuscitation 0.01 mg/kg/dose (0.1 mL/kg/dose of 1:10,000 solution) IV/IO q3–5min prn	1 mg (10 mL) IV/IO	
	IV infusion: 0.1–1 mcg/kg/min via continuous IV infusion		
	Inhalation: (1:1000, 1 mg/mL solution) *<5 kg:* 0.5 mg/dose *≥5 kg:* 2.5–5 mg/dose Dilute dose to 2.5 or 3 mL in 0.9% NaCl, give via nebulizer prn to max q1h as above		

(continued)

***Refer to legend on p. 889.

Table IV.1 Drug Dosage Guidelines for Neonates* (Where Specified), Infants, and Older Children (continued)

Drug†‡§	Dose	Dose Limit	Comments
Epoetin alfa Inj preloaded 1000, 2000, 3000, 4000, 10,000 units Inj 20,000 units/vial	**Anemia of chronic renal failure** Initial dose: 50 units/kg/d IV/SC 3 × weekly		Titrate dose according to hemoglobin
Erythromycins Base: tab 250 mg Estolate: susp 50 mg/mL Lactobionate: inj 0.5, 1 g/vial	*Neonates:* **Lactobionate** 20–40 mg/kg/d IV ÷ q6h **Estolate** <2 kg, 0–7 d: 20 mg/kg/d PO ÷ q12h <2 kg, >7 d: 30 mg/kg/d PO q8h ≥2 kg, 0–7 d: 20 mg/kg/d PO ÷ q12h ≥2 kg, >7 d: 30–40 mg/kg/d PO ÷ q8h		Assess risk–benefit in full-term infants <14 d of age due to association with infantile hypertrophic pyloric stenosis; dose reduction in renal impairment: severe, 50–75% of dose; estolate contraindicated in patients with hepatic dysfunction; use other erythromycins with caution in these patients; clearance of drugs including cyclosporine, tacrolimus, and carbamazepine will be decreased; use base for patients with cystic fibrosis; give PO on empty stomach (1 h ac or 2 h pc) unless GI upset occurs
	Infants and older children: **Base** 30–50 mg/kg/d PO ÷ q6h	2 g/d PO	
	Estolate 30–50 mg/kg/d PO ÷ q6–12h	2 g/d PO	
	Lactobionate 20–50 mg/kg/d IV ÷ q6h	4 g/d IV	
Esmolol Inj 10 mg/mL, 250 mg/mL	Bolus/loading dose: 100–500 mcg/kg IV over 1 min Maintenance: 100–300 mcg/kg/min IV as continuous infusion		Max concentration for PIV administration: 10 mg/mL; for concentrations >10 mg/mL, administer via central venous line

Ethambutol Tab 100, 400 mg	**Tuberculosis** 15 mg/kg/d PO as single daily dose or 50 mg/kg/dose PO twice weekly	2.5 g/dose	Give with food if GI upset occurs; dose interval adjustment in renal impairment: moderate, q24–36h; severe, q48h and/or reduce dose Regular ophthalmic examinations recommended in patients receiving >15 mg/kg/d; less risk of optic neuritis at 15 mg/kg/d Bacteriostatic at 15 mg/kg/d, but will help prevent development of resistance; bacteriocidal at 25 mg/kg/d
Ethosuximide Syrup 50 mg/mL Cap 250 mg	15 mg/kg/d PO as single daily dose or ÷ bid; increase gradually q3d prn to max dose	1.5 g/d or 40 mg/kg/d, whichever is less	Reduce dose in liver impairment; monitoring of serum drug concentration recommended; give with food or milk
Fentanyl Inj 50 mcg/mL Transdermal patch: 25, 50, 75, 100 mcg/h	*Neonates:* **Sedation/Analgesia** 1 mcg/kg/dose IV, then 0.5–2 mcg/kg/h IV infusion; titrate upward Mean required dose: *GA <34 wk:* 0.64 mcg/kg/h *GA ≥34 wk:* 0.75 mcg/kg/h **Rapid sequence intubation** 2 mcg/kg/dose IV *Infants and older children:* Continuous IV infusion: 0.5–2 mcg/kg/h Patch: >12 yr, initial: 25 mcg/h		Reduce dose in renal or hepatic failure; patch is not for acute pain; use only for established pain and in patients with stable opioid requirements
Ferrous sulfate/ferrous fumarate	See iron		

†‡§Refer to legend on p. 889.

(continued)

Pediatric Drug Dosing Guidelines

IV

Table IV.1 Drug Dosage Guidelines for Neonates* (Where Specified), Infants, and Older Children (continued)

Drug†§	Dose	Dose Limit	Comments
Filgrastim (G-CSF) Inj 300 mcg/mL	5 mcg/kg/d SC/IV as single daily dose; if response marginal after a cycle of chemotherapy, increase dose to 10 mcg/kg/d SC/IV as single daily dose after next and subsequent cycles	10 mcg/kg/d	
Flecainide Susp (HSC) 20 mg/mL Tab 100 mg	**Supraventricular tachycardia** Initial dose: 1-3 mg/kg/d PO ÷ tid OR 50-100 mg/m²/d PO ÷ tid	8 mg/kg/d or 200 mg/m²/d	Dose adjustment in renal impairment: CrCl <20 mL/min/1.73 m², give 50-75% of usual dose Use with caution in patients with underlying structural heart disease Avoid concurrent administration with milk or milk-based formulas; use caution when diet changes to decreased consumption of milk or milk-based formulas as increased absorption may occur
Fluconazole Susp 10 mg/mL Tab 50, 100 mg Inj 200 mg/vial	*Neonates:* Loading dose: 12 mg/kg IV/PO on day 1 Maintenance dose: 6 mg/kg IV/PO, as per intervals below: <30 wk GA and 0-14 d PNA: q72h <30 wk GA and >14 d PNA: q48h 30-36 wk GA and 0-14 d: q48h 30-36 wk GA and >14 d: q24h 37-44 wk GA and 0-14 d: q48h 37-44 wk GA and >14 d: q24h >45 wk GA and all PNAs: q24h *Infants and older children:* 3-12 mg/kg/d PO/IV as single daily dose	400 mg/d	Use with caution in patients with liver impairment; interval adjustment in renal impairment: moderate, q48h; severe, q72h OR adjust dose (not interval); moderate, 50% usual dose; severe, 25% usual dose; hemodialysis: dose after each dialysis May decrease clearance of tacrolimus, cyclosporine, phenytoin, and other medications; monitor carefully in patients also taking warfarin

Oropharyngeal candidiasis 3 mg/kg/d PO once daily	200 mg/d PO	
Esophageal candidiasis 6–12 mg/kg/d PO once daily	400 mg/d PO	
Secondary prophylaxis of candidiasis in HIV-infected patients 3–5 mg/kg/d PO once daily		
BMT prophylaxis 5 mg/kg/d PO/IV as daily dose beginning day 0 and continuing until ANC ≥ 0.5×10^9 (usually day +14 to day +21)	400 mg/d	
Flucytosine Inj (HSC) 10 mg/mL (Special Access drug)	*Neonates:* 50–150 mg/kg/d IV ÷ q6h *Infants and older children:* 100–150 mg/kg/d IV ÷ q6h	Dose interval adjustment in renal failure: moderate, q12–24h; severe, q24–48h; monitoring of serum drug concentration recommended
Fludrocortisone Tab 0.1 mg	**Salt-losing hypoadrenalism** 0.05–0.2 mg/d PO ÷ q12h	Give with food or milk; monitor BP, serum electrolytes; dosage must be individualized; infants have relatively higher dosage requirements
Fluticasone Inhalation 50, 125, 250 mcg/puff	Moderate dose: 250–500 mcg/d ÷ bid High dose: >500 mcg/d ÷ bid	High doses not recommended beyond 14 d unless under the care of an asthma specialist because of risk of adrenal insufficiency Monitor for signs of systemic corticosteroid adverse effects
Fomepizole Inj 1000 mg/mL	Loading dose: 15 mg/kg IV Maintenance dose: 10 mg/kg/dose IV q12h × 4 doses, then 15 mg/kg/dose IV q12h	Consult toxicologists or poison center for management of patients with methanol or ethylene glycol intoxication; dose adjustment required for dialysis patients; must be diluted for administration

(continued)

*†‡§Refer to legend on p. 889.

Table IV.1 Drug Dosage Guidelines for Neonates* (Where Specified), Infants, and Older Children (continued)

Drug††§	Dose	Dose Limit	Comments
Fosphenytoin Inj 50 mg PE/mL	**Status epilepticus** Loading dose: 15–20 mg PE/kg IV/IM × 1 Maintenance: 4–6 mg PE/kg IV/IM q24h		Calculate loading dose using effective body weight; fosphenytoin should be prescribed in PE units; fosphenytoin 1.5 mg = phenytoin 1 mg = fosphenytoin 1 mg PE Reduce dose in liver failure; monitoring of serum drug concentration recommended
Furosemide Liquid 10 mg/mL Tab 20, 40 mg Inj 10 mg/mL	*Neonates:* 1–2 mg/kg/dose IV/PO given as required or q12–24h *Infants and older children:* 1–2 mg/kg/d PO; may increase to 3–8 mg/kg/d PO ÷ q6–8h prn; 0.5–2 mg/kg/dose IV/IM	6 mg/kg/dose PO 80 mg/dose PO/IM/IV	Use with caution in patients with hypokalemia, hypovolemia; monitor fluid balance and serum electrolytes, especially potassium; may displace bilirubin in neonates
Gabapentin Cap 100, 300, 400 mg Susp (HSC) 100 mg/mL Tab 600 mg	Initial dose: 20–30 mg/kg/d PO ÷ tid, increase dose gradually over 3–7 d Maintenance dose: 20–50 mg/kg/d PO ÷ tid *Adolescents, adults:* Initial dose: 300 mg PO once on day 1, 300 mg PO bid on day 2, 300 mg PO tid on day 3 Maintenance dose: 900–1800 mg/d PO ÷ tid	3600 mg/d (short-term) 2400 mg/d (long-term)	Dose adjustment in renal impairment: mild, 50% standard dose; moderate, 25% standard dose; severe, 12.5% standard dose
Ganciclovir Inj 50 mg/mL	**CMV infection** Treatment: 10 mg/kg/d IV ÷ q12h **Allogenic bone marrow transplant prophylaxis** Day −8 to day 0: 10 mg/kg/d IV ÷ q12h		Handle as a biohazard; discontinue in BMT patients if ANC <0.5 × 10⁹ consult product monograph for dose and interval adjustment in impaired renal function

	Posttransplantation when ANC ≥1 5 mg/kg/d IV once daily **Solid organ transplant prophylaxis, EBV/CMV high risk** 10 mg/kg/d IV + q12h × 14 d, then 5 mg/kg/d IV + q24h × 10 wk	
Gentamicin Inj 10 mg/mL, 40 mg/mL	*Neonates PCA:* 0–7 d, <34 wk PCA: 3 mg/kg/dose IV q24h 0–7 d, ≥34 wk PCA: 3 mg/kg/dose IV q18h >7 d, ≤1 kg: 3.5 mg/kg/dose IV q24h >7 d, >1 kg, <37 wk PCA: 2.5 mg/kg/dose IV q12h >7 d, >1 kg, ≥37 wk PCA: 2.5 mg/kg/dose IV q8h	Monitoring of serum drug concentration recommended
	Gut sterilization: 10–15 mg/kg/d PO + q8h *Infants and older children:* 7.5 mg/kg/d IV/IM + q8h **Fever and neutropenia** 1 mo–<9 yr: 10 mg/kg/dose IV/IM q24h 9–12 yr: 8 mg/kg/dose IV/IM q24h ≥12 yr: 6 mg/kg/dose IV/IM q24h	120 mg/dose before TDM	Dose interval adjustment in renal impairment for infants and older children: mild–moderate, q12h; severe, q24–48h Calculate dose according to effective body weight
Glucagon Inj 1 mg/vial	*Neonates:* 0.5–1 mg/d IV via continuous infusion; if IV access not available, may give 0.1 mg/kg/dose IM q3–4h to max total dose of 1 mg/d		For neonates, dilute in D5W or D10W to 24 mL

(continued)

***§Refer to legend on p. 889.

Table IV.1 — Drug Dosage Guidelines for Neonates* (Where Specified), Infants, and Older Children (continued)

Drug†‡§	Dose	Dose Limit	Comments
Glucagon—cont'd	*Infants and older children:* **Hypoglycemia** ≤20 kg: 0.02–0.03 mg/kg/dose IM/IV/SC; max 0.5 mg >20 kg: 1 mg/dose IM/IV/SC May repeat in 20 min prn		
GoLYTELY	See PEG electrolyte		
Granisetron Inj 1 mg/mL	20 mcg/kg/dose IV/PO prechemotherapy and q12h		Use with caution in hepatic impairment
Growth hormone 5 mg/vial	0.06 mg/kg/dose IM/SC 3 × weekly		
Haloperidol Solution 2 mg/mL Tab 0.5, 1, 2, 5 mg Inj 5 mg/mL	*Children 3–12 yr (15–40 kg):* Initial: 0.25–0.5 mg/d PO + bid-tid; increase by 0.25–0.5 mg q5-7d Maintenance: **Agitation/hyperkinesia** 0.01–0.03 mg/kg/d PO once daily **Tourette disorder** 0.05–0.075 mg/kg/d PO + bid-tid **Psychotic disorder** 0.05–0.15 mg/kg/d PO + bid-tid 6–12 yr: IM (lactate) 1–3 mg/dose q4-8h	0.15 mg/kg/d: adult dose, 0.5–5 mg/dose; usual max 30 mg/d PO 0.15 mg/kg/d IM	Use with caution in cardiac disease because of hypotension and in patients with epilepsy (lowers seizure threshold) Extrapyramidal side effects in patients 6–12 yr; switch to oral therapy as soon as able

Heparin Inj 100 units/mL, 1000 units/mL, 10,000 units/mL	*Neonates:* **Maintenance of indwelling lines** ≤1800 g: 0.5 unit/mL >1800 g: 1 unit/mL	Monitor PTT and/or anti-factor Xa and titrate infusion rate accordingly; avoid concurrent use of ASA or other antiplatelet drugs; antidote: protamine sulfate
	Thrombosis Loading dose: 50-100 units/kg IV Maintenance: 20-30 units/kg/h IV via continuous infusion *Infants and older children:* Loading dose: 75 units/kg IV over 10 min Initial maintenance dose: ≤1 yr: 28 units/kg/h IV >1 yr: 20 units/kg/h IV	Guidelines for Unfractionated Heparin Therapy (Thrombosis Guidelines)
Hydralazine Inj 20 mg/mL Oral solution (HSC) 1 mg/mL Tab 10, 25, 50 mg	*Neonates:* 1.7-3.5 mg/kg/d IV ÷ q4-6h 0.75-5 mg/kg/d PO ÷ q6h *Infants and older children:* Initial dose: 0.15-0.8 mg/kg/dose IV q4-6h OR 1.5 mcg/kg/min IV Maintenance: 0.75-7 mg/kg/d PO ÷ q6h	20 mg/dose IV 7 mg/kg/d PO or 200 mg/d PO, whichever is less	Interval adjustment in renal impairment: mild to moderate, q8h; severe, q8-24h; associated with development of drug-induced lupus
Hydrochlorothiazide Susp (HSC) 5 mg/mL Tab 25, 50 mg	2-4 mg/kg/d PO ÷ q12h	Usual adult dose: 25- 100 mg/dose PO as single daily dose, bid or q2d	Ineffective when GFR <30 mL/min

(continued)

***Refer to legend on p. 889.

Pediatric Drug Dosing Guidelines

IV

Table IV.1 Drug Dosage Guidelines for Neonates* (Where Specified), Infants, and Older Children (continued)

Drug[++§]	Dose	Dose Limit	Comments
Hydrocortisone Susp (HSC) 1 mg/mL Tab 10, 20 mg Hydrocortisone sodium succinate inj 100, 250, 500, 1000 mg/vial	**Acute asthma** 4–6 mg/kg/dose IV q4–6h **Anaphylaxis** 5–10 mg/kg IV **Hypoadrenalism** (Normal endogenous production = 10 ± 3 mg/m²/d) Maintenance dose: 20 mg/m²/d PO ÷ tid 12 mg/m²/d IV ÷ q6h Preop: 100 mg/m² IV × 1 preoperatively, then 100 mg/m²/d IV ÷ q6h **Acute adrenal crisis** 100 mg/m² IV, then 100 mg/m²/d IV ÷ q6h		Triple the maintenance dose during concurrent illness or stress; in congenital adrenal hyperplasia (CAH), administer ½ daily dose at bedtime to suppress A.M. surge of ACTH; to suppress A.M. surge of ACTH; give PO with food or milk; to discontinue in patients receiving therapy ≥10 d, reduce dose by 50% q48h until 10 ± 3 mg/m²/d achieved, then reduce by 50% q10–14d
Hydromorphone Inj 2 mg/mL, 10 mg/mL Syrup: 1 mg/mL Tablet: 2, 4, 8 mg Cap CR 3, 6, 12, 18, 24, 30 mg	Intermittent IV: 15–20 mcg/kg/dose IV q2–4h Continuous infusion: 4–6 mcg/kg/h IV *Children ≤50 kg:* 0.04–0.08 mg/kg/dose PO q3–4h prn *Children >50 kg:* 2–4 mg/dose PO q3–4h prn; patients with prior opiate exposure may tolerate higher doses	2–4 mg/dose PO (up to 8 mg/ dose PO has been used)	Reduce dose in renal or hepatic impairment Administer with or after food to decrease GI upset; if oral liquid spills on skin, remove contaminated clothing and rinse area with cool water
Hydroxyzine Syrup 2 mg/mL Cap 10, 25 mg	2 mg/kg/d PO ÷ tid or qid **Chronic urticaria** 2–4 mg/kg/d PO ÷ tid or qid	400 mg/d	

Ibuprofen		
Susp 20 mg/mL	**Antipyretic**	40 mg/kg/d; max adult dose: 2400 mg/d	Do not use in patients with renal impairment; use with caution in patients with hepatic impairment, compromised cardiac function, or hypertension (may cause fluid retention, edema), or history of GI bleeding or ulcers; may inhibit platelet aggregation (duration of effect, ~5–10 h); monitor closely patients who may be adversely affected by prolonged bleeding times; give with food to minimize GI upset; may increase serum concentrations of digoxin, methotrexate, lithium; recommended as antipyretic for children with fever unresponsive to maximal doses of acetaminophen or in children intolerant to acetaminophen
Tab 200, 300, 400, 600 mg	<6 *mo:* 5 mg/kg/dose PO q8h		
	6 *mo–12 yr:* 5–10 mg/kg/dose PO q6-8h		
	Analgesic		
	6 *mo–12 yr:* 5–10 mg/kg/dose PO q6-8h		
	Anti-inflammatory (rheumatology)		
	20–40 mg/kg/d PO ÷ tid–qid		

Immune globulin (human, IV)		
Inj 5%, 10%	**Hypogammaglobulinemia**		
	600 mg/kg/dose IV once monthly		
	BMT		
	200–500 mg/kg/dose IV once weekly		
	Idiopathic thrombocytopenic purpura		
	0.8–1 g/kg/dose IV × 1 and reassess in 24–48 h		
	Kawasaki disease		
	2 g/kg IV as single dose	70 g	
	Polymyositis, dermatomyositis		
	1 g/kg/dose IV once daily × 2 subsequent days monthly		
	Guillain-Barré syndrome		
	1 g/kg/dose IV once daily × 2 d		

***Refer to legend on p. 889.**

(continued)

Pediatric Drug Dosing Guidelines

IV

931

Table IV.1 Drug Dosage Guidelines for Neonates* (Where Specified), Infants, and Older Children (*continued*)

Drug†§	Dose	Dose Limit	Comments
	JIA 1.5 g/kg/d IV once monthly **Perinatal AIDS** 400 mg/kg/dose IV once monthly	70 g	
Indomethacin Susp (HSC) 5 mg/mL Cap 25, 50 mg Inj 1 mg/vial	*Neonates:* **Patent ductus arteriosus** 0.2 mg/kg/dose IV q12h × 3 doses		Reduce doses of aminoglycosides and digoxin to half until good urine output returns; infuse over 20 min; in patients with renal impairment, dose at 0.1 mg/kg/dose IV q24h × 5–6 doses
	Infants and older children: 1.5–3 mg/kg/d PO ÷ tid with meals	200 mg/d	Give with food or milk
Infliximab Inj 100 mg/vial	**Active or refractory Crohn disease (with or without fistulas)** 5 mg/kg IV given as induction at 0, 2, and 6 wk followed by maintenance of 5 mg/kg IV q8wk If incomplete response, dose can be increased to 10 mg/kg		Infuse over 2–3 h to prevent acute infusion reactions
Insulin Lispro insulin inj 100 units/mL	*Neonates:* **Hyperglycemia** 0.01–0.02 unit/kg/h IV via continuous infusion **Hyperkalemia** 0.3 unit/g of dextrose IV		Titrate infusion according to blood glucose; use regular insulin only for infusions

	Infants and older children:	
	Diabetes	
	SC or IV as needed (see Endocrinology section)	
Iodine Lugol solution 126 mg elemental iodine/mL (as 100 mg/mL potassium iodide, 50 mg/mL iodine)	**Radiation protection** 30 mg elemental iodine/d PO as single daily dose	100 mg elemental iodine daily	Dilute in 1 glassful of water, juice, or milk; give with food or milk; duration of treatment depends on type of radiation exposure
Ipratropium Metered-dose aerosol (HFA) 20 mcg/puff Inhalation solution 250 mcg/mL	*Neonates:* 0.125 mg (0.5 mL)/dose tid-qid prn via nebulizer		Dilute to a total of 3 mL with normal saline if required; may be mixed with salbutamol and/or budesonide solutions immediately before administration
	Infants and older children: **Metered-dose aerosol** 20–40 mcg tid or qid via inhalation **Inhalation solution** 250 mcg/dose, given in 3 mL 0.9% NaCl via nebulizer tid–qid prn; in severe acute asthma, may be given q20min	Metered-dose aerosol: 240 mcg/d Usual adult dose: 250–500 mcg/dose in 3 mL 0.9% NaCl via nebulizer q4–6h prn	
Iron Susp 60 mg/mL ferrous fumarate (20 mg elemental iron/mL) Tab 300 mg ferrous sulfate (60 mg elemental iron)	*Neonates:* **Supplementation** (prematurity, long-term PN) *Birth weight (BW)* ≥ *1000 g:* 2–3 mg elemental iron/kg/d PO daily *BW < 1000 g:* 3–4 mg elemental iron/kg/d PO daily		Supplementation for preterm infants usually begins at 6–8 wk PNI; iron-fortified formula (instead of iron drops/syrup) is recommended for bottle-fed infants; some TPN solutions do not contain iron, and patients on long-term PN may require supplementation

(continued)

***†††§Refer to legend on p. 889.

933

Table IV.1 Drug Dosage Guidelines for Neonates* (Where Specified), Infants, and Older Children (continued)

Drug[‡§]	Dose	Dose Limit	Comments
Iron—cont'd	*Infants and older children:* **Treatment** 6 mg elemental iron/kg/d PO once daily or ÷ tid **Prophylaxis** 0.5–2 mg elemental iron/kg/d PO once daily or ÷ bid-tid	60 mg/dose	Before administration, dilute susp in glass of juice or water and mix thoroughly; administer tabs with ½–1 glass water or juice; administer 1 h before or 2 h after dairy products, eggs, tea, or whole-grain bread or cereal
Iron sucrose Inj 100 mg/5 mL (20 mg elemental iron/mL)	**Hemodialysis** If TSAT is 20–50% and ferritin is 100–800 mcg/L, 2 mg/kg/dose IV once weekly If TSAT <20% or if ferritin <100 mcg/L, 7 mg/kg/dose IV once weekly × 1 wk, then 2 mg/kg/dose IV once weekly If TSAT >50% or ferritin >800 mcg/L, discontinue iron sucrose and restart when one of the above criteria is met	100 mg/dose 200 mg/dose 100 mg/dose	TSAT (transferrin saturation) = iron ÷ (2 × transferrin) Oral iron absorption decreased with iron sucrose; wait at least 5 d after IV iron therapy before initiating PO iron
Isoniazid Syrup 10 mg/mL Tab 300 mg	**Tuberculosis** 10–20 mg/kg/d PO once daily or ÷ q12h or 20–30 mg/kg/dose PO twice weekly (regimens for treatment and prophylaxis vary; consult specialty references for more information)	CNS disease: 500 mg/d Twice-weekly regimen: 900 mg/d Other: 300 mg/d	Pyridoxine supplementation recommended in adolescents, children with nutritional deficiencies, breastfed infants, and pregnant or lactating women; given on an empty stomach (1 h ac or 2 h pc) unless GI upset occurs; monitor liver function tests periodically
Isoproterenol Inj 0.2 mg/mL	*Neonates, infants, and older children:* 0.05–1 mcg/kg/min IV as continuous infusion		≤33 kg: 0.15 × wt (kg) = dose (mg) added to crystalloid to make 50 mL; 1 mL/h = 0.05 mcg/kg/min; in neonates, stop or slow infusion if HR >200/min

Itraconazole Cap 100 mg Liquid 10 mg/mL	**Oropharyngeal candidiasis treatment or secondary prophylaxis** 2–5 mg/kg/d PO once daily **Other fungal infections** 5–10 mg/kg/d PO as single daily dose or ÷ bid	400 mg/d	Caution regarding drug interactions including cisapride, cyclosporine, tacrolimus; may cause hepatic dysfunction; reduce dose in liver impairment; oral solution and caps are not interchangeable; oral solution should be administered on an empty stomach; caps must be swallowed whole and given after a full meal; avoid giving within 2 h of antacids; in patients with achlorhydria or taking acid-suppressing agents, administer with a cola beverage
Kaletra (lopinavir/ ritonavir) Caps 133.3 mg lopinavir + 33.3 mg ritonavir Tab 200 mg lopinavir + 50 mg ritonavir Solution 80 mg/mL lopinavir + 20 mg/mL ritonavir	**Postexposure prophylaxis, in combination with lamivudine and zidovudine, and in HIV infection in combination therapy** < 6 mo: 600 mg lopinavir/m² /d PO ÷ bid 6 mo–12 yr: 460–600 mg lopinavir/m² /d PO ÷ bid > 12 yr or > 50 kg: 800 mg lopinavir/d PO ÷ bid	800 mg lopinavir/d	Plasma levels may be increased in patients with hepatic impairment Oral solution contains 42.4% v/v alcohol 5 mL oral solution = 3 caps Many potential drug interactions; give with food; absorption enhanced with high-fat meal
Kayexalate	See sodium polystyrene sulfonate		
Ketoconazole Susp (HSC) 20 mg/mL	5–10 mg/kg/d PO as single daily dose or ÷ q12h	400 mg/d	Give with food; may interact with many other medications including cisapride, cyclosporine, tacrolimus, sirolimus; consult product monograph or pharmacy; avoid giving within 2 h of antacids; in patients with achlorhydria or taking acid-suppressing agents, administer with a carbonated beverage
Ketorolac tromethamine Inj 30 mg/mL	**Postoperative pain** 0.5 mg/kg/dose IV q6h prn	< 16 yr: 15 mg/dose ≥ 16 yr: 30 mg/dose	Max duration of IV therapy is 2 d; do not use in tonsillectomy patients because of increased risk of bleeding; do not use in patients with impaired renal function

(continued)

†‡§Refer to legend on p. 889.

Pediatric Drug Dosing Guidelines

IV

935

Table IV.1 Drug Dosage Guidelines for Neonates* (Where Specified), Infants, and Older Children (continued)

Drug†‡§	Dose	Dose Limit	Comments
Labetalol Inj 5 mg/mL	**Hypertension** 1 mg/kg/h by continuous IV infusion **Acute hypertension** 1-3 mg/kg IV	3 mg/kg/h	Reduce dose in liver impairment
Lactulose Syrup 667 mg/mL	**Constipation** Initial dose: 5-10 mL/d PO once daily; double daily dose until stool is produced **Hepatic encephalopathy** *<1 yr:* 2.5 mL PO bid *Older children and adolescents:* 10-30 mL PO tid	*<1 yr:* 2.5 mL PO qid; usual adult dose: 15-30 mL/d (constipation)	For hepatic encephalopathy: decrease/discontinue if severe diarrhea develops; treatment is effective if stool is soft with pH <5.5; hypernatremia and/or hypokalemia may occur
Lamivudine Tab 150 mg Liquid 10 mg/mL	**HIV-infected children (in combination therapy for treatment or postexposure prophylaxis)** *>3 mo–16 yr:* 8 mg/kg/d PO ÷ bid *≥16 yr and ≥50 kg:* 150 mg PO bid or 300 mg PO as single daily dose	300 mg/d	Reduce dose in renal impairment; may cause pancreatitis, peripheral neuropathy; oral solution contains sugar
Lamotrigine Tab 25, 100, 150 mg Chew/disperse tab 2, 5 mg	*Children 2–12 yr, taking VPA ± enzyme-inducing agents:* Weeks 1 and 2: 0.15 mg/kg/d PO in 1-2 divided doses Weeks 3 and 4: 0.3 mg/kg/d PO in 1-2 divided doses, then titrate dose, increasing by 0.3 mg/kg q1-2wk Usual maintenance: 1-5 mg/kg/d PO daily or ÷ bid	200 mg/d	Use with caution in patients with impaired renal or hepatic function and patients taking VPA; monitor for rash (may be sign of serious toxicity)
	Children 2–12 yr, taking enzyme-inducing agents but not VPA:	400 mg/d	

Weeks 1 and 2: 0.3 mg/kg/dose PO bid Weeks 3 and 4: 0.6 mg/kg/dose PO bid, then titrate dose, increasing by 1.2 mg q1–2wk Usual maintenance: 5–15 mg/kg/d ÷ bid	
Children >12 yr, taking enzyme-inducing agents but not VPA: *Initial:* 25 mg PO bid for 2 wk, then increase to 50 mg PO bid × 2 wk, then titrate dose Usual maintenance: 300–500 mg/d PO ÷ bid	500 mg/d
Children >12 yr, taking VPA but not enzyme-inducing agents: *Initial:* 25 mg/dose PO every other day × 2 wk, then increase dose to 25 mg PO daily × 2 wk, then titrate dose Usual maintenance: 50–100 mg/dose PO bid	200 mg/d
Children >12 yr, taking enzyme-inducing agents with VPA: Initial dose: 25 mg/dose PO daily × 2 wk, then increase dose by 25–50 mg/d q1–2wk Usual maintenance: 50–100 mg/dose PO bid	200 mg/d
Lansoprazole Cap 15, 30 mg Tab, ODT 15, 30 mg	*<10 kg:* 7.5 mg PO once daily *10–30 kg:* 15 mg PO once daily *≥30 kg:* 30 mg PO once daily	1.6 mg/kg/d or 30 mg/d, whichever is less	Administer before food; for oral use, give caps whole, whenever possible; consult pharmacy for administration for patients who cannot take caps or ODT tabs

***§§Refer to legend on p. 889.

(continued)

Table IV.1 Drug Dosage Guidelines for Neonates* (Where Specified), Infants, and Older Children *(continued)*

Drug†‡§	Dose	Dose Limit	Comments
Levetiracetam Tab 250, 500 mg	Initial dose: 5–10 mg/kg/d PO ÷ bid May increase dose q1–2wk to 20–40 mg/kg/d PO ÷ bid	60 mg/kg/d or 3000 mg/d, whichever is less	Dose adjustment in renal impairment (adults); mild, 500–1000 mg PO bid; moderate, 250–750 mg PO bid; severe, 250–500 mg PO bid
Levocarnitine (carnitine, L-carnitine) Inj 200 mg/mL Liquid 100 mg/mL Tab 330 mg	**Metabolic crisis** Loading dose: 50–300 mg/kg IV, then same dose IV over next 24 h ÷ q4h Maintenance: 50–100 mg/kg/d PO/IV ÷ q4–6h	Usual adult dose: 4 g/d ÷ bid–tid	
Levothyroxine Tab 25, 50, 75, 88, 100, 112, 125, 150, 175, 200 mcg	*Neonates:* 10–12 mcg/kg/d PO		In neonates, measure TSH and free T₄ 2 wk after initiation of therapy and then at 2, 3, 6, 9, and 12 mo of age; titrate to normalize TSH and free T₄ at 4–6 wk after any dosage adjustment; infants: start with half the dose for 4–8 wk if TSH >100; in older children, measure TSH and free T₄ q6–12wk and titrate dose to normalize
	Infants and older children: 2–3 mcg/kg/d PO	Average adult dose: 100–200 mcg/d	
Lidocaine Inj 20 mg/mL (2%)	*Infants and older children:* **Resuscitation** 1 mg/kg/dose IV/IO over at least 2 min (0.05 mL/kg/dose); max single dose = 100 mg (5 mL); may repeat up to a max total dose of 3 mg/kg (0.15 mL/kg) 2–3 mg/kg/dose ETT (0.1–0.15 mL/kg/dose) Infusion: 20–50 mcg/kg/min IV as continuous infusion		For infusion: 60 × wt (kg) = dose (mg) added to crystalloid to make 50 mL → 1 mL/h = 20 mcg/kg/min

Loperamide Solution 0.2 mg/mL Tab 2 mg	**Acute diarrhea** (initial dose in first 24 h) 2-5 yr: 1 mg/dose PO tid 6-8 yr: 2 mg/dose PO bid 8-12 yr: 2 mg/dose PO tid	2 mg/dose	After initial dosing, 0.1 mg/kg/dose after each loose stool, not exceeding initial dose
	Chronic diarrhea 0.08-0.24 mg/kg/d PO ÷ bid or tid	2 mg/dose	
Loratadine Tab 10 mg Liquid 1 mg/mL	2-9 yr and/or <30 kg: 5 mg PO daily ≥10 yr and/or ≥30 kg: 10 mg PO daily		
Lorazepam Sublingual tab 0.5, 1, 2 mg Inj 4 mg/mL	*Neonates:* **Seizures** 0.05-0.1 mg/kg/dose IV/PR; may repeat once prn	Max cumulative dose: 4 mg	For PR administration, dilute injection to 2 mg/mL in D5W or 0.9% NaCl
	Infants and older children: **Preoperative/procedural sedation** 0.05 mg/kg/dose SL 0.03-0.05 mg/kg/dose IV **Status epilepticus** 0.1 mg/kg/dose IV/PR (max 4 mg), may repeat once prn **Antiemetic for breakthrough nausea and vomiting with antineoplastics** 0.025-0.05 mg/kg/dose IV/PO/SL q6h prn	4 mg/dose; 8 mg/12 h or 0.1 mg/kg/12 h, whichever is less	May give SL tablets PO; for sublingual/buccal administration, dry saliva in region to ensure tab dissolves and is absorbed in mucous membrane

**§Refer to legend on p. 889.

(continued)

Table IV.1 Drug Dosage Guidelines for Neonates* (Where Specified), Infants, and Older Children (continued)

Drug†‡§	Dose	Dose Limit	Comments
Lorazepam—cont'd	**Antiemetic for anticipatory nausea and vomiting with antineoplastics** *5–10 yr:* 0.5 mg/dose PO *>10 yr:* 1 mg/dose PO Give doses the night before chemotherapy and/or the morning of chemotherapy		
Losartan Tab 25, 50, 100 mg Susp (HSC) 2.5 mg/mL	**Hypertension, proteinuria** Initial: 0.5–1 mg/kg/d PO once daily	1.5 mg/kg/d up to 100 mg/d	Monitor serum potassium and renal function (especially when patients are on combined ACE inhibitor and losartan)
Magnesium Solution: 100 mg/mL magnesium glucoheptonate = 5 mg elemental magnesium/mL = 0.21 mmol elemental magnesium/mL 15 g/300 mL magnesium citrate Susp: 80 mg/mL magnesium hydroxide = 33 mg elemental magnesium/mL	*Neonates:* **Hypomagnesemia** Initial: 25–100 mg/kg/dose of magnesium sulfate (0.1–0.4 mmol elemental magnesium/kg/dose) given by IV infusion over 30–60 min q8–12h × 2–3 doses Maintenance: 30–60 mg/kg/d of magnesium sulfate IV (0.12–0.24 mmol elemental magnesium/kg/d)		Injection must be diluted before administration; titrate dose according to serum magnesium level; use with caution in renal impairment Neonates: for bolus infusions, dilute injection to 10 mg/mL magnesium sulfate (0.04 mmol/mL elemental magnesium) by adding 1 part magnesium sulfate to 49 parts diluent

mL = 1.4 mmol elemental
magnesium/mL

Tab:
420 mg magnesium
oxide = 252 mg elemental
magnesium = 10.6 mmol
elemental magnesium

Inj:
500 mg/mL magnesium
sulfate (50%) = 50 mg
elemental magnesium/
mL = 2 mmol elemental
magnesium/mL

Infants and older children:
Hypomagnesemia
Oral therapy: 20–40 mg elemental magnesium/kg/d
PO ÷ tid (0.8–1.6 mmol magnesium/kg/d PO ÷ tid)
IV therapy: initial dose: 5–10 mg elemental magnesium/
kg/dose IV (0.21–0.42 mmol magnesium/kg/dose IV)
Continuous infusion: 2.9 mg elemental magnesium/kg/d
IV (0.12 mmol magnesium/kg/d IV)

10 mmol/dose IV (250 mg
elemental magnesium)

Infants and older children: large doses of oral magnesium may cause
diarrhea; magnesium hydroxide tabs may be swallowed whole,
chewed, or dispersed in water for administration; magnesium oxide
tabs must not be given by G tube

Cathartic
Magnesium citrate: 4 mL/kg/dose PO
Magnesium hydroxide: 0.5 mL/kg/dose PO

Citrate: 300 mL/dose
Hydroxide: usual adult dose:
30–60 mL

(continued)

***§Refer to legend on p. 889.

Table IV.1 Drug Dosage Guidelines for Neonates* (Where Specified), Infants, and Older Children (continued)

Drug‡‡§	Dose	Dose Limit	Comments
Magnesium—cont'd	**Bronchodilation (adjunctive treatment in moderate to severe asthma)** 25–50 mg magnesium sulfate/kg/dose IV × 1 (2.5–5 mg elemental magnesium/kg/dose IV × 1) (0.1–0.2 mmol magnesium/kg/dose IV × 1)	2.5 g magnesium sulfate/dose (250 mg elemental magnesium/dose) (10 mmol magnesium/dose)	Administer as IV bolus over 20 min
Malarone (atovaquone/proguanil) Adult tab: atovaquone 250 mg + proguanil base 85.6 mg (100 mg proguanil HCl) Pediatric (ped) tab: atovaquone 62.5 mg + proguanil base 21.8 mg (25 mg proguanil HCl)	**Treatment of resistant *Falciparum* malaria** 5–8 *kg*: 2 ped tabs PO daily × 3 d 9–10 *kg*: 3 ped tabs PO daily × 3 d 11–20 *kg*: 1 adult tab PO daily × 3 d 21–30 *kg*: 1 adult tab PO daily × 3 d 31–40 *kg*: 3 adult tabs PO daily × 3 d >40 *kg (adult dose)*: 4 adult tabs PO daily × 3 d	Adult dose: 4 tabs PO daily × 3 d	Dose should be administered as single daily dose Give with food or milk; if vomiting occurs within 1 h of dosing, repeat the dose
Mannitol Inj 10% (100 g/1000 mL), 20% (100 g/500 mL), 25% (12.5 g/50 mL)	*Neonates:* 1 g/kg/dose IV (5 mL of 20% solution/kg/dose) *Infants and older children:* **Test for oliguria** 0.2 g/kg IV over 10 min × 1	Test dose: 12.5 g/dose	Contraindicated in patients with anuria or impaired renal function who do not respond to test dose with adequate urine output; monitor fluid and electrolyte balance

	Diuresis, reduction of ICP, reduction of intraocular pressure 0.2–2 g/kg/dose IV push or as IV infusion over up to 6 h	
Mebendazole Tab 100 mg	**Pinworm** 100 mg PO × 1 dose; repeat in 2 wk **Other nematodes** 200 mg/d PO ÷ bid × 3 d	Do not use for children <2 yr
Mefloquine Tab 250 mg	**Prophylaxis** Start 1 wk before travel; continue once weekly during travel and for 4 wk after leaving area 5–20 *kg*: 62.5 mg (¼ tab) PO once weekly >20–30 *kg*: 125 mg (½ tab) PO once weekly >30–45 *kg*: 187.5 mg (¾ tab) PO once weekly >45 *kg*: 250 mg (1 tab) PO once weekly	Plasma concentrations may be increased in patients with impaired hepatic function; consult product monograph for drug interactions; may cause various disturbances of peripheral and central nervous system; use with caution in patients with cardiac disease; pediatric experience limited in children <3 mo and/or <5 kg

Total treatment dose

Wt	Nonimmune	Semi-immune
<20 kg	20–25 mg/kg	15 mg/kg
20–30 kg	500–750 mg	375–500 mg
30–45 kg	750–1000 mg	500–750 mg
45–60 kg	1250 mg	750 mg
>60 kg	1500 mg	1000 mg

Treatment dose may be divided into 2–3 doses given 6–8 h apart; give larger portion as first dose (½–¾ total)

Semi-immune patients are those who have resided in malaria-endemic areas and who have previous history of malarial infection with the same species of parasite

Mefloquine does not eliminate hepatic phase of *Plasmodium vivax*; additional therapy required

Round dose to nearest ¼ tab, if possible. Administer with food and at least 240 mL liquid; tabs may be crushed and mixed with small amount of liquid or swallowed whole

Repeated dose recommended if patient vomits <30 min after administration; repeated ½ dose recommended if patient vomits 30–60 min after administration

(continued)

Pediatric Drug Dosing Guidelines

IV

Table IV.1 — Drug Dosage Guidelines for Neonates* (Where Specified), Infants, and Older Children (continued)

Drug†‡§	Dose	Dose Limit	Comments
Meperidine Solution (HSC) 10 mg/mL Tab 50 mg Inj 50, 100 mg/mL	**Analgesic** 1–1.5 mg/kg/dose IV/SC/PO q3–4h prn **Preoperatively** 1–2 mg/kg/dose IM/SC/PO 60 min preoperatively **Continuous infusion** 0.5–1 mg/kg IV loading dose; 0.3 mg/kg/h initial rate; may require 0.5–0.7 mg/kg/h IV	2 mg/kg/dose or 100 mg/dose IV/SC, whichever is less 4 mg/kg/dose or 150 mg/dose PO, whichever is less	Dosage adjustment required in renal or hepatic impairment; avoid in severe renal impairment; may cause constipation, respiratory or CNS depression; dose is cumulative; metabolite may cause seizures; IM route not recommended for analgesia; infusion only used in select cases; skin reactions and itching often respond to antihistamines and usually do not imply allergy
Meropenem Inj 500 mg, 1 g/vial	*Neonates:* **Meningitis** 40 mg/kg/dose IV q12h **Other** 20 mg/kg/dose IV q12h		Dose may need to be adjusted for renal impairment
	Infants and older children: **Meningitis, lower respiratory tract infections in patients with cystic fibrosis** 120 mg/kg/d IV ÷ q8h **Fever/neutropenia** 60 mg/kg/d IV ÷ q8h **Other** 60 mg/kg/d IV ÷ q8h	6 g/d 3 g/d 3 g/d	Dose and interval adjustment in renal impairment: mild, usual dose q12h; moderate, 50% dose q12h; severe, 50% dose q24h; dose after dialysis
Mesalamine (5-ASA, 5-aminosalicylic acid) Tab (enteric-coated) 400,	**Ulcerative colitis, Crohn disease** *Children:* 30–50 mg/kg/d PO ÷ bid-qid *Adolescents, adults:* 2400–4800 mg/d PO ÷ tid-qid,	4.8 g/d PO or 4 g/d PR	For best results, rectal susp should be retained for as long as possible 500-mg tab may be dispersed in water to ease swallowing or may be split along score line

500 mg Rectal susp 4 g/60 g	then reduce to lowest possible maintenance dose *Rectal susp:* 1–4 g PR qhs × 3–6 wk, then reduce to lowest possible dose and frequency for maintenance	
Metformin Tab 500 mg	*Adolescents:* 500 mg/dose PO daily	1000 mg PO bid	Contraindicated in liver impairment
Methadone Solution 1 mg/mL	**Opioid-naive patients ≥2 yr** 0.2–0.4 mg/kg/d PO ÷ bid or tid, titrated to effect **Opioid-tolerant patients ≥2 yr** Use a fixed dose equivalent to ⅒ of the total 24-hr PO morphine dose administered orally as required but not more frequently than q3h, to a max of 30 mg/dose On day 6, the total amount of methadone taken over previous 2 d is calculated and averaged per day and converted to a q12h regimen If prn medication is still required, increase the dose of methadone by ⅓ q4–6d	Initial dose limit in opioid-tolerant patient: 30 mg/dose	Dose adjustment in renal impairment: CrCl <10 mL/min, 50–75% Dose and frequency should be reduced with repeated use because of the cumulative effects of methadone Discontinuation of chronic therapy with opioids should be carried out gradually to avoid precipitating withdrawal symptoms In Canada, restricted to physicians who have methadone prescribing privileges; consult your local drug regulatory body
Methimazole Tab 5 mg	Initial: 0.4–0.7 mg/kg/d PO ÷ q8–12h; increase up to 1.5 mg/kg/d if no improvement within 2–3 wk Maintenance: 0.2 mg/kg/d PO ÷ q8–12h or once daily	Initial: 60 mg/d Maintenance: 30 mg/d	Give at same time in relation to meals every day; reduce dose in liver impairment; may cause agranulocytosis
Methotrexate Tab 2.5 mg Inj 25 mg/mL	**Rheumatologic disorders** 10–15 mg/m²/dose PO/SC once weekly; may increase by 1 mg/kg/wk to max 25 mg/wk	Initial: 10–15 mg/wk Maintenance: 25 mg/wk	Reduce dose in renal impairment; handle as a biohazard; give folic acid (usual dose, 1 mg/d); avoid concurrent use with cotrimoxazole; high-dose penicillins may inhibit renal clearance of methotrexate

(continued)

Table IV.1 Drug Dosage Guidelines for Neonates* (Where Specified), Infants, and Older Children *(continued)*

Drug†‡§	Dose	Dose Limit	Comments
Methylprednisolone Inj 40, 125, 500, 1000 mg/vial	**Acute asthma** 2–4 mg/kg/d IV ÷ q6h **Pulse therapy** (rheumatology, immunology) 10–30 mg/kg/dose IV over 1 h **Idiopathic thrombocytopenic purpura** 30 mg/kg/dose IV daily × 1–3 d	1 g/dose	Consider use of oral prednisone in less severe cases
Metoclopramide Liquid 1 mg/mL Tab 5, 10 mg Inj 5 mg/mL	*Neonates:* Initial: 0.1 mg/kg/d PO/IV ÷ q8h *Infants and older children:* **Small-bowel intubation** 0.1 mg/kg/dose PO/IM/IV	0.5 mg/kg/d	Extrapyramidal side effects may be reversed with diphenhydramine 1 mg/kg/dose IV; may alter absorption of other drugs; when used as antiemetic, concomitant diphenhydramine is recommended
	GERD 0.4–0.8 mg/kg/d PO/IM/IV ÷ qid **Acute chemotherapy-induced nausea and vomiting** 1.5–2 mg/kg/dose IV prechemotherapy and q2–4h prn **Delayed chemotherapy-induced nausea and vomiting** 0.1–0.2 mg/kg/dose PO/IV q6h	GERD adult dose: 10–15 mg qid Antiemetic therapy: 10 mg/kg/d	
Metolazone Tab 2.5, 5 mg Susp (HSC) 1 mg/mL	0.2–0.4 mg/kg/d PO ÷ q12–24h	10 mg/dose	
Metoprolol Tab 50 mg Susp (HSC) 10 mg/mL	1–5 mg/kg/d PO ÷ bid	400 mg/d	

Metronidazole	*Neonates:*			
Susp (HSC) 15 mg/mL	**Weight (g)**	**Age (d)**	**Dosage**	Dose adjustment in renal impairment: severe, 50% of standard dose;
Tab 250 mg	*<1200 g*		7.5 mg/kg/dose IV q48h	dose *after* dialysis; reduce dose in liver impairment; use IV formulation
Inj 5 mg/mL	*1200–2000 g*	≤7 d	7.5 mg/kg/dose IV q24h	of metronidazole for gut sterilization in infants with short-bowel
	1200–2000 g	>7 d	7.5 mg/kg/dose IV q12h	syndrome; give PO with food or milk; avoid alcohol; suspension
	>2000 g	≤7 d	7.5 mg/kg/dose IV q12h	is chocolate-cherry flavored but very bitter tasting
	>2000 g	>7 d	15 mg/kg/dose IV q12h	
	Gut sterilization: 15 mg/kg/d PO ÷ q8h			
	Infants and older children:			
	Anaerobes, including Clostridium difficile			
	15–30 mg/kg/d PO ÷ tid		2 g/d PO	
	30 mg/kg/d IV ÷ q6-8h		4 g/d IV	
	Giardiasis			
	15 mg/kg/d PO ÷ tid × 5 d or single daily dose as follows:		750 mg/d	
	<25 kg: 35 mg/kg/d PO × 3 d			
	25–40 kg: 50 mg/kg/d PO × 3 d			
	>40 kg: 2 g/d PO × 3 d			
	Amebiasis			
	35–50 mg/kg/d PO ÷ tid × 5–10 d		2.25 g/d	
	Trichomonas vaginalis			
	>13 yr: 2 g PO stat			For *T. vaginalis*, partner must also be treated

(continued)

947

Table IV.1   Drug Dosage Guidelines for Neonates* (Where Specified), Infants, and Older Children (continued)

Drug†‡§	Dose	Dose Limit	Comments
Metronidazole—cont'd	**Gut sterilization** 10 mg/kg/dose PO at 1300h, 1400h, and 2300h, starting day before surgery		
	Ulcerative colitis, Crohn disease 10–20 mg/kg/d PO ÷ tid pc	1 g/d	
	Helicobacter pylori-associated ulcer _Infants and children:_ 15–20 mg/kg/d PO ÷ bid, in combination with at least one other agent active against _H. pylori_ _Adolescents:_ 250–500 mg PO tid, in combination with at least one other agent active against _H. pylori_	1 g/d	
Mexiletine Cap 100, 200 mg Solution (HSC) 10 mg/mL or Dissolve 'n' Dose system	Loading dose: 6–8 mg/kg PO Maintenance: 6–16 mg/kg/d PO ÷ tid or qid	1500 mg/d 1200 mg/d; usual adult dose: 600 mg/d PO ÷ tid	Reduce dose in renal impairment: severe, give 50–75% of standard dose; reduce dose in hepatic impairment; give with food, milk, or antacids
Midazolam Inj 5 mg/mL Syrup (HSC) 3 mg/mL	_Neonates:_ Loading: 0.05–0.1 mg/kg IV (over 5 min) Maintenance: 0.01–0.06 mg/kg/h IV via continuous infusion		Use with caution in patients with hepatic or renal impairment, CHF, pulmonary disease; adjust doses of both drugs when used in combination with other CNS depressants; do not discontinue abruptly in patients receiving prolonged midazolam infusions; calculate dose according to ideal body weight

Milrinone Inj 1 mg/mL	*Infants and older children:* *<20 kg:* 0.5–0.75 mg/kg/dose PO *≥20 kg:* 0.3–0.5 mg/kg/dose PO administered 15–30 min before procedure or surgery 0.05 mg/kg/dose IV for sedation; repeat × 1 prn 0.1–0.2 mg/kg/dose IV preoperatively Loading dose: 0.05 mg/kg IV over ≥10 min, given undiluted or in appropriate diluent Maintenance: 0.375–0.75 mcg/kg/min continuous IV infusion	20 mg/dose PO, except when ordered by anesthesia for preop 0.15 mg/kg/dose IV 1.13 mg/kg/d	Reduce dose in renal impairment; half-life may be prolonged in patients with CHF and renal impairment
Mineral oil (heavy) Liquid	1 mL/kg/dose PO qhs	Usual adult dose: 15–45 mL PO as single dose	Because of risk of aspiration, avoid in children <1 yr and in neurologically impaired children
Montelukast Chew tabs 4, 5, 10 mg	*1–5 yr:* 4 mg PO once daily *6–14 yr:* 5 mg PO once daily *>14 yr:* 10 mg PO once daily		Administer in the evening; chew tabs contain phenylalanine; use with caution in patients with phenylketonuria
Morphine Syrup 1 mg/mL Tab 5, 10 mg Tab SR 15, 30, 60, 100 mg Cap SR 10, 30, 60 mg Suppos 5, 10 mg Inj 2, 10, 25, 50 mg/mL Inj epidural 5 mg/10 mL	*Neonates:* Loading dose: 0.05–0.1 mg/kg IV Maintenance: 0.005–0.01 mg/kg/h IV via continuous infusion *Infants and older children:* **Moderate sedation** 0.05–0.1 mg/kg IV; may repeat × 1 in 15 min prn; 0.3 mg/kg PO 30–60 min before procedure		Reduce dose in renal impairment: moderate, 75% of dose; severe, 50% of dose; reduce dose in liver impairment Formula for dilution: (wt [kg] × 0.5) mg in 50 mL IV fluid at 1 mL/h = 10 mcg/kg/h For patients being converted from parenteral to oral therapy, IM/IV:PO ratio = 1:3

*†‡§Refer to legend on p. 889.

(continued)

Pediatric Drug Dosing Guidelines

IV

Table IV.1 Drug Dosage Guidelines for Neonates* (Where Specified), Infants, and Older Children (continued)

Drug†‡§	Dose	Dose Limit	Comments
Morphine—cont'd	**Preoperative sedation** 0.05–0.2 mg/kg/dose IM 30–60 min preoperatively		
	Analgesia Intermittent dosing: 0.2–0.4 mg/kg/dose PO/PR q4h or 0.05–0.1 mg/kg/dose IV/SC q2–4h Continuous infusion: 0.1–0.2 mg/kg IV loading dose, then 0.01–0.04 mg/kg/h IV/SC infusion; 0.02–0.05 mg/kg/dose IV/SC q4h prn for breakthrough pain; increase infusion rate q8h prn in increments ≤25% of previous infusion rate	Analgesia: 15 mg/dose IV/SC; no dose limit for palliative care	Caps may be opened and contents sprinkled on soft food; pellets should not be chewed; IM route should not be used for analgesia Continuous IV/SC infusion is preferred for management of prolonged pain requiring frequent or high-dose morphine administration; do not adjust maintenance infusion dose until current dose has been running for at least 8 h; if a maintenance dose of >0.1 mg/kg/h or additional boluses seem to be required, consider consulting pain management service
	Vaso-occlusive crisis in sickle cell disease Loading dose: 0.15 mg/kg IV over 5 min Maintenance: 0.04 mg/kg/h IV; increase dose q8h prn in increments of 0.02 mg/kg/h up to max of 0.1 mg/kg/h	*Vaso-occlusive crisis:* Loading dose: 7.5 mg Maintenance: 0.1 mg/kg/h	
Mycophenolate mofetil Susp 200 mg/mL Cap 250 g Tab 500 g Inj (HSC) 6 mg/mL	**Renal transplantation** 600–1200 mg/m²/dose PO ÷ q12h **GVHD** 10–40 mg/kg/d IV ÷ q12h	3 g/d	Initial dose may be lower or dose may be divided tid to allow for tolerance to GI irritation Oral to IV conversion as follows: BMT: 1.25:1 Other patients: 1:1

Nabilone Cap 0.5, 1 mg	*<18 kg:* 0.5 mg PO prechemotherapy and q12h *18–30 kg:* 1 mg PO prechemotherapy and q12h *>30 kg:* 1 mg PO prechemotherapy and q8–12h		Reduce dose in liver impairment
Nadolol Susp (HSC) 10 mg/mL Tab 40, 80 mg	**Hypertension** 1 mg/kg/d PO once daily or ÷ bid; increase dose by 1 mg/kg/d q3–4d prn	4 mg/kg/d or 320 mg/d, whichever is less	Reduce dose in renal impairment: moderate, 50% of dose; severe, 25% of dose
Naloxone Inj 0.4 mg/mL	*Neonates:* 0.1 mg/kg/dose IV/ETT; repeat prn		
	Infants and older children: **Resuscitation** Titrate to effect with 0.01 mg/kg/dose IV/ETT increments or 0.1 mg/kg/dose IV/ETT, repeat prn	2 mg/dose	Whenever possible, titration of naloxone dose is more desirable; in sedated patients, administration of naloxone should be reserved for emergency use (i.e., severe obtundation and respiratory depression); following administration of naloxone, patients must be cared for in a constant care setting and discharged only when fully awake and a minimum 3 h has elapsed
	Partial narcotic reversal for sedated patients 0.001–0.01 mg/kg/dose IV prn **Management of adverse opioid effects** 1–10 mcg/kg/dose; observe and repeat q10min prn to max total of 100 mcg/kg		

*†§Refer to legend on p. 889.

(continued)

Pediatric Drug Dosing Guidelines

IV

Table IV.1   Drug Dosage Guidelines for Neonates* (Where Specified), Infants, and Older Children (continued)

Drug[††‡]	Dose	Dose Limit	Comments
Naproxen Susp 25 mg/mL Tab 125, 250, 375 mg Suppos 500 mg	10–20 mg/kg/d PO ÷ bid 25–49 kg: 250 mg/dose PR ≥50 kg: 500 mg/dose PR	1 g/d	Reduce dose in liver impairment; use with caution and monitor closely in patients with impaired renal function; avoid in patients with severe renal impairment
Nelfinavir Tab 250, 625 mg	2–13 yr: 90–110 mg/kg/d PO ÷ bid >13 yr: 1250 mg PO bid	Adult usual dose: 1250 mg PO bid	Reduce dose in liver impairment; administer with meal or light snack; tabs may be dissolved in small amount of water or crushed and mixed with pudding
Neostigmine Inj 0.5 mg/mL	**Supraventricular tachycardia** 0.01–0.04 mg/kg/dose IV **Curare antagonism** 0.02–0.08 mg/kg/dose IV	2.5 mg/dose	Have atropine at hand
Nevirapine Susp (Special Access drug) 10 mg/mL Tab 200 mg	Initial dose: 120 mg/m²/dose PO as single daily dose × 14 d Maintenance dose: 120–200 mg/m²/dose PO q12h	200 mg/d initial 400 mg/d maintenance	
Nifedipine Cap 5, 10 mg Tab (prolonged action) 10, 20 mg Tab XL (24-h action) 30, 60 mg	**Hypertension** Initial: 0.5 mg/kg/d PO ÷ q8h (min., 1.25 mg/dose); increase gradually prn to 1–1.5 mg/kg/d PO **prn dosing (short-acting cap)** 0.125–0.25 mg/kg/dose PO; may repeat × 1	Usual adult dose: 10–30 mg/dose (of PA or XL tab) prn dose: 10 mg/dose (of short-acting cap)	PA tabs may be given q12h; do not crush or split XL tabs; for more rapid action, direct patient to bite and swallow cap Caution with prn dosing in patients with coronary artery disease or disease of the head and neck vessels (e.g. Takayasu or moyamoya) where a sudden drop in BP could cause stroke or MI

Nitrazepam Susp (HSC) 1 mg/mL Tab 5 mg	Initial: 0.25 mg/kg/d PO once daily or ÷ tid, increase gradually prn to 1.2 mg/kg/d PO	Reduce dose in liver impairment; give with food or milk
Nitrofurantoin Macrocrystals, cap 50, 100 mg Tab 50 mg Susp (HSC) 10 mg/mL	**Treatment** 5–7 mg/kg/d PO ÷ q6h *Prophylaxis:* usual adult dose: 50–100 mg qhs	Give with food or milk; do not give to infants <1 mo; avoid if GFR is <50 mL/min; may discolor urine rust-yellow to brown; has also been given on an alternate-day schedule
	UTI prophylaxis 1–2 mg/kg/d PO daily	
	400 mg/d or 10 mg/kg/d, whichever is less	
Nitroglycerin Inj 5 mg/mL	0.5–10 mcg/kg/min via continuous IV infusion	
Nitroprusside Inj 50 mg/3mL	0.5–10 mcg/kg/min via continuous infusion	Caution regarding cyanide toxicity
Norepinephrine Inj 2 mg/mL norepinephrine bitartrate = 1 mg/mL norepinephrine base	0.02–0.1 mcg/kg/min via continuous IV infusion (as norepinephrine base)	Avoid extravasation; administer via central line, when possible
Nystatin Drops 100,000 units/mL Tab 500,000 units	**Oral candidiasis prophylaxis and treatment** 400,000–2,400,000 units/d PO ÷ qid	2.5 mg/kg/d cumulative dose

*†‡§Refer to legend on p. 889.

(continued)

Table IV.1 Drug Dosage Guidelines for Neonates* (Where Specified), Infants, and Older Children *(continued)*

Drug‡‡§	Dose	Dose Limit	Comments
Octreotide Inj 50, 500, 1000 mcg/mL	**Chylothorax** Continuous infusion: 1–4 mcg/kg/h IV infusion Intermittent dosing: 10–40 mcg/kg/d IV/SC ÷ q8h; increase dose by 5–10 mcg/kg/d q72–96h **Portal hypertensive GI bleeding** 1–2 mcg/kg IV bolus, then 1–5 mcg/kg/h IV infusion	10 mcg/kg/h	Reduce dose in renal impairment; regular monitoring for glucose tolerance, biliary tract abnormalities, and hypothyroidism is required
Olanzapine Tab 2.5, 10 mg Tab (ODT) 5 mg	2.5–5 mg/dose PO once daily Titrate weekly by 2.5 or 5 mg/wk	Usual target dose: 15–20 mg/d	Consider dose adjustment in renal or hepatic impairment; clinical experience in organ dysfunction is lacking
Omeprazole Delayed-release tab 10, 20 mg Susp (HSC) 2 mg/mL	Initial: 0.7–1.4 mg/kg/d PO once daily ***Helicobacter pylori*–associated ulcer** *Adolescents, adults:* 20 mg/dose PO bid × 1 wk with clarithromycin and amoxicillin or metronidazole	Usual adult dose: initial therapy 20–40 mg PO daily	Reduce dose in liver impairment
Ondansetron Tab 4, 8 mg Tab ODT 4, 8 mg Inj 2 mg/mL Liquid 0.8 mg/mL	**Antiemetic with antineoplastics** IV dosing: *Highly or very highly emetogenic regimens:* 5 mg/m² IV prechemotherapy and q8h *Moderately emetogenic regimens:* 5 mg/m²/dose IV prechemotherapy and q12h *Mildly emetogenic regimens:* 3 mg/m²/dose IV prechemotherapy × 1 Alternate oral dosing in the above regimens: BSA <0.3 m²: 1 mg/dose	8 mg/dose	

0.3–0.6 *m²*: 2 mg/dose 0.61–1.5 *m²*: 4 mg/dose >1.5 *m²*: 8 mg/dose		
Postoperative nausea and vomiting Prophylaxis: 0.1 mg/kg × 1 dose preoperatively or intraoperatively	Usual adult dose: 4 mg/dose IV or 8 mg/dose PO; max: 0.15 mg/kg/dose or 8 mg/dose PO or IV	Literature supports prophylactic use for postoperative nausea/vomiting; little support exists for rescue dosing; giving a second dose to patients who do not achieve adequate control after a single dose will not provide additional control
Nausea and vomiting due to gastroenteritis 0.15 mg/kg/dose PO × 1 dose 8–≤15 *kg*: 2 mg PO × 1 dose 15–≤30 *kg*: 4 mg PO × 1 dose >30 *kg*: 8 mg PO × 1 dose 0.15 mg/kg/dose IV	Max 8 mg/dose	
Opium and belladonna Suppos 65 mg opium and 15 mg belladonna extract	**Ureteral spasm** 8–16 *kg*: ¼ suppos PR q4–6h prn 16–32 *kg*: ½ suppos PR q4–6h prn ≥32 *kg*: 1 suppos PR q4–6h prn	Min dose: ¼ suppos
Oseltamivir Cap 75 mg Susp 12 mg/mL	**Treatment of influenza A or B** ≤15 *kg*: 30 mg/dose PO bid × 5 d >15–≤23 *kg*: 45 mg/dose PO bid × 5 d 23–≤40 *kg*: 60 mg/dose PO bid × 5 d >40 *kg*: 75 mg/dose PO bid × 5 d	Usual adult dose: 75 mg PO bid × 5 d	Dose interval adjustment in renal impairment: moderate, q24h; no recommendation available for end-stage renal disease Do not use in children less than 1 yr of age

(continued)

*†‡§Refer to legend on p. 889.

Pediatric Drug Dosing Guidelines

IV

Table IV.1   Drug Dosage Guidelines for Neonates* (Where Specified), Infants, and Older Children (continued)

Drug†‡§	Dose	Dose Limit	Comments
Oxcarbazepine Tab 150, 300, 600 mg Susp 60 mg/mL	**Adjunctive therapy** >6 yr: 8-10 mg/kg/d PO ÷ bid for first 2 wk **Maintenance** 20-29 kg: 900 mg/d PO ÷ bid 29.1-39 kg: 1200 mg/d PO ÷ bid >39 kg: 1800 mg/d PO ÷ bid **Monotherapy** 20-24 kg: 600-900 mg/d PO ÷ bid 25-34 kg: 900-1200 mg/d PO ÷ bid 35-44 kg: 900-1500 mg/d PO ÷ bid 45-49 kg: 1200-1500 mg/d PO ÷ bid 50-59 kg: 1200-1800 mg/d PO ÷ bid	Usual adult adjunctive therapy dose: 1200 mg/d Usual adult monotherapy dose: 2400 mg/d	Dose adjustment in renal impairment: CrCl <30 mL/min, start at 300 mg/d and titrate slowly Cross-sensitivity with carbamazepine in 25-30% of patients
Oxybutynin Syrup 1 mg/mL Tab 5 mg	**Neurogenic bladder** 1-5 yr: 0.2 mg/kg/dose PO ÷ bid-qid >5 yr: 5 mg/dose PO bid, up to 5 mg/dose PO qid		
Pamidronate Inj 30 mg/10 mL	**Hypercalcemia** 0.5-1 mg/kg/dose; may repeat in 1 wk **Osteogenesis imperfecta, McCune-Albright syndrome** <2 yr: 0.5 mg/kg/dose IV over 3-4 h × 3 d q2mo 2-3 yr: 0.75 mg/kg/dose IV over 3-4 h × 3 d q2mo >3 yr: 1 mg/kg/dose IV over 3-4 h × 3 d q2mo Reduce first dose (day 1, cycle 1) by 50%		Use with caution in renal impairment; maintain hydration and urine output during treatment

		Do not chew or crush cap contents; titrate dose to stool fat content

Pancrelipase
Cap: lipase 8000 USP units, amylase 30,000 USP units, protease 30,000 USP units
ECS-8: lipase 8000 USP units, amylase 30,000 USP units, protease 30,000 USP units
ECS-20: lipase 20,000 USP units, amylase 55,000 USP units, protease 55,000 USP units

Infants:
1 regular cap/120 mL of formula

Children and adults:
Regular caps: 6 per meal, 2 per snack
ECS (enteric-coated) caps: 3 per meal, 1 per snack

Pancuronium
Inj 1 mg/mL

Neonates:
0.05–0.1 mg/kg/dose IV prn
Older children:
0.1–0.15 mg/kg/dose IV prn

Reduce dose in renal impairment

Pantoprazole
Inj 40 mg/vial

Indications (GERD, acid suppression requiring a proton pump inhibitor, and oral proton pump inhibitor is not feasible)
1–1.5 mg/kg/d IV once daily

40 mg/dose

For indications other than GI bleeding, gastric pH may be monitored as clinically necessary

***†§Refer to legend on p. 889.**

(continued)

Table IV.1 Drug Dosage Guidelines for Neonates* (Where Specified), Infants, and Older Children *(continued)*

Drug†‡§	Dose	Dose Limit	Comments
Pantoprazole—cont'd	**Upper GI bleeding** 5–15 kg: 2 mg/kg/dose IV × 1 and then 0.2 mg/kg/h IV >15–40 kg: 1.8 mg/kg/dose IV × 1 and then 0.18 mg/kg/h IV >40 kg: 80 mg/dose IV × 1 and then 8 mg/h IV	Bolus: 80 mg/dose Max rate: 8 mg/h Max infusion duration: 72 h	For upper GI bleeding, gastric pH should be monitored to maintain pH >6
Paraldehyde Inj 1 g/mL (Special Access drug)	*Neonates:* 150 mg/kg/h (3 mL of 5% solution/kg/h) IV over 2 h once daily 300 mg/kg (0.3 mL undiluted paraldehyde/kg) × 1 PR diluted in olive oil or 0.9% NaCl to make 30–50% solution *Infants and older children:* 200–400 mg/kg/dose (0.2–0.4 mL undiluted paraldehyde/kg/dose) PR q4-8h; give PR as a 30–50% solution in oil or 0.9% NaCl	PR: 10 g/dose	Reduce dose in liver impairment To make a 5% solution, add 1.75 mL of paraldehyde to D5W to make total volume of 35 mL in a syringe
PEG electrolyte liquid (GoLYTELY, PegLyte, etc.) Oral powder	25 mL/kg/h PO/NG until rectal effluent is clear *Adolescents:* 240 mL PO q10min until rectal effluent is clear	2 L/h, 4 L total	Use with caution in patients with renal insufficiency; for PO administration, product is more palatable when chilled
Penicillin G Na (1.68 mmol Na/MU) Inj 1, 5, 10 MU/vial	*Neonates:* **Meningitis** 0–7 d, ≤2000 g: 100,000 IU/kg/d IV/IM ÷ q12h 0–7 d, >2000 g: 150,000 IU/kg/d IV/IM ÷ q8h >7 d, <1200 g: 100,000 IU/kg/d IV/IM ÷ q12h >7 d, 1200–2000 g: 150,000 IU/kg/d IV/IM ÷ q8h >7 d, >2000 g: 200,000 IU/kg/d IV/IM ÷ q6h		600 mg = 1 million units Reduce dose interval in renal impairment; moderate q8-12h, severe q12-18h

Group B streptococcal meningitis
0–7 d: 250,000–450,000 IU/kg/d IV/IM ÷ q8h
Congenital syphilis
0–7 d: 100,000 IU/kg/d IV/IM ÷ q12h
Other:
0–7 d, ≤2000 g: 50,000 IU/kg/d IV/IM ÷ q12h
0–7 d, >2000 g: 75,000 IU/kg/d IV/IM ÷ q8h
>7 d, <1200 g: 50,000 IU/kg/d IV/IM ÷ q12h
>7 d, >1200–2000 g: 75,000 IU/kg/d IV/IM ÷ q8h
>7 d, >2000 g: 100,000 IU/kg/d IV/IM ÷ q6h

Infants and older children:
Mild to moderate infections
50,000 IU/kg/d IM/IV ÷q6h

Severe infections
250,000–400,000 IU/kg/d IM/IV ÷ q4–6h

	20 million units/d	Dose interval adjustment in renal impairment: moderate, q8–12h; severe, q12–18h
	24 million units/d	600 mg = 1 million units
Meningitis 400,000 IU/kg/d IV/IM ÷ q4–6h	24 million units/d	
Penicillin VK Susp 60 mg/mL Tab 300 mg	**Streptococcal infection** (mild to moderate infections) 25–50 mg/kg/d PO ÷ bid × 10 d	1.5 g/d	Reduce dose in renal impairment: moderate, 75% of dose; severe, 25–50% of dose; may be given with food 300 mg = 480,000 units Prophylaxis in asplenic patients <6 mo: use cotrimoxazole; alternate agent for patients 2–5 yr is amoxicillin; note that penicillin-resistant organisms are becoming more prevalent and prophylactic drug of choice may change

(continued)

Table IV.1 Drug Dosage Guidelines for Neonates* (Where Specified), Infants, and Older Children (continued)

Drug†‡§	Dose	Dose Limit	Comments
Penicillin VK—cont'd	**Other infections** 50–100 mg/kg/d PO ÷ q6–8h	3 g/d	Note that penicillin-resistant organisms are becoming more prevalent and prophylactic drug choice may change
	Rheumatic fever Treatment: 125–300 mg PO tid–qid × 10 d Prophylaxis >5 yr: 125–300 mg PO bid **Prophylaxis in asplenic patients** 6 mo–5 yr: 125 or 150 mg PO bid >5 yr: 250 or 300 mg PO bid		
Pentamidine isethionate Inj 300 mg/vial	**Pneumocystis pneumonia** Treatment: 4 mg/kg/d IM/IV as single daily dose for 14–21 d Prophylaxis: 4 mg/kg/dose IV q2wk; 300 mg/dose by inhalation every month		Dose interval adjustment in renal impairment: moderate, q24–36h; severe, q48h; IV preferred over IM administration; dose of inhaled pentamidine should be individualized for younger uncooperative children (600 mg/dose)
Pentobarbital (Nembutal) (Special Access drug) Inj 50 mg/mL	2.5 mg/kg (max 50 mg) IV over 1 min, wait 1 min, then 1.25 mg/kg (max 25 mg) IV over 30 s, wait 1 min, then 1.25 mg/kg (max 25 mg) over 30 s, wait 1 min and, if required, an additional dose of 1 mg/kg (max 20 mg) may be given OR Give IM only if no IV access <15 kg: 6 mg/kg/dose IM ≥15 kg: 5 mg/kg/dose IM 20–30 min preprocedure	Cumulative dose: 6 mg/kg or 200 mg IV, whichever is less 200 mg/dose IM	Too rapid IV administration may cause respiratory depression, apnea, laryngospasm, and hypotension Injection may be given orally undiluted or mixed with water Reduce dose in liver impairment

Phenobarbital
Elixir 5 mg/mL
Tab 15, 30 mg
Inj 30 mg/mL, 120 mg/mL

Preoperative sedative
≥8 yr: 2–4 mg/kg/dose PO 60–120 min preoperatively

Neonates:
Loading dose:
<37 wk PCA: 10–20 mg/kg IV; may repeat 5–10 mg/kg IV up to max total dose of 25 mg/kg
≥37 wk PCA: 10–20 mg/kg IV; may repeat 10 mg/kg IV up to max of 30 mg/kg
Maintenance: 4–6 mg/kg/d IV/PO daily

Reduce dose in liver impairment; administer IV undiluted at a rate not to exceed 1 mg/kg/min or 60 mg/min, whichever is less; monitoring of serum drug concentration recommended; calculate loading dose according to total body weight; calculate maintenance dose according to ideal body weight

Infants and older children:
Status epilepticus
20 mg/kg IV × 1
Antiepileptic maintenance
<3 mo: 5–6 mg/kg/d PO once daily or ÷ bid
≥3 mo: 3–5 mg/kg/d PO once daily or ÷ bid
Adolescents: 2–4 mg/kg/d PO once daily or ÷ bid

1g/dose

Maintenance dose: 200 mg/d

Phenoxybenzamine
(Special Access drug)
Cap (HSC) 0.5, 1, 2 mg
Cap 10 mg
Inj 50 mg/mL

Loading dose: 0.25–1 mg/kg IV over 1 h
Maintenance: 0.5–2 mg/kg/d IV as a continuous infusion or IV/PO ÷ q6–12h

***§Refer to legend on p. 889.

(continued)

Table IV.1 Drug Dosage Guidelines for Neonates* (Where Specified), Infants, and Older Children (continued)

Drug††§	Dose	Dose Limit	Comments
Phentolamine Inj 10 mg/mL	**Treatment of extravasation of vasoactive drug** (e.g., dopamine) Prepare solution of 5 mg in 10 mL 0.9% NaCl and use SC to infiltrate area of extravasation	5 mg	
Phenylephrine Inj 10 mg/mL	**Supraventricular tachycardia (SVT)** Initial: 0.01 mg/kg/dose IV; increase in increments of 0.01 mg/kg up to 0.1 mg/kg/total dose **Tetralogy of Fallot spell** 5 mcg/kg/dose IV followed by continuous IV infusion of 0.1–4 mcg/kg/min		For SVT and tetralogy of Fallot spells, the final dose should be based on a successful result or a 50% increase in BP over baseline
Phenytoin Susp 25 mg/mL Chew tab 50 mg Cap 100 mg Inj 50 mg/mL	*Neonates:* Loading: 20 mg/kg IV Maintenance: 4–8 mg/kg/d IV/PO once daily or ÷ bid *Infants and older children:* **Status epilepticus** 20 mg/kg IV **Antiepileptic** Maintenance dose: 0.5–3 yr: 7–9 mg/kg/d PO ÷ q8–12h 4–6 yr: 6.5 mg/kg/d PO ÷ q8–12h	Loading dose: 1 g	Poorly absorbed after oral administration in neonates; reduce dose in liver impairment; administer at rate not to exceed 1 mg/kg/min or 50 mg/min, whichever is less; monitoring of serum drug concentration recommended; calculate loading dose according to total body weight; calculate maintenance dose according to ideal body weight; injection and caps are the sodium salt form of phenytoin (equivalent to 92% phenytoin)

		Monitor serum phosphate
	7–9 yr: 6 mg/kg/d PO ÷ q8–12h *10–16 yr:* 3–5 mg/kg/d PO ÷ q8–12h **Arrhythmia** Loading dose: 15 mg/kg/dose IV over 1 h; simultaneously give 3 mg/kg/dose PO × 1, then 6 h later give 2 mg/kg/dose PO × 1; start maintenance 6 h later OR 5 mg/kg/dose PO q6h × 4 doses, then 2.5 mg/kg/ dose PO q6h × 4 doses Maintenance: 5–6 mg/kg/d PO ÷ q12h	
Phosphate Inj sodium phosphate 3 mmol phosphate/mL (4 mmol sodium/mL) Oral solution sodium phosphate USP 4.2 mmol elemental phosphate/mL Effervescent tab (Phosphate Novartis) 500 mg elemental phosphate (16 mmol phosphate)	**Hypophosphatemia** (moderate) Oral therapy: 1–2 mmol/kg/d PO ÷ bid-qid **Hypophosphatemic rickets:** 1–3 mmol/kg/d PO ÷ qid	
	Hypophosphatemia (moderate to severe) IV therapy: 1–2 mmol phosphate/kg/d IV or 0.042–0.083 mmol phosphate/kg/h IV as a continuous infusion	Max rate of infusion: 0.125 mmol/kg/h

†‡§Refer to legend on p. 889.

(continued)

Table IV.1 Drug Dosage Guidelines for Neonates* (Where Specified), Infants, and Older Children (continued)

Drug††‡§	Dose	Dose Limit	Comments
Phosphate—cont'd	**Bowel preparation** (oral solution USP) (give dose with 120 mL water followed by 240 mL water) *<4 yr:* no dosage information *4–6 yr:* 10 mL PO *7–9 yr:* 20 mL PO *≥10 yr:* 45 mL PO	45 mL	Bowel preparation: sodium phosphate not recommended in patients with renal failure, electrolyte imbalance, advanced liver disease, ascites, poorly compensated CHF or ileus; if a repeat dose is required, monitoring of fluids and electrolytes may be warranted
Phytonadione (vitamin K₁) Inj 1 mg/0.5 mL, 10 mg/mL Tab 5 mg (Special Access drug)	*Neonates:* **Hemorrhagic disease of the newborn** Prophylaxis: 0.5–1 mg IM/SC at birth Treatment: 1 mg/dose IM/IV		Administer IV at a rate not to exceed 1 mg/min
	Infants and older children: **Warfarin antidote** No bleeding, future need for warfarin: 0.5–2 mg/dose PO No bleeding, no future need for warfarin: 2–5 mg/dose PO or IV Significant bleeding, not life threatening: 2–5 mg/dose PO or IV Significant bleeding, life threatening: 5 mg/dose IV over 10–20 min		Injection may be given by mouth, undiluted; oral tabs available by Special Access Program for long-term patients; severe anaphylactoid reactions have occurred with IV administration; give IV in emergency situations only
	Acute fulminant hepatic failure Infants: 1–2 mg/dose IV Children: 5–10 mg/dose IV		
	Malabsorption 2.5–5 mg/dose PO given 1–7 d/wk (titrate dose and frequency to effect); 1–2 mg/dose IV	25 mg/dose PO	

Piperacillin Inj 3, 4 g/vial	*Neonates:* <2 kg, 0–7 d: 150 mg/kg/d IV ÷ q12h <2 kg, >7 d: 225 mg/kg/d IV ÷ q8h ≥2 kg, 0–7 d: 225 mg/kg/d IV ÷ q8h ≥2 kg, >7 d: 300 mg/kg/d IV ÷ q6h		In neonates, reduce dose in renal impairment
	Infants and older children: 200–300 mg/kg/d IM/IV ÷ q4–6h **CF patients** 300 mg/kg/d IV/IM ÷ q4–6h	24 g/d	For infants and older children, dose interval adjustment in renal impairment: moderate, q6–8h; severe, q8h
Potassium chloride Solution 1.33 mmol/mL Cap SR 600 mg (8 mmol) Inj 2 mmol/mL	**Prevention of hypokalemia during diuretic therapy** 1–2 mmol/kg/d PO daily or ÷ bid **Treatment of hypokalemia** 2–5 mmol/kg/d PO/IV in divided doses		Give PO with food; dilute oral solution in water or juice and give over 5–10 min; cap may be opened and contents sprinkled on soft food for administration (pellets should not be chewed)
Prednisolone, prednisone Prednisolone liquid 1 mg base/mL Prednisone Susp (HSC) 5 mg/mL Tab 1, 5, 50 mg (1 mg prednisolone base = 1 mg prednisone)	**Asthma** 1–2 mg/kg/d PO daily × 5 d	60 mg/d	Individualize dose according to response. (see Table IV.3 for steroid equivalents); give with food or milk; to discontinue in patients receiving therapy for ≥10 d, reduce dose by 50% q48h until 2.5 ± 0.8 mg/m² /d is achieved, then reduce dose by 50% q10–14d except in pneumocystis pneumonia, as noted; for patients requiring oral liquid (which is very bitter), consider prednisolone liquid (commercially available as Pediapred 1 mg base/mL) or dexamethasone liquid (prepared by pharmacy, 1 mg/mL)

(continued)

Table IV.1 Drug Dosage Guidelines for Neonates* (Where Specified), Infants, and Older Children (continued)

Drug‡§	Dose	Dose Limit	Comments
Prednisolone, prednisone —cont'd	**Nephrotic syndrome** *Initial:* 60 mg/m²/d PO as single daily dose or in divided doses **Juvenile Idiopathic Arthritis (JIA)** *Initial:* 2 mg/kg/d PO daily or in divided doses		
	Idiopathic Thrombocytopenic Purpura (ITP) 3–4 mg/kg/d PO in divided doses; taper to 1–2 mg/kg/d once platelet count >30 × 10⁹/L		ITP: For life-threatening bleeding, consider IV methylprednisolone 30 mg/kg/dose (max 1 g) daily × 1–3 if patient is unable to tolerate oral therapy
	Pneumocystis pneumonia 1.6 mg/kg/d PO ÷ bid × 5 d, then 0.8 mg/kg/d as a single daily dose × 5 d, then 0.4 mg/kg/d as single daily dose × 11 d	40 mg PO bid × 5 d, then 40 mg PO daily × 5 d, then 20 mg PO daily × 11 d	
Primaquine phosphate 15 mg base/tab	**Plasmodium vivax or Plasmodium ovale (prevention of relapse)** 0.6 mg base/kg/d PO as single daily dose × 14 d **Patients with mild G6PD deficiency (10–60%)** 0.8 mg base/kg/d PO once weekly for 8 wk	Adult dose: 15 mg base/d Adult dose: 45 mg base/wk	26.3 mg primaquine phosphate = 15 mg primaquine base; check G6PD level before use
Primidone Susp (HSC) 50 mg/mL Tab 125, 250 mg	**0–8 yr / >8 yr** Starting dose: 125 mg PO qhs / 250 mg PO qhs ↑ on day 7 to 125 mg PO bid / 250 mg PO bid ↑ on day 14 to 125 mg PO tid / 250 mg PO tid ↑ on day 21 to 10–25 mg/kg/d / 750–1500 mg/kg/d PO ÷ tid–qid / PO ÷ tid–qid		Dose interval adjustment in renal impairment: moderate, q8–12h; severe, q12–24h; reduce dose in liver impairment; monitor serum concentrations of primidone and phenobarbital

Procainamide Inj 100 mg/mL	Loading dose ≤1 yr: 3–7 mg/kg/dose IV over 30–60 min >1 yr: 7–15 mg/kg/dose IV over 30–60 min	2 g/d IV	Dose interval adjustment in renal impairment: moderate: q6–12h; severe, q8–24h; IV loading dose should be switched to maintenance infusion rate before completion
Propafenone Tab 10, 150, 300 mg Inj 3.5 mg/mL (10-mg tabs and inj are Special Access drugs)	Maintenance 20–80 mcg/kg/min via continuous IV infusion 200–600 mg/m²/d PO ÷ tid–qid	500 mg/dose PO 900 mg/d; usual adult dose: 450–600 mg/d PO ÷ q8–12h	Reduce dose in renal or liver impairment; give with food or milk; reduce digoxin dose by 50% when initiating concurrent propafenone therapy
Propofol Inj 10 mg/mL	Induction: 3 mg/kg IV Maintenance: 0.25–0.3 mg/kg/min IV		Not approved for long-term sedation; carefully weigh risks vs. benefits when prescribing
Propranolol Susp (HSC) 1 mg/mL Tab 10, 40 mg Inj 1 mg/mL	Neonates: Resuscitation 0.01–0.1 mg/kg/dose IV Arrhythmia Initial: 2–3 mg/kg/d PO ÷ q6h; 0.01–0.15 mg/kg/dose IV Other 0.5–1 mg/kg/d PO ÷ q6h; 0.01–0.15 mg/kg/dose IV q6–8h, titrate dose slowly		Reduce dose in liver impairment; give IV only under electrocardiographic monitoring, undiluted over 2–10 min, at a rate not exceeding 1 mg/min

***§Refer to legend on p. 889.

(continued)

Table IV.1 Drug Dosage Guidelines for Neonates* (Where Specified), Infants, and Older Children (continued)

Drug†‡§	Dose	Dose Limit	Comments
Propranolol—cont'd	*Infants and older children:* **Arrhythmia** 0.01–0.15 mg/kg/dose IV q6–8h prn OR 2–3 mg/kg/d PO ÷ q6–8h **Antihypertensive** 0.5–4 mg/kg/d PO ÷ tid or qid **Tetralogy of Fallot spells** 0.05–0.1 mg/kg/dose IV over 10 min Maintenance: 1–6 mg/kg/d PO ÷ tid–qid **Wolff-Parkinson-White syndrome** 2–10 mg/kg/d PO ÷ tid or qid	3 mg/dose IV	
Propylthiouracil Tab 50 mg	Initial dose: 150 mg/m²/d PO ÷ q8h OR 10 mg/kg/d PO ÷ q8h	Initial dose: *6–10 yr:* 150 mg/d *>10 yr:* 300 mg/d; higher doses can be used when necessary	Reduce dose in liver impairment; give at same time in relation to meals every day; once patient is euthyroid, reduce dose to minimum required (usually ⅓–½ of initial dose); may cause agranulocytosis or hepatic dysfunction
Prostaglandin E₁	See alprostadil		
Protamine sulfate Inj 10 mg/mL	*From last dose* <30 min 30–60 min 61–120 min >120 min	*Per 100 units of unfractionated heparin (max 50 mg/dose)* 1 mg 0.5–0.75 mg 0.375–0.5 mg 0.25–0.375 mg	Protamine sulfate should be administered in a concentration of 10 mg/mL at a rate not to exceed 5 mg/min; or may cause cardiovascular collapse; hypersensitivity risk in those with fish allergy, those who received protamin-containing insulin or previous protamin therapy

Pseudoephedrine Syrup 6 mg/mL Tab 60 mg	<2 yr: 4 mg/kg/d PO ÷ q6h prn 2-5 yr: 15 mg/dose PO q6h prn 6-12 yr: 30 mg/dose PO q6h prn	Usual adult dose: 60 mg/dose PO q4-6h prn	Use with caution in hypertensive patients and children <2 yr; dose combination products according to pseudoephedrine content
Pyrazinamide Tab 500 mg Susp (HSC) 100 mg/mL	15-30 mg/kg/d PO daily OR ÷ q12h or 50-70 mg/kg/ dose PO twice weekly Regimens for treatment and prophylaxis vary; consult specialty references or local Infectious Diseases service for more information	2 g/d; 2 g/dose twice/wk	Dose reduction may be required in hepatic impairment; dose reduction in severe renal impairment: 50-100%
Pyridoxine (vitamin B₆) Inj 100 mg/mL Solution (HSC) 1 mg/mL Tab 25, 100, 250 mg	*Neonates, infants, and older children:* **Pyridoxine-dependent seizures** Initial: 10-100 mg/dose IV/PO Maintenance: 50-100 mg/d PO **Drug-induced neuritis** Treatment: 10-50 mg/d PO Prophylaxis: 1-2 mg/kg/d PO		Monitor EEG concurrently
Quetiapine Tab 25, 100, 200 mg	*Children:* Initial dose: 12.5 mg/dose PO once daily or bid *Adolescents:* Initial: 25 mg/dose PO once daily or bid	Usual adult target dose: 300-600 mg/d	Reduce dose in liver impairment; to achieve maintenance dose, increase by 25-50 mg q2d
Quinidine Sulfate (83% quinidine base) Solution (HSC) 10 mg/mL	**Dysrhythmia** 15-60 mg (base)/kg/d PO ÷ q4-6h	500 mg/dose	Reduce dose to 30% in severe liver impairment; dose may require reduction in severe CHF; digoxin maintenance dose requires reduction during concurrent quinidine therapy
Quinine sulfate (83% quinine base) Cap 200 mg sulfate = 166 mg base	**Severe plasmodium** (all types) 20 mg/kg IV loading dose over 4 h, followed by 10 mg/kg IV over 2-4 h q8h (max 1800 mg/d) until oral therapy can be started	1.5 g (base)/d	If >48 h of parenteral treatment required, quinine dose should be reduced by ⅓ to ½; give with food or milk; chloroquine-resistant strains generally require total of 7 d of treatment with quinine or quinidine and a second drug

(continued)

***Refer to legend on p. 889.

969

Table IV.1 — Drug Dosage Guidelines for Neonates* (Where Specified), Infants, and Older Children (continued)

Drug††§	Dose	Dose Limit	Comments
Quinine—cont'd 300 mg sulfate = 249 mg base **Dihydrochloride** Inj 600 mg dihydrochloride/ 2 mL (300 mg/mL dihydrochloride = 245 mg/mL quinine) (injection is Special Access drug)	**Uncomplicated falciparum** or sequential oral therapy 22.5 mg (base)/kg/d PO ÷ tid × 3–7 d		
Ranitidine Solution 15 mg/mL Tab 75, 150 mg Inj 25 mg/mL	*Neonates:* 1.25–1.9 mg/kg/d IV ÷ q6–12h 2.5–3.8 mg/kg/d PO ÷ q12h *Infants and older children:* 2–6 mg/kg/d IV ÷ q6–12h **Peptic ulcer, GERD** Treatment: 5–8 mg/kg/d PO ÷ q12h × 8 wk Maintenance: 2.5–5 mg/kg/d PO once daily	300 mg/d except in Zollinger-Ellison syndrome; usual adult dose: 300 mg/d as single hs dose or ÷ q12h	Reduce dose in renal impairment For infants and older children, moderate: 75% usual dose; severe: 50% usual dose Monitor gastric pH in patients requiring IV therapy
Rasburicase Inj (HSC) 1.5 mg/mL	0.2 mg/kg/dose IV over 30 min q24h		Contraindicated in G6PD deficiency; do not give for longer than 7 d
Rifampin Susp (HSC) 25 mg/mL Cap 150, 300 mg	*Neonates:* 10–20 mg/kg/d IV once daily or ÷ bid 20 mg/kg/d PO ÷ q12h		Reduce dose in liver impairment; may discolor urine, sweat, saliva, tears; give on an empty stomach (1 h ac or 2 h pc) unless GI upset occurs; monitor liver function tests periodically; may reduce serum

			concentration of many other medications, including anticoagulants, tacrolimus, cyclosporine, and oral contraceptives
Inj 300 mg/vial (available through Special Access Program)	*Infants and older children:* **Tuberculosis** 10–20 mg/kg/d PO once daily or ÷ q12h OR 10–20 mg/ kg/dose PO twice weekly (regimens for treatment and prophylaxis vary; consult Infectious Diseases service for more information)	600 mg/d	
	Meningococcal prophylaxis 20 mg/kg/d PO ÷ q12h × 2 d	600 mg/d	
	Haemophilus influenzae prophylaxis 20 mg/kg/d PO once daily × 4 d	600 mg/d	
Risperidone Liquid 1 mg/mL Tab 0.25, 1, 2 mg	*Children:* Initial dose: 0.25–0.5 mg/dose PO once daily OR 0.25 mg/dose PO bid *Adolescents:* Initial dose: 1 mg/dose PO once daily OR 0.5–1 mg/dose PO bid Titrate dose upward based on clinical response	Usual adult target dose: 4–6 mg/d	Reduce dose in renal or liver impairment; to achieve maintenance dose, increase by 0.5–1 mg q3-4d

(continued)

†‡§Refer to legend on p. 889.

971

Table IV.1 Drug Dosage Guidelines for Neonates* (Where Specified), Infants, and Older Children (continued)

Drug[†§]	Dose	Dose Limit	Comments
Ritonavir Liquid 80 mg/mL Cap 100 mg	500 mg/m²/d PO + bid × 2 d, then 600 mg/m²/d PO + bid × 2 d, then 700 mg/m²/d PO + bid × 2 d, then 800 mg/m²/d PO + bid	Adult dose: 1200 mg/d	Liquid is unpalatable: give after popsicle or frozen juice (to dull taste buds); give with high-fat snack or meal (ice cream, high-fat dairy products); may develop resistance if only a few doses are missed; liquid contains 43% alcohol v/v
Rituximab Inj 100 mg/10 mL	375 mg/m²/dose IV weekly	375 mg/m²/dose	Premedication with acetaminophen and diphenhydramine is recommended
Salbutamol Oral solution 0.4 mg/mL Inhalation solution 5 mg/mL Metered-dose aerosol 100 mcg/puff Inj 1 mg/mL	*Neonates:* 0.25 mL/dose via nebulizer q4–12h prn, up to q2h max *Infants and older children:* **Acute asthma** *Inhalation solution:* 0.01–0.03 mL/kg/dose in 3 mL 0.9% NaCl via nebulizer q½–4h prn; in severe cases, give initial dose of 0.03 mL/kg/dose q20min via nebulizer *Infusion:* initial rate, 1 mcg/kg/min IV; increase by 1 mcg/kg/min q15min prn up to max of 10 mcg/min **Maintenance therapy for asthma** 100–200 mcg/dose prn, max frequency q4h via metered-dose aerosol/Diskhaler 0.03 mL/kg/dose in 3 mL 0.9% NaCl via nebulizer prn, max q4h 0.3 mg/kg/d PO ÷ tid or qid **Hyperkalemia** 4 mcg/kg IV over 20 min	Inhalation solution: min. 0.2 mL/dose; max 1 mL/dose Oral dose: 16 mg/d	Monitor for tachycardia, hypokalemia; limit nebulized salbutamol to 4 × per day for outpatients

Senna Syrup 1.7 mg/mL Tab 8.6 mg	Syrup: 2–5 yr: 3–5 mL/dose PO qhs 6–12 yr: 5–10 mL/dose PO qhs Tab: 6–12 yr: 1–2 tabs/dose PO qhs	Have patient drink plenty of fluids; effects occur within 6–24 h after PO dosing; avoid prolonged use
	Usual adult dose: 2–4 tabs qhs	
Sevelamer Tab 800 mg	Initial: 400 mg PO bid; titrate dose to serum phosphorus Usual dose: 800–1600 mg PO tid with meals; additional doses may be required with snacks	Tabs should not be split or chewed; separate administration from that of other medications whenever possible, administering them at least 1 h before or 3 h after sevelamer; if calcium supplements required, give sevelamer qhs; monitor serum calcium and phosphate at least q1–3wk until target concentrations are achieved
Simethicone Oral drops 40 mg/mL	<2 yr: 20 mg PO qid 2–12 yr: 40 mg PO qid >12 yr: 40–250 mg PO qid	500 mg/d
		Administer after meals and at bedtime; may be mixed with water or other liquids
Sirolimus Liquid 1 mg/mL Tab 1 mg	Loading dose (de novo transplant recipient): 0.42 mg/kg/d PO Initial maintenance dose: 0.14 mg/kg/d PO once daily	15 mg/dose
		Reduce dose in liver impairment; maintenance dose individualized based on disease state, type of transplant, and time since transplant; tabs should not be cut or crushed; liquid must be further diluted with water or orange juice (not grapefruit juice); sirolimus may interact with many other medications
Sodium bicarbonate Inj 4.2% (0.5 mmol/mL), 8.4% (1 mmol/mL) Oral solution (HSC) 1 mmol/mL	*Neonates:* **Correction of metabolic acidosis** IV dose (mmol HCO_3) = weight (kg) × 0.3 × HCO_3 deficit (mmol/L) Administer half the calculated dose for half correction and assess need for remainder; complete correction not recommended	Dilute the 8.4% strength 1:1 with sterile water or use the 4.2% strength undiluted; give over 5–10 min Incompatible with epinephrine, calcium, atropine

(continued)

Pediatric Drug Dosing Guidelines

IV

Table IV.1 — Drug Dosage Guidelines for Neonates* (Where Specified), Infants, and Older Children (continued)

Drug†‡§	Dose	Dose Limit	Comments
Sodium bicarbonate —cont'd	**Mild asphyxia** 1–3 mmol/kg/dose IV over 5 min **Severe asphyxia** 3–5 mmol/kg/dose IV over 5 min *Infants and older children:* **Resuscitation** 1–2 mmol/kg/dose IV/IO; repeat 1–2 mmol/kg/dose prn as per blood gases and clinical response		
Sodium polystyrene sulfonate (Kayexalate) Powder Susp 250 mg/mL Enema 30 g/120 mL	*Neonates:* 1 g/kg/dose in water or D5W PO/PR *Infants and older children:* 1 g/kg/dose PO q6h prn 1 g/kg/dose PR q2–6h prn	Usual adult oral dose: 15 g/dose	Exchanges approximately 1 mmol K⁺/ g of resin Administer rectally in appropriate volume of tap water, D10W, or equal parts tap water and 2% methylcellulose; moisten resin with honey or jam for PO use
Sorbitol Syrup 70%	**Cathartic** 1.5–2 mL/kg/dose PO	150 mL/dose	
Sotalol Susp (HSC) 5 mg/mL Tab 80, 160 mg	**Arrhythmias** 2–5 mg/kg/d PO ÷ q12h–q8h	480 mg/d; usual adult dose: 320 mg/d PO ÷ bid	Dose reduction in renal impairment: moderate, 30% standard dose; severe, 15–30% standard dose; reduce dose in hepatic impairment
Spironolactone Susp (HSC) 5 mg/mL Tab 25, 100 mg	*Neonates:* 2–4 mg/kg/d PO ÷ q12h *Infants and older children:* 1–4 mg/kg/d PO given once daily–qid	Usual adult dose: 25–200 mg/d	Avoid when creatinine clearance <10 mL/min; for spironolactone combined with hydrochlorothiazide, see aldactazide

Stavudine Cap 15 mg Liquid 1 mg/mL (Special Access drug)	*<30 kg:* 2 mg/kg/d PO ÷ q12h *30-50 kg:* 30 mg PO bid (may initiate at 15 mg PO bid) *≥60 kg:* 40 mg PO bid (may initiate at 20 mg PO bid)	40 mg/dose	Adjust dose in renal impairment: moderate, 50% of usual dose q12-24h; severe, 50% of usual dose q24h
Sterculia Granules 7 g/packet	*<12 yr:* ½ packet PO daily; may increase to ½ packet PO bid *≥12 yr:* 1-2 packets PO as a single daily dose or ÷ bid		Granules should not be chewed; avoid giving within 2 h of other medications
Sucralfate Susp 200 mg/mL Tab 1 g	*1-10 kg:* 250 mg/dose PO q6h *>10-20 kg:* 500 mg/dose PO q6h *>20 kg:* 1 g/dose PO q6h	Adult dose: 4 g/d PO ÷ qid (1 h ac + qhs)	
Sulfasalazine Susp (HSC) 100 mg/mL Tab 500 mg EC tab 500 mg	**Juvenile Idiopathic Arthritis (JIA)** 40-60 mg/kg/d PO ÷ bid-qid		For JRA: begin with ½ recommended dose and increase q2d to max required dose; reduce dose in renal impairment; give with food; maintain fluid intake; may discolor skin, tears, and urine orange yellow; monitor for blood dyscrasias; caution in patients with hypersensitivity to salicylates or sulfonamides and in patients with G6PD deficiency
	Ulcerative colitis *Acute:* 40-70 mg/kg/d PO ÷ tid-qid pc	6 g/d	
	Maintenance: 20-50 mg/kg/d PO ÷bid-qid	2 g/d	
Surfactant (BLES) 3, 5 mL vial	*Neonates:* 5 mL/kg/dose; may be repeated q6-12h × 2 doses		

*†‡§Refer to legend on p. 889.

(continued)

Table IV.1   Drug Dosage Guidelines for Neonates* (Where Specified), Infants, and Older Children (continued)

Drug[†‡§]	Dose	Dose Limit	Comments
Sumatriptan Solution, nasal spray 5, 20 mg	*20–39 kg:* 5–10 mg inhaled ×1 *≥40 mg or >12 yr:* 20 mg inhaled ×1 May repeat dose × 1 after 2 h if headache returns or if only partial response to first dose	40 mg/24 h	
Tacrolimus Inj 5 mg/mL Cap 0.5, 1, 5 mg Susp (HSC) 0.5 mg/mL	Initial dose before TDM **Cardiac transplantation** 0.01 mg/kg/d as continuous IV infusion or ÷ q12h 0.2 mg/kg/d PO/NG ÷ q12h **Liver transplantation** 0.2 mg/kg/d PO/NG ÷ q12h **Renal transplantation** 0.2 mg/kg/d PO/NG ÷ q12h **Various indications** 0.05–0.3 mg/kg/d PO ÷ q12h; adjust dose by TDM		Maintenance dose should be individualized based on factors such as disease state, type of transplant, and time since transplantation; measure initial trough concentration within 48 h and adjust dose as necessary; to switch from cyclosporine to tacrolimus, discontinue cyclosporine and start tacrolimus 24 h later; tacrolimus may interact with many other medications; tacrolimus should always be taken with the same beverage (not grapefruit juice); cap should be used in patients with short gut
Tazocin (piperacillin/ tazobactam) Inj 3.375 g (piperacillin 3 g + tazobactam 0.375 g) 4.5 g (piperacillin 4 g + tazobactam 0.5 g)	240 mg piperacillin/kg/d IV ÷ q8h	100 mg piperacillin/kg/dose OR 4 g piperacillin/dose, whichever is less	Dose and interval adjustment in renal impairment: moderate, decrease dose by 30% and give q6h; severe, decrease dose by 30% and give q8h
Tetracycline Cap 250 mg	25–50 mg/kg/d PO ÷ q6h **As alternative agent for *Helicobacter pylori* eradication** 50 mg/kg/d PO ÷ bid-qid	3 g/d 1 g bid	Dose interval adjustment in renal impairment: moderate, q12-24h; avoid in severe renal impairment; use with caution in patients with hepatic insufficiency; do not use in children ≤8 yr as may cause

Theophylline Liquid 5.3 mg/mL Inj 0.8 mg/mL, 4 mg/mL	**For patients not currently receiving aminophylline or theophylline** Loading dose: 6 mg/kg IV Initial maintenance dose: 2–6 mo: 0.4 mg/kg/h IV 6–11 mo: 0.7 mg/kg/h IV 1–12 yr: 0.8 mg/kg/h IV 12–16 yr: 0.7 mg/kg/h IV >16 yr (nonsmoker): 0.6 mg/kg/h IV Cardiac decompensation, cor pulmonale, liver dysfunction: 0.2 mg/kg/h IV **Prevention of contrast-induced nephropathy** 3–5 mg/kg IV × 1, 30–45 min before procedure (reserved for urgent procedures)	Max. maintenance dose before TDM: 4 wk–1 yr: 0.2 [age in wk] + 5 mg/kg/d PO ÷ q6-8h 1–9 yr: 20 mg/kg/d PO ÷ q8-12h 9–12 yr or smokers: 16 mg/kg/d PO ÷ q8-12h 12–16 yr (nonsmoker): 13 mg/kg/d PO ÷ q8-12h >16 yr (nonsmoker): 10 mg/kg/d PO ÷ q8-12h or 900 mg/d, whichever is less Cardiac decompensation, cor pulmonale, liver dysfunction: 5 mg/kg/d PO ÷ q8-12h or 400 mg/d, whichever is less	permanent discoloration of teeth, enamel hypoplasia, and (usually reversible) retardation of skeletal development; give on an empty stomach; do not administer with dairy products, milk formulas, antacids, bismuth, or iron products; enhances effects of warfarin; may cause photosensitivity Reduce dose in liver impairment; monitoring of serum drug concentration recommended; calculate loading dose according to effective body weight; calculate maintenance dose according to ideal body weight; administer IV at a rate not to exceed 20 mg/min; IV doses are conservative; titrate dose according to serum concentration; oral doses in patients ≥1 yr apply to sustained-release products, which are preferred for chronic dosing; max oral doses should be attained in stepwise fashion to prevent intolerance in patients not being converted from IV therapy; begin at 50% of recommended doses; give PO on empty stomach (1 h ac or 2 h pc) unless GI upset occurs

(continued)

†‡§Refer to legend on p. 889.

Table IV.1 — Drug Dosage Guidelines for Neonates* (Where Specified), Infants, and Older Children *(continued)*

Drug†‡§	Dose	Dose Limit	Comments
Tobramycin Inj 10 mg/mL, 40 mg/mL	*Neonates:* 0–7 d, <34 wk PCA: 3 mg/kg/dose IV q24h 0–7 d, ≥34 wk PCA: 3 mg/kg/dose IV q18h >7 d, ≤1 kg: 3.5 mg/kg/dose IV q24h >7 d, >1 kg, <37 wk PCA: 2.5 mg/kg/dose IV q12h >7 d, >1 kg, ≥37 wk PCA: 2.5 mg/kg/dose IV q8h		Calculate dose according to effective body weight; in neonates, reduce dose in renal impairment; for infants and older children, adjust dose interval in renal impairment: moderate, q12h; severe, q24–48h; monitoring of serum drug concentration recommended; peripheral venous sampling to be done in patients on concurrent inhaled and IV tobramycin
	Infants and older children: 7.5 mg/kg/d IV/IM ÷ q8h	120 mg/dose before TDM	
	CF patients (for non–lung transplant patients only) *Females >14 yr:* 7 mg/kg/d IV q24h *All other patients:* 9 mg/kg/d IV q24h 80 mg tid via inhalation	CF: no max single dose	
Topiramate Tabs: 25, 100 mg Sprinkle caps: 15, 25 mg	*>2–16 yr:* Initial dose: 1–3 mg/kg/d PO as single daily dose hs or ÷ bid	Initial dose: 25 mg	Dose or interval adjustment in renal impairment: moderate, q36h or give 75% of standard dose; severe, q48h or give 50% of standard dose
	Increase dose at 1–2-wk intervals by 1–3 mg/kg/d ÷ bid Maintenance dose: 5–9 mg/kg/d ÷ bid	Max increase: 50 mg	Give PO dose with food; tabs may be split; sprinkle caps may be opened, sprinkled on small amount (5 mL) of soft food and swallowed (not chewed)
	≥17 yr: Initial dose: 50 mg PO daily Increase dose at weekly intervals by 50 mg/d ÷ bid Usual maintenance dose: 200–400 mg/d PO ÷ bid	Max maintenance dose: 600 mg/d	

Tranexamic acid Inj 100 mg/mL Tab 500 mg Mouth rinse (HSC) 4.8 mg/mL	**Before procedures for dental surgery in patients with coagulopathy** 7–10 mg/kg/dose IV preprocedure and tid-qid afterward until able to take PO medications 25 mg/kg/dose PO tid-qid, beginning 1 d before procedure and for up to 6–8 d afterward **Cardiac surgery** Pediatric dose not well established; 50–100 mg/kg IV at beginning of procedure; an infusion of 10 mg/kg/h intraoperatively has been used	Adjust interval in renal impairment: mild, q12h; moderate, q24h; severe, q48h OR adjust dose: mild, 50% usual dose; moderate, 25% usual dose; severe, 10% usual dose; may give injection undiluted over at least 5 min or at max rate of 100 mg/min; faster infusion may cause hypotension Contraindicated in patients with history or risk of thrombosis unless also receiving anticoagulation Ophthalmic assessment recommended before and during chronic therapy (e.g., treatment several weeks in duration)
Trimethoprim Susp (HSC) 10 mg/mL Tab 100 mg	**Treatment** 4–6 mg/kg/d PO ÷ q12h **UTI prophylaxis** (including neonates) 2 mg/kg/d PO ÷ bid or as single daily dose	Usual adult dose: 200 mg/d Interval adjustment in renal impairment: moderate, q18h; severe, avoid; may be given with food
Ursodiol Tab 250 mg Susp (HSC) 50 mg/mL	10–20 mg/kg/d PO ÷ bid-tid	45 mg/kg/d

*†‡§Refer to legend on p. 889.

(continued)

Table IV.1 Drug Dosage Guidelines for Neonates* (Where Specified), Infants, and Older Children (continued)

Drug‡‡§	Dose	Dose Limit	Comments
Valproic acid Syrup 50 mg/mL Cap 250 mg Tab (divalproex) 125, 250, 500 mg Inj 100 mg/mL (available through Special Access Program)	Initial dose: 15 mg/kg/d PO once daily or ÷ q8–12h; increase dose weekly prn by 5–10 mg/kg/d up to 30–60 mg/kg/d PO ÷ tid or qid	60 mg/kg/d	Reduce dose in liver impairment; monitoring of serum drug concentration recommended; dose conversion from PO to IV is 1:1; whereas total daily IV dose equals total daily PO dose, IV dose should be divided q6h
Vancomycin Cap 125 mg Liquid (HSC) 100 mg/mL Inj 500 mg: 1, 5, 10 g/vial	*Neonates:* <800 g or <27 wk PCA: 27 mg/kg/dose IV q36h 800–1200 g or 27–30 wk PCA: 24 mg/kg/dose IV q24h 1200–2000 g or 31–36 wk PCA: 18 mg/kg/dose IV q12h OR 27 mg/kg/dose IV q18 h >2000 g or ≥37 wk PCA: 22.5 mg/kg/dose IV q12h		Monitoring of serum drug concentration recommended
	Infants and older children: **Mild to moderate infections** 40 mg/kg/d IV ÷ q6h	2 g/d	Calculate doses according to effective body weight; injection may be used for oral dosing; dose interval adjustment in renal impairment: mild, q8–18h; moderate, q18–72h; severe, q3–7d
	Severe infections 40–60 mg/kg/d IV ÷ q6h	4 g/d	
	Unstable neutropenic patient with fever 60 mg/kg/d IV ÷ q6h	4 g/d	

	Meningitis 60 mg/kg/d IV ÷ q6h	4 g/d	
	Pseudomembranous colitis 50 mg/kg/d PO ÷ q6h	500 mg/dose	
	Cardiac surgery prophylaxis 20 mg/kg/dose IV q12h × 2 doses	1 g/dose	
	Sickle cell disease 60 mg/kg/d IV ÷ q6h	4 g/d	
Verapamil Susp (HSC) 8 mg/mL Tab 80, 120 mg Inj 2.5 mg/mL	0–2 yr: 0.1–0.2 mg/kg/dose IV 2–15 yr: 0.1–0.3 mg/kg/dose IV; may repeat × 1 in 30 min prn	Repeat dose: 10 mg/dose IV	Administer IV under electrocardiographic monitoring; avoid use in early postcardiosurgical period, in severe CHF, or in presence of β-blockers
	Maintenance: 4–10 mg/kg/d PO ÷ tid or qid	Usual adult dose: 240–480 mg/d	
Vigabatrin Tab 500 mg	Initial dose: 30 mg/kg/d PO as single daily dose or ÷ bid, increase weekly	Initial: 1 g/d	Reduce dose in renal impairment; may be given with food; concurrent use of vigabatrin may decrease serum phenytoin levels; regular ophthalmologic monitoring required
	Usual maintenance dose: 60 mg/kg/d PO as single daily dose or ÷ bid	Maintenance: 100 mg/kg/d or 4 g/d	
	Infantile spasms Day 1:100 mg/kg/d PO ÷ bid Day 2:125 mg/kg/d PO ÷ bid Day 3 and onward: 150 mg/kg/d PO ÷ bid		

*†‡§Refer to legend on p. 889.

Table IV.1 Drug Dosage Guidelines for Neonates* (Where Specified), Infants, and Older Children (continued)

Drug‡‡§	Dose	Dose Limit	Comments
Vitamin K₁	See phytonadione		
Warfarin Tab 1, 2, 2.5, 3, 5 mg Solution (HSC) Dissolve 'n' Dose System	For dosing guidelines, see Guidelines for Warfarin Therapy, p. xx		May interact with many medications; consider consulting pharmacist regarding patients taking multiple medications
Zidovudine Liquid 10 mg/mL Cap 100 mg Combination tab (Combivir): 300 mg zidovudine + 150 mg lamivudine	**Postexposure prophylaxis, in combination with lamivudine ± Kaletra and HIV infection, in combination therapy** 6 wk–12 yr: 360–480 mg/m²/d PO ÷ bid OR 480 mg/m²/d PO ÷ tid >12 yr or ≥50 kg: 600 mg/d PO ÷ bid–tid	600 mg/d	Reduce dose in renal or liver impairment
Zinc sulfate Solution (HSC) 10 mg/mL elemental zinc as zinc sulfate Inj 10 mg elemental zinc/10 mL	**Supplementation** 0.5–1 mg elemental zinc/kg/d PO ÷ bid–tid	15 mg elemental zinc/d	Give with food to reduce GI irritation
	Acrodermatitis enteropathica 1–2 mg elemental zinc/d PO ÷ bid–tid	45 mg elemental zinc/d	

*‡‡§Refer to legend on p. 889.

Table IV.2 Therapeutic Drug Monitoring

Drug	Time for First TDM*	Ideal Sampling Time†	Optimal Concentration Range	Comments
Acetaminophen		≥4 h after ingestion		Toxicology only; see nomogram, p. 67
Amikacin: traditional dosing	On day 4 of therapy (or in selected patients,‡ after the third or fourth dose)	*Trough:* (IV) 0–30 min before dose *Peak:* (IV) 30–60 min after finish of drug flush	Trough: 2.5–10 mg/L Peak: 20–35 mg/L	Half-life may be prolonged in patients with renal dysfunction; both clearance and volume of distribution may be increased in CF
Amikacin: once-daily dosing	"Special" concentrations 3 h and 6 h after the first dose		Peak: 60–80 mg/L Drug-free interval (where concentration <4 mg/L) = 4 h	Restricted to febrile neutropenia in hematology/oncology/ hematopoietic progenitor cell transplant (bone marrow transplant) patients
ASA: see salicylate				
Caffeine	1 wk (then weekly)	*Trough:* 0–4 h before dose	30–100 μmol/L	Half-life up to 100 h in premature neonates
Carbamazepine	Initial dose: 1 wk (then twice/ wk until stable) *Dose change:* 3 d	*Trough:* 0–1 h before dose 10,11-epoxide, trough: 0–1 h before dose	17–50 μmol/L (active metabolite carbamazepine-not routine but may be of assistance) 5–12 μmol/L	Because of enzyme autoinduction, half-life during chronic dosing may be considerably shorter than after first dose; consequently, within first 2–4 wk of therapy, dose may need to be increased

Under certain circumstances, it may be necessary to collect samples for monitoring at times that do not coincide with normal "peak" and "trough" assessment; such samples are referred to as "special" concentrations. Special drug concentrations may have to be obtained when

- patients are receiving peritoneal dialysis, hemodialysis, or CVVH
- patients have unstable or poor renal function
- therapy has been stopped after previous high drug concentration

(continued)

Table IV.2 Therapeutic Drug Monitoring (continued)

Drug	Time for First TDM*	Ideal Sampling Time†	Optimal Concentration Range	Comments
Cyclosporine	*Continuous infusion:* 2 d *Intermittent (IV or PO):* 5 doses	*Continuous infusion:* no restrictions *Intermittent:* *Trough:* 0–60 min before dose	Optimal concentration range dependent on clinical status of patient, type of transplant, time since transplant, and assay matrix	Monitoring considered mandatory to avoid extremely low or high levels that may precipitate therapeutic failure or nephrotoxicity
Digoxin	*After load:* 48 h *Maintenance:* 5 d (2 d if risk factors: poor therapeutic response, symptoms of toxicity, renal or hepatic impairment, drug interactions [e.g., amiodarone, propafenone])	*Trough:* 0–60 min before dose (or at least 8 h after last dose)	1–2.5 nmol/L	Half-life may be prolonged in renal impairment; in infants and children, concentration–effect relationship somewhat imprecise; if level normal on day 5 without clinical problems, repeat level on weekly basis as inpatient and every 3 mo as outpatient
Ethosuximide	7 d	*Trough:* 0–60 min before dose	280–710 μmol/L	Selected patients may tolerate and benefit from levels that are higher than recommended max level
Flucytosine	3 d	*Peak:* 2 h after PO dose or 1 h after IV dose	50–100 mg/L	
Gentamicin: traditional dosing	On day 4 of therapy (or in selected patients,‡ after the third or fourth dose)	*Trough:* 0–30 min before dose *Peak:* 30–60 min after end of infusion	*Trough:* 0.6–2 mg/L *Peak:* 5–10 mg/L	Target peak concentration for indication UTI: 3–5 mg/L Pyelonephritis, cellulitis: 5–7 mg/L Pneumonia, wound infection: 6–8 mg/L Positive culture with neutropenia: 7–9 mg/L

Gentamicin: once-daily dosing	"Special" concentrations 3 h and 6 h after the first dose	Peak: 20–25 mg/L Drug-free interval (where concentration <2 mg/L) = 4 h	Risk factors should prompt closer monitoring (neutropenia, positive cultures, persistent fever, concurrent therapy with a nephrotoxic agent, unstable renal function or fluid imbalance, abnormal cardiac status, prematurity, severe burns) Frequency of continued monitoring depends on clinical status and renal function; however, in stable patients, creatinine and trough concentrations are usually obtained approximately every 7 d; consult pharmacist regarding monitoring in dialysis patients
Lithium	*Trough:* 12 h after dose	0.5–1.5 mmol/L	Restricted to febrile neutropenia in hematology/oncology/ hematopoietic progenitor cell transplant (bone marrow transplant) patients Must be clotted sample
Methotrexate (high dose)	Dependent on treatment protocol	Folinic acid stopped once levels are <0.08 μmol/L (higher concentrations may be acceptable according to protocol)	Concentrations elevated by impairment of renal filtration or secretion
	4–6 d	Dependent on treatment protocol	
Mycophenolic acid (MPA) MMF metabolite	*Trough:* 0–60 min before dose	Optimal concentration range dependent on clinical status of patient, type of transplant, time since transplant, and assay matrix	
	3 d		

(continued)

Table IV.2 Therapeutic Drug Monitoring (continued)

Drug	Time for First TDM*	Ideal Sampling Time†	Optimal Concentration Range	Comments
Phenobarbital	*IV loading:* no restrictions *Maintenance:* 4 d (7 d for steady state)	*IV loading:* At least 1 h after load *Maintenance:* Trough: 0–60 min before dose	65–170 µmol/L	Specific patients tolerate and may benefit from serum levels that are significantly higher than "recommended maximum limit"
Phenytoin	*IV loading:* no restrictions *Maintenance:* 3 d (then twice/wk until stable)	*IV loading:* At least 1 h after load *Maintenance:* Trough: 0–1 h before dose	40–80 µmol/L Free: 4–8 µmol/L	Simultaneous monitoring of free phenytoin levels not routine but may be of assistance
Primidone	3 d	Trough: 0–1 h before dose	23–55 µmol/L	Phenobarbital is major metabolite; therefore, take concurrent level; expected parent drug-to-metabolite ratio varies from 1:4 to 1:2
Salicylate, ASA	Toxicology: no restrictions Therapeutic: 3 d	Toxicology: At least 6 h after ingestion Therapeutic: Trough: 0–1 h before dose	JIA: 1.1–2.2 mmol/L Kawasaki disease, pericarditis: <2.2 mmol/L	Time to peak varies and is prolonged with enteric-coated product Overdose: see p. 64
Sirolimus	5 d	Trough: 0–30 min before dose	5–15 mcg/L (optimal concentration range may vary according to clinical status of patient, type of transplant, time since transplant, and assay matrix)	

		Trough: 0–30 min before dose	5–15 mcg/L (optimal concentration range may vary according to clinical status of patient, type of transplant, time since transplant, and assay matrix)	
Tacrolimus	3 d			
Theophylline	Loading: no restrictions Continuous IV infusion: after 12–24 h Intermittent (PO or IV): 24–48 h	Loading: at least 1 h postload Continuous IV infusion: no restrictions Intermittent (PO or IV): Trough: 0–30 min before dose Peak: (a) 1–2 h after IV or Theolair (b) 3–7 h after sustained-release preparations	55–110 μmol/L	
Tobramycin: traditional dosing	On day 4 of therapy (or in selected patients,‡ after the third or fourth dose)	Trough: 0–30 min before dose Peak: 30–60 min after end of infusion	Trough: 0.6–2 mg/L Peak: 5–10 mg/L	See comments for gentamicin Consult pharmacist regarding monitoring in dialysis patients
Valproic acid	2 d	Trough: 0–1 h before dose	350–700 μmol/L	Half-life may be prolonged in patients with hepatic disease and may be shortened in patients receiving other anticonvulsant drugs

(continued)

Table IV.2 Therapeutic Drug Monitoring (continued)

Drug	Time for First TDM*	Ideal Sampling Time†	Optimal Concentration Range	Comments
Vancomycin	Fourth or fifth dose (earlier if significant renal impairment or dosing intervals ≥q12h)	*Trough:* 0–30 min before dose *Peak:* 60–90 min after end of 1-h infusion	*Trough:* CNS infections: 10–15 mg/L Other infections: 5–12 mg/L *Peak:* 24–40 mg/L	Peak routinely determined *only* for patients who may have altered pharmacokinetics (febrile neutropenic patients, burn patients, neonates); peak concentrations are of no utility when drug is infused for > 1 h and do not correlate with toxicity or effectiveness; additional trough monitoring required for dosage adjustment, treatment > 7 d in duration, addition of nephrotoxic drugs, high minimum inhibitory concentration (MIC) isolate, renal insufficiency/failure; consult pharmacist regarding monitoring in dialysis patients

*Time for first therapeutic drug monitoring (TDM): refers to first routine opportunity for sampling after new order or order change: normally represents attainment of steady state. Routine drug levels should not be measured before attainment of steady-state conditions unless failure of therapeutic response or onset of toxicity suspected.

†Ideal sampling time permits direct comparison with optimal concentration range: results of tests conducted on samples collected at other than ideal times must be interpreted cautiously.

‡Renal impairment, premature infants, term infants <7 d, documented infections where therapy continues >72 h, therapy >7 d, concurrent nephrotoxic drugs (i.e., amphotericin, cyclosporine), severe burns.

DOSE EQUIVALENTS OF COMMOMLY USED STEROIDS

Table IV.3	Dose Equivalents of Commonly Used Steroids	
Drug	Glucocorticoid Effect Equivalent to Cortisol 100 mg PO	Mineralocorticoid Effect Equivalent to Fludrocortisone Acetate (Florinef) 0.1 mg*
Cortisone	125	20
Hydrocortisone	100	20
Prednisone	25	50
Prednisolone	20–25	50
Methylprednisone	15–20	No effect
Triamcinolone	10–20	No effect
9-alpha-Fluorocortisol	6.5	0.1
Dexamethasone	1.5–3.75	No effect

*Total physiologic replacement for salt retention is usually 0.1 mg fludrocortisone acetate (Florinef) regardless of patient's size.

ENDOCARDITIS PROPHYLAXIS

Box IV.1 | Cardiac Conditions in Which Prophylaxis Is Recommended

Based on the balance of risk vs. benefit, antibiotic prophylaxis is no longer recommended for dental procedures based solely on an increased lifetime risk of infective endocarditis (IE). Prophylaxis is only recommended for patients with the highest risk of adverse outcomes from IE, including patients with the following cardiac conditions:

- Prosthetic cardiac valves, including bioprosthetic and homograft valves
- Previous bacterial endocarditis
- Congenital heart disease (CHD)
  1. Unrepaired cyanotic CHD, including palliative shunts and conduits
  2. Completely repaired congenital heart defect with prosthetic material or device, whether placed by surgery or catheter intervention, during the first 6 mo after the procedure
  3. Repaired CHD with residual defects at the site or adjacent to the site of a prosthetic patch or prosthetic device
- Cardiac transplant recipients who develop cardiac valvulopathy
- Rheumatic heart disease

Box IV.2 | Dental Procedures Requiring SBE Prophylaxis

Procedures in Which Endocarditis Prophylaxis is Recommended*
All dental procedures involving the manipulation of gingival tissue or the periapical region of the teeth or perforation of the oral mucosa including tooth extraction, biopsies, suture removal, and placement of orthodontic bands

*Prophylaxis is recommended only for patients with the high-risk cardiac conditions listed in Box IV.1.

Table IV.4 — Recommended Prophylactic Regimens for Dental Procedures

Situation	First-Line Agent	Alternative Agent(s)
Standard general prophylaxis	Amoxicillin 50 mg/kg (max 2 g) PO 1 h before procedure	
Unable to take oral medications	Ampicillin 50 mg/kg (max 2 g) IM/IV 30 min before procedure	Cefazolin or ceftriaxone 50 mg/kg (max 1 g) IM/IV 30 min before procedure
Allergic to penicillins	Clarithromycin or azithromycin 15 mg/kg (max 500 mg) PO 1 h before procedure	Clindamycin 20 mg/kg (max 600 mg) PO 1 h before procedure
Allergic to penicillin and unable to take oral medications	Clindamycin 20 mg/kg (max 600 mg) IM/IV 30 min before procedure	

Box IV.3 — Other (Nondental) Procedures Requiring SBE Prophylaxis

Antibiotic prophylaxis is not necessary for the sole purpose of preventing IE in nondental procedures. Various nondental procedures reportedly cause transient bacteremia and have been anecdotally associated with endocarditis. Listed below are some examples of procedures for which IE prophylaxis can be considered:

Oral or respiratory tract procedures:
Invasive procedures of the respiratory tract that involve incision or biopsy of the respiratory mucosa:

- Tonsillectomy/adenoidectomy
- Surgical procedures on the upper respiratory tract
- Nasal packing and nasal intubation
- Cosmetic piercing of the tongue or involving oral mucosa

Gastrointestinal/genitourinary procedures:

- Sclerotherapy for esophageal dilatation
- Esophageal stricture dilatation
- Endoscopic retrograde cholangiopancreatography (ERCP)
- Hepatic/biliary operations
- Surgical operations involving intestinal mucosa
- Cystoscopy
- Urethral dilatation

In patients who would normally receive standard perioperative antibiotic prophylaxis or in patients with an established infection at the procedure site, the antibiotic regimen should be modified to include an agent active against the most common causes of IE in the procedure:

- Viridans group streptococci for oral or respiratory tract procedures (see Table IV.4)
- Enterococci for gastrointestinal, hepatic/biliary, or genitourinary procedures (e.g., ampicillin, piperacillin, or vancomycin, ± low-dose gentamicin for synergy) (see Table IV.5)
- Staphylococci and β-hemolytic streptococci for procedures on infected skin, skin structure, or musculoskeletal tissue (e.g., cephalexin, cefazolin, clindamycin, or vancomycin ± low-dose gentamicin for synergy) (see Table IV.6)

Table IV.5	Recommended Prophylactic Regimens for Genitourinary and Gastrointestinal (Excluding Esophageal) Procedures	
Situation	**Agent***	**Regimen**
High-risk patients	Ampicillin plus gentamicin	Ampicillin 50 mg/kg (max 2 g) IV plus gentamicin 2.5 mg/kg (max 120 mg) within 30 min before starting procedure; then 6 h later, ampicillin 50 mg/kg (max 2 g) IV
High-risk patient allergic to ampicillin	Vancomycin plus gentamicin	Vancomycin 20 mg/kg (max 1 g) IV over 1–2 h plus gentamicin 2.5 mg/kg (max 120 mg) IV; complete injection/infusion within 30 min before starting procedure

*No second dose of vancomycin or gentamicin is recommended.

Table IV.6	Recommended Prophylactic Regimens for Procedures on Infected Tissues*	
Situation	**Agent**	**Regimen**
Standard antistaphylococcal prophylaxis (e.g., abscess, cellulitis, osteomyelitis, septic arthritis)	Cefazolin	30 mg/kg (max 2 g) IV within 30 min before starting procedure
Antistaphylococcal prophylaxis in patient allergic to penicillin	Clindamycin	15 mg/kg (max 600 mg) IV within 30 min before starting procedure
Patient known to have methicillin-resistant *Staphylococcus aureus*	Vancomycin	20 mg/kg (max 1 g) IV infusion over 1–2 h; complete infusion within 30 min before starting procedure

*Patients at high risk of endocarditis.

GUIDELINES FOR WARFARIN THERAPY

- See Hematology chapter, p. 467 for heparin therapy
- General:
  - Loading period 3–5 d
  - Must be taking full enteral feeds, including solids
  - Avoid in infants <12 mo
  - If formula-fed, consider formula with least amount of vitamin K
  - Multiple drug interactions (consult pharmacist)
- Loading dose Day 1: 0.2 mg/kg PO × 1 dose (max 5 mg). Reduce dose to 0.1 mg/kg if liver dysfunction, Fontan, or severe renal dysfunction
- Loading dose Days 2–4

If your response is an INR of:		
INR	1.1–1.3	Repeat initial loading dose
INR	1.4–3.0	50% of initial loading dose
INR	3.1–3.5	25% of initial loading dose
INR	>3.5	Hold until INR <3.5, then restart at 50% less than the previous dose

- Long-term warfarin maintenance dose guidelines

(INR should be monitored at least monthly in stable patients)

			Mechanical Value
INR	1.1–1.4	Check for compliance. If compliant, increase by 20% of dose	1.1–2.0
INR	1.5–1.7	Increase by 10% of dose	2.0–2.2
INR	1.8–3.2	No change	2.3–3.7
INR	3.3–3.5	Decrease dose by 10%	N/A
INR	3.6–4.0	Administer one dose at 50% less than maintenance dose Then decrease maintenance dose by 20%	3.8–4.0
INR	4.1–5.0	Hold × 1 dose then restart at 20% less than maintenance dose	N/A
INR	>5.0	Contact the Thrombosis Service	>4.0

- See p, 470 for reversal of warfarin therapy

ALTERNATIVE MEDICINE INTERACTIONS

Table IV.7	Interactions Between Commonly Used Alternative Medications and Commonly Prescribed Medications
Alternative Medication	**Drug Interactions**
Alfalfa	Cyclosporine/steroids: may have immune stimulating effects Hypoglycemic medications: may cause further hypoglycemia Warfarin: ↑↓INR: may contain warfarin constituents or ↓ effect because of vitamin K content in herb
Aloe	Digoxin, thiazide diuretics: ↑ cardiac toxicity due to electrolyte imbalance
Anise	MAOIs: herb may ↑ risk of hypertensive crisis Warfarin ↑INR: may contain warfarin constituents
Bitter melon	Additive hypoglycemic effects in combination with antidiabetic agents such as insulin or oral hypoglycemics
Bitter orange (synephrine)	Caution with QT interval–prolonging drugs (amiodarone, procainamide, quinidine, sotalol, thioridazine) Increases levels and adverse effects of midazolam MAOIs: increased blood pressure, hypertensive crisis CNS stimulants: increased risk of hypertension and adverse cardiovascular effects
Capsicum	MAOIs: ↑ risk of hypertensive crisis ACE inhibitor: may ↑ cough Theophylline: oral administration of capsicum may ↑ theophylline absorption
Cascara	Various medications: ↓ absorption because of increased GI transit time Digoxin/thiazides/steroids: may potentiate hypokalemia
Chamomile	Warfarin: ↑INR: may contain warfarin constituents Iron: contains tannic acids that may ↓ iron absorption

(continued)

Table IV.7	Interactions Between Commonly Used Alternative Medications and Commonly Prescribed Medications (continued)
Alternative Medication	**Drug Interactions**
Chromium picolinate	Nephrotoxic drugs: may ↑ renal failure and rhabdomyolysis Hypoglycemics: may cause hypoglycemia
Coenzyme Q10 (ubiquinone)	β-Blockers: may counteract negative inotropic effects Antihypertensive drugs: may have additive blood pressure–lowering effects Warfarin ↓INR: may decrease effect of warfarin
Dandelion	Diuretics and lithium: may ↑ diuretic effect and ↑ lithium toxicity Warfarin: ↓INR: ↓ effect due to vitamin K content in the herb
Echinacea	Immunosuppressant drugs (e.g., corticosteroids, cyclosporine): echinacea has immunostimulant effects that may interfere with these drugs Hepatotoxic drugs (e.g., ketoconazole, isoniazid, methotrexate, terbinafine): herb may have additive hepatotoxicity if used for >8 wk Hypoglycemic drugs: may cause hypo/hyperglycemia Midazolam (IV): reduced levels and effect Warfarin: ↑INR
Feverfew	Antiplatelets: increased risk of bleeding
Flaxseed	Warfarin ↑INR: may ↑ bleeding time
Garlic	Antiplatelet and anticoagulant drugs (e.g., aspirin, NSAIDs, clopidogrel, dipyridamole, warfarin, heparin, low molecular weight heparins): increased risk of bleeding Isoniazid, saquinavir: reduced plasma levels with garlic May reduce levels and effects of the following drugs by ↑ metabolism (P450 3A4 inducer): azole antifungals (ketoconazole, itraconazole), calcium channel blockers, chemotherapy drugs (etoposide, paclitaxel, vinblastine, vincristine, vindesine), cyclosporine, HIV protease inhibitors and NNRTIs (nevirapine, efavirenz), midazolam, oral contraceptives
Ginger	Antihypertensives: may ↑ or ↓ effect with these medications Hypoglycemics: may cause hypoglycemia Antiplatelet and anticoagulant drugs: excessive amounts of ginger could increase bleeding risk
Ginkgo	Anticonvulsant drugs: may lower seizure threshold Antiplatelet and anticoagulant drugs (e.g., aspirin, NSAIDs, clopidogrel, dipyridamole, warfarin, heparin, low molecular weight heparins): increased risk of bleeding
Ginseng	Corticosteroids: may affect steroid concentrations Cardiac and antihypertensive medications: have negative chronotropic and inotropic activity and may cause possible ↓ blood pressure Estrogens/corticosteroids: may have possible additive effects Furosemide: may reduce effect of furosemide Hypoglycemics: may have additive hypoglycemic effect MAOIs, mood stabilizers: ↑ tremor/mania Warfarin: ↑ ↓INR

(continued)

Table IV.7	Interactions Between Commonly Used Alternative Medications and Commonly Prescribed Medications (continued)
Alternative Medication	**Drug Interactions**
Glucosamine	Hypoglycemics/insulin: may cause insulin resistance Doxorubicin and etoposide: may cause resistance to these drugs
Goldenseal	Cardiac and antihypertensive medications: can have variable effects on the heart and blood pressure Heparin: can counteract effect of heparin Sedatives: may have additive sedative effects
Hawthorn	Digoxin and antihypertensives: may interfere with these medications MAOIs: may contain tyramine: ↑ risk of hypertensive crisis
Horse chestnut	Warfarin: ↑INR
Licorice	Antihypertensives/digoxin/diuretics: may cause hypokalemia and sodium and fluid retention which can ↑ blood pressure (i.e., pseudoaldosteronism) Corticosteroids: may ↑ systemic and topical steroid effects Digoxin: herb may interfere with effect of digoxin Hypoglycemics: may cause ↓ glucose tolerance Oral contraceptives: may lead to hypertension, edema, and ↓ potassium Warfarin: herb may inhibit platelet activity
Melatonin	Anticonvulsant medications: may lower seizure threshold Drugs affecting metabolism of melatonin through CYP1A2 may alter its effects (*increased effect*: amiodarone, ciprofloxacin, fluoxetine, fluvoxamine; *decreased effect*: carbamazepine, phenobarbital, phenytoin, rifampin, ritonavir) Hypoglycemic medications: may have ↓ effect Nifedipine: ↑ blood pressure and heart rate with melatonin Other antihypertensive drugs: additive effects Warfarin: ↑ ↓INR
Milk thistle	Hypoglycemics: herb may have additive hypoglycemic effect
Nettle	Contains tannic acids that may ↓ iron absorption Warfarin ↓INR: may contain vitamin K
Passionflower	MAOIs/SSRIs/TCAs: may ↑ risk of serotonin syndrome Warfarin ↑INR: herb may contain warfarin constituents
Royal jelly	Asthma medications: may cause bronchospasm
Senna	Digoxin/thiazides/steroids: may potentiate hypokalemia Various medications: ↓ absorption due to increased GI transit time

(continued)

Table IV.7	Interactions Between Commonly Used Alternative Medications and Commonly Prescribed Medications *(continued)*
Alternative Medication	**Drug Interactions**
St. John wort (SJW)	Reduces levels and effects of the following drugs by ↑ metabolism (P450 3A4 inducer): azole antifungals (ketoconazole, itraconazole), calcium channel blockers, chemotherapy drugs (etoposide, imatinib, irinotecan, paclitaxel, vinblastine, vincristine, vindesine), cyclosporine, digoxin, HIV protease inhibitors, midazolam, nevirapine, omeprazole, oral contraceptives, phenobarbital, phenytoin, sumatriptan, theophylline, warfarin Increases activity of clopidogrel SSRIs, TCAs, MAOIs, meperidine, sumatriptan: increased risk of serotonin syndrome
Valerian	Sedatives: may have additive sedative effects

MAOIs, monoamine oxidase inhibitors; *NNRTIs*, nonnucleoside reverse transcriptase inhibitors; *SSRIs*, selective serotonin reuptake inhibitors; *TCAs*, tricyclic antidepressants.

DRUG INFUSION CALCULATIONS

Table IV.8	Drug Infusion Calculations
Desired Concentration	**Dose (mg) in 50 mL**
0.33 mcg/kg/min = 1 mL/h	$1 \times$ wt (kg)
1 mcg/kg/min = 1 mL/h	$3 \times$ wt (kg)
10 mcg/kg/h = 1 mL/h	$0.5 \times$ wt (kg)
0.25 mg/kg/h = 1 mL/h	$12.5 \times$ wt (kg)
1 mg/kg/d = 1 mL/h	$2 \times$ wt (kg)
	Dose (units) in 50 mL
0.0001 unit/kg/min = 1 mL/h	$0.3 \times$ wt (kg)
10 units/kg/h = 1 mL/h	$10 \times 50 \times$ wt (kg)

FURTHER READING

Bezchlibnyk-Butler KZ, Virani AS. *Clinical Handbook of Psychotropic Drugs for Children and Adolescents.* Cambridge, Mass: Hogrefe and Huber; 2004.

Bradley JS, Nelson JD. *2006–2007 Nelson's Pocket Book of Pediatric Antimicrobial Therapy.* 16th ed. Philadelphia, Pa: Lippincott Williams & Wilkins; 2007.

Pickering LK, ed. *2006 Red Book: Report of the Committee on Infectious Diseases.* 28th ed. Elk Grove Village, Ill: American Academy of Pediatrics; 2006.

Taketomo CK, Hodding JH, Kraus DM. *Pediatric Dosage Handbook.* 14th ed. Hudson, Ohio: Lexi-Comp; 2007.

Young TE, Mangum B, eds. *Neofax.* Raleigh, NC: Acorn; 2005. Available at: www.neofax.com.

USEFUL WEB SITES

American Academy of Pediatrics. Available at: **www.aap.org**

CAMLINE – The Evidence-Based Complementary and Alternative Medicine Website for Healthcare Professionals. Available at: **www.camline.ca**

Canadian Paediatric Society (CPS). Available at: **www.cps.ca**

HerbMed. Available at: **www.herbmed.org**

Hospital for Sick Children pharmacy manufacturing department. Available at: **www.sickkids.ca/pharmacy/**

Longwood Herbal Task Force. Available at: **www.longwoodherbal.org**

Medline Plus. Available at: **www.nlm.nih.gov/medlineplus/druginfo/herb_All.html**

Pediatric Pharmacy Advocacy Group (PPAG). Available at: **www.ppag.org**

Index

Page numbers followed by b indicate boxes; f, figures; t, tables. Page number as ibc indicates inside back cover; ifc indicates inside front cover.

Index

Index

Index

Index

Index

Index

Index

Resuscitation Drugs in Infants and Older Children— Intermittent Doses

SUPPLIED	DOSE	COMMENTS

ADENOSINE
Injection:
6 mg/2 mL vial
3 mg/mL
	0.1 mg/kg/dose IV/IO
	Maximum 1st dose: 6 mg (2 mL)
	If no effect, repeat q2min at
	  0.2 mg/kg/dose
	Maximum repeated dose: 12 mg (4 mL)
		Administer by rapid IV/IO bolus over
		  1-2 s followed by 0.9% NaCl flush
		Record continuous rhythm strip ECG during
		  adenosine administration

AMIODARONE
Injection:
150 mg/3 mL ampule
50 mg/mL
	5 mg/kg/dose IV/IO
	Maximum dose: 300 mg (6 mL)
	May repeat up to 15 mg/kg
	Maximum repeated dose: 150 mg (3 mL)
		For pulseless ventricular fibrillation, ventricular
		  tachycardia: consider administration by
		  IV bolus diluted to 3 mg/mL with D5W
		Dilute in D5W
		Administer over 1 h
		Use non-PVC tubing
		See below for continuous infusion
		Adjust administration rate to urgency; give
		  more slowly when perfusing rhythm present
		Record continuous rhythm strip ECG and
		  monitor blood pressure during amiodarone
		  administration
		Use caution when administering with other
		  drugs that prolong QT (consider expert
		  consultation)

ATROPINE
Injection:
0.5 mg/5 mL syringe
0.1 mg/mL
	0.02 mg/kg/dose
	  (0.2 mL/kg/dose) IV/IO
	0.03 mg/kg/dose
	  (0.3 mL/kg/dose) ETT*
	Repeat once if needed
	Minimum single dose:
	  0.1 mg (1 mL)
	Maximum single dose:
	  Child 0.5 mg (5 mL)
	  Adolescent 1 mg (10 mL)
		Incompatible with sodium bicarbonate
		Higher or repeated doses may be used
		  with organophosphate poisoning

CALCIUM CHLORIDE
Injection 10%:
1 g/10 mL syringe
100 mg CaCl$_2$/mL
(0.68 mmol Ca^{2+}/mL)
	20 mg/kg/dose IV/IO q10-20min prn
	  (0.2 mL/kg/dose)
	Maximum single dose:
	  1 g (10 mL)
		Incompatible with sodium bicarbonate
		Avoid extravasation
		Administer slowly

EPINEPHRINE
Injection **1:10,000**
1 mg/10 mL syringe
0.1 mg/mL
Injection **1:1000**
1 mg/1 mL ampule,
30 mg/30 mL
  multidose vial
1 mg/mL
	0.01 mg/kg/dose IV/IO
	  (0.1 mL/kg/dose of **1:10,000**)
	q3-5min prn
	Maximum dose:
	  1 mg (10 mL) IV/IO
	ETT* route:
	0.1 mg/kg (0.1 mL/kg of **1:1000**)
	  ETT q3-5min prn
	Maximum dose:
	  10 mg (10 mL) ETT
	Anaphylaxis without shock:
	0.01 mg/kg/dose
	  (0.01 mL/kg/dose of **1:1000**)
	  IM q10-20min prn
	Minimum dose: 0.1 mg (0.1 mL) IM
	Maximum dose: 0.5 mg (0.5 mL) IM
		Incompatible with sodium bicarbonate
		See inside front cover and Table 1.1 for
		  continuous infusion

(continued)